Diabetes in Women

CONTEMPORARY DIABETES

ARISTIDIS VEVES, MD, DSc
SERIES EDITOR

Diabetes in Women

Edited by

Agathocles Tsatsoulis, MD, PHD, FRCP
Department of Endocrinology, University of Ioannina Medical School, Ioannia, Greece

Jennifer Wyckoff, MD
Division of Endocrinology, Metabolism, and Diabetes, Department of Internal Medicine, University of Michigan, Ann Arbor, MI

Florence M. Brown, MD
Harvard Medical School, Department of Medicine, Joslin Diabetes Center, Boston, MA, USA

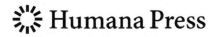 Humana Press

Editors

Agathocles Tsatsoulis, MD, PHD, FRCP
Department of Endocrinology
University of Ioannina Medical School
Ioannia
Greece

Jennifer Wyckoff, MD
Division of Endocrinology, Metabolism and Diabetes
Department of Internal Medicine
University of Michigan
Ann Arbor, MI
USA

Florence M. Brown, MD
Harvard Medical School
Department of Medicine,
Joslin Diabetes Center
Boston, MA
USA

ISBN 978-1-60327-249-0   e-ISBN 978-1-60327-250-6
DOI 10.1007/978-1-60327-250-6
Springer New York Dordrecht Heidelberg London

Library of Congress Control Number: 2009926313

Printed on acid-free paper

Springer is part of Springer Science+Business Media (www.springer.com)

"The Book is dedicated to my wife Mary for her understanding and support, and to all women with Diabetes"

Agathocles Tsatsoulis

" I would like to dedicate this work to all my patients who are my inspiration and to my family who are my strength."

Jennifer Ann Wyckoff

"This book is dedicated to Suzanne Ghiloni, RN, CDE, and Breda Curran for their combined service of over 45 years to the Joslin Diabetes in Pregnancy Program."

Florence M. Brown

Preface

This book is devoted to women with diabetes and to women at risk of diabetes. The primary aim is to provide up-to-date information on current topics pertaining to diabetes and cardiometabolic risk in women throughout the lifecycle.

The concept behind this book arises from the understanding that gender differences impact the pathophysiology and clinical burden of diabetes in women. The fundamental differences between men and women are primarily attributed to sex hormones, which define not only the sexually dimorphic traits but also play an important role in regulating energy metabolism, body composition, and vascular function.

The book is structured into five main sections with a total of 23 chapters. The first section, "Sex Differences in Cardiometabolic Risk", reviews the differences between the sexes in energy balance and body composition, the impact of menopause on these parameters, and the clinical expression and burden of cardiovascular disease in women with diabetes. There is also special reference to the cardiometabolic risk in women with PCOS and the concept of fetal programming of PCOS by androgen excess. Section 2 focuses on the "Impact of Diabetes on Women's Health". It includes a chapter that explores the impact of poverty and globalization on the emerging epidemic of obesity in developing countries. Other chapters review depression, eating disorders, sexual health, and contraception in women with diabetes. Fertility and pregnancy in women with PCOS is also reviewed with a special focus on the metabolic aspects of the syndrome. "Diabetes and Pregnancy" is covered in Section 3. The diagnosis and treatment of gestational diabetes, nutrition in pregnancy, prepregnancy counseling, obstetrical and medical care of women with diabetes, preeclampsia, and the use of ultrasound in the management of gestational and preexisting diabetes in pregnancy are reviewed. The increasing burden of diabetes and gestational diabetes in developing nations is highlighted in Chapter 12. Section 4 is devoted to the "Offspring of the Diabetic Mother", and reviews the phenomenon of metabolic imprinting as well as the genetic basis of the various forms of diabetes and the issue of breastfeeding. Lastly, Section 5 summarizes in a chapter "The Disease Management of Women with Diabetes".

The book *Diabetes in Women* is meant for physicians with an interest in diabetes: endocrinologists, obstetricians, and gynecologists, generalists as well as medical students and those training in these areas of health care. The text will also be of interest to clinical and basic scientists in the field. We hope that the topics in the book will help improve the knowledge of diabetes in women and serve as a stimulus for further research in this important area.

Each chapter was written by authors who are prominent in their respective fields. Without their contribution this book would not have materialized. We are, therefore, indebted to all the authors, who contributed their chapters to this volume.

We want also to extend our appreciation and gratitude to Paul Dolgert, Kevin Wright, and Gina Impallomeni of Springer for their help throughout the preparation of the book. We owe special thanks to Dr. Aris Veves, who inspired us with the idea for such a volume and guided us in our joint effort of editing the book.

Ioannina, Greece   **Agathocles Tsatsoulis**
Ann Arbor, MI   **Jennifer Wyckoff**
Boston, MA   **Florence M. Brown**

Contents

Contributors

PATRICIA AGUIRRE, PhD • *Institute of High Social Studies, Universidad Nacional de San Martín, Buenos Aires, Argentina*

ALLISON L. COHEN, MD • *Joslin Diabetes Center, One Joslin Place, Boston, MA*

DANA DABELEA, MD, PhD • *Dept. of Preventive Medicine and Biometrics, Denver, CO*

ASSIAMIRA FERRARA, MD, PhD • *Division of Research, Kaiser Permanente, Oakland, CA*

DILYS FREEMAN, PhD • *Reproductive and Maternal Medicine, University of Glasgow, Royal Infirmary, Glasgow UK*

CATHERINE KIM, MD, MPH • *Depts. of Medicine and Obstetrics & Gynecology, University of Michigan, Ann Arbor, MI*

SIRI L. KJOS, MD • *Dept. of OB/GYN, Harbor UCLA Medical Center., Torrance, CA*

JOHN E. NESTLER, MD • *Division of Endocrinology and Metabolism, Virginia Commonwealth University, , Richmond, VA*

RENATO PASQUALI, MD • *Division of Endocrinology, Dept. of Internal Medicine, S. Orsola-Malpighi Hospital, Bologna, Italy*

CONSTANTIN POLYCHRONAKOS • *The McGill University Health Center, Montreal Children's Hospital, Montréal, Canada*

JO-ANNE M. RIZZOTTO, MEd, RD, LDN, CDE • *Joslin Clinic/Joslin Diabetes Center, Boston, MA*

GARY RODIN, MD • *Princess Margaret Hospital, Toronto, ON, Canada*

S.M. SADIKOT, MD • *Dept. of Endocrinology and Metabolic Disorders, Jaslok Hospital and Research Centre, Mumbai, India*

ANDREA SALONIA, MD • *Dept. of Urology, University Vita-Salute San Raffaele, Milan, Italy*

UTE SCHAEFER-GRAF, MD • *Gynäkologin und Diabetologin DDG, Oberärztin, Berliner Diabeteszentrum für Schwangere, Klinik für Gynäkologie und Geburtshilfe, St. Joseph Krankenhaus, Berlin Bundesrepublik Deutschland*

ELLEN W. SEELY, MD • *Division of Endocrinology, Diabetes and Hypertension, Brigham and Women's Hospital, Harvard Medical School, Boston, MA*

JAMES R. SOWERS, MD, FACE, FACP, ASCI • *Division of Endocrinology, Diabetes and Metabolism, University of Missouri – Columbia, Columbia, MO*

TAMARA C. TAKOUDES, MD • *Harvard Medical School, Joslin Diabetes in Pregnancy Program, Maternal-Fetal Medicine, Dept. of Obstetrics and Gynecology, Beth Israel Deaconess Medical Center, Boston, MA*

JULIE SCOTT TAYLOR, MD, MSC, IBCLC • *Dept. of Family Medicine, Memorial Hospital of Rhode Island, Pawtucket, RI*

ANDRÉ TCHERNOF, PhD • *Molecular Endocrinology and Oncology, Laval University Medical Research Center, Department of Nutrition, Laval University, , Quebec City, QC, Canada*

AGATHOCLES TSATSOULIS, MD, PhD, FRCP • *Dept. of Endocrinology, University of Ioannina Medical School, Ioannina, Greece*

ANGELINA L. TRUJILLO, MD • *Sansum Diabetes Research Institute, Santa Barbara, CA*

JENNIFER WYCKOFF, MD • *Division of Endocrinology, Metabolism, and Diabetes, Dept. of Internal Medicine, University of Michigan, Ann Arbor, MI*

1 Sex Differences in Energy Balance, Body Composition, and Body Fat Distribution

André Tchernof

CONTENTS

ABSTRACT

Human males and females differ greatly in their body composition and body fat distribution. However, in both sexes, excess accumulation of adipose tissue within the abdominal cavity, termed visceral obesity, has emerged as a determinant of obesity-related metabolic alterations known to increase type 2 diabetes and cardiovascular disease risk. Although there are sex-related differences in both energy expenditure and food intake, these variations cannot by themselves explain the rather pronounced and systematic body composition and body fat distribution dimorphism. Mechanisms involving glucocorticoids, androgens, and estrogens likely play a critical role in the establishment of these patterns. Specific characteristics of each fat depot including fat cell size and metabolism, storage capacity, adipokine secretion, and, more generally, gene expression can help delineate some of the plausible links between excess visceral fat accumulation and metabolic disorders eventually leading to type 2 diabetes and cardiovascular disease.

Key words: Obesity; Visceral fat; Sex hormones; Sex dimorphism; Androgens; Glucocorticoids.

From: *Diabetes in Women: Pathophysiology and Therapy*
Edited by: A. Tsatsoulis et al. (eds.), DOI 10.1007/978-1-60327-250-6_1
© Humana Press, a part of Springer Science+Business Media, LLC 2009

INTRODUCTION

Human males and females differ greatly in terms of body composition and body fat distribution. In fact, such substantial gross anatomical differences attributable to regional adipose tissue partitioning are practically unique to this species *(1)*. Vague *(2, 3)* first documented this sex difference in relation to disease risk, stating that men are usually characterized by a body fat distribution pattern that he termed "android," with adipose accumulation in the abdominal region, whereas women often display a body fat distribution pattern that he termed "gynoid," with a greater proportion of their adipose tissue in the gluteal and femoral regions (Fig. 1). One of the seminal articles by Vague in 1956 concluded that "android obesity, with upper body predominance and pronounced muscle-blood development, leads to metabolic disturbances. It not only is associated with premature atherosclerosis and diabetes, but it is also the usual cause of diabetes in the adult in 80 to 90 per cent of the cases" *(3)*.

Over the past 20 years, consistent with these initial observations, large accumulation of abdominal adipose tissue has emerged as a critical determinant of obesity-related metabolic alterations, which are known to increase the risk of type 2 diabetes and cardiovascular disease in both males and females *(4–6)*. The amount of fat located inside the abdominal cavity on anatomical structures such as the greater omentum and mesentery, also termed intra-abdominal or visceral fat, can be quantified using computed tomography (Fig. 2) or magnetic resonance imaging. Studies using these techniques have shown that excess visceral fat accumulation is now recognized as the most prevalent manifestation of the metabolic syndrome and represents an essential feature of the current worldwide obesity epidemic *(7)*.

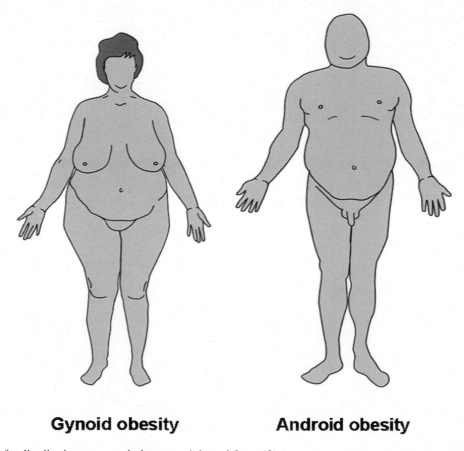

Gynoid obesity   **Android obesity**

Fig. 1. Body fat distribution patterns in humans. Adapted from *(3)*.

The present chapter will provide an overview of the existing sex differences in energy balance, body composition, and body fat distribution in humans. The link between visceral adipose tissue accumulation and metabolic alterations as well as the teleological significance and mechanisms underlying this sex dimorphism will also be discussed.

SEX DIFFERENCES IN ENERGY BALANCE

Before addressing sex differences in body composition and body fat distribution, sex differences in the determinants of energy balance, that is, energy expenditure and food intake, will be briefly examined.

One of the major determinants of basal or resting metabolic rate and total energy expenditure is body composition, more specifically fat-free mass *(8)*. Thus, because of higher fat-free mass, men generally have higher energy expenditure measurements on an absolute basis than women. Analyses where body composition differences were controlled for indicate, however, that resting and 24-h energy expenditure may be higher in men than in women, independent of body composition *(9)*. This difference is relatively small, but can be detected in elderly individuals as well as prepubescent boys and girls, suggesting that it is independent of hormonal status *(10)*.

Regarding food intake, sex differences are not apparent in infancy and childhood and seem to surface during adolescence. The difference in body composition dramatically influences energy requirements leading men to consume more calories than women *(11)*. Similar to energy expenditure, there seems to be a significantly higher energy intake in men than in women, even when body weight and height are controlled for *(12)*. With increasing age, however, a greater decrease in energy intake is apparent in men than in women *(11, 12)*. Cyclic hormonal variations in women have been shown to impact significantly on food intake *(13)*. Specifically, energy intake is higher in the postovulatory (luteal) or premenstrual phase of the cycle than in the preovulatory or follicular phase *(13)*. These differences are greatly attenuated in women using oral contraceptives, in women with anovulatory cycles *(13, 14)*, or in women with

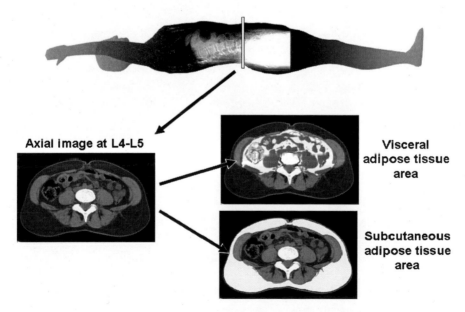

Fig. 2. Computed tomography measure of visceral and subcutaneous adipose tissue areas at the L4–L5 vertebrae level in a female subject. Areas of interest were delineated using the interface of the image analysis software, and adipose tissue within these regions was identified using a defined Hounsfield unit range. Visceral and subcutaneous adipose tissue areas are identified on the *right panels* in *light gray*. Methodological details can be found in *(199, 200)*.

restrained eating patterns *(13, 15)*. Studies on macronutrient selection during the hormonal cycle are much less consistent, and it has been suggested that they may reflect general increases in appetite rather than specific intake of a particular macronutrient *(13)*. Thus, the premenstrual phase can be considered as a time when women are especially vulnerable to overconsumption and food cravings.

Social and cultural influences also exert greater influence with the onset of adolescence and could impact sex differences in food intake. Women are generally less satisfied with their body shape and weight than men *(11)*. Accordingly, dieting is particularly common in women. Estimates have shown that 53.8% of young women were dieting vs. 23.8% of young men in a survey of American students performed from 1995 to 2005 *(16)*. Eating behavior, eating style, and the response to variety in the diet may also differ between sexes, which could contribute to increase the susceptibility of women to eating and body-weight disorders *(11)*.

In summary, there are documented sex differences in both energy expenditure and food intake that appear to be independent of body weight or composition. However, from available studies in humans, it is difficult to clearly pinpoint sex-related differences in energy expenditure, food intake or eating patterns that could readily and systematically explain the very clear and relatively constant sex differences observed in body composition and body fat distribution. Mechanisms involving the hormone-dependent partition of substrates toward lean and fat mass accretion as well as fat depot-specific characteristics likely contribute to explain these sex differences in the presence of a given energy imbalance.

SEX DIFFERENCES IN BODY COMPOSITION AND BODY FAT DISTRIBUTION

Weight gain is slightly higher in boys than in girls over the course of childhood. Total body fat-free mass seems to be relatively similar in boys and girls, although boys have approximately 1 kg more fat-free mass before puberty. Total body fat mass is comparable between boys and girls before the age of 7, after which girls accumulate fat mass slightly more rapidly to reach values higher than that of boys by approximately 2 kg *(17, 18)*. Thus, differences in body composition exist but are relatively small in magnitude before puberty.

With puberty, boys accumulate approximately twice as much fat-free mass compared with girls (33 kg vs. 16 kg, respectively) in the period extending from 10 to 20 years of age *(19)*. Conversely, total body fat mass increases proportionately more in girls than in boys *(19)*. As a result, adult women have significantly higher fat mass values and relatively lesser fat-free mass than men *(18, 20)*. Average percent body fat mass is around 10–15% for men and 20–30% for women in healthy subjects, and the values can obviously reach higher levels in other populations *(18, 19)*. With aging, women tend to have a slightly higher propensity to gain fat mass than men *(18)*.

The sex dimorphism in body fat distribution also becomes apparent at puberty. Despite higher percent body fat masses than men, women generally have significantly lower visceral adipose tissue accumulations than men. For example, cross-sectional data from the Quebec Family Study *(21)* and the Heritage Family study *(22)* enabled us to examine the sex dimorphism in Caucasian populations. In a Quebec Family Study subsample (Table 1), the sex dimorphism in body composition is readily apparent with 32% fat in women vs. 23% in men. Conversely, fat-free mass is at 61 kg in men vs. 46 kg in women. Despite this highly significant difference, men have a higher computed tomography-measured visceral adipose tissue area than women (Table 1). Very similar differences can be observed in other Caucasian populations *(22, 23)*. Other ethnicities also generally show this pattern of sex differences, although there are marked ethnicity-related disparities in total adiposity and the propensity to store visceral fat. For example, in African American individuals *(24)*, a lower proportion of visceral fat is observed for a given total body fat mass, suggesting a reduced susceptibility to visceral obesity in black individuals. The opposite is true for other ethnic groups such as the South East Asians and Canadian Aboriginals *(23, 25, 26)*.

Table 1
Adiposity Measures Including Underwater Weighing Measures of Body Fat Mass, Body Fat-Free Mass, and Body Fat Percentage as well as Computed Tomography-Measured Abdominal Adipose Tissue Areas in a Sample of Caucasian Men (n = 203) and Women (n = 219)

	Men	Women
Age (year)	42 ± 15	39 ± 18*
Weight (kg)	80.7 ± 15.2	69.4 ± 17.5**
BMI (kg/m²)	27.0 ± 4.8	27.0 ± 7.2
Body fat mass (kg)	19.5 ± 10.0	23.5 ± 13.2**
Body fat-free mass (kg)	61.2 ± 7.6	46.0 ± 6.2**
Body fat percentage (%)	23.1 ± 8.2	31.7 ± 10.7**
Visceral adipose tissue area (cm²)	127 ± 75	93 ± 59**
Subcutaneous adipose tissue area (cm²)	219 ± 130	328 ± 184**

Values are mean ± SD; *p< 0.05 and **p < 0.001 for the sex difference; adapted from (21)

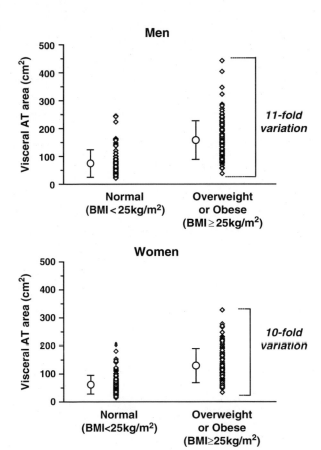

Fig. 3. Interindividual variability in computed tomography-measured visceral adipose tissue (AT) area in a sample of Caucasian men (n = 203) and women (n = 219) stratified according to their BMI values. Adapted from (21).

A most striking feature is the very large interindividual variability in visceral adipose tissue area in both men and women. As shown in Fig. 3, high interindividual variability can be observed in computed tomography-measured visceral adipose tissue accumulation in the normal weight and overweight/obese category of both sexes. Thus, despite a generally lower visceral adipose tissue accumulation on average in women, relatively important and physiologically significant visceral fat accumulations can still be observed in this sex, even in the normal BMI range (Fig. 3).

FAT DEPOT-SPECIFIC CHARACTERISTICS: A KEY TO THE LINK BETWEEN VISCERAL FAT ACCUMULATION AND DISEASE OUTCOME

Specific features of the visceral adipose tissue depots, which include the omental, mesenteric, and retroperitoneal fat compartments, have been shown to be closely related or even lead to metabolic alterations. This section will provide an overview of how the biological nature of visceral adipose tissue and the visceral adipocyte may explain the link between visceral obesity and the metabolic disturbances generally associated with this condition.

Adipocyte Size

The mature adipocyte population of a given depot shows important differences in cell size according to the volume of the triglyceride droplet located in each cell. Adipocyte size varies as a function of sex, adiposity level, nutritional status, and anatomical location of the adipose tissue depot (Fig. 4) *(27–31)*. In both sexes, omental and subcutaneous adipocytes become larger with obesity, but adipocyte size reaches a plateau in massively obese subjects *(28, 31)*. In normal weight to obese women, omental adipocytes are 20–30% smaller than subcutaneous adipocytes *(28, 31)*. Omental and subcutaneous adipocytes actually reach a similar size at very elevated BMI values (>60 kg/m^2) *(28, 31)*. In men, omental and subcutaneous adipocytes have a similar cell size through most of the adiposity range. In addition, maximal adipocyte size is lower in men (approximately 120 µm) than in women (approximately 140 µm) *(27)*. Since fat cell size is a critical determinant of adipocyte function *(27)*, these sex-, depot-, and adiposity-related differences likely play a critical role in the variation of adipose cell function in various fat compartments (Fig. 4).

	MEN		WOMEN		
	Subcutaneous adipose tissue	Omental adipose tissue	Subcutaneous adipose tissue	Omental adipose tissue	
LEAN	105 µm	95 µm	90 µm	70 µm	Average adipocyte size and number
	++	+++	+++	+	LPL activity[a]
	++	++	++	+	Free fatty acid release[b]
	++	++	++	+++	Responsiveness to positive lipolytic stimulus[b]
	++*	++*	++	++	Adiponectin release[b]
	−	−	−	−	Macrophage infiltration[a]
	++	+++	++	+++	IL-6 release[a]
OBESE	105 µm	110 µm	115 µm	105 µm	Average adipocyte size and number
	+++	+++	++++	+++	LPL activity[a]
	+++	+++	+++	++	Free fatty acid release[b]
	+++	+++	+++	++++	Responsiveness to positive lipolytic stimulus[b]
	+*	+*	++	+	Adiponectin release[b]
	++	+++	++	+++	Macrophage infiltration[a]
	+++	++++	+++	++++	IL-6 release[a]

* Hypothesized

Fig. 4. Representation of average adipocyte size and number in omental and subcutaneous adipose tissue of lean and obese subjects of both sexes and semiquantitative comparison of depot-, sex-, and obesity-related differences in several adipocyte phenotypes. a: Tissue-based measurement and; b: isolated adipocyte measurement.

Adipocyte Metabolism

The response of adipose tissue to lipolytic agonists is known to be different in the visceral and subcutaneous compartments *(28, 31–34)*. One of the main determinants of these regional differences is adipocyte size *(27, 28, 31)*. Studies assessing differences in adipocyte metabolism between small and large adipocytes from the same adipose tissue depot of a given individual showed that lipolysis, lipid synthesis, and glucose uptake *(27, 35, 36)* as well as gene expression *(37)* were strongly influenced by adipocyte size. Larger adipocyte size in a given adipose tissue depot appears to be associated with increased lipid synthesis, increased lipolysis, and, therefore, increased fatty acid flux across the cell membrane *(38)*. Consistent with the smaller adipocyte size in the omental than in the subcutaneous depot in women, lipolysis in the absence of hormonal stimulation (basal state) is lower in cells from the former than the latter fat depot *(31–34)*. Thus, in women and possibly in very lean men, visceral adipose tissue is not believed, at least in the basal condition, to be a major contributor to the pool of circulating free fatty acids (FFA) *(39)*. However, compared with the subcutaneous adipose tissue depot, lipolysis in omental fat was found to be more responsive to β-adrenergic agonist stimulation *(31–34)* and less to insulin suppression *(40, 41)*. In men, lipolytic activity is higher than that observed in women, although no regional difference is observed in isoproterenol-stimulated lipolysis *(28, 31)*. In absolute terms, however, more FFAs are released into the portal circulation by visceral adipose tissues in men *(39)*. Compared with that in women, this may increase the impact of omental adipose tissue on the metabolism and lead to a greater cardiovascular disease risk *(28)*.

Accumulation of triglycerides in adipose tissue relies mainly on the hydrolysis of triglyceride-rich lipoproteins by lipoprotein lipase (LPL) and on triglyceride synthesis inside the adipocyte. The regional differences in the rate of these processes are also tightly associated with adipocyte size. Some studies including both sexes failed to find differences in omental vs. subcutaneous LPL activity *(42, 43)*. However, higher LPL activity in subcutaneous adipose tissue was observed in studies including mostly women *(31, 41, 44)* and the opposite was observed in studies that included mostly men *(28, 44, 45)*. Thus, we propose that regional differences in LPL activity are sex-specific and likely reflect the propensity of each compartment to accumulate lipids in each sex. Concordant with these observations, triglyceride synthesis in women is reduced in omental adipose tissue *(32, 46)* and is similar in abdominal subcutaneous and omental adipose tissue in men *(32)*.

In summary, adipocyte metabolism seems to favor greater accumulation of lipids in the visceral fat compartment and higher release of FFA in the portal vein of men than in women. Adipocyte size appears to be a major determinant of these differences (Fig. 4).

The physiological mechanisms underlying the relationship between adipocyte function and the metabolic abnormalities of visceral obesity have been extensively studied. Hepatic VLDL synthesis is a central factor in the dyslipidemic state of abdominal obesity *(47, 48)*. In fact, the hypertriglyceridemic state of this condition is primarily due to VLDL overproduction, while the concomitant low HDL-cholesterol levels and predominance of small, dense LDL particles appear to be consequences of high triglyceride levels *(47–49)*. Availability of fatty acids in the liver is recognized as the primary determinant of reduced Apo B degradation and VLDL overproduction *(48)*. Thus, an increased fatty acid flux from visceral adipose tissue to the liver could potentially explain abdominal obesity-related hypertriglyceridemia *(50)*.

The activity of the enzyme LPL is responsible for the catabolism of triglyceride-rich lipoproteins such as chylomicrons and VLDL. Its activity measured in postheparin plasma has been reported to be lower in visceral obese patients *(51)*, which could contribute to the reduction in the catabolism of triglyceride-rich particles and to elevated plasma triglyceride concentrations. The high concentrations of triglyceride-rich lipoproteins found in visceral obesity could also favor increased lipid transfer by the cholesterol ester transfer protein (CETP) between VLDL particles and LDL as well as

HDL particles. HDL particles then become relatively depleted in cholesterol esters and enriched in triglycerides. Triglycerides can also be transferred to LDL by CETP, and this phenomenon also reduces the cholesterol to triglyceride ratio in LDL particles. Since hepatic triglyceride lipase (HL) activity has been reported to be increased in visceral obesity *(51, 52)*, triglyceride-rich HDL and LDL particles are then submitted to hydrolysis by this enzyme, generating on the one hand small, dense LDL and HDL particles and, as a consequence, reduced HDL-cholesterol levels, especially in the HDL_2 subfraction.

With respect to insulin resistance, excess FFA release through the portal system to the liver may be associated with reduced hepatic insulin extraction *(53, 54)*, which could partly contribute to the hyperinsulinemic state of this condition *(50, 55)*. It may also be associated with increased hepatic gluconeogenesis, leading to elevated hepatic glucose production, which could contribute to the deterioration in glucose tolerance *(52, 56)*. Current literature suggests that excess systemic FFA release is involved in skeletal muscle insulin resistance through inhibition of insulin signaling and glucose transport, as well as inhibition of glycogen synthase, pyruvate dehydrogenase, and hexokinase *(57–60)*. Results on lipodystrophic mice and ectopic fat accumulation have led to the suggestion that the appearance of insulin resistance in a high dietary fat intake context may be due to increased lipid burden on skeletal muscle and liver resulting from reduced capacity for excess lipid handling and storage when facing caloric excess *(61–64)*. Increased muscle lipid content is closely associated with insulin resistance *(65, 66)*. Moreover, in mice overexpressing either liver or skeletal muscle LPL, insulin resistance specific to the tissue overexpressing LPL was observed, suggesting a direct and causative relationship between the accumulation of intracellular fatty acids and insulin resistance *(67)*. According to this hypothesis, insulin resistance could be due not only to lipids released from fat, but also to a reduced capacity for excess lipid handling and storage *(62, 67, 68)*.

To examine the relative capacity of each abdominal fat compartment to store excess lipids through fat cell hypertrophy and hyperplasia, we examined a sample of women in which we performed measures of abdominal adipose tissue areas by computed tomography and also obtained omental and subcutaneous adipose tissue samples by surgery to characterize adipocyte size and adipogenic gene expression *(69)*. We observed a marked difference in, on the one hand, the regression of adipocyte size to total body fat mass, and on the other, the regressions of adipose tissue areas and total body fat mass. The fact that the regression slopes of subcutaneous and omental fat cell size were parallel showed that obese women have proportionately larger adipocytes in both fat compartments than lean women. Conversely, the fact that the regression of subcutaneous adipose tissue area was much steeper than that of visceral adipose tissue area with total body fat mass suggested that subcutaneous fat is hyperplastic in obese women. Thus, in women, hyperplasia is predominant in the subcutaneous fat depot, whereas fat cell hypertrophy is observed both in the omental and subcutaneous compartments *(69)*. Considering that adipocyte number and anatomical localization are major determinants of metabolic consequences related to obesity *(38)*, we suggest that a higher storage capacity of the subcutaneous compartment in women could theoretically prevent fat accumulation in the visceral compartment and explain the lower prevalence of metabolic disturbances in women than in men.

Adipokines

In addition to its lipid storage function, adipose tissue is known to produce a number of cytokines, also termed adipokines, as well as many other factors involved in the regulation of biological processes *(70)*. Adipokines are mainly secreted by adipocytes or preadipocytes, but also, especially in obesity, by macrophages invading the tissue *(70)*. Recent studies have observed that visceral and subcutaneous adipose tissues do not equally contribute to the secretion of these factors *(71–74)*. The literature also suggests that adipocyte size has an important influence on the secretion pattern of these factors *(75)*.

Similar to adipocyte metabolism, sex- and depot-specific differences in adipocyte size may modulate the secretion pattern of some adipokines (Fig. 4).

Circulating concentrations of adiponectin, an adipokine with insulin-sensitizing and anti-inflammatory properties, are inversely associated to adiposity levels (76). The decrease in adiponectin concentration with obesity is believed to have negative consequences on whole-body glucose homeostasis (76). Studies suggest that visceral adipose tissue accumulation assessed by computed tomography is an independent predictor of circulating adiponectin levels (77, 78). Omental adipose tissue also seems to be a critical determinant of serum adiponectin levels. Indeed, omental adipocyte adiponectin secretion is primarily reduced in obesity, while subcutaneous adipocyte adiponectin secretion is similar in abdominally obese women (79).

Interleukin-6 (IL-6), a proinflammatory cytokine, is positively associated with obesity and especially with visceral fat accumulation (80, 81). IL-6 is also tightly linked to C-reactive protein (CRP) production and other markers of cardiovascular disease (82). As adipose tissue accounts for a third of IL-6 production, it is suggested that adipose tissue-derived IL-6 has systemic effects on metabolism (82). In addition, local production and accumulation of this cytokine can alter lipid metabolism in adipose tissue (75, 82, 83). Indeed, elevated plasma IL-6 is associated with increased omental fat cell β-adrenergic lipolytic responsiveness (84), and β-adrenergic-dependent lipolysis is increased by high levels of IL-6 (85). Moreover, LPL activity is reduced by half in subcutaneous and omental adipose tissue depots by chronic IL-6 treatment (85, 86). Although metabolism of both adipose tissue depots is affected by IL-6, this effect may be more pronounced in visceral fat since this tissue releases two to three times more IL-6 than subcutaneous fat (83). Increased secretion of IL-6 in obesity could alter lipid metabolism of visceral adipose tissue and possibly increase its FFA release (82).

Tumor necrosis factor alpha (TNF-α) is a proinflammatory cytokine mainly secreted by immune cells such as macrophages (82). Obesity is associated with increased circulating and adipose tissue TNF-α (73). This increase is mainly attributed to infiltration of macrophages in adipose tissue and to increased secretion by adipocytes (75, 87). In addition to its role in immunity, chronically high levels of TNF-α tend to reduce fat mass accumulation through the induction of lipolysis and the impairment of insulin-induced lipogenesis and glucose uptake (88, 89). Moreover, TNF-α may be associated with insulin resistance in muscle through the induction of nitric oxide production (90). TNF-α could alter fat partitioning between the visceral and subcutaneous compartment through the regulation of adipocyte metabolism (91, 92). However, this remains controversial (81, 88) as studies measuring regional expression differences in TNF-α and its receptor failed to find consistent results (72, 88), and the alteration of fat disposal by this cytokine seems to be greater in subcutaneous adipose tissue (88).

Impairment of fibrinolysis by an enhanced plasma activity of the plasminogen activator inhibitor-1 (PAI-1) may be involved in the development of cardiovascular disease (93). PAI-1 is expressed by hepatocytes and endothelial cells, although preadipocytes and mature adipocytes also secrete significant amounts of PAI-1 (93). The release of this cytokine in omental adipose tissue is higher than in subcutaneous adipose tissue and this regional difference is more pronounced in obesity (74, 94, 95). Indeed, strong positive correlations have been observed between plasma PAI-1 levels and measures of visceral obesity (96). Specific accumulation of visceral adipose tissue may contribute to increased plasma levels of PAI-1 and consequently to the impaired fibrinolysis associated with abdominal obesity (93). Hence, PAI-1 secretion by the visceral adipocyte could contribute to visceral obesity-associated metabolic disturbances.

As described earlier, adipose tissue can secrete several adipokines that can alter metabolic pathways and lead to an increased risk of developing metabolic diseases. Several studies support the hypothesis that visceral adipocyte hypertrophy is accompanied with deleterious changes in the expression and/or secretion pattern of some key adipokines such as adiponectin, IL-6, TNF-α, and PAI-1.

These studies tend to confirm that visceral obesity is characterized by a proinflammatory and proathero-genic state, at least partly created by abnormal adipokine secretion.

Genomics and Gene Expression

Few studies have compared gene expression profiles of visceral and subcutaneous adipose tissue to highlight the intrinsic properties of abdominal adipocytes and other cell types found within these fat depots (97–100). It appears that the interindividual variability of gene expression within each depot is relatively low even if physiological, metabolic, and environmental factors are not controlled for (97). Moreover, less than 10% of the genes are differentially expressed in omental vs. subcutaneous adipose tissue (98). This highly similar expression pattern suggests that the primary characteristics of adipose tissue are generally conserved regardless of anatomical localization and habitus of the individual in whom the sample is taken (97, 98). However, specific biological functions, including cell differentiation, lipolysis, and cytokine secretion, show clear differential regulation in visceral vs. subcutaneous adipose tissue (98, 99). Furthermore, the identification of genes specifically prone to high interindividual variation led to pathways of the inflammatory response, cell death regulation, and lipid metabolism (100). None of the available genomic studies have assessed the consequences of obesity on gene expression patterns in visceral and subcutaneous adipose tissue. Jernas et al. (37) have identified gene expression differences in large compared with small adipocytes. In the latter study, immune and structure-related genes showed higher expression levels in larger adipocytes. Thus, on the basis of the increase in mean adipocyte size with obesity, we suggest that adipocyte gene expression patterns would also change with obesity. Macrophage infiltration in adipose tissue of obese individuals could also significantly affect gene expression patterns (87). Future studies will be necessary to better evaluate the contribution of nonadipocyte cells and the impact of obesity on adipose tissue gene expression profiles.

In summary, the greater negative impact of the visceral fat depot on metabolic pathways appears to be attributable, at least partly, to the physiological and metabolic nature of visceral adipose tissue (Fig. 4). Visceral adipocyte lipolysis is more sensitive to β-adrenergic agonists and less to its suppression by insulin. Even if this visceral fat is not a major contributor to whole-body FFA production, its altered lipolytic responsiveness, amplified by the release of FFA directly in the portal vein of abdominally obese individuals, may play a significant role. As previously described, visceral adipocytes and other cells contained in the visceral fat depots reveal a distinct secretion pattern of pro- and anti-inflammatory adipokines compared with cells located in subcutaneous adipose tissue. The greater proinflammatory potential of the visceral adipocyte may alter local and systemic metabolism. Visceral adipocytes and surrounding cells secrete more proinflammatory adipokines such as TNF-α, IL-6, and PAI-1, which can alter lipolysis, insulin sensitivity, and fibrinolysis. Moreover, in abdominally obese individuals, this depot apparently secretes less adiponectin, which acts as an anti-inflammatory and insulin-sensitizing molecule. Taken together, the proinflammatory adipokine profile and altered lipolysis in visceral adipose tissue may contribute to metabolic alterations observed in abdominally obese individuals and subse-quently to the increased risk of developing type 2 diabetes and cardiovascular disease.

TELEOLOGICAL SIGNIFICANCE

The sex difference in body composition, with females having greater body fat accumulation than men, seems to transcend culture and time (101). Moreover, such a marked sex dimorphism in body fat distribution is rather unique to the human species (1). The evolutionary mechanisms underlying these dimorphisms and their teleological significance will be briefly discussed in this section.

Hoyenga put forward a theory stating that through sexually dimorphic natural selection, females were placed under more pressure to survive in times of short food supplies than men *(101)*. According to this theory, females would have evolved ways to conserve calories and withstand starvation, leading them to accumulate more fat in times of abundant food supplies. Though very interesting, this theory could, however, be better extended by focusing on mechanisms of *sexual* selection, which involve reproductive success, rather than mechanisms of *natural* selection, which involve likelihood of survival. Darwin's original natural selection theory could not explain extravagant traits that actually decrease survival ability (e.g., peacock's tail), and this led him to reason that in a sexually reproducing species, any heritable trait that could help compete for sexual mates would tend to spread through the species, even if they somewhat compromise survival *(102)*. According to this concept, mate choice and competition for mates could have shaped organic form to maximize reproductive success. According to Miller *(102)*, some traits would have evolved as aesthetic displays and sometimes also as indicators of fertility. The pattern of body composition and fat distribution may be one of these sexual selection-driven traits.

In this regard, reproductive roles possibly represent the origin of the body composition and fat distribution dimorphism in humans. Trivers *(103)* defined the concept of parental investment as "any investment by the parent in an individual offspring's chance of surviving (and hence reproductive success) at the cost of the parent's ability to invest in other offspring." This concept includes metabolic investment in generating gametes, gestation, and feeding and guarding the offspring *(103)*. According to this theory, women would have evolved to maximize reproductive success through parental investment. The presence of larger body fat reserves in women is consistent with these reproductive roles, which are very demanding from the energetic standpoint. Peripheral subcutaneous adipose cells are also fairly stable in response to physiological lipolytic stimuli *(31)*, which is consistent with these depots being able to provide energy supplies in the long term (Fig. 5).

According to Trivers *(103)*, the sex whose typical parental investment is highest becomes the limiting resource, and individuals of the sex investing less will compete among themselves to breed with

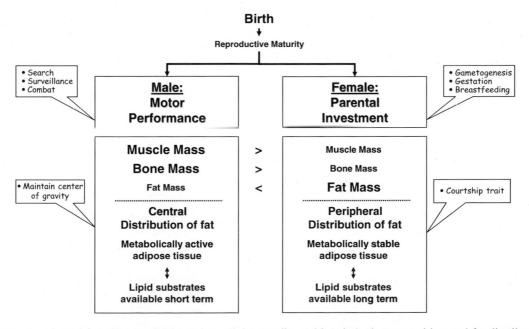

Fig. 5. Human male and female reproductive roles and the sex dimorphism in body composition and fat distribution.

members of the sex investing more. Quite consistently, male gamete production is not an energy demanding, nor limiting process. Rather, typical male reproductive roles involve searching, fighting, and competing for mates *(102–104)*. Hence, men would have evolved to maximize reproductive success through better motor performance. This is consistent with a higher body fat-free mass/body fat mass ratio in men *(105)*. The presence of central, visceral fat depots that are rapidly mobilized due to high responsiveness to catecholamine stimulation is also consistent with these reproductive roles (Fig. 5). In addition to providing readily available energy resources, the predominance of central fat depots would have only a modest effect on the center of gravity *(1)*.

These traits apparently coevolved in males and females both as courtship traits (e.g., breasts and buttocks in females, upper-body mass in males) and indicators of nutritional/reproductive status, in a context where males compete for females, who in turn select mates among the males that they attract *(102)*.

STEROID HORMONES AND BODY FAT DISTRIBUTION PATTERNS

We still know little about the etiological factors leading to preferential deposition of intra-abdominal fat in the presence of excess energy intake. It is widely believed that sex hormones and more generally steroid hormones play a key role in the regulation of body fat distribution *(106)*. However, their specific influence on fat cells has remained elusive, especially in humans. The following section will address the role of steroid hormones, namely cortisol, androgens, and estrogens in the appearance of sex-specific adiposity patterns.

Cortisol

Increased exposure of fat tissue to cortisol may influence its mass and distribution *(107)*. This is clearly evident in Cushing's syndrome, in which alterations of the hypothalamic–pituitary–adrenal axis leading to cortisol hypersecretion create a phenotype of abdominal obesity, dyslipidemia, insulin resistance, and hypertension *(108)*. Common abdominal obesity obviously shares the latter features, although more subtle alterations of cortisol activity have been documented. Specifically, plasma cortisol levels are normal in abdominal obese subjects *(107)*, but the sensitivity and drive of the hypothalamic–pituitary–adrenal axis have been shown to be increased in some studies *(109, 110)*. Urinary free cortisol levels are also elevated and the cortisol circadian rhythm is flattened *(111)*. In addition to these features, increased peripheral cortisol synthesis by 11β-hydroxysteroid dehydrogenase (HSD) is now clearly emerging as perhaps the most significant hormonal alteration in patients with idiopathic abdominal obesity *(112, 113)*.

Following the discovery of 11β-HSD activity and initial cloning of 11β-HSD types 1 and 2, the classical view was that these enzymes were responsible for cortisol inactivation and glucocorticoid clearance. However, in original purifications, 11β-HSD-1 activity was shown to be bidirectional, either converting active cortisol to inactive cortisone (dehydrogenase activity) or inactive cortisone to active cortisol (oxoreductase activity). In vivo, oxoreductase activity may be predominant over reductase activity, making this enzyme a glucocorticoid-activating enzyme in the tissue where it is expressed *(112)*. Current data obtained in adipose tissue have now clearly shown that 11β-HSD-1, indeed, acts as a local (peripheral) regulator of cortisol action by modulating cellular concentrations of cortisol at the prereceptor level *(114, 115)*.

An important study by Masuzaki et al. *(113)* demonstrated that increased local cortisol production by 11β-HSD-1 is one of the causal factors in the etiology of visceral obesity. Transgenic mice selectively overexpressing the enzyme in adipose tissue had increased adipose tissue levels of corticosterone (the active glucocorticoid in mice) and developed intra-abdominal obesity that was exaggerated by a high-fat diet *(113)*. The strong conclusion of this article reflects the potential importance of this enzyme in abdominal obesity: "Increased expression of 11β-HSD-1 in abdominal adipose tissue may represent a common molecular etiology for visceral obesity and the metabolic syndrome" *(113)*.

In humans, only a few studies have tried to relate peripheral cortisol homeostasis and 11β-HSD-1 to abdominal obesity phenotypes. Although some studies on urinary cortisol metabolites support a critical role for 11β-HSD-1 in abdominal obesity, results on the enzyme itself are not unanimous. Some studies examining activity and mRNA abundance of the enzyme in whole adipose tissue samples have found increased levels in obesity *(107, 116–119)*. However, data from Tomlinson have shown no association between either omental or subcutaneous adipose tissue 11β-HSD-1 activity or mRNA and BMI in women *(120)*. This study also showed no difference in 11β-HSD-1 expression in omental compared with subcutaneous adipose tissue *(120)*. The inconsistent nature of the fat depot difference and the low level association between obesity and 11β-HSD-1 mRNA observed in women may be considered surprising given the postulated importance of this enzyme as a determining factor for abdominal obesity. However, studies examining 11β-HSD-1 activity in cultured preadipose cells generated larger depot differences and stronger correlations with obesity *(120)*. Other in vitro evidence regarding 11β-HSD-1 in the various cell types of human adipose tissue remains limited, but studies have suggested that in stromal cells that are not yet committed to the adipocyte lineage, 11β-HSD1 predominantly inactivates cortisol by forming cortisone (dehydrogenase activity). However, in preadipocytes that are committed to the adipocyte lineage, the same enzyme generates active cortisol from cortisone (oxoreductase activity) *(121, 122)*. Since cortisol inhibits cell proliferation and stimulates cell differentiation, it is currently believed that the predominant inactivation of cortisol in uncommitted stromal cells has a proliferative effect, whereas the generation of active cortisol in committed preadipocytes stimulates fat storage and adipogenesis. Thus, 11β-HSD-1 has been suggested to act as a molecular switch regulating the link between cell proliferation and cell differentiation/adipogenesis *(122)*.

Androgens

In men, abdominal obesity has usually been associated with low plasma testosterone levels in cross-sectional *(123)* as well as in longitudinal studies *(124, 125)*. Waist circumference and waist-to-hip ratio are also inversely associated with plasma sex hormone-binding globulin (SHBG) levels *(123–125)*. Many studies that have measured abdominal fat areas using imaging techniques such as computed tomography or magnetic resonance have confirmed that low plasma testosterone concentrations are often found with elevated visceral fat accumulation *(126–131)*. The fact that both SHBG and total testosterone are reduced in abdominally obese men *(132)* and methodological limitations in free-testosterone measurement *(133, 134)* have made it difficult to detect obesity-related differences in free androgen levels. Nevertheless, androgen treatment in hypogonadal men generally leads to a decrease in abdominal fat accumulation *(135)*. These effects appear to be dose-dependent *(136)* and lead to concomitant improvements of glucose–insulin homeostasis *(135, 137)* while having neutral effects on the lipid profile *(138)*. These effects are observed when the androgen levels reached during treatment remain within the physiological range *(106)*. Supraphysiological androgen treatment has a different set of effects including increased visceral fat accumulation and insulin resistance [e.g., in female-to-male transsexuals *(139, 140)*] and dramatic alterations of the lipid profile [e.g., anabolic steroid users *(141)*]. Thus, when examining physiologically relevant data in men, low circulating androgen levels are associated with increased abdominal adiposity, and restoration of physiological levels leads to reduced abdominal fat *(106)*.

In women, the association between circulating androgens and abdominal obesity is more complex. In contrast to men, it is generally thought that abdominal obese women are hyperandrogenic *(132)*.

This belief is largely based on the observation that women with the polycystic ovary syndrome (PCOS) show hyperandrogenism often associated with abdominal obesity and hyperinsulinemia *(142)*. Interesting developments in our understanding of the pathophysiology of PCOS indicate that the elevated androgens of these women are not the cause of abdominal obesity, but the result of a hyperinsulinemic/insulin resistant state often associated with excess visceral fat *(142)*. Indeed, insulin-sensitizing treatments such as diazoxide, metformin, troglitazone *(143–145)*, or weight loss *(146, 147)* all lead to reduced androgen secretion through improved insulinemia in PCOS women. A specific sensitivity of ovarian steroidogenesis to insulin is thought to be present in PCOS women and is maintained even in insulin-resistant states *(142)*. Outside PCOS-related hyperandrogenism, however, the association between circulating androgen levels and abdominal obesity in women remains unclear. Some reported high plasma testosterone (total or free) in women with visceral obesity *(148, 149)*, but few studies are available and results are not always consistent *(150, 151)*. Some studies actually found negative associations between plasma testosterone levels and visceral fat accumulation *(152–154)*. Further studies are needed to clarify the link between endogenous androgens and visceral obesity in non-PCOS women.

Significant androgen binding in adipose tissue (and adipocytes) has long been established *(155–161)*. These findings are supported by our own analyses of fat tissue steroid content and androgen-receptor expression *(162, 163)*. Numerous studies investigated the effects of androgens on adipocyte/adipose tissue function using various models. We recently performed a detailed review of these studies *(106)*. Overall, the most consistent effect of androgens observed on fat cell function is a stimulation of lipolysis that is receptor-dependent and may affect the lipolysis cascade at different levels. These data are concordant with observations in androgen-receptor null mice, which show a late-onset obesity phenotype likely attributable to impaired lipolysis *(164)*. Additional data seem to indicate that testosterone inhibits adipose tissue LPL activity in human fat cells *(165)*, consistent with an inhibitory effect of androgens on lipid accumulation.

In rats *(166)* or in the 3T3-L1 cell line *(167)*, androgens (testosterone and DHT) were found to inhibit preadipocyte differentiation. Castration was found to increase differentiation in preadipocytes from the perirenal fat depot in rats *(168)*. However, castration was also found to inhibit differentiation of epididymal preadipocytes *(169)*. In addition, it was reported in human fat cells that testosterone had no effect, in any region, on glycerol-3-phosphate dehydrogenase activity, a late marker of differentiation *(170)*. Androgen responsiveness was found to be more pronounced in deep fat depots (visceral) in comparison to subcutaneous adipose compartments in other studies *(161, 166, 168, 171)*. Thus, available data seem to suggest that androgens inhibit fat cell differentiation, although further studies are needed to clearly establish this effect in humans.

Previous results from our group *(163, 172–177)* have suggested that prereceptor modulation of androgen action by aldo-keto reductases from the 1C family (AKR1C) may be related to abdominal obesity. Our original studies suggesting increased circulating androgen metabolite levels in abdominal obese males *(172–174)* have recently been confirmed in a large cohort study by a Swedish group *(178)*. Our work has also shown that the conversion of dihydrotestosterone, the most potent natural androgen, to the inactive androgen metabolite 5α-androstane-3α,17β-diol (3α-diol) was detected in the fat tissue of both men and women *(163, 176, 177)*. Activity was higher in subcutaneous fat than in omental fat, and, most importantly, androgen inactivation rates in omental fat were positively correlated with measures of obesity including BMI, fat cell size, and visceral adipose tissue area assessed by computed tomography *(163, 176, 177)*. The enzyme responsible for most of the dihydrotestosterone-to-3α-diol conversion in humans is AKR1C2 or 3α-HSD-3. Despite having rather distinct substrate specificities *(179)* compared with other AKR1C enzymes of the same family such as AKR1C1 (20α-HSD) and AKR1C3 (17β-HSD-5) *(179–182)*, these enzymes are highly homologous (e.g., 97.8% amino acid identity between 1C1 and 1C2), suggesting that they have diverged very recently in evolution *(181)*.

We have shown that omental AKR1C enzyme mRNA expression in adipose tissue was specifically and positively associated with visceral adipose tissue area in women *(176)*. Depot differences were similar to those observed with activity measures, and significant positive correlations were found between AKR1C mRNA expression and androgen inactivation rates *(176)*. We suggest that increased androgen inactivation by AKR1C enzymes, especially AKR1C2, may lead to reduced local exposure of fat cells to androgens, which could remove some of the inhibitory effects of this hormone on adipocyte differentiation. Additional experiments will further establish the importance of prereceptor androgen metabolism in the etiology of visceral obesity.

Estrogens

Studies have shown that estrogens may exert significant regulatory effects on adipocyte metabolism. The presence of both estrogen receptor isoforms α and β in human adipose tissue is well established *(183–186)*. Moreover, studies have reported evidence for regional differences in estrogen receptor levels and regulation *(186–188)*. A study by Price and O'Brien *(189)* showed that transdermal estradiol treatment significantly decreased gluteal adipose tissue LPL activity, and that this phenomenon was attributable to posttranscriptional modification of protein levels. In vitro studies also support an important regulatory role of estradiol on adipocyte function and metabolism. Estradiol has been shown to stimulate the proliferation of subcutaneous adipocytes from female rats *(166)*. Moreover, Palin et al. *(190)* found that high doses (10^{-7} M) of estradiol decreased LPL and increased hormone-sensitive lipase protein levels in human abdominal subcutaneous isolated adipocytes. Interestingly, lower estradiol doses had the opposite effect, which suggests a biphasic action of the hormone at the cellular level *(190)*.

Previous studies have suggested a direct effect of estrogens on lipolysis *(190, 191)*. We also reported a significant ovarian status-related difference in basal lipolysis in one of our studies *(192)*. However, we also reported no difference in agonist-stimulated glycerol release over basal, which suggests an unaltered adrenoreceptor and postadrenoreceptor lipolytic pathway. Accordingly, a study by Jensen et al. *(191)* demonstrated that although estrogen deficiency was associated with a 10–20% increase in adipose tissue FFA release, these differences did not appear to be attributable to changes in the adrenergic regulation of lipolysis *(191)*.

A most elegant study on the impact of estradiol on adipose tissue and fuel partitioning has been performed in rats *(193)*. This study demonstrated clearly that estrogen replacement in ovariectomized rats leads to a reduction in adipose tissue mass, a decrease that was significant only for periovarian, perirenal, and mesenteric or omental fat. Adipocyte size and adipogenic gene expression were also reduced in these tissues, whereas increased lipolytic responsiveness was also observed in response to estradiol. These effects appeared to be independent of the central effects of estrogens on food intake since estrogen-replaced rats were pair-fed with placebo-replaced animals. Results from this study clearly suggest a predominant role of estradiol in the modulation of body fat distribution, independent of food-intake regulation *(193)*.

Finally, although this is beyond the scope of the present chapter, sex differences in the control of energy homeostasis through hypothalamic neuroendocrine signaling involve estradiol *(194–196)*. Elegant work from Deborah Clegg's group has clearly established that adiposity signals such as leptin and insulin may act in a sex-specific manner *(197, 198)*. In rats, the female brain appears to be more sensitive to leptin, a close correlate of subcutaneous fat accumulation, whereas the male brain appears to be more sensitive to insulin, a close correlate of visceral fat accumulation *(197, 198)*.

Interestingly, these signals appear to be conditioned by sex hormones *(194, 195)*. Specifically, estradiol has been shown to increase the brain's sensitivity to leptin and decrease sensitivity to insulin, thereby favoring the signal from subcutaneous fat over that of visceral fat *(195)*. Moreover, estradiol inhibits the orexigenic action of ghrelin in females *(196)*. Future studies will help establish how differential sensitivity to adiposity signals affects body fat partitioning.

In summary, in addition to intrinsic properties of adipocytes and other cell types located in each fat compartment, cortisol, androgens, and estrogens all have significant influences on adipose tissue function and metabolism. All three categories of steroids may actually be closely involved in determining the sex dimorphism in both body composition and body fat distribution. While we have a growing understanding of how each hormone may influence fat tissue function, more studies are needed to better integrate how these steroid hormones interact in each specific fat depot, especially in humans. Prereceptor glucocorticoid and androgen metabolism within adipose tissue clearly represents an interesting research avenue in this respect.

CONCLUSION

A sexually dimorphic body composition and, most importantly, body fat distribution patterning are an especially striking feature of the human race. These marked anatomic differences between males and females may have arisen from each sex's reproductive roles through mechanisms of sexual selection. Women have higher body fat masses than men, while men have higher muscle masses and larger visceral fat accumulations than women. Specific characteristics of each fat depot including fat cell size and metabolism, storage capacity, adipokine secretion, and, more generally, gene expression, can help delineate some of the possible links between excess visceral fat accumulation and metabolic disorders eventually leading to type 2 diabetes and cardiovascular disease. It is difficult to clearly identify sex-related differences in energy expenditure, food intake, or eating patterns that could readily and systematically explain the very clear and relatively constant sex differences observed in body composition and body fat distribution. Mechanisms involving the modulation of fuel partitioning by glucocorticoids, androgens, and estrogens as well as region-specific adipose tissue depot characteristics likely contribute to explain these sex differences in the presence of a given energy imbalance.

REFERENCES

1. Pond CM 1992 An evolutionary and functional view of mammalian adipose tissue. Proc Nutr Soc 51:367–377
2. Vague J 1947 La différenciation sexuelle, facteur déterminant des formes de l'obésité. Presse Med 30:339–340
3. Vague J 1956 The degree of masculine differentiation of obesities: a factor determining predisposition to diabetes, atherosclerosis, gout and uric calculous disease. Am J Clin Nutr 4:20–34
4. Kissebah AH, Krakower GR 1994 Regional adiposity and morbidity. Physiol Rev 74:761–811
5. Després JP, Moorjani S, Ferland M, Tremblay Y, Lupien PJ, Nadeau A, Pinault S, Thériault G, Bouchard C 1989 Adipose tissue distribution and plasma lipoprotein levels in obese women: importance of intra-abdominal fat. Arteriosclerosis 9:203–210
6. Yusuf S, Hawken S, Ôunpuu S, Bautista L, Franzosi MG, Commerford P, Lang CC, Rumboldt Z, Onen CL, Lisheng L, Tanornsup S, Wangai P, Jr, Razak F, Sharma AM, Anand SS, INTERHEART Study Investigators 2005 Obesity and the risk of myocardial infarction in 27 000 participants from 52 countries: a case-control study. Lancet 366:1640–1649
7. Després JP, Lemieux I 2006 Abdominal obesity and metabolic syndrome. Nature 444:881–887
8. Carpenter WH, Poehlman ET, O'Connell M, Goran MI 1995 Influence of body composition and resting metabolic rate on variation in total energy expenditure: a meta-analysis. Am J Clin Nutr 61:4–10
9. Ferraro R, Lillioja S, Fontvieille AM, Rising R, Bogardus C, Ravussin E 1992 Lower sedentary metabolic rate in women compared with men. J Clin Invest 90:780–784
10. Goran MI 1995 Variation in total energy expenditure in humans. Obes Res 3(Suppl 1):59–66

11. Rolls BJ, Fedoroff IC, Guthrie JF 1991 Gender differences in eating behavior and body weight regulation. Health Psychol 10:133–142

12. Basiotis PP, Thomas RG, Kelsay JL, Mertz W 1989 Sources of variation in energy intake by men and women as determined from one year's daily dietary records. Am J Clin Nutr 50:448–453

13. Dye L, Blundell JE 1997 Menstrual cycle and appetite control: implications for weight regulation. Hum Reprod 12:1142–1151

14. Barr SI, Janelle KC, Prior JC 1995 Energy intakes are higher during the luteal phase of ovulatory menstrual cycles. Am J Clin Nutr 61:39–43

15. Schweiger U, Tuschl RJ, Platte P, Broocks A, Laessle RG, Pirke KM 1992 Everyday eating behavior and menstrual function in young women. Fertil Steril 57:771–775

16. Chao YM, Pisetsky EM, Dierker LC, Dohm FA, Rosselli F, May AM, Striegel-Moore RH 2008 Ethnic differences in weight control practices among U.S. adolescents from 1995 to 2005. Int J Eat Disord 41:124–133

17. Veldhuis JD, Roemmich JN, Richmond EJ, Rogol AD, Lovejoy JC, Sheffield-Moore M, Mauras N, Bowers CY 2005 Endocrine control of body composition in infancy, childhood, and puberty. Endocr Rev 26:114–146

18. Wells JC 2007 Sexual dimorphism of body composition. Best Pract Res Clin Endocrinol Metab 21:415–430

19. Van Loan MD 1996 Total body composition: birth to old age. In: Roche AF, Heymsfield SB, Lohman TG (eds.) Human body composition. Human Kinetics: Champaign, IL, pp. 205–215

20. Siervogel RM, Demerath EW, Schubert C, Remsberg KE, Chumlea WC, Sun S, Czerwinski SA, Towne B 2003 Puberty and body composition. Horm Res 60:36–45

21. Hajamor S, Després JP, Couillard C, Lemieux S, Tremblay A, Prud'homme D, Tchernof A 2003 Relationship between sex hormone-binding globulin levels and features of the metabolic syndrome. Metabolism 52:724–730

22. Desmeules A, Couillard C, Tchernof A, Bergeron J, Rankinen T, Leon AS, Rao DC, Skinner JS, Wilmore JH, Després JP, Bouchard C 2003 Post-heparin lipolytic enzyme activities, sex hormones and sex hormone-binding globulin (SHBG) in men and women: the HERITAGE Family Study. Atherosclerosis 171:343–350

23. Lear SA, Humphries KH, Frohlich JJ, Birmingham CL 2007 Appropriateness of current thresholds for obesity-related measures among Aboriginal people. Can Med Assoc J 177:1499–1505

24. Després JP, Couillard C, Gagnon J, Bergeron J, Leon AS, Rao DC, Skinner JS, Wilmore JH, Bouchard C 2000 Race, visceral adipose tissue, plasma lipids, and lipoprotein lipase activity in men and women: the Health, Risk Factors, Exercise Training, and Genetics (HERITAGE) family study. Arterioscler Thromb Vasc Biol 20:1932–1938

25. Lear SA, Humphries KH, Kohli S, Chockalingam A, Frohlich JJ, Birmingham CL 2007 Visceral adipose tissue accumulation differs according to ethnic background: results of the Multicultural Community Health Assessment Trial (M-CHAT). Am J Clin Nutr 86:353–359

26. Sniderman AD, Bhopal R, Dorairaj P, Sarrafzadegan N, Tchernof A 2007 Why might South Asians be so susceptible to central obesity and its atherogenic consequences? The adipose tissue compartment hypothesis. Int J Epidemiol 36:220–225

27. Farnier C, Krier S, Blache M, Diot-Dupuy F, Mory G, Ferre P, Bazin R 2003 Adipocyte functions are modulated by cell size change: potential involvement of an integrin/ERK signalling pathway. Int J Obes 27:1178–1186

28. Boivin A, Brochu G, Marceau S, Marceau P, Hould FS, Tchernof A 2007 Regional differences in adipose tissue metabolism in obese men. Metabolism 56:533–540

29. Fried SK, Kral JG 1987 Sex differences in regional distribution of fat cell size and lipoprotein lipase activity in morbidly obese patients. Int J Obes 11:129–140

30. Salans LB, Cushman SW, Weismann RE 1973 Studies of human adipose tissue. Adipose cell size and number in non-obese and obese patients. J Clin Invest 52:929–941

31. Tchernof A, Bélanger C, Morisset AS, Richard C, Mailloux J, Laberge P, Dupont P 2006 Regional differences in adipose tissue metabolism in women: minor effect of obesity and body fat distribution. Diabetes 55:1353–1360

32. Edens NK, Fried SK, Kral JG, Hirsch J, Leibel RL 1993 In vitro lipid synthesis in human adipose tissue from three abdominal sites. Am J Physiol 265:E374–E379

33. Reynisdottir S, Dauzats M, Thörne A, Langin D 1997 Comparison of hormone-sensitive lipase activity in visceral and subcutaneous human adipose tissue. J Clin Endocrinol Metab 82:4162–4166

34. Richelsen B, Pedersen SB, Mollcr-Pedersen T, Bak JF 1991 Regional differences in triglyceride breakdown in human adipose tissue: effects of catecholamines, insulin, and prostaglandin E_2. Metabolism 40:990–996

35. Zinder O, Shapiro B 1971 Effect of cell size on epinephrine- and ACTH-induced fatty acid release from isolated fat cells. J Lipid Res 12:91–95

36. Franck N, Stenkula KG, Ost A, Lindstrom T, Stralfors P, Nystrom FH 2007 Insulin-induced GLUT4 translocation to the plasma membrane is blunted in large compared with small primary fat cells isolated from the same individual. Diabetologia 50:1716–1722

37. Jernas M, Palming J, Sjoholm K, Jennische E, Svensson PA, Gabrielsson BG, Levin M, Sjogren A, Rudemo M, Lystig TC, Carlsson B, Carlsson LM, Lonn M 2006 Separation of human adipocytes by size: hypertrophic fat cells display distinct gene expression. FASEB J 20:1540–1542

38. Smith J, Al-Amri M, Dorairaj P, Sniderman A 2006 The adipocyte life cycle hypothesis. Clin Sci 110:1–9

39. Nielsen S, Guo Z, Johnson M, Hensrud DD, Jensen MD 2004 Splanchnic lipolysis in human obesity. J Clin Invest 113: 1582–1588

40. Zierath JR, Livingston JN, Thorne A, Bolinder J, Reynisdottir S, Lonnqvist F, Arner P 1998 Regional difference in insulin inhibition of non-esterified fatty acid release from human adipocytes: relation to insulin receptor phosphorylation and intracellular signalling through the insulin receptor substrate-1 pathway. Diabetologia 41:1343–1354

41. Mauriège P, Marette A, Atgie C, Bouchard C, Theriault G, Bukowiecki LK, Marceau P, Biron S, Nadeau A, Després JP 1995 Regional variation in adipose tissue metabolism of severely obese premenopausal women. J Lipid Res 36:672–684

42. Fried SK, Russell CD, Grauso NL, Brolin RE 1993 Lipoprotein lipase regulation by insulin and glucocorticoid in subcutaneous and omental adipose tissue of obese men and women. J Clin Invest 92:2191–2198

43. Panarotto D, Poisson J, Devroede G, Maheux P 2000 Lipoprotein lipase steady-state mRNA levels are lower in human omental versus subcutaneous abdominal adipose tissue. Metabolism 49:1224–1227

44. Rebuffé-Scrive M, Andersson B, Olbe L, Björntorp P 1989 Metabolism of adipose tissue in intraabdominal depots of nonobese men and women. Metabolism 38:453–458

45. Mårin P, Andersson B, Ottosson M, Olbe L, Chowdhury B, Kvist H, Holm G, Sjöström L, Björntorp P 1992 The morphology and metabolism of intraabdominal adipose tissue in men. Metabolism 41:1242–1248

46. Maslowska MH, Sniderman AD, MacLean LD, Cianflone K 1993 Regional differences in triacylglycerol synthesis in adipose tissue and in cultured preadipocytes. J Lipid Res 34:219–228

47. Lewis GF, Carpentier A, Adeli K, Giacca A 2002 Disordered fat storage and mobilization in the pathogenesis of insulin resistance and type 2 diabetes. Endocr Rev 23:201–229

48. Lewis GF 1997 Fatty acid regulation of very low density lipoprotein production. Curr Opin Lipidol 8:146–153

49. Lamarche B, Rashid S, Lewis GF 1999 HDL metabolism in hypertrygliceridemic states: an overview. Clin Chim Acta 286:145–161

50. Björntorp P 1990 "Portal" adipose tissue as a generator of risk factors for cardiovascular disease and diabetes. Arteriosclerosis 10:493–496

51. Després JP, Ferland M, Moorjani S, Nadeau A, Tremblay A, Lupien PJ, Thériault G, Bouchard C 1989 Role of hepatic-triglyceride lipase activity in the association between intra-abdominal fat and plasma HDL-cholesterol in obese women. Arteriosclerosis 9:485–492

52. Després JP, Marette A 1994 Relation of components of insulin resistance syndrome to coronary disease risk. Curr Opin Lipidol 5:274–289

53. Hennes M, Shrago E, Kissebah AH 1990 Receptor and postreceptor effects of FFA on hepatocyte insulin dynamics. Int J Obes 14:831–841

54. Svedberg J, Björntorp P, Smith V, Lonnroth P 1990 FFA inhibition of insulin binding, degradation, and action in isolated hepatocytes. Diabetes 39:570–574

55. Després JP 1991 Obesity and lipid metabolism: relevance of body fat distribution. Curr Opin Lipidol 2:5–15

56. Björntorp P 1992 Metabolic abnormalities in visceral obesity. Ann Med 24:3–5

57. Kelley DE, Mokan M, Simoneau JA, Mandarino LJ 1993 Interaction between glucose and free fatty acid metabolism in human skeletal muscle. J Clin Invest 92:91–98

58. Griffin ME, Marcucci MJ, Cline GW, Bell K, Barucci N, Lee D, Goodyear LJ, Kraegen EW, White MF, Shulman GI 1999 Free fatty acid-induced insulin resistance is associated with activation of protein kinase C theta and alterations in the insulin signaling cascade. Diabetes 48:1270–1274

59. Thompson AL, Cooney GJ 2000 Acyl-CoA inhibition of hexokinase in rat and human skeletal muscle is a potential mechanism of lipid-induced insulin resistance. Diabetes 49:1761–1765

60. Boden G, Chen X, Ruiz J, White JV, Rossetti L 1994 Mechanisms of fatty acid-induced inhibition of glucose uptake. J Clin Invest 93:2438–2446

61. Gray SL, Vidal-Puig AJ 2007 Adipose tissue expandability in the maintenance of metabolic homeostasis. Nutr Rev 65:S7–S12

62. Frayn KN 2002 Adipose tissue as a buffer for daily lipid flux. Diabetologia 45:1201–1210

63. Medina-Gomez G, Virtue S, Lelliott C, Boiani R, Campbell M, Christodoulides C, Perrin C, Jimenez-Linan M, Blount M, Dixon J, Zahn D, Thresher RR, Aparicio S, Carlton M, Colledge WH, Kettunen MI, Seppanen-Laakso T, Sethi JK, O'Rahilly S, Brindle K, Cinti S, Oresic M, Burcelin R, Vidal-Puig A 2005 The link between nutritional status and insulin sensitivity is dependent on the adipocyte-specific peroxisome proliferator-activated receptor-gamma2 isoform. Diabetes 54:1706–1716

64. Reitman ML, Mason MM, Moitra J, Gavrilova O, Markus-Samuels B, Eckhaus M, Vinson C 1999 Transgenic mice lacking white fat: models for understanding human lipoatrophic diabetes. Ann N Y Acad Sci 892:289–296

65. Goodpaster BH, Thaete FL, Simoneau JA, Kelley DE 1997 Subcutaneous abdominal fat and thigh muscle composition predict insulin sensitivity independently of visceral fat. Diabetes 46:1579–1585

66. Goodpaster BH, Kelley DE 2002 Skeletal muscle triglyceride: marker or mediator of obesity-induced insulin resistance in type 2 diabetes mellitus? Curr Diab Rep 2:216–222

67. Kim JK, Fillmore JJ, Chen Y, Yu C, Moore IK, Pypaert M, Lutz EP, Kako Y, Velez-Carrasco W, Goldberg IJ, Breslow JL, Shulman GI 2001 Tissue-specific overexpression of lipoprotein lipase causes tissue-specific insulin resistance. Proc Natl Acad Sci U S A 98:7522–7527

68. Nadler ST, Stoehr JP, chueler KL, Tanimoto G, Yandell BS, Attie AD 2000 The expression of adipogenic genes is decreased in obesity and diabetes mellitus. Proc Natl Acad Sci U S A 97:11371–11376

69. Drolet R, Richard C, Sniderman AD, Mailloux J, Fortier M, Huot C, Rhéaume C, Tchernof A 2008 Hypertrophy and hyperplasia of abdominal adipose tissues in women. Int J Obes 32:283 291

70. Trayhurn P, Wood IS 2005 Signalling role of adipose tissue: adipokines and inflammation in obesity. Biochem Soc Trans 33:1078–1081

71. Drolet R, Bélanger C, Fortier M, Huot C, Mailloux J, Légaré D, Tchernof A 2009 Fat depot-specific impact of visceral obesity on adipocyte adiponectin release in women. Obesity 17:424–430

72. Hube F, Birgel M, Lee YM, Hauner H 1999 Expression pattern of tumour necrosis factor receptors in subcutaneous and omental human adipose tissue: role of obesity and non-insulin-dependent diabetes mellitus. Eur J Clin Invest 29:672–678

73. Hotamisligil GS, Arner P, Caro JF, Atkinson RL, Spiegelman BM 1995 Increased adipose tissue expression of tumor necrosis factor-alpha in human obesity and insulin resistance. J Clin Invest 95:2409–2415

74. He G, Pedersen SB, Bruun JM, Lihn AS, Jensen PF, Richelsen B 2003 Differences in plasminogen activator inhibitor 1 in subcutaneous versus omental adipose tissue in non-obese and obese subjects. Horm Metab Res 35:178–182

75. Skurk T, Alberti-Huber C, Herder C, Hauner H 2007 Relationship between adipocyte size and adipokine expression and secretion. J Clin Endocrinol Metab 92:1023–1033

76. Whitehead JP, Richards AA, Hickman IJ, Macdonald GA, Prins JB 2006 Adiponectin--a key adipokine in the metabolic syndrome. Diabetes Obes Metab 8:264–280

77. Cnop M, Havel PJ, Utzschneider KM, Carr DB, Sinha MK, Boyko EJ, Retzlaff BM, Knopp RH, Brunzell JD, Kahn SE 2003 Relationship of adiponectin to body fat distribution, insulin sensitivity and plasma lipoproteins: evidence for independent roles of age and sex. Diabetologia 46:459–469

78. Park KG, Park KS, Kim M-J, Kim H-S, Suh Y-S, Ahn JD, Park K-K, Chang Y-C, Lee I-K 2004 Relationship between serum adiponectin and leptin concentrations and body fat distribution. Diabetes Res Clin Pract 63:135–142

79. Motoshima H, Wu X, Sinha MK, Hardy E, Rosato EL, Barbot DJ, Rosato FE, Goldstein BJ 2002 Differential regulation of adiponectine secretion from cultured human omental and subcutaneous adipocytes: effects of insulin and rosiglitazone. J Clin Endocrinol Metab 87:5662–5667

80. Bastard JP, Jardel C, Bruckert E, Blondy P, Capeau J, Laville M, Vidal H 2000 Elevated levels of interleukin 6 are reduced in serum and subcutaneous adipose tissue of obese women after weight loss. J Clin Endocrinol Metab 85:3338–3342

81. Fenkci S, Rota S, Sabir N, Sermez Y, Guclu A, Akdag B 2006 Relationship of serum interleukin-6 and tumor necrosis factor alpha levels with abdominal fat distribution evaluated by ultrasonography in overweight or obese postmenopausal women. J Invest Med 54:455–460

82. Wisse BE 2004 The inflammatory syndrome: the role of adipose tissue cytokines in metabolic disorders linked to obesity. J Am Soc Nephrol 15:2792–2800

83. Fried SK, Bunkin DA, Greenberg AS 1998 Omental and subcutaneous adipose tissues of obese subjects release interleukin-6: depot difference and regulation by glucocorticoid. J Clin Endocrinol Metab 83:847–850

84. Morisset AS, Huot C, Légaré D, Tchernof A 2008 Circulating IL-6 concentrations and abdominal adipocyte isoproterenol-stimulated lipolysis in women. Obesity 16:1487–1492

85. Trujillo ME, Sullivan S, Harten I, Schneider SH, Greenberg AS, Fried SK 2004 Interleukin-6 regulates human adipose tissue lipid metabolism and leptin production in vitro. J Clin Endocrinol Metab 89:5577–5582

86. Greenberg AS, Nordan RP, McIntosh J, Calvo JC, Scow RO, Jablons D 1992 Interleukin 6 reduces lipoprotein lipase activity in adipose tissue of mice in vivo and in 3T3-L1 adipocytes: a possible role for interleukin 6 in cancer cachexia. Cancer Res 52:4113–4116

87. Weisberg SP, McCann D, Desai M, Rosenbaum M, Leibel RL, Ferrante AW, Jr 2003 Obesity is associated with macrophage accumulation in adipose tissue. J Clin Invest 112:1796–1808

88. Good M, Newell FM, Haupt LM, Whitehead JP, Hutley LJ, Prins JB 2006 TNF and TNF receptor expression and insulin sensitivity in human omental and subcutaneous adipose tissue--influence of BMI and adipose distribution. Diab Vasc Dis Res 3:26–33

89. Grunfeld C, Feingold KR 1991 The metabolic effects of tumor necrosis factor and other cytokines. Biotherapy 3:143–158

90. Perreault M, Marette A 2001 Targeted disruption of inducible nitric oxide synthase protects against obesity-linked insulin resistance in muscle. Nat Med 7:1138–1143

91. Park HS, Park JY, Yu R 2005 Relationship of obesity and visceral adiposity with serum concentrations of CRP, TNF-alpha and IL-6. Diabetes Res Clin Pract 69:29–35

92. Tsigos C, Kyrou I, Chala E, Tsapogas P, Stavridis JC, Raptis SA, Katsilambros N 1999 Circulating tumor necrosis factor alpha concentrations are higher in abdominal versus peripheral obesity. Metabolism 48:1332–1335

93. Alessi MC, Juhan-Vague I 2006 PAI-1 and the metabolic syndrome: links, causes, and consequences. Arterioscler Thromb Vasc Biol 26:2200–2207

94. Gottschling-Zeller H, Birgel M, Rohrig K, Hauner H 2000 Effect of tumor necrosis factor alpha and transforming growth factor beta 1 on plasminogen activator inhibitor-1 secretion from subcutaneous and omental human fat cells in suspension culture. Metabolism 49:666–671

95. Alessi MC, Peiretti F, Morange P, Henry M, Nalbone G, Juhan-Vague I 1997 Production of plasminogen activator inhibitor 1 by human adipose tissue: possible link between visceral fat accumulation and vascular disease. Diabetes 46:860–867

96. Kockx M, Leenen R, Seidell J, Princen HM, Kooistra T 1999 Relationship between visceral fat and PAI-1 in overweight men and women before and after weight loss. Thromb Haemost 82:1490–1496

97. van Beek EA, Bakker AH, Kruyt PM, Hofker MH, Saris WH, Keijer J 2007 Intra- and interindividual variation in gene expression in human adipose tissue. Pflugers Arch 453:851–861

98. Vohl MC, Sladek R, Robitaille J, Gurd S, Marceau P, Richard D, Hudson TJ, Tchernof A 2004 A survey of genes differentially expressed in subcutaneous and visceral adipose tissue in men. Obes Res 12:1217–1222

99. Montague CT, Prins JB, Sanders L, Zhang J, Sewter CP, Digby J, Byrne CD, O'Rahilly S 1998 Depot-Related gene expression in human subcutaneous and omental adipocytes. Diabetes 47:1384–1391

100. Zhang Y, Bossé Y, Marceau P, Biron S, Lebel S, Richard D, Vohl MC, Tchernof A 2007 Gene expression variability in subcutaneous and omental adipose tissue of obese men. Gene Expr 14:35–46

101. Hoyenga KB, Hoyenga KT 1982 Gender and energy balance: sex differences in adaptations for feast and famine. Physiol Behav 28:545–563

102. Miller GF 1998 A review of sexual selection and human evolution: how mate choice shaped human nature. In: Crawford C, Krebs D (eds.) Handbook of evolutionary psychology: ideas, issues, and applications. Lawrence Erlbaum: New Jersey, pp. 87–130

103. Trivers RL 1972 Parental investment and sexual selection. In: Campbell B (ed.) Sexual selection and the descent of man. Aldine: Chicago, pp. 136–179

104. Dixson A, Dixson B, Anderson M 2005 Sexual selection and the evolution of visually conspicuous sexually dimorphic traits in male monkeys, apes, and human beings. Annu Rev Sex Res 16:1–19

105. Thomas JR, French KE 1985 Gender differences across age in motor performance a meta-analysis. Psychol Bull 98:260–282

106. Blouin K, Boivin A, Tchernof A 2008 Androgens and body fat distribution. J Steroid Biochem Mol Biol 108:272–280

107. Rask E, Walker BR, Söderberg S, Livingstone DEW, Eliasson M, Johnson O, Andrew R, Olsson T 2002 Tissue-specific changes in peripheral cortisol metabolism in obese women: increased adipose 11β-hydroxysteroid dehydrogenase type 1 activity. J Clin Endocrinol Metab 87:3330–3336

108. Beaulieu EE, Kelly PA 1990 Hormones: from molecules to disease, ed. 1. Hermann Publishers in Arts and Science, Chapman and Hall, New York and London

109. Duclos M, Gatta B, Corcuff JB, Rashedi M, Pehourcq F, Roger P 2001 Fat distribution in obese women is associated with subtle alterations of the hypothalamic-pituitary-adrenal axis activity and sensitivity to glucocorticoids. Clin Endocrinol (Oxf) 55:447–454

110. Mårin P, Darin N, Anemiya T, Andersson B, Jern S, Björntorp P 1992 Cortisol secretion in relation to body fat distribution in obese premenopausal women. Metabolism 41:882–886

111. Putignano P, Giraldi FP, Cavagnini F 2004 Tissue-specific dysregulation of 11β-hydroxysteroid dehydrogenase type 1 and pathogenesis of the metabolic syndrome. J Endocrinol Invest 27:969–974

112. Seckl JR, Walker BR 2001 11β-hydroxysteroid dehydrogenase type 1 – a tissue specific amplifier of glucocorticoid action. Endocrinology 142:1371–1376

113. Masuzaki H, Paterson J, Shinyama H, Morton NM, Mullins JJ, Seckl JR, Flier JS 2001 A transgenic model of visceral obesity and the metabolic syndrome. Science 294:2166–2170

114. Bujalska IJ, Kumar S, Stewart PM 1997 Does central obesity reflect "Cushing's disease of the omentum"? Lancet 349:1210–1213

115. Katz JR, Mohamed-Ali V, Wood PJ, Yudkin JS, Coppack SW 1999 An in vivo study of the cortisol-cortisone shuttle in subcutaneous abdominal adipose tissue. Clin Endocrinol 50:63–68

116. Rask E, Olsson T, Soderberg S, Andrew R, Livingstone DE, Johnson O, Walker BR 2001 Tissue-specific dysregulation of cortisol metabolism in human obesity. J Clin Endocrinol Metab 86:1418–21

117. Lindsay RS, Wake DJ, Nair S, Bunt J, Livingstone DE, Permana PA, Tataranni PA, Walker BR 2003 Subcutaneous adipose 11β-hydroxysteroid dehydrogenase type 1 activity and messenger ribonucleic acid levels are associated with adiposity and insulinemia in Pima Indians and Caucasians. J Clin Endocrinol Metab 88:2738–2744

118. Paulmyer-Lacroix O, Boullu S, Oliver C, Alessi MC, Grino M 2002 Expression of the mRNA coding for 11β-hydroxysteroid dehydrogenase type 1 in adipose tissue from obese patients: an in situ hybridization study. J Clin Endocrinol Metab 87:2701–2705

119. Stewart PM, Boulton A, Kumar S, Clark PM, Shackleton CH 1999 Cortisol metabolism in human obesity: impaired cortisone-cortisol conversion in subjects with central adiposity. J Clin Endocrinol Metab 84:1022–1027

120. Tomlinson JW, Sinha B, Bujalska I, Hewison M, Stewart PM 2002 Expression of 11β-hydroxysteroid dehydrogenase type 1 in adipose tissue is not increased in human obesity. J Clin Endocrinol Metab 87:5630–5635

121. Bujalska IJ, Walker EA, Tomlinson JW, Hewison M, Stewart PM 2002 11Beta-hydroxysteroid dehydrogenase type 1 in differentiating omental human preadipocytes: from de-activation to generation of cortisol. Endocr Res 28:449–461

122. Bujalska IJ, Walker EA, Hewison M, Stewart PM 2002 A switch in dehydrogenase to reductase activity of 11β-hydroxysteroid dehydrogenase type 1 upon differentiation of human omental adipose stromal cells. J Clin Endocrinol Metab 87:1205–1210

123. Pasquali R, Casimirri F, Cantobelli S, Melchionda N, Morselli Labate AM, Fabbri R, Capelli M, Bortoluzzi L 1991 Effect of obesity and body fat distribution on sex hormones and insulin in men. Metabolism 40:101–104

124. Khaw KT, Barrett-Connor E 1992 Lower endogenous androgens predict central adiposity in men. Ann Epidemiol 2:675–682

125. Gapstur SM, Gann PH, Kopp P, Colangelo L, Longcope C, Liu K 2002 Serum androgen concentrations in young men: a longitudinal analysis of associations with age, obesity, and race. The CARDIA male hormone study. Cancer Epidemiol Biomarkers Prev 11:1041–1047

126. Seidell JC, Björntorp P, Sjöström L, Kvist H, Sannrstedt R 1990 Visceral fat accumulation in men is positively associated with insulin, glucose, and C-peptide levels, but negatively with testosterone levels. Metabolism 39:897–901

127. Couillard C, Gagnon J, Bergeron J, Leon AS, Rao DC, Skinner JS, Wilmore JH, Després JP, Bouchard C 2000 Contribution of body fatness and adipose tissue distribution to the age variation in plasma steroid hormone concentrations in men: the HERITAGE family study. J Clin Endocrinol Metab 85:1026–1031

128. Tchernof A, Després JP, Bélanger A, Dupont A, Prud'homme D, Moorjani S, Lupien PJ, Labrie F 1995 Reduced testosterone and adrenal C19 steroid levels in obese men. Metabolism 44:513–519

129. Garaulet M, Pérez-Llamas F, Fuente T, Zamora S, Tebar FJ 2000 Anthropometric, computed tomography and fat cell data in an obese population: relationship with insulin, leptin, tumor necrosis factor-alpha, sex hormone-binding globulin and sex hormones. Eur J Endocrinol 143:657–666

130. Tsai EC, Matsumoto AM, Fujimoto WY, Boyko EJ 2004 Association of bioavailable, free, and total testosterone with insulin resistance: influence of sex hormone-binding globulin and body fat. Diabetes Care 27:861–868

131. Phillips GB, Jing T, Heymsfield SB 2003 Relationships in men of sex hormones, insulin, adiposity, and risk factors for myocardial infarction. Metabolism 52:784–790

132. Tchernof A, Després JP 2000 Sex steroid hormones, sex hormone-binding globulin, and obesity in men and women. Horm Metab Res 32:526–536

133. Vermeulen A, Verdonck L, Kaufman JM 1999 A critical evaluation of simple methods for the estimation of free testosterone in serum. J Clin Endocrinol Metab 84:3666–3672

134. Rosner W, Auchus RJ, Azziz R, Sluss PM, Raff H 2007 Position statement: utility, limitations, and pitfalls in measuring testosterone: an Endocrine Society position statement. J Clin Endocrinol Metab 92:405–413

135. Boyanov MA, Boneva Z, Christov VG 2003 Testosterone supplementation in men with type 2 diabetes, visceral obesity and partial androgen deficiency. Aging Male 6:1–7

136. Woodhouse LJ, Gupta N, Bhasin M, Singh AB, Ross R, Phillips J, Bhasin S 2004 Dose-dependent effects of testosterone on regional adipose tissue distribution in healthy young men. J Clin Endocrinol Metab 89:718–726

137. Mårin P, Holmäng S, Jönsson L, Sjöström L, Kvist H, Holm G, Lindstedt G, Björntorp P 1992 The effects of testosterone treatment on body composition and metabolism in middle-aged and obese men. Int J Obes 16:991–997

138. Gruenewald DA, Matsumoto AM 2003 Testosterone supplementation therapy for older men: potential benefits and risks. J Am Geriatr Soc 51:101–115

139. Elbers JMH, Asscheman H, Seidell JC, Megens JA, Gooren LJG 1997 Long-term testosterone administration increases visceral fat in female to male transsexuals. J Clin Endocrinol Metab 82:2044–2047

140. Elbers JMH, Giltay EJ, Teerlink T, Scheffer PG, Asscheman H, Seidell JC, Gooren LJG 2003 Effects of sex steroids on components of the insulin resistance syndrome in transsexual subjects. Clin Endocrinol 58:562–571
141. Glazer G 1991 Atherogenic effects of anabolic steroids on serum lipid levels. A literature review. Arch Intern Med 151:1925–1933
142. Dunaif A 1997 Insulin resistance and the polycystic ovary syndrome: mechanism and implications for pathogenesis. Endocr Rev 18:774–800
143. Nestler JE, Barlascini CO, Matt DW, Steingold KA, Plymate SR, Clore JN, Blackard WG 1989 Suppression of serum insulin by diazoxide reduces serum testosterone levels in obese women with polycystic ovary syndrome. J Clin Endocrinol Metab 68:1027–1032
144. Dunaif A, Scott D, Finegood D, Quintana B, Whitcomb R 1996 The insulin-sensitizing agent troglitazone improves metabolic and reproductive abnormalities in the polycystic ovary syndrome. J Clin Endocrinol Metab 81:3299–3306
145. Velazquez EM, Mendoza S, Hamer T, Sosa F, Glueck CJ 1994 Metformin therapy in polycystic ovary syndrome reduces hyperinsulinemia, insulin resistance, hyperandrogenemia, and systolic blood pressure, while facilitating normal menses and pregnancy. Metabolism 43:647–654
146. Bates GW, Whitworth NS 1982 Effect of body weight reduction on plasma androgens in obese, infertile women. Fertil Steril 38:406–409
147. Kiddy DS, Hamilton-Fairley D, Bush A, Short F, Anyaoku V, Reed MJ, Franks S 1992 Improvement in endocrine and ovarian function during dietary treatment of obese women with polycystic ovary syndrome. Clin Endocrinol 36:105–111
148. Evans DJ, Barth JH, Burke CW 1988 Body fat topography in women with androgen excess. Int J Obes 12:157–162
149. Seidell JC, Cigolini M, Charzewska J, Ellsinger BM, DiBiase G, Björntorp P, Hautvast JGA, Contaldo F, Szostak V, Scuro LA 1990 Androgenicity in relation to body fat distribution and metabolism in 38-year-old women-the European fat distribution study. J Clin Epidemiol 43:21–32
150. Ivandic A, Prpic-Krizevac I, Sucic M, Juric M 1998 Hyperinsulinemia and sex hormones in healthy premenopausal women: relative contribution of obesity, obesity type, and duration of obesity. Metabolism 47:13–19
151. Kaye SA, Folsom AR, Soler JT, Prineas RJ, Potter JD 1991 Associations of body mass and fat distribution with sex hormone concentrations in postmenopausal women. Int J Epidemiol 20:151–156
152. de Pergola G, Triggiani V, Giorgino F, Cospite MR, Garruti G, Cignarelli M, Guastamacchia E, Giorgino R 1994 The free testosterone to dehydroepiandrosterone sulphate molar ratio as a marker of visceral fat accumulation in premenopausal obese women. Int J Obes 18:659–664
153. Armellini F, Zamboni M, Castelli S, Robbi R, Mino A, Todesco T, Bergamo-Andreis IA, Bossello O 1994 Interrelationship between intraabdominal fat and total serum testosterone levels in obese women. Metabolism 43:390–395
154. Turcato E, Zamboni M, de Pergola G, Armellini F, Zivelonghi A, Bergamo-Andreis IA, Giorgino R, Bosello O 1997 Interrelationships between weight loss, body fat distribution and sex hormones in pre- and postmenopausal obese women. J Intern Med 241:363–372
155. Deslypere JP, Verdonck L, Vermeulen A 1985 Fat tissue: a steroid reservoir and site of steroid metabolism. J Clin Endocrinol Metab 61:564–570
156. Fehér T, Bodrogi L 1982 A comparative study of steroid concentrations in human adipose tissue and the peripheral circulation. Clin Chim Acta 126:135–141
157. Fehér T, Halmy L, Bodrogi L, Kazik MH 1976 dehydroepiandrosterone concentration in adipose tissue of normal and overweight subjects. Horm Metab Res 8:372–374
158. Szymczak J, Milewicz A, Thijssen JHH, Blankenstein MA, Daroszewski J 1998 Concentrations of sex steroids in adipose tissue after menopause. Steroids 63:319–321
159. Borg W, Shackelton CHL, Pahuja SL, Hochberg RB 1995 Long-lived testosterone esters in the rat. Proc Natl Acad Sci U S A 92:1545–1549
160. de Pergola G, Xu X, Yang S, Giorgino R, Björntorp P 1990 Up-regulation of androgen receptor binding in male rat fat pad adipose precursor cells exposed to testosterone: study in a whole cell assay system. J Steroid Biochem Mol Biol 4:553–558
161. Joyner J, Hutley L, Cameron D 2002 Intrinsic regional differences in androgen receptors and dihydrotestosterone metabolism in human preadipocytes. Horm Metab Res 34:223–228
162. Bélanger C, Hould FS, Lebel S, Biron S, Brochu G, Tchernof A 2006 Omental and subcutaneous adipose tissue steroid levels in obese men. Steroids 71:674–682
163. Blouin K, Richard C, Brochu G, Hould FS, Lebel S, Marceau S, Biron S, Luu-The V, Tchernof A 2006 Androgen inactivation and steroid-converting enzyme expression in abdominal adipose tissue in men. J Endocrinol 191:637–649
164. Fan W, Yanase T, Nomura M, Okabe T, Goto K, Sato T, Kawano H, Kato S, Nawata H 2005 Androgen receptor null male mice develop late-onset obesity caused by decreased energy expenditure and lipolytic activity but show normal insulin sensitivity with high adiponectin secretion. Diabetes 54:1000–1008

165. Mårin P, Lönn L, Andersson B, Odén B, Olbe L, Bengtsson BA, Björntorp P 1996 Assimilation of triglycerides in subcutaneous and intraabdominal adipose tissues in vivo in men: effects of testosterone. J Clin Endocrinol Metab 81:1018–1022

166. Dieudonne MN, Pecquery R, Leneveu MC, Giudicelli Y 2000 Opposite effects of androgens and estrogens on adipogenesis in rat preadipocytes: evidence for sex and site-related specificities and possible involvement of insulin-like growth factor 1 receptor and peroxisome proliferator-activated receptor gamma2. Endocrinology 141:649–656

167. Singh R, Artaza JN, Taylor WE, Braga M, Yuan X, Gonzalez-Cadavid NF, Bhasin S 2006 Testosterone inhibits adipogenic differentiation in 3T3-L1 cells: nuclear translocation of androgen receptor complex with beta-catenin and T-cell factor 4 may bypass canonical Wnt signaling to down-regulate adipogenic transcription factors. Endocrinology 147:141–154

168. Lacasa D, Garcia E, Henriot D, Agli B, Giudicelli Y 1997 Site-related specificities of the control by androgenic status of adipogenesis and mitogen-activated protein kinase cascade/c-fos signaling pathways in rat preadipocytes. Endocrinology 138:3181–3186

169. Lacasa D, Agli B, Moynard D, Giudicelli Y 1995 Evidence for a regional-specific control of rat preadipocyte proliferation and differentiation by the androgenic status. Endocrine 3:793

170. Dicker A, Ryden M, Näslund E, Muehlen IE, Wiren M, Lafontan M, Arner P 2004 Effect of testosterone on lipolysis in human pre-adipocytes from different fat depots. Diabetologia 47:420–428

171. Rodriguez-Cuenca S, Monjo M, Proenza AM, Roca P 2005 Depot differences in steroid receptor expression in adipose tissue: possible role of the local steroid milieu. Am J Physiol Endocrinol Metab 288:E200–E207

172. Tchernof A, Labrie F, Bélanger A, Prud'homme D, Bouchard C, Tremblay A, Nadeau A, Després JP 1997 Androstane-3α, 17β-diol glucuronide as a steroid correlate of visceral obesity in men. J Clin Endocrinol Metab 82:1528–1534

173. Pritchard J, Després JP, Gagnon J, Tchernof A, Nadeau A, Tremblay A, Bouchard C 1998 Plasma adrenal, gonadal and conjugated steroids before and after long term overfeeding in identical twins. J Clin Endocrinol Metab 83:3277–3284

174. Pritchard J, Després JP, Gagnon J, Tchernof A, Nadeau A, Tremblay A, Bouchard C 1999 Plasma adrenal, gonadal, and conjugated steroids following long--term exercise-induced negative energy balance in identical twins. Metabolism 48:1120–1127

175. Tchernof A, Lévesque E, Beaulieu M, Couture P, Després JP, Hum DW, Bélanger A 1999 Expression of the androgen metabolizing enzyme UGT2B15 in adipose tissue and relative expression measurement using a competitive RT-PCR method. Clin Endocrinol 50:637–642

176. Blouin K, Blanchette S, Richard C, Dupont P, Luu-The V, Tchernof A 2005 Expression and activity of steroid aldoketoreductases 1C in omental adipose tissue as positive correlates of adiposity in women. Am J Physiol Endocrinol Metab 288:E398–E404

177. Blouin K, Richard C, Bélanger C, Dupont P, Daris M, Laberge P, Luu-The V, Tchernof A 2003 Local androgen inactivation in abdominal visceral adipose tissue. J Clin Endocrinol Metab 88:5944–5950

178. Vandenput L, Mellstrom D, Lorentzon M, Swanson C, Karlsson MK, Brandberg J, Lonn L, Orwoll E, Smith U, Labrie F, Ljunggren O, Tivesten A, Ohlsson C 2007 Androgens and glucuronidated androgen metabolites are associated with metabolic risk factors in men. J Clin Endocrinol Metab 92:4130–4137

179. Zhang Y, Dufort I, Rheault P, Luu-The V 2000 Characterization of a human 20alpha-hydroxysteroid dehydrogenase. J Mol Endocrinol 25:221–228

180. Dufort I, Rheault P, Huang XF, Soucy P 1999 Characteristics of a highly labile human type 5 17β-hydroxysteroid dehydrogenase. Endocrinology 140:568–574

181. Dufort I, Labrie F, Luu-The V 2001 Human types 1 and 3 3α-hydroxysteroid dehydrogenases: differential lability and tissue distribution. J Clin Endocrinol Metab 86:841–846

182. Dufort I, Soucy P, Labrie F, Luu-The V 1996 Molecular cloning of human type 3 3 alpha-hydroxysteroid dehydrogenase that differs from 20 alpha-hydroxysteroid dehydrogenase by seven amino acids. Biochem Biophys Res Commun 228:474–479

183. Crandall DL, Busler DE, Novak TJ, Weber RV, Kral JG 1998 Identification of estrogen receptor β RNA in human breast and abdominal subcutaneous adipose tissue. Biochem Biophys Res Commun 248:523–526

184. Mizutani T, Nishikawa Y, Adachi H, Enomoto T, Ikegami H, Kurachi H, Nomura T, Miyake A 1994 Identification of estrogen receptor in human adipose tissue and adipocytes. J Clin Endocrinol Metab 78:950–954

185. Price TM, O'Brien SN 1993 Determination of estrogen receptor messenger ribonucleic acid (mRNA) and cytochrome P450 aromatase mRNA levels in adipocytes and adipose stromal cells by competitive polymerase chain reaction amplification. J Clin Endocrinol Metab 77:1041–1045

186. Dieudonne MN, Leneveu MC, Giudicelli Y, Pecquery R 2004 Evidence for functional estrogen receptors alpha and beta in human adipose cells: regional specificities and regulation by estrogens. Am J Physiol Cell Physiol 286:C655–C661

187. Pedersen SB, Borglum JD, Eriksen EF, Richelsen B 1991 Nuclear estradiol binding in rat adipocytes. Regional variations and regulatory influences of hormones. Biochim Biophys Acta 1093:80–86

188. Watson GH, Manes JL, Mayes JS, McCann JP 1993 Biochemical and immunological characterization of oestrogen receptor in the cytosolic fraction of gluteal, omental and perirenal adipose tissue from sheep. J Endocrinol 139:107–115

189. Price TM, O'Brien SN, Welter BH, George R, Anandjiwala J, Kilgore M 1998 Estrogen regulation of adipose tissue lipoprotein lipase – possible mechanism of body fat distribution. Am J Obstet Gynecol 178:101–107

190. Palin SL, McTernan PG, Anderson LA, Sturdee DW, Barnett AH, Kumar S 2003 17Beta-estradiol and anti-estrogen ICI:compound 182,780 regulate expression of lipoprotein lipase and hormone-sensitive lipase in isolated subcutaneous abdominal adipocytes. Metabolism 52:383–388

191. Jensen MD, Martin ML, Cryer PE, Roust LR 1994 Effects of estrogen on free fatty acid metabolism in humans. Am J Physiol 266:E914–E920

192. Tchernof A, Desmeules A, Richard C, Laberge P, Daris M, Mailloux J, Rheaume C, Dupont P 2004 Ovarian hormone status and abdominal visceral adipose tissue metabolism. J Clin Endocrinol Metab 89:3425–3430

193. D'Eon TM, Souza SC, Aronovitz M, Obin MS, Fried SK, Greenberg AS 2005 Estrogen regulation of adiposity and fuel partitioning: evidence of genomic and non-genomic regulation of lipogenic and oxidative pathways. J Biol Chem 280:35983–35991

194. Clegg DJ, Riedy CA, Smith KA, Benoit SC, Woods SC 2003 Differential sensitivity to central leptin and insulin in male and female rats. Diabetes 52:682–687

195. Clegg DJ, Brown LM, Woods SC, Benoit SC 2006 Gonadal hormones determine sensitivity to central leptin and insulin. Diabetes 55:978–987

196. Clegg DJ, Brown LM, Zigman JM, Kemp CJ, Strader AD, Benoit SC, Woods SC, Mangiaracina M, Geary N 2007 Estradiol-dependent decrease in the orexigenic potency of ghrelin in female rats. Diabetes 56:1051–1058

197. Benoit SC, Clegg DJ, Seeley RJ, Woods SC 2004 Insulin and leptin as adiposity signals. Recent Prog Horm Res 59:267–285

198. Woods SC, Gotoh K, Clegg DJ 2003 Gender differences in the control of energy homeostasis. Exp Biol Med 228:1175–1180

199. Deschenes D, Couture P, Dupont P, Tchernof A 2003 Subdivision of the subcutaneous adipose tissue compartment and lipid-lipoprotein levels in women. Obes Res 11:469–476

200. Casey JL, Bouchard C, Wideman L, Kanaley J, Teates CD, Thorner MO, Hartman ML, Weltman A 1997 The influence of anatomical boundaries, age, and sex on the assessment of abdominal visceral fat. Obes Res 5:395–401

2 Menopause and Diabetes Mellitus

Emily D. Szmuilowicz and Ellen W. Seely

CONTENTS

ABSTRACT

Around the time of menopause, there are important changes in body composition and insulin sensitivity, which may impact both the risk for diabetes mellitus as well as glycemic control in individuals with established diabetes. Furthermore, these parameters may be affected by the use of hormone replacement therapy, a common treatment for menopausal vasomotor symptoms. Changes in body composition, beyond changes in weight, occur around the time of menopause, and these alterations in body composition have been correlated with changes in insulin resistance and glucose tolerance. Several studies have suggested that hormone therapy use reduces diabetes risk in postmenopausal women. Clinicians must keep these metabolic changes in mind when caring for postmenopausal women with and without diabetes.

Key words: Diabetes; Menopause; Insulin sensitivity; Body composition; Hormone therapy.

CHANGES IN GONADAL HORMONES AT MENOPAUSE

Menopause is defined as the cessation of menses for 12 months after the final menstrual period *(1)*, and it results from the depletion of ovarian follicles with resulting loss of ovarian sex hormone production. The average age at which women in the USA and Western Europe undergo natural menopause is 50–51 years *(2, 3)*. Women who undergo menopause before 40 years of age are considered to have premature ovarian failure *(4)*. In 2001, the Stages of Reproductive Aging Workshop (STRAW) was convened in order to develop a useful staging system for reproductive aging in women and to revise the often-confusing nomenclature used to describe this process. The menopausal transition was

From: *Diabetes in Women: Pathophysiology and Therapy*
Edited by: A. Tsatsoulis et al. (eds.), DOI 10.1007/978-1-60327-250-6_2
© Humana Press, a part of Springer Science+Business Media, LLC 2009

defined as the period beginning with the onset of irregular menstrual cycles (cycle length more than 7 days different from normal) and ending with the final menstrual period (which is recognized in retrospect, after 12 months of amenorrhea) *(1)*. Postmenopause was defined as the period spanning from the final menstrual period until death.

The normal process of reproductive aging is characterized by marked hormonal changes. The inhibins are peptides secreted from ovarian granulosa cells, which inhibit pituitary production of follicle-stimulating hormone (FSH) *(4)*. Decreased ovarian inhibin B production, the earliest marker of ovarian aging, begins during the late reproductive years *(5)*. This decrease in inhibin B production leads to a reciprocal rise in FSH, and thus the late reproductive stage is characterized by regular menstrual cycles associated with increased follicular-phase FSH levels *(5)*. Levels of estradiol, the predominant and most potent ovarian estrogen, are typically normal or elevated during this time, despite the decrease in ovarian follicle number. It has been hypothesized that the rise in FSH, which occurs during the late reproductive years, enables the maintenance of normal estradiol levels in the face of decreasing ovarian reserve *(6, 7)*.

The onset of the menopausal transition is marked by a shift from regular to irregular menstrual cycles *(1)*. Marked hormonal fluctuations occur during the menopausal transition *(5, 7)*. While FSH levels during the menopausal transition are higher than in the late reproductive phase, FSH levels may intermittently decrease to the normal premenopausal range *(5, 7)*. As a result of this hormonal variability, single measurements of estradiol or FSH are of little value in diagnosing the perimenopause *(5, 7)*.

After the final menstrual period, estradiol levels remain persistently low while FSH levels remain persistently high. In postmenopausal women, the main form of circulating estrogen is estrone *(8)*, which is formed via peripheral conversion of the androgen androstenedione and is less potent than estradiol.

Luteal phase progesterone levels have been reported to decrease during the late reproductive years *(9)*, and levels of urinary progesterone metabolites were found to be lower in perimenopausal than in premenopausal women *(10)*. In addition, there is a decrease in the frequency of ovulatory cycles (as indicated by a luteal phase increase in progesterone) as women near their final menstrual period *(8)*. After menopause, progesterone levels remain persistently low *(8)*.

The steepest decline in androgen levels occurs during the reproductive years (prior to menopause) *(11)*, in contrast with the sharp decline in estradiol that occurs around the time of menopause. While small decreases in testosterone and dehydroepiandrosterone sulfate (DHEAS) around the time of menopause have been reported *(8)*, several large studies have suggested that testosterone and DHEAS levels decrease with age but are not independently related to menopausal status *(7, 11, 12)*.

Little information is available about how the hormonal changes described earlier occur in women with diabetes. A small study of postmenopausal women with a history of regular menses and type 2 diabetes (DM2) demonstrated higher free testosterone levels than in women without diabetes after adjustment for body mass index (BMI) *(13)*. One explanation for these findings could be that the postmenopausal ovary remains responsive to insulin effect on thecal cells. Alternatively, hyperinsulinemia in the women with diabetes could lead to lower levels of sex hormone binding globulin (SHBG) and resulting higher levels of free testosterone in women with diabetes.

SYMPTOMS OF MENOPAUSE

Characteristic symptoms of menopause include vasomotor instability (hot flashes and sweating), vaginal dryness, urinary incontinence, and sleep disturbance *(3)*. The sleep disturbance is often due to hot flashes or night sweats that occur during sleep hours. Whether these symptoms differ in women with diabetes has not been systematically studied. Women with diabetes may attribute their menopausal hot flashes or sweats to hypoglycemia and inappropriately take in calories leading to weight gain. On the other hand, these women may also attribute sweating from hypoglycemia to menopause symptoms and not appropriately treat episodes of hypoglycemia. Urinary incontinence increases in frequency at menopause. In a study of over 1,000 postmenopausal women, there was no difference in urinary incontinence in women with diabetes as compared to those without. Severe incontinence was more common in women with diabetes although that may be in part explained by higher BMI *(14)*.

AGE OF MENOPAUSE

There are some data to suggest that women with both type 1 diabetes (DM1) *(15, 16)* and DM2 *(17)* may enter menopause a few years earlier than those without. Another study suggested no difference in age of menopause in women with DM2 *(18)*.

DM1 can also occur as part of the autoimmune polyglandular type 2 syndrome. The polyglandular type 2 syndrome is the most common of the immunoendocrinopathy syndromes and is inherited in an autosomal dominant pattern with variable penetrance *(19)*. Premature gonadal failure can be a manifestation of this syndrome. Women with DM1 and another autoimmune conditions or with a family history of the polyglandular failure syndrome should be informed and counseled about associated conditions. The association with premature gonadal failure may be important to women with DM1 for purposes of family planning.

CHANGES IN BODY COMPOSITION AT MENOPAUSE

Effects of Menopause on Body Composition

Although weight gain is a common occurrence around the time of menopause, the bulk of the evidence suggests that this weight gain is a function of aging rather than a change in menopausal status *(20)*. Yet several studies have demonstrated that several changes in body composition, beyond changes in overall body weight, are independently related to menopausal status *(21–29)*. Changes in body composition, including the amount and distribution of body fat, are important predictors of cardiovascular risk. In particular, increased abdominal fat (also referred to as android or upper body fat) is associated with increased coronary heart disease risk, independent of body mass index (BMI) and traditional cardiovascular risk factors *(30, 31)*.

Cross-sectional studies have shown that postmenopausal women compared with premenopausal women have increased fat mass *(21, 22, 29)*, increased abdominal fat *(21–24)*, and decreased lean body mass *(21, 25–27)*, independent of age. In addition, data from the Study of Women's Health Across the Nation (SWAN), a longitudinal study, suggested that ovarian aging (as reflected by increase in FSH level over time) was associated with increases in fat mass and waist circumference and decreases in lean body mass, independent of age *(28)*. This study suggests that ovarian aging may be directly related to menopause-associated changes in body composition, and future studies will be necessary to further explore this hypothesis.

While menopause is associated with adverse changes in body composition, it is important to note that increased physical activity is associated with lower BMI *(32)*, decreased percent body fat *(27)*, and decreased waist circumference *(27)* among midlife women. In addition, postmenopausal hormone replacement therapy (HRT) has been reported to have neutral or beneficial effects on the menopause-associated changes in body composition. A large observational study found that HRT use was not associated with significant differences in BMI, waist-to-hip ratio, or fat mass *(33)*.

Similarly, a randomized controlled trial concluded that HRT does not significantly affect body composition or fat distribution in postmenopausal women *(34)*. Some studies, however, have found that postmenopausal women assigned to HRT had reductions in weight *(35)*, abdominal fat *(36)*, and waist-to-hip ratio *(35, 36)*. Other randomized controlled trials found that postmenopausal HRT use attenuated the increases in weight *(37)* and abdominal fat *(38)* observed with placebo treatment. Furthermore, a meta-analysis of randomized controlled trials found that postmenopausal HRT decreased waist circumference and abdominal fat and increased lean body mass in comparison to placebo or no treatment *(39)*.

Effects of Changes in Body Composition on Insulin Sensitivity in Postmenopausal Women

The menopause-associated adverse changes in body composition are in turn associated with unfavorable effects on insulin sensitivity. It is well established that obesity, and particularly abdominal obesity, increases the risk of insulin resistance in the general population *(40)*. These relationships have not been as extensively studied in postmenopausal women. Abdominal obesity has been shown to be independently associated with decreased insulin sensitivity *(41)* and glucose tolerance *(42)* in postmenopausal women. A secondary analysis of women participating in the Postmenopausal Estrogen/Progestin Interventions (PEPI) study who were not taking estrogen revealed that increased BMI and waist-to-hip ratio were independently associated with increased glucose and insulin levels, both during fasting and after oral glucose *(43)*. Furthermore, an interventional study of obese postmenopausal women with DM2 showed that exercise training led to improvements in insulin sensitivity, and these improvements in insulin sensitivity were independently related to decreases in abdominal fat and increased muscle density *(44)*. Given the changes in body composition that occur at menopause, women with diabetes may have a deterioration in insulin sensitivity and rise in blood glucose levels. Measures to decrease abdominal adiposity including diet and exercise are important in this population.

RISK OF DIABETES IN POSTMENOPAUSAL WOMEN

The risk for diabetes increases with increasing age in both women and men. Whether menopause per se magnifies the risk for diabetes in women beyond that of age alone is not clear. The changes in body composition described earlier could contribute to increased diabetes risk following menopause. In addition, it is possible that hormonal changes that occur at menopause may affect diabetes risk. In the Multi-Ethnic Study of Atherosclerosis (MESA) study of 1,973 postmenopausal women of age 45–87 years, investigators found that higher levels of free testosterone were associated with a higher likelihood of impaired fasting glucose (IFG) but not diabetes. On the other hand, higher levels of estradiol were associated with both IFG and diabetes *(45)*. In the Rancho Bernardo study, higher levels of free testosterone were predictive of the future development of DM2 independent of adiposity in older women of age 55–89 years *(46)*.

HORMONE REPLACEMENT THERAPY

Hormone replacement therapy with estrogen remains the most effective and only FDA approved treatment for the vasomotor symptoms of menopause *(47)*. In women with a uterus, a progestin should be given to prevent endometrial hyperplasia. Vaginal estrogens that are not systemically absorbed can be effective for vaginal dryness *(48)*.

Effects of HRT on Glycemic Control in Women with Diabetes

Women with diabetes were found to use HRT less commonly than women without diabetes (49). Yet studies have suggested neutral or beneficial effects of HRT on glycemic control among postmenopausal women with diabetes. Large observational studies have shown that glycemic control is improved in postmenopausal women with diabetes who use HRT compared with those who do not use HRT. One large study of women with diabetes aged ≥50 years included in the Northern California Kaiser Permanente Diabetes Registry found that HRT use was associated with an approximate 0.5% reduction in hemoglobin A_{1c} (HbA_{1c}), independent of age, ethnicity, obesity, education, exercise, disease duration, treatment type, and monitoring practices (50). Another study examining postmenopausal women with diabetes who participated in the Third National Health and Nutrition Examination Survey (NHANES III) found that current users of HRT had significantly lower HbA_{1c} and fasting glucose levels than women who had never used HRT (51). These findings, however, must be considered in the context of the limitations inherent to all observational studies. The apparent improvements in glycemic control associated with HRT use in these studies may reflect that HRT use is associated with the practice of other beneficial health behaviors, which in turn improve glycemic control. That is, a causal relationship between HRT use and glycemic control cannot be inferred from these observational data, despite rigorous adjustment for conventional confounding factors.

Yet several randomized controlled trials have also suggested that HRT use improves glycemic control in postmenopausal women with DM2, consistent with the findings of these large observational trials. A randomized cross-over trial of postmenopausal women with DM2 showed that oral conjugated equine estrogen (CEE) treatment lowered fasting glucose, HbA_{1c}, and postprandial glucose in comparison to placebo treatment (52). Another randomized cross-over trial of postmenopausal women with DM2 showed that treatment with oral estradiol also led to reductions in fasting glucose and HbA_{1c} (53). A small placebo-controlled trial showed that treatment with oral estradiol led to significant improvements in hepatic insulin sensitivity as well as HbA_{1c} (54). In addition, a recent meta-analysis of randomized controlled trials comparing HRT to placebo or no treatment among postmenopausal women found that diabetic women assigned to HRT had decreased insulin resistance [as estimated by homeostasis model assessment (HOMA-IR)], fasting glucose, and fasting insulin levels (39).

Other studies have shown either neutral effects of HRT on glycemic control or have shown improvement in some but not all measures of glycemic control (55). A randomized cross-over trial found no significant effects of either CEE or combined CEE/medroxyprogesterone (MPA) treatment on fasting glucose or insulin levels among postmenopausal women with DM2 (56). One study that prospectively studied the effects of CEE alone followed by combined CEE/MPA treatment in overweight postmenopausal women with DM2 showed that CEE treatment improved HbA_{1c}, but there were no significant changes in fasting glucose (36). A longer term randomized cross-over trial showed that treatment with combined CEE/MPA for 6 months led to improvements in fructosamine levels (a blood marker used less commonly than HbA_{1c} to estimate glycemic control) but no significant changes in HbA_{1c} or fasting glucose in comparison to placebo treatment (57). It is possible that differences in hormone preparations, treatment duration, study populations, or study power have led to divergent findings among these various trials. Because of potential effects of HRT on glucose homeostasis, women with diabetes should increase glucose monitoring at the time of the initiation and cessation of such therapy.

Effects of HRT on Risk of Developing Diabetes

Given the suggestions of beneficial effects of hormone replacement on glucose homeostasis, the question has been asked as to whether HRT can impact the risk for the development of diabetes. Several observational studies have shown a decreased risk for diabetes in women on HRT (58, 59) although this reduction was not seen in all studies (60). In a post hoc analysis of the Heart and Estrogen/Progestin Replacement Study (HERS), a large randomized, double-blind placebo-controlled study, the use of CEE and MPA in postmenopausal women with documented coronary artery disease (CAD) was associated with a 35% reduction in the new diagnosis of DM2 over 4.1 years vs. placebo. Of interest, the decrease in risk was primarily due to lower levels of fasting blood glucose as opposed to BMI or waist circumference (35). However, the study was designed to determine whether HRT was of benefit in reducing myocardial infarction and death from CAD, and the study demonstrated no reduction of CV risk. Women in the study on HRT had a significant increase in deep venous thrombosis than those on placebo (61), which makes this regimen undesirable for diabetes prevention.

In the Women's Health Initiative (WHI), a large randomized placebo-controlled study of hormone replacement therapy (CEE and MPA) for primary prevention of cardiovascular disease, a lower risk for the development of DM2 in women on HRT was also seen again in a post hoc analysis. As compared with those women on placebo (cumulative incidence of type 2 DM 4.2%), women on HRT (cumulative incidence 3.5%) were 21% less likely to develop treated diabetes as defined by the self-report of diabetes treated with oral agents or insulin over 5.6 years. This finding held true after adjustment for common associates of diabetes such as BMI and waist circumference (62). As there was a significant decrease in HOMA-IR at 1 year, it is possible that HRT may reduce insulin resistance. However, this was no longer significant at 3 years. Given that the use of combined HRT in this study was associated with an increase in coronary heart disease, stroke, venous thromboembolism, and breast cancer, this regimen is undesirable for diabetes prevention. As the MPA component of combined HRT is associated with a potential increase in insulin resistance, it was expected that women in the WHI study who were randomized to estrogen alone would have an even greater reduction in risk for diabetes. However, the reduction in risk associated with use of CEE alone vs. placebo was smaller (12%) than that associated with combined HRT (63). In the estrogen-alone study, as in the study with combined HRT, there was an increase in overall adverse risk. While there was no increase in CHD, there was an increase in venous thromboembolism (64).

Whether other forms of estrogen demonstrate a similar reduction in the risk for diabetes is not as thoroughly studied. A nonrandomized study of transdermal 17 β-estradiol also demonstrated a decreased risk of diabetes as compared to placebo (58).

The mechanism by which estrogen may decrease diabetes risk is currently unknown. Estrogen may have direct effects on glucose homeostasis or may affect it indirectly, such as through effects on inflammation or via increased endothelial-dependent vasodilation leading to improved glucose delivery to muscle.

Data supporting the use of HRT for prevention of diabetes in postmenopausal women are currently outweighed by risk. Therefore, combined HRT or estrogen alone should not be used for diabetes prevention in postmenopausal women. As in women without diabetes, HRT (combined or estrogen alone) should not be used to decrease risk of heart disease in postmenopausal women with diabetes (65). The use of HRT for women symptomatic from hot flashes should be made on a case-by-case basis weighing risk vs. benefit (66).

Table 1
Associations of Menopause and Diabetes

Increased fat mass
Increased abdominal adiposity
Increased variability of blood glucose levels
Increased insulin resistance

Many pharmacological and nonpharmacologic alternatives to HRT for vasomotor symptoms have been studied with conflicting results in general populations of postmenopausal women (see reviews) *(3)*. None are currently approved for this indication. As discussed earlier, women with diabetes initiating such therapy should be aware of a potential impact in glucose control.

CONCLUSION

Menopause is associated with changes in body composition, including an increase in total fat mass and abdominal obesity, and these changes may increase risk for DM2. This change in body composition does not appear to be explained solely by an increase in body weight. The risk for DM2 increases with menopause, though how much of this increase in risk is due to the hormonal changes of menopause vs. the increase in BMI with aging is not clear. Existing studies support a decrease in risk for DM2 with HRT. Given the increase in cardiovascular risk with HRT, however, it should not be used for this indication. The mechanism for this decrease in risk is unclear at present. Future studies are needed to define whether the symptoms and pattern of hormonal changes characteristic of menopause differ in women with DM2. Women with DM2 and their caregivers should be aware that menopause and its treatments may affect diabetes risk as well as glucose control in women with DM2.

REFERENCES

1. Soules MR, Sherman S, Parrott E, et al. Executive summary: Stages of Reproductive Aging Workshop (STRAW). Fertil Steril 2001;76:874–8.
2. Gold EB, Bromberger J, Crawford S, et al. Factors associated with age at natural menopause in a multiethnic sample of midlife women. Am J Epidemiol 2001;153:865–74.
3. Nelson HD. Menopause. Lancet 2008;371:760–70.
4. Bulun SE, Adashi EY. The physiology and pathology of the female reproductive axis. In: Larsen PR, Kronenberg HM, Melmed S, Polonsky KS, eds. Williams textbook of endocrinology. 10th ed. Philadelphia, PA: Saunders, 2003:587–664.
5. Hall JE. Neuroendocrine physiology of the early and late menopause. Endocrinol Metab Clin North Am 2004;33:637–59.
6. Welt CK, Jimenez Y, Sluss PM, Smith PC, Hall JE. Control of estradiol secretion in reproductive ageing. Hum Reprod 2006;21:2189–93.
7. Burger HG, Dudley EC, Robertson DM, Dennerstein L. Hormonal changes in the menopause transition. Recent Prog Horm Res 2002;57:257–75.
8. Rannevik G, Jeppsson S, Johnell O, Bjerre B, Laurell-Borulf Y, Svanberg L. A longitudinal study of the perimenopausal transition: altered profiles of steroid and pituitary hormones, SHBG and bone mineral density. Maturitas 1995;21:103–13.
9. Welt CK, McNicholl DJ, Taylor AE, Hall JE. Female reproductive aging is marked by decreased secretion of dimeric inhibin. J Clin Endocrinol Metab 1999;84:105–11.
10. Santoro N, Brown JR, Adel T, Skurnick JH. Characterization of reproductive hormonal dynamics in the perimenopause. J Clin Endocrinol Metab 1996;81:1495–501.
11. Davison SL, Bell R, Donath S, Montalto JG, Davis SR. Androgen levels in adult females: changes with age, menopause, and oophorectomy. J Clin Endocrinol Metab 2005;90:3847–53.
12. Basaria S, Dobs AS. Clinical review: controversies regarding transdermal androgen therapy in postmenopausal women. J Clin Endocrinol Metab 2006;91:4743–52.
13. Korytkowski MT, Krug EI, Daly MA, Deriso L, Wilson JW, Winters SJ. Does androgen excess contribute to the cardiovascular risk profile in postmenopausal women with type 2 diabetes? Metabolism 2005;54:1626–31.
14. Jackson SL, Scholes D, Boyko EJ, Abraham L, Fihn SD. Urinary incontinence and diabetes in postmenopausal women. Diabetes Care 2005;28:1730–8.
15. Dorman JS, Steenkiste AR, Foley TP, et al. Menopause in type 1 diabetic women: is it premature? Diabetes 2001;50:1857–62.
16. Strotmeyer ES, Steenkiste AR, Foley TP, Jr, Berga SL, Dorman JS. Menstrual cycle differences between women with type 1 diabetes and women without diabetes. Diabetes Care 2003;26:1016–21.
17. Malacara JM, Huerta R, Rivera B, Esparza S, Fajardo ME. Menopause in normal and uncomplicated NIDDM women: physical and emotional symptoms and hormone profile. Maturitas 1997;28:35–45.
18. Lopez-Lopez R, Huerta R, Malacara JM. Age at menopause in women with type 2 diabetes mellitus. Menopause 1999;6:174–8.
19. Eisenbarth GS, Gottlieb PA. Autoimmune polyendocrine syndromes. N Engl J Med 2004;350:2068–79.

20. Carr MC. The emergence of the metabolic syndrome with menopause. J Clin Endocrinol Metab 2003;88:2404–11.
21. Svendsen OL, Hassager C, Christiansen C. Age- and menopause-associated variations in body composition and fat distribution in healthy women as measured by dual-energy X-ray absorptiometry. Metabolism 1995;44:369–73.
22. Ley CJ, Lees B, Stevenson JC. Sex- and menopause-associated changes in body-fat distribution. Am J Clin Nutr 1992;55:950–4.
23. Tremollieres FA, Pouilles JM, Ribot CA. Relative influence of age and menopause on total and regional body composition changes in postmenopausal women. Am J Obstet Gynecol 1996;175:1594–600.
24. Panotopoulos G, Ruiz JC, Raison J, Guy-Grand B, Basdevant A. Menopause, fat and lean distribution in obese women. Maturitas 1996;25:11–9.
25. Douchi T, Yamamoto S, Nakamura S, et al. The effect of menopause on regional and total body lean mass. Maturitas 1998;29:247–52.
26. Wang Q, Hassager C, Ravn P, Wang S, Christiansen C. Total and regional body-composition changes in early postmenopausal women: age-related or menopause-related? Am J Clin Nutr 1994;60:843–8.
27. Sternfeld B, Bhat AK, Wang H, Sharp T, Quesenberry CP, Jr. Menopause, physical activity, and body composition/fat distribution in midlife women. Med Sci Sports Exerc 2005;37:1195–202.
28. Sowers M, Zheng H, Tomey K, et al. Changes in body composition in women over six years at midlife: ovarian and chronological aging. J Clin Endocrinol Metab 2007;92:895–901.
29. Guo SS, Zeller C, Chumlea WC, Siervogel RM. Aging, body composition, and lifestyle: the Fels Longitudinal Study. Am J Clin Nutr 1999;70:405–11.
30. Iribarren C, Darbinian JA, Lo JC, Fireman BH, Go AS. Value of the sagittal abdominal diameter in coronary heart disease risk assessment: cohort study in a large, multiethnic population. Am J Epidemiol 2006;164:1150–9.
31. Rexrode KM, Carey VJ, Hennekens CH, et al. Abdominal adiposity and coronary heart disease in women. JAMA 1998;280:1843–8.
32. Progetto Menopausa Italia Study Group. Determinants of body mass index in women around menopause attending menopause clinics in Italy. Climacteric 2003;6:67–74.
33. Kritz Silverstein D, Barrett-Connor E. Long-term postmenopausal hormone use, obesity, and fat distribution in older women. JAMA 1996;275:46–9.
34. Sites CK, L'Hommedieu GD, Toth MJ, Brochu M, Cooper BC, Fairhurst PA. The effect of hormone replacement therapy on body composition, body fat distribution, and insulin sensitivity in menopausal women: a randomized, double-blind, placebo-controlled trial. J Clin Endocrinol Metab 2005;90:2701–7.
35. Kanaya AM, Herrington D, Vittinghoff E, et al. Glycemic effects of postmenopausal hormone therapy: the Heart and Estrogen/progestin Replacement Study. A randomized, double-blind, placebo-controlled trial. Ann Intern Med 2003;138:1–9.
36. Samaras K, Hayward CS, Sullivan D, Kelly RP, Campbell LV. Effects of postmenopausal hormone replacement therapy on central abdominal fat, glycemic control, lipid metabolism, and vascular factors in type 2 diabetes: a prospective study. Diabetes Care 1999;22:1401–7.
37. Espeland MA, Stefanick ML, Kritz-Silverstein D, et al. Effect of postmenopausal hormone therapy on body weight and waist and hip girths. Postmenopausal Estrogen-Progestin Interventions Study Investigators. J Clin Endocrinol Metab 1997;82:1549–56.
38. Haarbo J, Marslew U, Gotfredsen A, Christiansen C. Postmenopausal hormone replacement therapy prevents central distribution of body fat after menopause. Metabolism 1991;40:1323–6.
39. Salpeter SR, Walsh JM, Ormiston TM, Greyber E, Buckley NS, Salpeter EE. Meta-analysis: effect of hormone-replacement therapy on components of the metabolic syndrome in postmenopausal women. Diabetes Obes Metab 2006;8:538–54.
40. Despres JP, Lemieux I. Abdominal obesity and metabolic syndrome. Nature 2006;444:881–7.
41. Sites CK, Calles-Escandon J, Brochu M, Butterfield M, Ashikaga T, Poehlman ET. Relation of regional fat distribution to insulin sensitivity in postmenopausal women. Fertil Steril 2000;73:61–5.
42. Campbell AJ, Busby WJ, Horwath CC, Robertson MC. Relation of age, exercise, anthropometric measurements, and diet with glucose and insulin levels in a population aged 70 years and over. Am J Epidemiol 1993;138:688–96.
43. Barrett-Connor E, Schrott HG, Greendale G, et al. Factors associated with glucose and insulin levels in healthy postmenopausal women. Diabetes Care 1996;19:333–40.
44. Cuff DJ, Meneilly GS, Martin A, Ignaszewski A, Tildesley HD, Frohlich JJ. Effective exercise modality to reduce insulin resistance in women with type 2 diabetes. Diabetes Care 2003;26:2977–82.
45. Golden SH, Dobs AS, Vaidya D, Szklo M, Gapstur S, Kopp P, Liu K, Ouyang P. Endogenous sex hormones and glucose tolerance status in postmenopausal women. J Clin Endocrinol Metab 2007;92:1289–95.
46. Oh JY, Barrett-Connor E, Wedick NM, Wingard DL, Rancho Bernardo Study. Endogenous sex hormones and the development of type 2 diabetes in older men and women: the Rancho Bernardo study. Diabetes Care 2002;25:55–60.
47. Stefanick ML. Estrogens and progestins: background and history, trends in use, and guidelines and regimens approved by the US Food and Drug Administration. Am J Med 2005;118(Suppl 12B):64–73.
48. North American Menopause Society. The role of local vaginal estrogen for treatment of vaginal atrophy in postmenopausal women: 2007 position statement of The North American Menopause Society. Menopause 2007;14:355,69; quiz 370–1.
49. Keating NL, Cleary PD, Rossi AS, Zaslavsky AM, Ayanian JZ. Use of hormone replacement therapy by postmenopausal women in the United States. Ann Intern Med 1999;130:545–53.

50. Ferrara A, Karter AJ, Ackerson LM, Liu JY, Selby JV, Northern California Kaiser Permanente Diabetes Registry. Hormone replacement therapy is associated with better glycemic control in women with type 2 diabetes: The Northern California Kaiser Permanente Diabetes Registry. Diabetes Care 2001;24:1144–50.

51. Crespo CJ, Smit E, Snelling A, Sempos CT, Andersen RE, NHANES III. Hormone replacement therapy and its relationship to lipid and glucose metabolism in diabetic and nondiabetic postmenopausal women: results from the Third National Health and Nutrition Examination Survey (NHANES III). Diabetes Care 2002;25:1675–80.

52. Friday KE, Dong C, Fontenot RU. Conjugated equine estrogen improves glycemic control and blood lipoproteins in postmenopausal women with type 2 diabetes. J Clin Endocrinol Metab 2001;86:48–52.

53. Andersson B, Mattsson LA, Hahn L, et al. Estrogen replacement therapy decreases hyperandrogenicity and improves glucose homeostasis and plasma lipids in postmenopausal women with noninsulin-dependent diabetes mellitus. J Clin Endocrinol Metab 1997;82:638–43.

54. Brussaard HE, Gevers Leuven JA, Frolich M, Kluft C, Krans HM. Short-term oestrogen replacement therapy improves insulin resistance, lipids and fibrinolysis in postmenopausal women with NIDDM. Diabetologia 1997;40:843–9.

55. Palin SL, Kumar S, Sturdee DW, Barnett AH. HRT in women with diabetes – review of the effects on glucose and lipid metabolism. Diabetes Res Clin Pract 2001;54:67–77.

56. Manwaring P, Morfis L, Diamond T, Howes LG. The effects of hormone replacement therapy on plasma lipids in type II diabetes. Maturitas 2000;34:239–47.

57. Manning PJ, Allum A, Jones S, Sutherland WH, Williams SM. The effect of hormone replacement therapy on cardiovascular risk factors in type 2 diabetes: a randomized controlled trial. Arch Intern Med 2001;161:1772–6.

58. Rossi R, Origliani G, Modena MG. Transdermal 17-beta-estradiol and risk of developing type 2 diabetes in a population of healthy, nonobese postmenopausal women. Diabetes Care 2004;27:645–9.

59. Manson JE, Rimm EB, Colditz GA, et al. A prospective study of postmenopausal estrogen therapy and subsequent incidence of non-insulin-dependent diabetes mellitus. Ann Epidemiol 1992;2:665–73.

60. Gabal LL, Goodman-Gruen D, Barrett-Connor E. The effect of postmenopausal estrogen therapy on the risk of non-insulin-dependent diabetes mellitus. Am J Public Health 1997;87:443–5.

61. Hulley S, Grady D, Bush T, et al. Randomized trial of estrogen plus progestin for secondary prevention of coronary heart disease in postmenopausal women. Heart and Estrogen/progestin Replacement Study (HERS) Research Group. JAMA 1998;280:605–13.

62. Margolis KL, Bonds DE, Rodabough RJ, et al. Effect of oestrogen plus progestin on the incidence of diabetes in postmenopausal women: results from the Women's Health Initiative Hormone Trial. Diabetologia 2004;47:1175–87.

63. Bonds DE, Lasser N, Qi L, et al. The effect of conjugated equine oestrogen on diabetes incidence: the Women's Health Initiative randomised trial. Diabetologia 2006;49:459–68.

64. Hsia J, Langer RD, Manson JE, et al. Conjugated equine estrogens and coronary heart disease: the Women's Health Initiative. Arch Intern Med 2006;166:357–65.

65. Mosca L, Appel LJ, Benjamin EJ, et al. Evidence-based guidelines for cardiovascular disease prevention in women. American Heart Association scientific statement. Arterioscler Thromb Vasc Biol 2004;24:e29–50.

66. North American Menopause Society. Recommendations for estrogen and progestogen use in peri-and postmenopausal women: October 2004 position statement of The North American Menopause Society. Menopause 2004;11:589–600.

3

Cardiovascular Disease in Women with Diabetes

Sonia Gajula, Ashwini Reddy, L. Romayne Kurukulasuriya, Camila Manrique, Guido Lastra, and James R. Sowers

CONTENTS

ABSTRACT

Cardiovascular disease (CVD) is the leading cause of morbidity and mortality in women in the USA. Women with diabetes are at a greater risk of CVD than men with diabetes. In this chapter we review the various mechanisms by which hyperglycemia potentiates this increased CVD risk, including coagulation abnormalities as well as endothelial dysfunction. Where applicable, sex-specific differences in these mechanisms are highlighted. Finally, the impact and burden of diabetes on CVD as well as screening for CVD in women are discussed.

Key words: Diabetes mellitus; Coagulation abnormalities; Hyperglycemia; Endothelial dysfunction; Insulin resistance; Oxidative stress; Metabolic syndrome; Cardiovascular disease; Sex differences.

From: *Diabetes in Women: Pathophysiology and Therapy*
Edited by: A. Tsatsoulis et al. (eds.), DOI 10.1007/978-1-60327-250-6_3
© Humana Press, a part of Springer Science+Business Media, LLC 2009

INTRODUCTION

Cardiovascular disease (CVD) is the most important single cause of death among women world-wide, accounting for roughly one-third of all causes of mortality *(1)*. Available literature suggests the existence of gender-related differences influencing the relationship between cardiovascular risk factors and CVD.

Importantly, the impact of risk factor modification interventions has been translated in clinical benefits mainly for diabetic men, while cardiovascular mortality in female diabetics remains largely unchanged *(2)*. Few studies have specifically addressed CVD in women, and even fewer have been focused on women with both type 2 diabetes mellitus (DM2) and CVD *(3)*. Early clinical and experimental data underscore the cardioprotective effects of estrogens, and it is accepted that the loss of female sex hormones after menopause contributes, in part, to the increased incidence of CVD experienced by postmenopausal women *(4)*. In addition, the presence of DM2 in women appears to abrogate the cardiovascular protective effects of endogenous estrogens before menopause *(5)*. In this chapter we address the impact of DM2 on CVD in women, focusing on platelet and coagulation abnormalities and endothelial dysfunction in women with DM2 as well as screening for coronary heart disease (CHD) in female diabetic patients.

IMPACT AND BURDEN OF DIABETES ON CARDIOVASCULAR DISEASE IN WOMEN

Gender-Specific Differences in CVD

The disparity between the incidence of CHD in age-matched premenopausal nondiabetic women and men suggests that endogenous sex hormones such as estrogen, progesterone, and/or both may have a significant influence on the vasculature. Specific estrogen receptors (ER) located in endothelial and vascular smooth muscle cells (VSMC) modulate vascular tissue function *(6–8)*. Studies using postmortem coronary artery specimens obtained from pre- and postmenopausal women have linked expression of ER to reduced atherosclerotic changes in premenopausal women. This suggests that estrogen signaling through these receptors plays an important role in coronary protection from atherosclerosis. In this context, estrogen has been shown to increase endothelial nitric oxide synthase (eNOS) activity and associated increases in nitric oxide (NO) bioavailability. Since NO attenuates platelet aggregation, expression of endothelial cell (EC) adhesion molecules, and vascular smooth muscle cell (VSMC) proliferation, this might be one mechanism by which estrogen exerts its antiatherogenic effects. Also, estrogens may promote both antihypertensive and antiatherogenic effects, in part, via decreasing VSMC intracellular calcium (Ca^{2+}) levels and Ca^{2+} sensitization *(7)*.

Loss of Estrogen Protection in Diabetic Women

The mechanism by which DM2 abrogates the protective effect of estrogens in premenopausal women is incompletely understood. Increased CVD in diabetics has been linked to several factors, including enhanced platelet aggregation, hypercoagulability, decreased fibrinolysis, endothelial dysfunction, lipoprotein abnormalities, increased oxidative stress and inflammation, and enhanced vascular growth factor stimulation. Both hyperglycemia and insulin resistance/hyperinsulinemia abrogate "estrogen protection" in premenopausal diabetic women by interfering with one or more of the earlier mechanisms.

Experimental studies have shown that 17β-estradiol reduces the synthesis and activity of inducible nitric oxide synthase (iNOS) in response to inflammatory mediators in rat aortic VSMC. iNOS activation leads to rapid production of large amounts of NO, which causes various pathological effects including excessive vasodilation. In diabetic women reductions in estradiol receptor expression and the ability of estrogen to modulate iNOS contribute to diabetic vascular dysfunction (2). This impairment in estrogen modulation of both eNOS and iNOS activity appears to be related to abnormalities in receptor function and cell signaling (9). Indeed hyperglycemia decreases estradiol-mediated eNOS activation and NO production from cultured ECs. This may be contributing to the loss of "estrogen protection" in diabetic females. Since NO reduces vascular growth, vascular tone, and platelet aggregation, this could explain why premenopausal women with DM2 have a higher prevalence of hypertension (HTN), platelet abnormalities, and premature atherosclerosis than their nondiabetic counterparts (2).

CVD Morbidity and Mortality in Diabetic Women: The Evidence

Well-designed population-based studies have shown an increased risk for fatal and nonfatal CVD among women with DM. Analysis of data from the Framingham Heart Study and the Framingham Offspring Study evaluated the gender-specific effect of DM and established CHD on subsequent mortality in adults. Risk for CHD was adjusted for age, hypertension (HTN), cholesterol levels, tobacco use, and body mass index (BMI). The increased risk ratios for death from CHD were 2.1 in men with diabetes only, and 4.2 in men with CHD only, compared with nondiabetic men without CHD. The diabetes-related increased ratio for CHD death was 3.8 in women with diabetes and 1.9 in women with CHD. Thus, these data indicate that men with established CHD have higher risk for CHD mortality than diabetic men. In contrast, in women the presence of DM was associated with a greater risk than established CHD for subsequent CHD mortality (10).

The Copenhagen City Heart Study followed-up 13,105 subjects for 20 years. In this population-based study, DM2 was associated with increased risk for myocardial infarction and stroke. The risk associated with diabetes was independent of other CVD risk factors and was markedly higher in diabetic women than in men (11).

The Nurses Health Study examined the prospective impact of DM2 and history of prior CHD on mortality from all causes and CHD among 121,046 women aged 30–55 years between 1976 and 1996. The age-adjusted relative risks (RR) of overall mortality were 3.39 for women with a history of DM and no CHD at baseline, 3.00 for women with a history of CHD and no DM at baseline, and 6.84 for women with both conditions at baseline, compared with that for women without DM2 or CHD at baseline. The corresponding age-adjusted RRs of fatal CHD in these four groups were 1.0, 8.70, 10.6, and 25.8, respectively. The combination of prior CHD and DM for over 15 years was associated with a 30-fold increased risk of fatal CHD (12).

The Rancho Bernardo Study reported the 14 year gender-specific effects of DM2 on the risk of fatal CHD in a geographically defined population of men and women aged 40–79 years. This study included 207 men and 127 women with DM2. Control population was composed of 2,137 euglycemic adults with negative personal and family history of diabetes. The relative hazard of CHD-related death in diabetics vs. nondiabetics was 1.9 and 3.3 for men and women, respectively, after adjusting for age, systolic blood pressure, cholesterol, BMI, and cigarette smoking (13).

A recent analysis from the National Health and Nutrition Examination Surveys (NHANES 1971–2000) found that among diabetic men, the all-cause mortality rate decreased by 18.2 annual deaths per 1,000 persons (from 42.6 to 24.4, $p = 0.03$) between 1971–1986 and 1988–2000. Similarly, CVD mortality decreased from 26.4 annual deaths per 1,000 men in the period 1971–1986 to 12.8 in 1988–2000 ($p = 0.06$). On the other hand, in diabetic women, all-cause mortality doubled than in women without diabetes (14). Classically, it was considered that female gender protects against CVD, but in women with diabetes this advantage seems to be minimized or nonexistent.

A large prospective study in Norway following a population older than 20 years for 18 years and using gender-specific analyses showed a stronger association of diabetes with CHD mortality in women (HR 2.71, CI 2.33–3.16) than in men (HR 1.98, CI 1.70–2.30, $P = 0.01$) (15). Similarly, based on a recently published meta-analysis, pooling data from 37 prospective cohort studies it was concluded that diabetes poses a greater increase in the risk of death from CHD among women than among men, with a 50% higher RR of fatal CAD in females. In the same analysis women with diabetes had higher levels of lipids and blood pressure than males (16).

Low levels of high density lipoprotein (HDL) and high very low density lipoprotein (VLDL) have also been previously postulated as a cause for the excess mortality seen in diabetic women, secondary to CHD (17). Another meta-analysis of ten prospective studies reported that the increased risk for coronary death seen in women persisted after adjustment for classical cardiac risk factors and after exclusion of patients with a history of coronary events, suggesting that additional factors are involved in the enhanced mortality risk in women with diabetes. A higher incidence of CAD in women with diabetes may also be due, in part, to lower HDL and an abnormal coagulation *milieu* (18,19).

Treatment of CVD Risk Factors in Diabetic Women: Are We Achieving the Goals?

A gender comparison of 2,788 diabetics at three urban and two suburban clinics showed that fewer women than men achieved a low density lipoprotein (LDL) level of less than 100 mg/dl. In parallel, women were less likely to receive standard screening for diabetic retinopathy and nephropathy. There were no gender differences in the percentage of patients who achieved a goal blood pressure of <130/80 and an A1C of <7%. This suggests that women are likely receiving less aggressive cardiovascular risk factor modification therapy, which may be contributing to increased prevalence of CVD (20). In concert with this notion, a cross-sectional analysis of 3,849 patients revealed that women were less likely to receive treatment well known to modify CVD outcomes (such as aspirin and statin), and if treatment was prescribed, goals such as A1C and LDL were less frequently achieved. These authors proposed that the less frequent use of lipid-lowering agents was at least partially related to the perception by physicians that the higher HDL levels seen in women were protective (21). More recently, a cross-sectional analysis from a cohort of patients with diabetes sampled from managed care health plans in the USA found that diabetic women with CVD were more likely to have uncontrolled systolic blood pressure and LDL cholesterol than their male counterparts. Correspondingly, when hypercholesterolemia was treated, women were less likely to receive intensive medical therapy (22).

In contrast, a meta-analysis of 16 studies showed that the relative increased cardiovascular risk seen in diabetic women was no longer significant after adjustment for HTN, total cholesterol, and tobacco use (23). Nevertheless, most available data suggest that increased CVD morbidity and mortality in diabetic women is related to a less than ideal control of modifiable CVD risk factors.

In summary, the higher morbidity and mortality of CVD in women can be partially explained by the fact that diabetic women are less likely to receive aggressive CVD risk factor modification: less use of aspirin, less frequent screening and treatment for dyslipidemia, and less stringent HTN treatment. Biological differences such as lower HDL and enhanced coagulation pathways can also play a role as cardiovascular risk factors (19, 24).

PLATELET AND COAGULATION ABNORMALITIES IN DIABETES

Micro- and macrovascular complications in DM2 are associated with platelet dysfunction and imbalance between coagulation and fibrinolysis, which in turn contribute to the generation of a prothrombotic state.

Table 1
Platelet Dysfunction in Diabetes [Source: *(2)*]

Increased platelet adhesiveness
Increased platelet aggregation
Decreased platelet survival
Increased platelet generation of vasoconstrictor prostanoids
Reduced platelet generation of prostacyclin and other vasodilator prostanoids
Altered platelet divalent cation homeostasis (i.e., decreased [Mg^{2+}] and increased [Ca^{2+}])
Increased nonenzymatic glycosylation of platelet proteins
Decreased platelet polyphosphoinositide content
Decreased platelet production of nitric oxide
Increased platelet myosin light chain phosphorylalion
Increased platelet adhesion to endothelium
Increased platelet surface glycoprotein's Mg^{2+}_i indicates intracellular magnesium
and Ca^{2+}_i indicates intracellular calcium

Platelet Mechanism of Action

Several factors stimulate platelet aggregation including thrombin, collagen, epinephrine, adenosine diphosphate (ADP), and thromboxane A2. Numerous abnormalities leading to increased platelet adhesion and aggregation contribute to enhanced thrombogenesis in diabetic patients (Table 1) *(25)*.

Intrinsic Platelet Abnormalities

It is unclear whether in DM2 platelet abnormalities are intrinsic or are a consequence of systemic metabolic abnormalities affecting platelet function. It has been postulated that platelet sensitivity and response to a variety of aggregating agents such as ADP, thrombin, and collagen is increased in persons and animal models with diabetes. In animal models of diabetes, enhanced platelet aggregation and thromboxane A2 synthesis is detected even before there is evidence of CVD *(26)*. Both exaggerated intracellular Ca^{2+} responses to agonists and decreased platelet intracellular magnesium contribute to enhanced platelet aggregation as seen in DM2 *(2, 27)*.

Increased Platelet Surface Glycoproteins

Platelet activation results in changes in the expression of platelet surface glycoproteins (GP) that are involved in platelet aggregation. For example, GPIIb-IIIa complexes serve as receptors for adhesive proteins while GPIb functions as a receptor for von Willebrand factor (VWF). Increased number of GP receptors and increases in VWF levels have been noted in both type 1 diabetes (DM1) and DM2 *(28)*.

Decreased Production of NO and Prostacyclin

Prostacyclin (PGI_2) and NO attenuate platelet adhesion to the endothelium as well as platelet aggregation. Upon binding of PGI_2 to its G-protein-coupled cell surface receptor, an increment in the intraplatelet concentration of cyclic adenosine monophosphate (cAMP) is seen. Contemporaneously, as NO diffuses across the platelet membrane it activates guanylate cyclase and increases cyclic guanosine monophosphate (cGMP) concentrations. These inhibitory pathways culminate in the phosphorylation of cAMP and cGMP-dependent protein kinases and inactivation of myosin light chain kinase involved in platelet aggregation *(25, 27)*. In patients with diabetes, platelets have been shown to have a decreased response to NO and PGI_2 inhibitory signals *(29)*.

Increased Advance Glycation End Products and Metabolic Alterations

Advance glycation end products (AGE) are the terminal products of nonenzymatic reaction between glucose and the amino group of proteins. They accumulate at an accelerated rate in the tissues of diabetic patients. Proteins of the platelet membrane are also subject to glycation, which reduces membrane fluidity and alters the lipid membrane dynamics contributing to enhanced platelet hyperfunction *(30, 31)*.

Similarly, hyperglycemia causes an increase in glycated LDL (GlycLDL), which makes this lipoprotein more susceptible to oxidative stress. GlycLDL modifies platelet biology by decreasing NO production and increasing intracellular calcium concentrations as well as inhibiting membrane Na^+/K^+-adenosine triphosphatase (Na^+/K^+-ATPase) and Ca^{2+}-ATPase activities *(32)*. Other lipid abnormalities seen in hyperglycemia include glycation of HDL, which enhances HDL clearance, and glycation of Apolipoprotein B that results in impaired recognition of LDL by hepatocyte receptors and prolonged LDL half-life. The resulting lipoprotein profile is that of elevated plasma VLDL, LDL, and lipoprotein(a) and low HDL *(33)*. This metabolic dyslipidemia may, in turn, enhance the sensitivity of platelets to aggregating agents, thereby contributing to the hypercoagulable state in diabetic patients (Fig. 1).

Insulin Action on Platelets

Platelets have been shown to be a target of insulin action as they have functional receptors capable of triggering a phosphorylation cascade in response to insulin. Stimulation through insulin receptors increases intracellular NO, reduces Ca^{2+}, and thus decreases platelet aggregation responses to ADP,

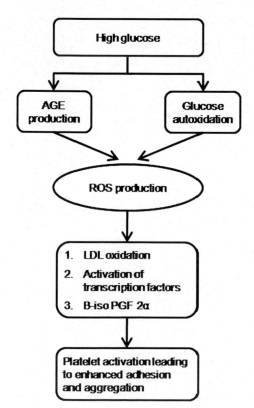

Fig. 1. Oxidative stress in diabetes and mechanisms of platelet activation. *AGE* advanced glycated end products, *ROS* reactive oxygen species, *LDL* low density lipoprotein, $PGF_{2\alpha}$ prostaglandin F 2α [Source: *(36)*].

thrombin, and collagen *(34)*. In this context, there is a diminished insulin platelet insulin receptor number and binding affinity, which might contribute to platelet hyperreactivity in DM2 *(35)*.

Oxidative Stress

Oxidative stress due to a number of metabolic abnormalities including chronic hyperglycemia plays an important role in the development of diabetic complications. The production of reactive oxygen species (ROS) is mediated directly through abnormal glucose metabolism and auto-oxidation and indirectly via formation of AGE.

Elevated levels of lipid hydroperoxidases and F 2-isoprostanes such as 8-iso-prostaglandin $(PG)F_{2\alpha}$ are seen in patients with diabetes. $8\text{-iso-PGF}_{2\alpha}$ is a nonenzymatic oxidation product of arachidonic acid as well as LDL. This superoxide product induces vasoconstriction and alters platelet function by enhancing activation and adhesive reactions *(36)*. In one interesting study, $8\text{-iso-PGF}_{2\alpha}$, as well as thromboxane A2 (TXA_2 – which is a marker for platelet hyperreactivity) production, was directly associated with poor glycemic control *(37)*. Furthermore, the levels of $8\text{-iso-PGF}_{2\alpha}$ and TXA_2 urinary metabolites decreased with improved glycemic control via insulin therapy. This led to the proposed notion that changes in the rate of arachidonate peroxidation and consequently produced biologically active iso-eicosanoids, such as 8-iso-PGF2a, may represent an important biochemical link between altered glycemic control, oxidant stress, and platelet activation in patients with diabetes.

Coagulation Abnormalities in Diabetes Mellitus

Eighty percent of the premature deaths in DM2 patients are secondary to thrombotic events, with 75% of these cases occurring in the cardiovascular system *(38)*. Diabetic patients are prone to enhanced thrombosis and platelet aggregation/adhesion, endothelial dysfunction, altered fibrinolysis, and lipid disorders *(2)*.

HEMOSTATIC MECHANISM

Hemostasis is the process of blood clot formation at the site of vessel injury. The coagulation system involves a complex cascade of proteins, which, after activation, lead to thrombin formation. Thrombin, in turn, is involved in the activation of fibrinogen and formation of a cross-linked fibrin clot. Plasmin is the main enzyme in the fibrinolytic system, which is activated by tissue plasminogen activator (t-PA). Plasminogen activator inhibitor-1 (PAI-1) is an inhibitor of fibrinolysis decreasing t-PA activity *(2, 27)*. The pathways of thrombin-stimulated fibrin clot formation and plasmin-induced clot lysis are linked and carefully regulated. When they work in coordinated harmony, a clot is laid down initially to stop bleeding, followed by eventual clot lysis and tissue modeling. In DM2 the balance is tilted to a procoagulatory state.

Fibrinolytic System in Diabetes Mellitus

PLASMINOGEN ACTIVATOR INHIBITOR

PAI-1, one of the inhibitors of the fibrinolytic system, is synthesized by hepatocytes, fibroblasts, adipocytes, and ECs and is stored within the platelet granules.

Elevated PAI-1 levels have been noted in patients with CAD and are strongly correlated with components of cardiometabolic syndrome (CMS) such as BMI, blood pressure, and triglycerides *(2, 27)*. Festa et al. examined the relationship between new-onset diabetes and dynamic changes of PAI-1 and fibrinogen *(39, 40)*. In nondiabetic, healthy individuals, increasing PAI-1 levels were associated with new cases of diabetes. Both fibrinogen and PAI-1 levels are elevated in prediabetic subjects; however, only PAI-1 levels further increased with rising glucose levels and the development of diabetes *(40)*. These investigators suggested that the findings in the Insulin Resistance Atherosclerosis Study (IRAS) population indicate that healthy individuals who have a hypofibrinolytic, proinflammatory, and procoagulant state as evidenced by high levels of PAI-1 and fibrinogen are at increased risk for development of diabetes *(40)*. Increases in both of these coagulation factors appear to be very early markers for the development of diabetes.

Clinical studies have shown that nonpharmacological and pharmacological interventions including diet, lifestyle, and weight reduction, as well as treatment with Metformin and ACE inhibitors, have been associated with reductions in PAI-1 levels *(41)*. Further prospective clinical trials are needed to prove if decreasing PAI-1 levels will prevent or delay the progression of diabetes (Fig. 2).

TISSUE PLASMINOGEN ACTIVATOR

t-PA is a serine protease synthesized and secreted by the ECs. The majority of t-PA circulates in the plasma bound to PAI-1. In the presence of a fibrin clot, t-PA and plasminogen bind to fibrin enhancing the formation of fibrin degradation products. Numerous studies have shown an association of insulin resistance and elevated PAI-1 and decreased t-PA activity. Furthermore, elevated PAI-1 levels may indicate long-standing EC damage as is commonly seen in insulin resistance *(27)*.

Alterations in Clotting Factor Levels

FIBRINOGEN

Fibrinogen is a heterodimer synthesized by the liver. It is involved in thrombogenesis and platelet aggregation. Several prospective epidemiological studies and clinical observations have shown that elevated fibrinogen is a risk factor for CVD *(42)*. There are several potential pathophysiological mechanisms by which elevated fibrinogen levels increase CVD risk. Fibrinogen is the substrate for thrombin and represents the final step in the coagulation cascade; it is essential for platelet aggregation, modulation of endothelial function, promotion of VSMC proliferation and migration, and interaction with the binding of plasmin to its receptor. In addition, it represents a major acute-phase protein. Elevated fibrinogen levels, as discussed earlier, can predict the development of DM2 in healthy individuals *(40)*.

Contradictory results regarding various diabetes treatment strategies and their impact on fibrinogen levels have been obtained. In the Veterans Affairs Cooperative Study in DM2, intensive insulin therapy transiently increased fibrinogen levels *(43)*. This increase in fibrinogen levels may have resulted from direct stimulation of fibrinogen synthesis by insulin. On the other hand, in another study, Metformin therapy resulted in a reduction of fibrinogen levels *(44)*.

Fibrinolytic Pathway

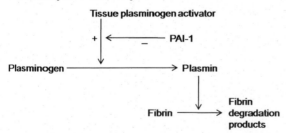

Fig. 2. Fibrinolytic pathway (Source: Created by Dr. Reddy).

FACTOR VIIC

Factor VIIc is a protein synthesized in the liver, which has been associated with increased cardiac incidents (27). The Prospective Cardiovascular Munster (PROCAM) study revealed a trend toward significance of higher factor VIIc levels in subjects who had fatal cardiovascular events (45). In concert with these data, another study of circulating tissue factor procoagulant activity found elevated factor VIIc, tissue factor, and thrombin complexes in patients with DM2 (46).

VON WILLEBRAND FACTOR AND FACTOR VIII

Von Willebrand Factor (VWF) is synthesized and secreted by vascular EC. It functions in primary hemostasis by forming an adhesive bridge between platelets and vascular subendothelial structures as well as between adjacent platelets at sites of endothelial injury. It also serves as a carrier protein for factor VIII, which has a greatly shortened half-life unless it is bound to VWF (27). Elevated levels of VWF may be a surrogate for endothelial dysfunction. Some studies have reported an association between elevated VWF and factor VIII and CVD (27). Elevated levels of factor VIII with hyperglycemia accelerate the rate of thrombin formation, which may contribute to occlusive vascular disease (3).

THROMBIN–ANTITHROMBIN COMPLEX

Thrombin plays a pivotal role in the coagulation system with multiple effects that result in formation of fibrin. Once activated, free thrombin is rapidly inactivated by combination with antithrombin. Thrombin–antithrombin complexes (TAT) subsequently circulate and are removed by the liver. Thus, elevated TAT levels are indicators of coagulation system activation. Multiple studies have documented elevated TAT in diabetes (2, 38).

Antithrombin III, Protein C, and Protein S

Antithrombin III inhibits the activity of multiple serine proteases of the coagulation pathway. Levels of antithrombin III have been shown to be diminished in patients with diabetes (38). Protein C and Protein S levels have been known to be decreased in patients with diabetes, predisposing them to thrombosis (2, 3).

LIPOPROTEIN(a) [LP(a)]

Lp(a) is a modified form of LDL in which a large glycoprotein, apolipoprotein(a), is covalently bound to apo B by a disulfide bridge. It is structurally similar to human plasminogen. Lp(a) competes with plasminogen and tissue-type plasminogen activator for fibrin binding. As a consequence, Lp(a) inhibits fibrinolysis and acts as a procoagulant (33). Elevated levels of Lp(a) have been associated with the CMS (Table 2).

Table 2
Coagulation Abnormalities in Diabetes [Source: (2)]

Increased plasma levels of factor VII, factor VIII, and von Willebrand factor
Increased fibrinogen levels
Increased lipoprotein(a) levels
Increased fibrinogen and plasminogen activator inhibitor-1 levels
Elevated thrombin–antithrombin complexes
Decreased antithrombin II, protein C, and protein S
Decreased plasminogen activators and fibrinolytic activity
Increased endothelial expression of adhesion molecules
Increased adhesion of platelets and leukocytes to the endothelium
Increased lipoprotein glycation

ENDOTHELIAL DYSFUNCTION

Atherosclerosis is the major contributor to CVD in diabetes. The initial lesion in atherosclerosis is endothelial cell dysfunction (ECD), which can be identified by the blunting of the NO-dependent vasodilation in response to acetylcholine and hyperemia *(47)*. ECD is not only important in the initiation of atherosclerosis, but also in its progression and the appearance of cardiovascular events. In diabetes, ECD is multifactorial, involving hyperglycemia and its biochemical sequelae, oxidative stress, over-expression of cytokines and growth factors, and abnormalities in coagulation fibrinolysis and lipid metabolism *(48)*. To understand the combined deleterious effects of these factors, it is important to appreciate the normal function of the EC and its critical role in overall homeostasis.

Normal Endothelial Cell Function

The endothelium is the biologically active inner layer of the vasculature *(47)*. It not only works as a physical barrier, but also serves as a guardian of the vasculature homeostasis. The EC role includes regulation of vascular tone, control of inflammatory response, vascular growth inhibition, and modulation of platelet aggregation and coagulation. These functions are integrated by complex interactions between several chemical mediators, including NO, endothelin, Angiotensin II (Ang II), aldosterone, growth factors, cytokines, and adhesion molecules to name a few. Via its interaction with plasma components and the VSMC, the EC maintains a balance of opposing forces in order to maintain proper blood flow and regulate inflammation and coagulation *(47)*.

NO as Mediator of Endothelial Cell Function

Endogenous NO is produced as a result of the conversion of L-arginine to L-citrulline in a reaction catalyzed by NOS. Several isoforms of NOS have been isolated. NOS-type III (isolated from EC) is termed "constitutive NOS" or eNOS, and produces picomolar levels of NO of which only a fraction needed to produce a physiological response. Several co-factors regulate NOS action, and these include Ca^{2+}–calmodulin with nicotinamide adenine dinucleotide phosphate-oxidase (NADPH), flavin adenine dinucleotide/mononucleotide (FAD/FMN), and tetrahydrobiopterin (BH_4) *(47)*.

eNOS (endothelial NOS-type III) is essential for the control of vascular tone in response to several stimuli, including mechanical (e.g., shear stress), receptor dependent (e.g., acetylcholine), and independent (e.g., calcium ionophore) *(49)*. Other isoforms of NOS have also been isolated and characterized. These include NOS types II and IV, which are isolated from macrophages and are Ca^{2+}–calmodulin independent, and are termed "inducible NOS" (iNOS), as their activation is promoted by cytotoxic effects of macrophages in response to cytokines *(47)*.

The EC produces NO by way of eNOS activation; resultant NO diffuses into the VSMC and activates guanylate cyclase, which in turn produces cGMP. cGMP reduces myosin light chain kinase activation, thus inducing muscle relaxation and thereby vasodilation. The continuous production of basal NO is responsible for the regulation of blood pressure. In addition to its vasodilating properties, NO contributes to the prevention of atherogenic process through cGMP-dependent inhibition of platelet aggregation and by regulation of VSMC proliferation *(50)*. In addition to regulating vascular tone, NO is also involved in vascular homeostasis and neuronal and immunological functions.

Angiotensin II

The EC also produces factors that mediate vasoconstriction, namely endothelin *(51)*, prostaglandins *(52)*, and Ang II *(53)*, and regulates vascular tone by balancing vasoconstriction (Ang II) and vasodilation (NO production). The EC membrane holds the angiotensin-converting enzyme (ACE) that, when overexpressed or overactivated, cleaves angiotensin I (Ang I) to produce Ang II. Ang I is produced by cleavage of a precursor molecule angiotensinogen by plasma renin, an enzyme produced by the juxta-glomerular apparatus in the kidney, in response to plasma volume. Ang II binds to specific receptors and regulates VSMC tone. Depending on the specific receptor type, Ang II can mediate vasoconstriction, growth, proliferation, and differentiation. In essence, Ang II actions antagonize those of NO.

As previously mentioned, NOS is regulated by specific activators and inhibitors. It is also modu-lated by local bradykinin (54), which acts via b2 receptors in the EC membrane to increase NO production via NOS activation. Local concentrations of bradykinin are regulated by ACE, which cleaves bradykinin into inactive peptides (55). Therefore, high ACE concentrations will antagonize NO activity not only by increasing Ang II levels, but also by decreasing bradykinin concentrations. High ACE activity will promote vasoconstriction. Moreover, sustained activity of ACE will also be associated with increase in growth, proliferation, and differentiation of VSMC, in addition to a decrease in local fibrinolysis and increased platelet aggregation. Aldosterone exerts many of the same effects as Ang II and may promote the atherogenic effects of Ang II.

REGULATION OF HEMOSTASIS

Besides regulating vascular tone, the EC also plays a key role in maintaining blood flow and restoring vessel wall integrity. The systems involved in maintaining hemostasis include vessel lumen, platelets, coagulation, and fibrinolysis. The coagulation cascade and the abnormalities associated with diabetes are covered elsewhere in this chapter. The EC plays a prominent role in regulating coagulation and fibrinolysis, and any injury to the endothelium will subsequently result in coagulation abnormalities with an increased propensity for atherosclerosis.

REGULATION OF VSMC GROWTH AND INFLAMMATION

The EC, in addition to regulating vasodilation, vasoconstriction, and hemostasis, also plays a promi-nent role in the growth and differentiation of VSMC through the release of various growth factors and/or inhibitors, thereby regulating vascular remodeling (56). Several factors have been implicated as promoting growth signals, including insulin-like growth factor-I (IGF-I), platelet growth factor (PGF), Ang II and aldosterone, and basic fibroblast growth factor (bFGF). Strong evidence suggests that pro-motion of VSMC growth is mediated by local production of PGF and Ang II (57). NO and PGI_2 are two mediators that have been proposed to antagonize these growth-promoting actions.

The EC also produces specific molecules that regulate inflammation, namely intracellular adhesion molecules (ICAM) and vascular cell adhesion molecules (VCAM) (58). These molecules are termed "adhesion molecules" as they attract and anchor those cells involved in the inflammatory reaction. It has been well documented that atherosclerosis is a condition that is associated with chronic low-grade inflammation (59).

Endothelial Dysfunction

As discussed earlier, the actions of EC are numerous and involve several systems. Therefore, alteration in EC function may affect one or more of these systems either simultaneously or at discrete periods. Endothelial dysfunction may be present when its properties, either in its basal state or after stimulation, have changed in a way that is inappropriate in preservation of organ function. As previously mentioned, endothelial dysfunction plays an important role not only in the initiation of atherosclerosis, but also in its progression and long-term sequelae. Risk factors for endothelial dysfunction include diabetes, hyperlipidemia, smoking, and HTN, among others.

Some examples of endothelial dysfunction include increased vascular permeability (60) and increased prothrombotic activity (61), in addition to blunting of the vasodilatory response to acetylcholine or hyperemia. At the cellular level, this translates into decreased NO bioavailability (either due to decreased production or increased degradation), increased production of ROS, increased production of Ang II, and elevated levels of growth factors and cytokines induced by inflammation, leading to increased expression of adhesion molecules resulting in a prothrombotic state and ultimately atherosclerosis.

MEASUREMENT OF ENDOTHELIAL DYSFUNCTION

Endothelial function cannot be measured directly in humans. Therefore, indirect methods are used to estimate endothelial function. Endothelium-dependent vasodilation, transcapillary escape rate of radiolabeled molecules, plasma levels of endothelium-derived regulatory proteins (e.g., NO, Ang II, endothelin, aldosterone, adhesion molecules, PAI-1), and microalbuminuria are some of the indirect markers of endothelial function *(62)* (see Table 3). Other vascular properties such as arterial stiffness and intima media thickness in the carotid artery, probably partially endothelium dependent, can be quantified. Available methods for examining blood flow and blood vessels in humans include intravascular catheters (using the Fick principle of chemical dilution and thermodilution), Doppler ultrasound, PET scans, laser Doppler flowmetry, and plethysmography *(47)*.

The validity of the earlier measurements is often questioned, as tests are based on certain assumptions. For example, tests intended to estimate NO-mediated endothelium-dependent vasodilation may also measure effects of other vasodilator mediators, such as PGI_2 and others, and may partly be confounded by impaired VSCM function. Furthermore, several of these testing procedures require expertise and are subject to observer variability. As such, these measurements can be reasonable estimates of endothelial function in humans but are by no means perfect for assessing endothelial biology.

Endothelial Dysfunction and Diabetes

Endothelial dysfunction as seen in diabetes is multifactorial. When the ECs are exposed to a diabetic environment, reduced generation of NO has been demonstrated both in vitro *(63)* and in vivo *(64)*. The EC is the target of the diabetic environment, and endothelial dysfunction plays an important role in the vasculopathy associated with diabetes. Several studies have demonstrated that the development of diabetic retinopathy, nephropathy, and atherosclerosis is closely associated with endothelial dysfunction in both DM1 and DM2 *(65)*. Along these lines, a recent growing body of evidence has accumulated, which suggests that perhaps the vessels are insulin responsive.

Table 3
Measurement of Endothelial Dysfunction in Humans [Source: *(62)*; Reproduced with permission of Portland Press LTD]

Measurement	Altered endothelial function
Impaired endothelium-dependent vasodilation	↓ Production of vasodilators ± ↑ production of vasoconstrictors
↑ Transcapillary escape rate of intravenous radio-labeled albumin, microalbuminuria	↑ Permeability to macromolecules
↑ Endothelin, ANG-II	↑ Production of vasoconstrictors
↓ NO	↓ Production of vasodilators
↑ t-PA, PAI-1	↓ Profibrinolytic activity
↑ ICAM, VCAM	↑ Adhesion of leukocytes and inflammation

NO nitric oxide, *ANG-II* angiotensin II, *t-PA* tissue plasminogen activator, *PAI* plasminogen activator inhibitor, *ICAM* intracellular adhesion molecule, *VCAM* vascular cell adhesion molecule

INSULIN EFFECTS ON THE ENDOTHELIUM

Presence of receptors for insulin has been demonstrated on micro- and macrovasculature *(66)* with binding characteristics similar to those of other cells. In addition, the ECs were also found to have receptors for insulin-like growth factor-I (IGF-I) and IGF-II, suggesting that perhaps there is a physiological role for these growth factors in the vascular complications associated with diabetes. Furthermore, a differential response to insulin was observed in ECs of micro- and macrovessels. Insulin-stimulated glucose disposal was increased in the retinal pericytes and endothelium than in aortic endothelium, suggesting that the retinal endothelium and pericytes are very insulin-sensitive tissues *(67)*. In the normally functioning endothelium, insulin and IGF-I stimulate NO production through the phosphatidylinositol 3-kinase (PI3K) and protein kinase B (Akt) pathways *(68)*, while under pathological conditions they stimulate migration and growth of vascular smooth muscle cells via the mitogen-activated protein kinase (MAPK) and other growth pathways.

Insulin deficiency and chronic hyperglycemia were associated with increased protein kinase C (PKC) activity and elevated levels of diacylglycerol (DAG) *(69)*. PKC activation leads to decreased NOS activity, decreased NO production, increased Ang II, production of ROS, and consequently endothelial dysfunction. Insulin administration resulting in subsequent euglycemia was shown to prevent activation of PKC and the resultant downstream events. More recently, investigators reported that physiological levels of insulin increased levels of eNOS messenger ribonucleic acid (mRNA) protein and its activity by twofold after 2–8 h of incubation of EC *(68)*. This effect of insulin was seen in microvasculature of lean Zucker insulin-sensitive rats but not in insulin-resistant Zucker obese rats. Hence, insulin may not only have acute vasodilatory effects but may also chronically modulate vascular tone. Furthermore, it may be that PKC activation in insulin-resistant states may be the primary event leading to endothelial dysfunction.

TYPE I DIABETES AND ENDOTHELIAL DYSFUNCTION

It is uncertain whether EC dysfunction in DM1 is a consequence of the diabetic milieu or a marker of vascular damage. In persons with DM1 of greater than 5–10 years duration without microalbuminuria, subtle increases in blood pressure, large-artery stiffness, some degree of endothelial dysfunction, and increased low-grade inflammation are commonly observed. All these abnormalities are worsened in the microalbuminuric stage *(70)*. It is unclear whether impaired endothelial function is a precursor or a consequence, but data exist to show that cardiovascular function, including endothelial function, does become impaired before the onset of microalbuminuria *(62)*. This is seen in DM2 and in those individuals in whom any increase in microalbuminuria is associated with an increased risk of atherosclerosis. Endothelial dysfunction thus occurs before the onset of microalbuminuria.

Some studies have shown that markers of EC dysfunction are not increased early in the disease, while others have demonstrated that the endothelium is impaired even in short-term uncomplicated DM1 and that hyperglycemia acutely injures the endothelium. In any case, the general consensus is that the presence of EC dysfunction in DM1 signifies a very high risk of micro- and macrovascular complications.

ENDOTHELIAL DYSFUNCTION IN DM2

In contrast to DM1, endothelial dysfunction is far more complex in DM2 presumably due to the interaction of several other factors that are characteristic of this disease entity, namely HTN, dyslipidemia, and, most importantly, insulin resistance. It is believed that endothelial dysfunction exists long before the development of overt DM2 and before microangiopathy becomes evident *(65)*. For us to better understand the complexity of endothelial dysfunction in DM2, it is important to recognize the effects of insulin resistance and chronic hyperglycemia at the cellular level.

Insulin Resistance: A Mediator of Endothelial Dysfunction

As discussed previously, insulin plays an important role in vasodilatory responses and in chronically modulating vascular tone. Moreover, insulin deficiency and chronic hyperglycemia lead to PKC activation, leading to decreased NO availability and production of ROS resulting in endothelial dysfunction. It is, therefore, reasonable to hypothesize that either insulin deficiency or even inefficient insulin action (i.e., insulin resistance) would lead to endothelial impairment. A large body of evidence has accumulated suggesting the coexistence of insulin resistance and endothelial dysfunction.

Obesity, being the human model of insulin resistance, has been clearly shown to be associated with elevated levels of endothelin (71) and PAI-1 levels; the levels of the latter were shown to decrease significantly with moderate weight loss (72). Women with polycystic ovarian syndrome were also found to have increased levels of PAI-1, which improved with interventions involving insulin sensitizers (73). Endothelial dysfunction observed in obesity is primarily facilitated by free fatty acids (FFA) (74) that are characteristically elevated in various forms of insulin resistance, that is, DM2, polycystic ovarian syndrome, and, in general, the CMS. Hence, there are sufficient data to support the hypothesis that metabolic derangements seen in insulin resistance may lead to endothelial dysfunction.

Insulin resistance and, in general, diabetes and the associated abnormalities in coagulation are discussed elsewhere in this chapter.

Mechanisms Underlying Endothelial Dysfunction in Diabetes

Endothelial dysfunction in diabetes stems from three main sources: chronic hyperglycemia, oxidative stress, and the increased production of cytokines and growth factors.

HYPERGLYCEMIA AND ITS IMMEDIATE BIOCHEMICAL SEQUELAE

High concentrations of glucose have been shown to be associated with endothelial dysfunction both in vivo (75) and in vitro (76). Underlying mechanisms contributing to this process include decreased activity and/or expression of eNOS, decreased activity and/or expression of the NO downstream target soluble guanylyl cyclase (sGC), and increased degradation of NO due to enhanced superoxide production (77).

It has been reported that in a hyperglycemic environment, expression of eNOS was upregulated, with resultant increases in NO production. Furthermore, they also found an overall decrease in the bioavailable NO, in concert with dramatic increases in superoxide production (78). It was postulated that, in a diabetic milieu, uncoupled eNOS becomes a significant source of superoxide. Other in vivo studies corroborated the earlier findings indicating that superoxide in diabetic vessels may either overwhelm NO production by the upregulated eNOS, or that the eNOS itself may be uncoupled, thereby contributing directly to the superoxide production (79).

Two conditions leading to uncoupling of eNOS have been described. These include BH_4 (eNOS co-factor) deficiency and intracellular L-arginine (eNOS substrate) depletion (77). In conditions of BH_4 deficiency, eNOS remains in an uncoupled state and preferentially produces superoxide rather than NO. NO in turn is thought to be a superoxide scavenger. Superoxide product peroxynitrite has been shown to rapidly oxidize the active eNOS cofactor BH_4 to inactive dihydrobiopterin (BH_2) (80). In addition, uncoupled eNOS and L-arginine depletion is characteristically found in conditions where high oxidative stress is encountered, as observed in patients with diabetes (77), hypercholesterolemia (81), and in chronic smokers (82). Thus, hyperglycemia-induced uncoupling of eNOS leads to increased formation of ROS resulting in increased oxidative stress, which has been shown to be a strong stimulus for PKC activation (see Fig. 3).

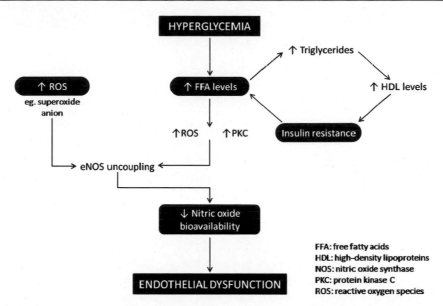

Fig. 3. Hyperglycemia and its biochemical sequelae. *ROS* reactive oxygen species, *FFA* free fatty acids, *HDL* high density lipoproteins, *PKC* protein kinase C, *eNOS* endothelial nitric oxide synthase (Source: Found on Web search; no source listed).

Hyperglycemia and Sex-specific Differences in EC Dysfunction

As discussed previously, hyperglycemia has also been shown to decrease estradiol-mediated NO production in women, perhaps contributing to the increased CVD risk in women than in men with diabetes. NO-dependent vascular tone and endothelial-dependent vasodilation are enhanced in nondiabetic premenopausal women than in men. The interaction between hyperglycemia and estradiol-mediated NO production has been well documented. Hyperglycemia decreases estradiol-mediated NO production from cultured EC *(83)*. Men with DM2 do not appear to have reduced endothelium-dependent vasodilation beyond that observed with obesity alone in contrast to women with DM2. Thus, hyperglycemia appears to negate the protective effects of estradiol in part by decreasing vascular and perhaps platelet NO production.

THE DAG/PKC PATHWAY

PKC activation in diabetes has been well established. It occurs primarily via increased levels of DAG, a common scenario in a hyperglycemic state *(84)*. A specific PKC isoform, the PKC-β, is implicated in hyperglycemia-induced endothelial dysfunction. The role of PKC in mediating endothelial dysfunction was evidenced by the observation that incubation of aortic rings with high glucose led to endothelial dysfunction, which improved by a simultaneous incubation with a PKC inhibitor *(76)*. Furthermore, a large body of evidence exists suggesting that PKC inhibition has beneficial effects on eNOS and has inhibitory effects on superoxide production, leading to a marked increase in NO bioavailability *(85)*.

The activity of the most important superoxide-producing enzyme in vascular tissue, NADPH oxidase, has been shown to be increased by fatty acid stimulation as well as by glucose, in a PKC-dependent manner *(86)*. This stimulation further increases the vascular superoxide burden. NADPH oxidase, as well as mitochondrial-formed superoxide, may combine with NO to form the highly reactive intermediate peroxynitrite, which as mentioned earlier, inactivates the eNOS cofactor BH_4, leading to eNOS uncoupling and perpetuating the vicious cycle of superoxide formation. The resultant increase in oxidative stress also leads to accumulation of asymmetrical dimethylarginine (ADMA), which is a competitive inhibitor of eNOS. Elevated levels of ADMA and intracellular BH_4 depletion act to maintain an environment of enhanced oxidative stress within the vascular tissue *(77)*.

HYPERGLYCEMIA-INDUCED OXIDATIVE STRESS AND VASCULAR DYSFUNCTION

Hyperglycemia-induced oxidative stress also involves the sorbitol and hexosamine pathways. These have been implicated in leading to a redox imbalance, simulating an environment similar to tissue hypoxia and augmented oxidative stress. The hexosamine pathway in particular has been associated with increased transcription of PAI-1 and TGF-β *(87)*, which are commonly associated with endothelial dysfunction.

The diabetic state, which is typified by an increased tendency for oxidative stress, leaves the EC very susceptible to damage. High levels of oxidized lipoproteins, fatty acids, and hyperglycemia have all been shown to induce oxidation of phospholipids and proteins, leading to impairment of EC function. ROS can affect many signaling pathways, including G proteins, protein kinases, ion channels, and transcription factors, which may modify endothelial function via various mechanisms. The end result is a decrease in the production of NO, VSMC hyperreactivity to vasoconstrictive stimuli, and an increase in proinflammatory and adhesion molecules, culminating in an extremely prothrombotic state. Oxidative stress is thought to be the final common pathway of hyperglycemia-induced endothelial dysfunction.

NONENZYMATIC GLYCATION

As mention earlier, chronic hyperglycemia has been shown to promote nonenzymatic glycation of proteins *(88)* and macromolecules, producing AGE. Nonenzymatic glycation of proteins is a condensation reaction of the carbonyl group of sugar aldehydes with the N-terminus of free amino acids of proteins *(62)*. Changes in the properties of protein and DNA have been documented to occur as a result of nonenzymatic glycation.

Formation of AGE may lead to endothelial activation. These products act to neutralize NO and increase the susceptibility of LDL to oxidation. The binding of the AGE to their receptors also activates the receptors for the cytokines interleukin-1 (IL-1), tumor necrosis factor-α (TNF-α), and growth factors, leading to the migration and proliferation of smooth muscle cells *(89)*. Furthermore, the introduction of AGE into the extracellular matrix can interfere with EC function. AGE-modified type I and IV collagen inhibit normal matrix formation and cross-linking and decrease arterial elasticity *(62)*. Hence, AGE may potentiate EC dysfunction by attracting proinflammatory factors including adhesion molecules as a result of immune-mediated damage, thereby disrupting the overall homeostasis of the vasculature.

THE ROLE OF GROWTH FACTORS AND CYTOKINES

Hyperglycemia and the associated state of oxidative stress results in excess production of cytokines and growth factors. Overexpression of growth factors has been implicated in diabetes-related proliferation of EC and VSM, resulting in increased angiogenesis *(90, 91)*. Among those studied include TGF-β, vascular endothelial growth factor (VEGF), and TNF-α. C-reactive protein (CRP), another marker of inflammation, has also been found to be significantly elevated in both DM1 and DM2 *(92)*.

TGF-β is increased via hyperglycemia-induced PKC stimulation, AGEs, Ang II, and other cytokines. TGF-β in particular has been proposed as the major candidate to mediate diabetic nephropathy *(93)*. VEGF is thought to be involved in differentiation, proliferation, and vascular permeability of the endothelium. This is likely mediated via Ang II as well. Elevated VEGF has been associated with proliferative diabetic retinopathy *(94)*. TNF-α is produced by neutrophils, macrophages, and adipocytes.

It is an important inflammatory cytokine, which also regulates the expression of CRP. These mediators have been implicated in inducing insulin resistance, thereby causing endothelial dysfunction and contributing to atherothrombosis.

Thus, endothelial dysfunction, caused by the deleterious effects of hyperglycemia, is the primary lesion leading to vascular complications associated with diabetes. The mechanisms are several, as outlined earlier, which culminate into a prothrombotic environment with an increased risk of atherosclerosis and CVD. This dysfunction is more pronounced in women with DM than in men, as suggested by several studies. Therapeutic interventions should, therefore, target various stages of the proposed mechanisms in an attempt to restore the overall homeostasis of the vasculature. Additionally screening, diagnosis, and treatment of CVD should be at least as aggressive in women with DM as it is in men.

SCREENING AND DIAGNOSIS OF CAD

No specific guidelines are available for screening of CVD or CAD in women with diabetes. If patients are symptomatic further testing is likely to be undertaken without delay. However, guidelines on screening asymptomatic individuals are not clearly defined. Recently the American Diabetes Association released a new expert panel recommendation regarding screening for CAD in diabetic patients based on recent evidence that did not support their previous recommendation of screening asymptomatic patients with two or more risk factors. The panel proposed several clinical markers aimed to identify a subgroup of diabetic patients at risk for silent myocardial ischemia. The mentioned markers that clinicians should look for to consider testing are presence of atherosclerosis in other vascular beds, existence of albuminuria and/or chronic kidney disease (CKD), evidence of abnormal resting electrocardiogram (Q waves, left bundle branch block, T wave inversion, and nonspecific ST-T wave changes); history of autonomic neuropathy and retinopathy, female gender and age >65 years, dyspnea of unclear origin, and the presence of multiple cardiac risk factors. As a first-line test, a cardiac CT scan to detect coronary artery calcification is proposed. If the calcium score is higher than 400, a myocardial stress test can be considered. The authors of the guidelines stress that age and CKD may alter the calcium scores (95).

Stable symptomatic diabetic women can be studied with noninvasive diagnostic methods (96). Despite the known limitations of exercise ECG testing (as false-positive ST-segment responses), the American Heart Association and the American College of Cardiology still considered exercise ECG testing as a feasible initial test for intermediate risk symptomatic women able to exercise with normal ECG at rest.

The accuracy of this testing modality is expected to improve when other parameters, as functional capacity, are added to the evaluation of the ST segment response (97). A positive ECG stress test result needs to be followed with further diagnostic modalities (96). Because diabetic women are considered to be at high risk for cardiovascular death, the current recommendations favor cardiac imaging as an initial diagnostic modality instead of exercise ECG testing (97).

The specificity of exercise echocardiography in women ranges from 81 to 86% and the sensitivity from 80 to 88%. False-negative results might be correlated with submaximal heart rate, single vessel CAD, and moderate stenosis. On the other hand, pharmacological stress echocardiography has a sensitivity ranging from 76 to 90% and specificity around 85% (97). Overall, exercise and pharmacological echocardiography are effective and accurate choices for detection of ischemic heart disease in women with an intermediate to high pretest likelihood of CAD. Exercise stress echocardiography is recommended for the symptomatic woman with an abnormal resting ECG, while dobutamine stress echocardiography is recommended for women with a normal or abnormal ECG who are incapable of exercise (97).

With the current available techniques, stress myocardial gated perfusion SPECT imaging is considered by the AHA as a modality with high diagnostic and prognostic accuracy for the evaluation of CAD in intermediate to high-risk symptomatic women. In addition, women with abnormal baseline ECG and unable to exercise can be also studied through this modality (97).

TREATMENT OF CVD IN WOMEN WITH DIABETES

The goals established for the prevention and management of cardiovascular disease in diabetic women do not differ from those established for men (98). Unfortunately, as mentioned earlier, diabetic women are less likely to have an adequate control of blood pressure, glycemia, and lipids and are also less likely to receive LDL-lowering therapy than males (99). Besides achieving a satisfactory glycemic control, practitioners should institute both an adequate pharmacological and nonpharmacological regimen aiming to achieve a blood pressure of <130/80 mmHg and a LDL cholesterol of <100 mg/dL (<70 mg/dL is indicated for patients with overt CVD). Frequently, multiple agents are required for blood pressure control, and the antihypertensive regimen should include at least one renin–angiotensin system blocking agent, angiotensin-converting enzyme inhibitor, or angiotensin receptor blocker. For patients older than 40 years of age with one more cardiovascular risk factor (family history of CVD, hypertension, smoking, dyslipidemia, or albuminuria) or with existent CVD, a statin should be added to their pharmacological treatment regardless of the baseline LDL. Furthermore, aspirin use is recommended as a secondary prevention strategy in those patients with diabetes and history of CVD. Additionally, for primary prevention purposes, aspirin is indicated for type 1 or 2 diabetes patients at increased cardiovascular risk, including those who are older than 40 years of age or who have additional risk factors (98).

Newer interventions, as mineralocorticoid blockade, present as an interesting and promising therapeutic strategy for modulation of diabetic cardiovascular disease.

SUMMARY

CVD is the leading cause of death in women in the USA, and in the female diabetic population the situation is no different. Even though during the last decade, a considerable amount of knowledge has been gained into the pathophysiology of diabetic CVD, the clinical outcomes for women remain far from acceptable. Premenopausal women have been classically considered protected against CVD secondary to a "hormonal effect"; unfortunately, in age-matched diabetic women this protective effect is blunted.

There are several factors that contribute to increased atherosclerotic disease and secondary CVD in the diabetic population. We have described how platelet dysfunction, low-grade inflammation, altered coagulation system, endothelial dysfunction, and oxidative stress result in a perfect environment for cardiovascular events.

Although sex-related biological differences may contribute to differences in morbidity and mortality in diabetic CVD, the current evidence points toward a poorer control of well-known cardiovascular risk factors in women with diabetes than in men with diabetes as an explanation for their increased risk of fatal and nonfatal cardiovascular events.

It is imperative to educate the public regarding symptoms of CVD in women as well as regarding effective strategies for prevention and treatment. On the other hand, health care providers should aggressively screen for cardiovascular risk factors and treat accordingly to obtain benefits from well-known pharmacological and nonpharmacological strategies. Ground-breaking studies focused specifically on women rather on diabetic men are very much needed in order to reduce the existing gap in terms of cardiovascular morbidity and mortality.

Acknowledgments The authors would like to thank Rieanne Brinkmann and Brenda Hunter for their assistance in the manuscript preparation. Dr. Sowers is a member of the Speakers' Bureau and has received grant funding from Novartis Pharmaceutical Company. Dr. Sowers is a member of the Speakers' Bureau for Merck Pharmaceutical Company. Dr. Sowers is on the Advisory Board and has received grant funding from Forest Research Institute.

REFERENCES

1. Mosca L, Banka CL, Benjamin EJ et al. Evidence-based guidelines for cardiovascular disease prevention in women: 2007 update. Circulation 2007; 115(11):1481–1501.
2. Sowers JR. Diabetes mellitus and cardiovascular disease in women. Archives of Internal Medicine 1998; 158(6):617–621.
3. Kaseta JR, Skafar DF, Ram JL, Jacober SJ, Sowers JR. Cardiovascular disease in the diabetic woman. Journal of Clinical Endocrinology & Metabolism 1999; 84(6):1835–1838.
4. Skafar DF, Xu R, Morales J, Ram J, Sowers JR. Clinical review 91: female sex hormones and cardiovascular disease in women. Journal of Clinical Endocrinology & Metabolism 1997; 82(12):3913–3918.
5. Hanes DS, Weir MR, Sowers JR. Gender considerations in hypertension pathophysiology and treatment. American Journal of Medicine 1996; 101(3A):10S–21S.
6. Horwitz KB, Horwitz LD. Canine vascular tissues are targets for androgens, estrogens, progestins, and glucocorticoids. Journal of Clinical Investigation 1982; 69(4):750–758.
7. Zhang F, Ram JL, Standley PR, Sowers JR. 17β-Estradiol attenuates voltage-dependent Ca2+ currents in A7r5 vascular smooth muscle cell line. American Journal of Physiology 1994; 266(4 Part 1):C975–C980.
8. Orimo A, Inoue S, Ikegami A et al. Vascular smooth muscle cells as target for estrogen. Biochemical & Biophysical Research Communications 1993; 195(2):730–736.
9. Maggi A, Cignarella A, Brusadelli A, Bolego C, Pinna C, Puglisi L. Diabetes undermines estrogen control of inducible nitric oxide synthase function in rat aortic smooth muscle cells through overexpression of estrogen receptor-beta. Circulation 2003; 108(2):211–217.
10. Natarajan S, Liao Y, Cao G, Lipsitz SR, McGee DL. Sex differences in risk for coronary heart disease mortality associated with diabetes and established coronary heart disease. Archives of Internal Medicine 2003; 163(14):1735–1740.
11. Almdal T, Scharling H, Jensen JS, Vestergaard H. The independent effect of type 2 diabetes mellitus on ischemic heart disease, stroke, and death: a population-based study of 13,000 men and women with 20 years of follow-up. Archives of Internal Medicine 2004; 164(13):1422–1426.
12. Hu FB, Stampfer MJ, Solomon CG et al. The impact of diabetes mellitus on mortality from all causes and coronary heart disease in women: 20 years of follow-up. Archives of Internal Medicine 2001; 161(14):1717–1723.
13. Barrett-Connor EL, Cohn BA, Wingard DL, Edelstein SL. Why is diabetes mellitus a stronger risk factor for fatal ischemic heart disease in women than in men? The Rancho Bernardo Study. JAMA 1991; 265(5):627–631.
14. Gregg EW, Gu Q, Cheng YJ, Venkat Narayan KM, Cowie CC. Mortality trends in men and women with diabetes, 1971 to 2000. Annals of Internal Medicine 2007; 147(3):149–155.
15. Dale AC, Nilsen TI, Vatten L, Midthjell K, Wiseth R. Diabetes mellitus and risk of fatal ischaemic heart disease by gender: 18 years follow-up of 74 914 individuals in the HUNT 1 Study. European Heart Journal 2007; 28(23):2924–2929.
16. Huxley R, Barzi F, Woodward M. Excess risk of fatal coronary heart disease associated with diabetes in men and women: meta-analysis of 37 prospective cohort studies. BMJ 2006; 332(7533):73–78.
17. Goldschmid MG, Barrett-Connor E, Edelstein SL, Wingard DL, Cohn BA, Herman WH. Dyslipidemia and ischemic heart disease mortality among men and women with diabetes. Circulation 1994; 89(3):991–997.
18. Lee WL, Cheung AM, Cape D, Zinman B. Impact of diabetes on coronary artery disease in women and men: a meta-analysis of prospective studies. Diabetes Care 2000; 23(7):962–968.
19. Ossei-Gerning N, Wilson IJ, Grant PJ. Sex differences in coagulation and fibrinolysis in subjects with coronary artery disease. Thrombosis and Haemostasis 1998; 79(4):736–740.
20. McFarlane SI, Castro J, Kaur J et al. Control of blood pressure and other cardiovascular risk factors at different practice settings: outcomes of care provided to diabetic women compared to men. Journal of Clinical Hypertension 2005; 7(2):73–80.
21. Kanaya AM, Grady D, Barrett-Connor E. Explaining the sex difference in coronary heart disease mortality among patients with type 2 diabetes mellitus: a meta-analysis. Archives of Internal Medicine 2002; 162(15):1737–1745.
22. Wexler DJ, Grant RW, Meigs JB, Nathan DM, Cagliero E. Sex disparities in treatment of cardiac risk factors in patients with type 2 diabetes. Diabetes Care 2005; 28(3):514–520.

23. Ferrara A, Mangione CM, Kim C et al. Gender disparities in control and treatment of modifiable cardiovascular disease risk factors among patients with diabetes: translating research into action for diabetes (TRIAD). Diabetes Care 2007; doi: 10.2337/dc07-1244.

24. Wenger NK. Heightened cardiovascular risk in diabetic women: can the tide be turned? Annals of Internal Medicine 2007; 147(3):208–210.

25. Vinik AI, Erbas T, Park TS, Nolan R, Pittenger GL. Platelet dysfunction in type 2 diabetes. Diabetes Care 2001; 24(8):1476–1485.

26. Gerrard JM, Stuart MJ, Rao GH et al. Alteration in the balance of prostaglandin and thromboxane synthesis in diabetic rats. Journal of Laboratory & Clinical Medicine 1980; 95(6):950–958.

27. Grant PJ. Diabetes mellitus as a prothrombotic condition. Journal of Internal Medicine 2007; 262(2):157–172.

28. Tschoepe D, Roesen P, Kaufmann L et al. Evidence for abnormal platelet glycoprotein expression in diabetes mellitus. European Journal of Clinical Investigation 1990; 20(2):166–170.

29. Akai T, Naka K, Okuda K, Takemura T, Fujii S. Decreased sensitivity of platelets to prostacyclin in patients with diabetes mellitus. Hormone & Metabolic Research 1983; 15(11):523–526.

30. Winocour PD, Watala C, Perry DW, Kinlough-Rathbone RL. Decreased platelet membrane fluidity due to glycation or acetylation of membrane proteins. Thrombosis & Haemostasis 1992; 68(5):577–582.

31. Winocour PD. Platelet abnormalities in diabetes mellitus. Diabetes 1992; 41(Suppl 2):26–31.

32. Ferretti G, Rabini RA, Bacchetti T et al. Glycated low density lipoproteins modify platelet properties: a compositional and functional study. Journal of Clinical Endocrinology & Metabolism 2002; 87(5):2180–2184.

33. McFarlane SI, Banerji M, Sowers JR. Insulin resistance and cardiovascular disease. Journal of Clinical Endocrinology & Metabolism 2001; 86(2):713–718.

34. Falcon C, Pfliegler G, Deckmyn H, Vermylen J. The platelet insulin receptor: detection, partial characterization, and search for a function. Biochemical & Biophysical Research Communications 1988; 157(3):1190–1196.

35. Udvardy M, Pfliegler G, Rak K. Platelet insulin receptor determination in non-insulin dependent diabetes mellitus. Experientia 1985; 41(3):422–423.

36. Ferroni P, Basili S, Falco A, Davi G. Platelet activation in type 2 diabetes mellitus. Journal of Thrombosis and Haemostasis 2004; 2(8):1282–1291.

37. Davi G, Ciabattoni G, Consoli A et al. In vivo formation of 8-iso-prostaglandin f2alpha and platelet activation in diabetes mellitus: effects of improved metabolic control and vitamin E supplementation. Circulation 1999; 99(2):224–229.

38. Carr ME. Diabetes mellitus: a hypercoagulable state. Journal of Diabetes & its Complications 2001; 15(1):44–54.

39. Festa A, D'Agostino R, Jr, Tracy RP, Haffner SM, Insulin Resistance AS. Elevated levels of acute-phase proteins and plasminogen activator inhibitor-1 predict the development of type 2 diabetes: the insulin resistance atherosclerosis study. Diabetes 2002; 51(4):1131–1137.

40. Festa A, Williams K, Tracy RP, Wagenknecht LE, Haffner SM. Progression of plasminogen activator inhibitor-1 and fibrinogen levels in relation to incident type 2 diabetes. Circulation 2006; 113(14):1753–1759.

41. Nagi DK, Yudkin JS. Effects of metformin on insulin resistance, risk factors for cardiovascular disease, and plasminogen activator inhibitor in NIDDM subjects. A study of two ethnic groups. Diabetes Care 1993; 16(4):621–629.

42. Koenig W. Fibrin(ogen) in cardiovascular disease: an update. Thrombosis & Haemostasis 2003; 89(4):601–609.

43. Emanuele N, Azad N, Abraira C et al. Effect of intensive glycemic control on fibrinogen, lipids, and lipoproteins: Veterans Affairs Cooperative Study in Type II Diabetes Mellitus. Archives of Internal Medicine 1998; 158(22):2485–2490.

44. Fanghanel G, Silva U, Sanchez-Reyes L, Sisson D, Sotres D, Torres EM. Effects of metformin on fibrinogen levels in obese patients with type 2 diabetes. Revista de Investigacion Clinica 1998; 50(5):389–394.

45. Heinrich J, Balleisen L, Schulte H, Assmann G, van de LJ. Fibrinogen and factor VII in the prediction of coronary risk. Results from the PROCAM study in healthy men. Arteriosclerosis & Thrombosis 1994; 14(1):54–59.

46. Boden G, Vaidyula VR, Homko C, Cheung P, Rao AK. Circulating tissue factor procoagulant activity and thrombin generation in patients with type 2 diabetes: effects of insulin and glucose. Journal of Clinical Endocrinology & Metabolism 2007; 92(11):4352–4358.

47. Calles-Escandon J, Cipolla M. Diabetes and endothelial dysfunction: a clinical perspective. Endocrine Reviews 2001; 22(1):36–52.

48. Calles-Escandon J, Garcia-Rubi E, Mirza S, Mortensen A. Type 2 diabetes: one disease, multiple cardiovascular risk factors. Coronary Artery Disease 1999; 10(1):23–30.

49. Furchgott RF. Introduction to EDRF research. Journal of Cardiovascular Pharmacology 1993; 22(Suppl 2):S1–S2.

50. Garg UC, Hassid A. Nitric oxide-generating vasodilators and 8-bromo-cyclic guanosine monophosphate inhibit mitogenesis and proliferation of cultured rat vascular smooth muscle cells. Journal of Clinical Investigation 1989; 83(5):1774–1777.

51. Cacoub P, Carayon A, Dorent R et al. Endothelin: the vasoconstrictor of the 1990's? Revue de Medecine Interne 1993; 14(4):229–232.

52. Goldin E, Casadevall M, Mourelle M et al. Role of prostaglandins and nitric oxide in gastrointestinal hyperemia of diabetic rats. American Journal of Physiology 1996; 270(4 Part 1):G684–G690.

53. Hsueh WA, Anderson PW. Systemic hypertension and the renin-angiotensin system in diabetic vascular complications. American Journal of Cardiology 1993; 72(20):14H–21H.

54. Busse R, Fleming I, Hecker M. Signal transduction in endothelium-dependent vasodilatation. European Heart Journal 1993; 14(Suppl I):2–9.

55. Mombouli JV. ACE inhibition, endothelial function and coronary artery lesions. Role of kinins and nitric oxide. Drugs 1997; 54(Suppl 5):12–22.

56. Cowan DB, Langille BL. Cellular and molecular biology of vascular remodeling. Current Opinion in Lipidology 1996; 7(2):94–100.

57. Natarajan R, Bai W, Lanting L, Gonzales N, Nadler J. Effects of high glucose on vascular endothelial growth factor expression in vascular smooth muscle cells. American Journal of Physiology 1997; 273(5 Part 2):H2224–H2231.

58. Biegelsen ES, Loscalzo J. Endothelial function and atherosclerosis. Coronary Artery Disease 1999; 10(4):241–256.

59. Tracy RP, Lemaitre RN, Psaty BM et al. Relationship of C-reactive protein to risk of cardiovascular disease in the elderly. Results from the Cardiovascular Health Study and the Rural Health Promotion Project. Arteriosclerosis, Thrombosis & Vascular Biology 1997; 17(6):1121–1127.

60. De Meyer GR, Herman AG. Vascular endothelial dysfunction. Progress in Cardiovascular Diseases 1997; 39(4):325–342.

61. Kario K, Matsuo T, Kobayashi H, Matsuo M, Sakata T, Miyata T. Activation of tissue factor-induced coagulation and endothelial cell dysfunction in non-insulin-dependent diabetic patients with microalbuminuria. Arteriosclerosis, Thrombosis & Vascular Biology 1995; 15(8):1114–1120.

62. Schalkwijk CG, Stehouwer CD. Vascular complications in diabetes mellitus: the role of endothelial dysfunction. Clinical Science 2005; 109(2):143–159.

63. Hattori Y, Kasai K, Nakamura T, Emoto T, Shimoda S. Effect of glucose and insulin on immunoreactive endothelin-1 release from cultured porcine aortic endothelial cells. Metabolism: Clinical & Experimental 1991; 40(2):165–169.

64. Cipolla MJ. Elevated glucose potentiates contraction of isolated rat resistance arteries and augments protein kinase C-induced intracellular calcium release. Metabolism: Clinical & Experimental 1999; 48(8):1015–1022.

65. Cosentino F, Luscher TF. Endothelial dysfunction in diabetes mellitus. Journal of Cardiovascular Pharmacology 1998; 32(Suppl 3):S54–S61.

66. Jialal I, Crettaz M, Hachiya HL et al. Characterization of the receptors for insulin and the insulin-like growth factors on micro- and macrovascular tissues. Endocrinology 1985; 117(3):1222–1229.

67. King GL, Buzney SM, Kahn CR et al. Differential responsiveness to insulin of endothelial and support cells from micro- and macrovessels. Journal of Clinical Investigation 1983; 71(4):974–979.

68. Kuboki K, Jiang ZY, Takahara N et al. Regulation of endothelial constitutive nitric oxide synthase gene expression in endothelial cells and in vivo: a specific vascular action of insulin. Circulation 2000; 101(6):676–681.

69. Inoguchi T, Xia P, Kunisaki M, Higashi S, Feener EP, King GL. Insulin's effect on protein kinase C and diacylglycerol induced by diabetes and glucose in vascular tissues. American Journal of Physiology 1994; 267(3 Part 1):E369–E379.

70. Vervoort G, Lutterman JA, Smits P, Berden JH, Wetzels JF. Transcapillary escape rate of albumin is increased and related to haemodynamic changes in normo-albuminuric type 1 diabetic patients. Journal of Hypertension 1999; 17(12 Part 2):1911–1916.

71. Ferri C, Bellini C, Desideri G et al. Circulating endothelin-1 levels in obese patients with the metabolic syndrome. Experimental & Clinical Endocrinology & Diabetes 1997; 105(Suppl 2):38–40.

72. Calles-Escandon J, Ballor D, Harvey-Berino J, Ades P, Tracy R, Sobel B. Amelioration of the inhibition of fibrinolysis in elderly, obese subjects by moderate energy intake restriction. American Journal of Clinical Nutrition 1996; 64(1):7–11.

73. Andersen P, Seljeflot I, Abdelnoor M et al. Increased insulin sensitivity and fibrinolytic capacity after dietary intervention in obese women with polycystic ovary syndrome. Metabolism: Clinical & Experimental 1995; 44(5):611–616.

74. Steinberg HO, Tarshoby M, Monestel R et al. Elevated circulating free fatty acid levels impair endothelium-dependent vasodilation. Journal of Clinical Investigation 1997; 100(5):1230–1239.

75. Ting HH, Timimi FK, Boles KS, Creager SJ, Ganz P, Creager MA. Vitamin C improves endothelium-dependent vasodilation in patients with non-insulin-dependent diabetes mellitus. Journal of Clinical Investigation 1996; 97(1):22–28.

76. Tesfamariam B, Brown ML, Cohen RA. Elevated glucose impairs endothelium-dependent relaxation by activating protein kinase C. Journal of Clinical Investigation 1991; 87(5):1643–1648.

77. Hink U, Tsilimingas N, Wendt M, Munzel T. Mechanisms underlying endothelial dysfunction in diabetes mellitus: therapeutic implications. Treat in Endocrinology 2003; 2(5):293–304.
78. Cosentino F, Hishikawa K, Katusic ZS, Luscher TF. High glucose increases nitric oxide synthase expression and super-oxide anion generation in human aortic endothelial cells. Circulation 1997; 96(1):25–28.
79. Hink U, Li H, Mollnau H et al. Mechanisms underlying endothelial dysfunction in diabetes mellitus. Circulation Research 2001; 88(2):E14–E22.
80. Milstien S, Katusic Z. Oxidation of tetrahydrobiopterin by peroxynitrite: implications for vascular endothelial function. Biochemical & Biophysical Research Communications 1999; 263(3):681–684.
81. Stroes E, Kastelein J, Cosentino F et al. Tetrahydrobiopterin restores endothelial function in hypercholesterolemia. Journal of Clinical Investigation 1997; 99(1):41–46.
82. Heitzer T, Brockhoff C, Mayer B et al. Tetrahydrobiopterin improves endothelium-dependent vasodilation in chronic smokers: evidence for a dysfunctional nitric oxide synthase. Circulation Research 2000; 86(2):E36–E41.
83. Sowers JR. Insulin and insulin-like growth factor in normal and pathological cardiovascular physiology. Hypertension 1997; 29(3):691–699.
84. Ishii H, Koya D, King GL. Protein kinase C activation and its role in the development of vascular complications in diabetes mellitus. Journal of Molecular Medicine 1998; 76(1):21–31.
85. Hirata K, Kuroda R, Sakoda T et al. Inhibition of endothelial nitric oxide synthase activity by protein kinase C. Hypertension 1995; 25(2):180–185.
86. Inoguchi T, Li P, Umeda F et al. High glucose level and free fatty acid stimulate reactive oxygen species production through protein kinase C – dependent activation of NAD(P)H oxidase in cultured vascular cells. Diabetes 2000; 49(11):1939–1945.
87. Du XL, Edelstein D, Rossetti L et al. Hyperglycemia-induced mitochondrial superoxide overproduction activates the hexo-samine pathway and induces plasminogen activator inhibitor-1 expression by increasing Sp1 glycosylation. Proceedings of the National Academy of Sciences of the United States of America 2000; 97(22):12222–12226.
88. King GL, Brownlee M. The cellular and molecular mechanisms of diabetic complications. Endocrinology & Metabolism Clinics of North America 1996; 25(2):255–270.
89. Guerci B, Bohme P, Kearney-Schwartz A, Zannad F, Drouin P. Endothelial dysfunction and type 2 diabetes, Part 2: altered endothelial function and the effects of treatments in type 2 diabetes mellitus. Diabetes & Metabolism 2001; 27(4 Part 1):436–447.
90. Border WA, Yamamoto T, Noble NA. Transforming growth factor beta in diabetic nephropathy. Diabetes/Metabolism Reviews 1996; 12(4):309–339.
91. Yamamoto T, Nakamura T, Noble NA, Ruoslahti E, Border WA. Expression of transforming growth factor beta is elevated in human and experimental diabetic nephropathy. Proceedings of the National Academy of Sciences of the United States of America 1993; 90(5):1814–1818.
92. McMillan DE. Increased levels of acute-phase serum proteins in diabetes. Metabolism: Clinical & Experimental 1989; 38(11):1042–1046.
93. Chen S, Hong SW, Iglesias-de la Cruz MC, Isono M, Casaretto A, Ziyadeh FN. The key role of the transforming growth factor-beta system in the pathogenesis of diabetic nephropathy. Renal Failure 2001; 23(3–4):471–481.
94. Aiello LP, Avery RL, Arrigg PG et al. Vascular endothelial growth factor in ocular fluid of patients with diabetic retinopathy and other retinal disorders. New England Journal of Medicine 1994; 331(22):1480–1487.
95. Bax JJ, Young LH, Frye RL, Bonow RO, Steinberg HO, Barrett EJ. Screening for coronary artery disease in patients with diabetes. Diabetes Care 2007; 30(10):2729–2736.
96. Stangl V, Witzel V, Baumann G, Stangl K. Current diagnostic concepts to detect coronary artery disease in women. European Heart Journal 2008; 29(6):707–717.
97. Mieres JH, Shaw LJ, Arai A et al. Role of noninvasive testing in the clinical evaluation of women with suspected coronary artery disease: Consensus statement from the Cardiac Imaging Committee, Council on Clinical Cardiology, and the Cardiovascular Imaging and Intervention Committee, Council on Cardiovascular Radiology and Intervention, American Heart Association. Circulation 2005; 111(5):682–696.
98. American Diabetes Association. Standards of medical care in diabetes – 2008. Diabetes Care 2008; 31(Suppl 1):S12–S54.
99. Gouni-Berthold I, Berthold HK, Mantzoros CS, Bohm M, Krone W. Sex disparities in the treatment and control of cardiovascular risk factors in type 2 diabetes. Diabetes Care 2008; 31(7):1389–1391.

4

Insulin Resistance, Diabetes, and Cardiovascular Risk in Women and the Paradigm of the Polycystic Ovary Syndrome

Renato Pasquali and Alessandra Gambineri

CONTENTS

ABSTRACT

There are many differences between the sexes in the susceptibility and the development of chronic metabolic and cardiovascular diseases, which may be partly explained by the disparate alterations of androgen balance particularly in the presence of obesity. Notably, available studies support the concept that the prevalence of insulin resistance, the metabolic syndrome, type 2 diabetes, and cardiovascular pathologies is different between the sexes. With respect to women, it is particularly evident from a recent meta-analysis that those with the abdominal phenotype of excess weight or obesity, who are characterized by a condition of relative hyperandrogenic state, are at high risk for a specific morbidity for these diseases. The paradigm of PCOS is a good example for investigating the relationship between hyperandrogenemia and insulin resistance and metabolic and cardiovascular disorders, since most affected women are overweight or obese, approximately two-thirds have insulin resistance and show a very high susceptibility to develop the metabolic syndrome and type 2 diabetes, even earlier than expected, based on trends reported in the general population. Therefore, reducing androgen levels in abdominally obese women with or without PCOS may represent a clinical challenge for treatment and, possibly, for preventive intervention strategies.

From: *Diabetes in Women: Pathophysiology and Therapy*
Edited by: A. Tsatsoulis et al. (eds.), DOI 10.1007/978-1-60327-250-6_4
© Humana Press, a part of Springer Science+Business Media, LLC 2009

Key words: Women; Insulin resistance; Abdominal obesity; Type 2 diabetes mellitus; Cardiovascular risk factors; Polycystic ovary syndrome.

THE BIOLOGY OF SEX DIFFERENCE IN HEALTH AND DISEASE

There is increasing evidence that there are many differences between the sexes in the susceptibility and development of chronic metabolic diseases and cardiovascular diseases (CVDs). This implies that mechanisms may partly differ in males and females, involving both endogenous and environmental factors. The fundamental differences between males and females are primarily attributed to hormones, which define the differentiation of secondary sex characteristics at puberty, regulate fertility, metabolism, and behavior, as well as play an important role in regulating many functions of nonreproductive tissues *(1)*. Androgens are fundamental examples of this sex-related hormonal function. They have different functions with typical genomic influences on protein synthesis mediated by transcription induced as a result of the binding of hormones to intracellular receptors and DNA, and by means of these actions they regulate body composition and fat metabolism as well as vascular function and metabolism *(1)*. Changes in the androgen balance have been found to be associated with a series of chronic metabolic diseases and CVDs, with different mechanisms according to sex *(2)*. There are also strong differences in the socioeconomic and cultural environment in which men and women live their daily lives, which are related to social, economic, and family roles; type of education and culture; and the influence of behavioral stereotypes conditioned by different traditions, religions, and political situations. The combination of these factors brings about specific adaptive behaviors that affect lifestyle, psychological, and cognitive attitudes and the ability to interact with environmental stressors, all factors which could play an important role in influencing the onset and evolution of metabolic diseases and CVDs.

We are faced with an increasing scientific interest in gender medicine, based on a clear definition of major biological differences according to sex, which not only involve hormones and genes, but also involve environmental factors, to which much more attention should be paid than was formerly believed necessary.

In this chapter, we will focus on some of the very complex aspects of the relationship between androgens and metabolic dysfunction, particularly insulin resistance, obesity, type 2 diabetes mellitus (T2D), and cardiovascular risk factors in women, in the general female population and particularly in women with the polycystic ovary syndrome (PCOS).

INSULIN RESISTANCE IN THE GENERAL FEMALE POPULATION

Insulin resistance is defined as a reduced biological effect of insulin for any given concentration of insulin. The definition and accurate quantification of insulin resistance is important, and a number of methods are available for its measurement *(3)*. Since there are basic mathematical principles common to various methods and each of them has well-known advantages and limitations, their use should depend on the major aim of each particular study. Insulin sensitivity can be evaluated in vivo by using either complex techniques or mathematical models based on simple tests. For in vivo assessment of the biological effect of insulin, the hyperinsulinemic euglycemic clamp technique represents the gold standard procedure *(4)*. With this technique, insulin concentrations are kept high by using a constant insulin infusion, and plasma glucose is maintained constant by a variable intravenous glucose infusion. The glucose infusion rate necessary to maintain euglycemia during the clamp represents the net effect of insulin on glucose metabolism. The average glucose infusion rate during the last hour of the clamp is often termed the *M*-value. An insulin resistant state is defined when the glucose disposal rate is reduced.

Insulin resistance can also be accurately measured by the minimal model. This is based on a complex computer modeling analysis of the glucose and insulin profiles obtained following the frequently sampled iv glucose tolerance test (FSIVGTT), which has undergone several modifications over the years *(4, 5)*. This test provides information on the biological effect of insulin, and on glucose effectiveness and early phase insulin secretion, as well as on glucose tolerance. Because of the complexity of these approaches, which are usually reserved for clinical research, great efforts have been made to identify simpler tests. In the last decade, most tests have in fact been produced as nondynamic measurements of insulin sensitivity, and because of their simplicity they have been widely used in both epidemiological and clinical studies. Most of these tests, which include fasting insulin alone, the homeostasis assessment method [(HOMA): (fasting glucose, mmol/L × fasting insulin, mIU/mL)/25] *(6)* and the quantitative insulin-sensitivity check index [QUICKI: 1/(log insulin fasting + log glucose fasting)], have been extensively reviewed *(7, 8)*. These tests are simple to perform, and are based on fasting insulin concentrations and glucose levels alone. However, even these simple procedures need to be carried out in carefully standardized conditions if reliable measurements of insulin resistance are to be obtained. Many factors must be controlled, such as the duration of sample storage before assay, processing of samples, and accuracy of the insulin assay performed *(3)*. It should also be emphasized that once a significant defect of insulin secretion exists, the value of these measurements is poor and can be misleading.

Sensitivity to insulin-mediated glucose disposal varies widely in the general population. Several studies have in fact demonstrated that, at least in apparently healthy nondiabetic individuals, insulin-mediated glucose disposal varies by approximately six- to eightfold and that, despite this great variability, insulin is secreted in sufficient amounts to prevent decompensation of glucose homeostasis *(9, 10)*. Increased β-cell insulin secretion represents an effort by the body to deal with the peripheral defect of insulin action, in order to preserve normal glucose tolerance. When insulin-resistant individuals cannot maintain the necessary degree of compensatory hyperinsulinemia to overcome the insulin resistant state, impaired glucose tolerance or DM2 develops.

A great deal of research has been carried out in the last two decades, focusing on the impact of insulin resistance on chronic metabolic disorders. In most cases, particularly in epidemiological studies, simple tests have been used, although in large clinical single-center studies complex tests have been used. Insulin resistance and compensatory hyperinsulinemia precede the development of DM2 in most women, particularly when obesity is present. Moreover, there is worldwide agreement that excess insulin concentration and reduced insulin sensitivity are associated with a greater risk of developing CVDs. Data supporting the concept that there is a substantial difference and heterogeneity between the sexes in the prevalence of the insulin resistance state are, however, very sparse and still inconsistent, at least from the epidemiological point of view *(9, 10)*. This is partly due to the fact that the majority of the studies did not segregate for sex in their analysis, but sex differences have usually been taken into consideration by controlling for sex in the statistical approach. In addition, in studies performed in adult populations, simple mathematical models to define insulin resistance have often been used, although they possess intrinsic limitations in this complex pathophysiological area. Nonetheless, available data support the suggestion that there is some difference in the prevalence of the metabolic syndrome, DM2, and CVD between the sexes, so the hypothesis that insulin resistance and associated hyperinsulinemia may be a sex trait is not arbitrary, although major determinants are not adequately understood.

The different prevalence in women and men may depend, at least in part, on the genetic background of the population studied, but susceptibility genes have still not been clearly defined *(11, 12)*. A history of insulin resistance could start during intrauterine life. Several findings are consistent with this. Girls are typically born lighter than boys. The consistency of this observation across different populations is striking, suggesting that it may have fundamental significance for those conditions linked with lower birth weight, such as insulin resistance or diabetes. However, previous hypotheses relating low birth weight to subsequent metabolic pathologies have addressed differences in insulin resistance within the sexes, not between them. It has recently been proposed that sex-specific genes affecting insulin sensitivity are responsible for the sex difference in birth weight. These genes may also render female subjects more susceptible to DM2, explaining why reports of this disorder in younger populations show a female preponderance. Sex-specific genes may therefore have a demonstrable impact on fetal growth and insulin resistance *(13–15)*. This hypothesis is consistent with studies showing that female newborns have higher insulin concentrations than male newborns, despite being small, suggesting intrinsic insulin resistance in girls *(16)*. Accordingly, another study showed that Caucasian girls aged 5 years are intrinsically more insulin resistant than boys *(17)*, and other studies confirm that this difference persists during puberty and adolescence *(18, 19)*.

Unfortunately, very few studies have been performed using the clamp technique to measure insulin resistance. In one study *(20)* it was found that women had higher fasting, glucose-stimulated insulin, insulin-to-glucose ratio, and lower insulin-stimulated glucose utilization measured by the euglycemic hyperinsulinemic clamp technique compared with men, and that these metabolic alterations were correlated with increased androgenicity in women. On the other hand, Ferrannini et al. *(21)* investigated 1,308 subjects (718 women and 590 men) participating in the European Group for the Study of Insulin Resistance (EGIR) and found that women were significantly leaner (BMI 24.0 ± 5.2) than men (BMI 26.0 + 4.4), were less insulin resistant, and had lower fasting insulin concentrations. This study, however, did not consider body composition, particularly lean body mass, that per se can account for differentiating insulin sensitivity between the sexes. In another study performed on 443 healthy volunteers selected from a database of individuals who had participated in various institutional review board-approved studies in the previous decade, Cheal et al. *(22)* did not find any difference in the presence of insulin resistance between men and women in relation to the presence of the metabolic syndrome. Finally, there are data suggesting that menopause does not seem to strictly relate to a decrease in insulin sensitivity, as postmenopausal women have been found to have the same insulin sensitivity as age-matched men. In the population studied by the EGIR, the best predictor of CVD was fasting insulin rather than insulin sensitivity measured as glucose disposal rate by the clamp technique *(23)*. Finally, in a further study performed in postmenopausal women with various degrees of glucose tolerance, it was found that only some of the women with menopause could be defined as having insulin resistance, its prevalence being significantly dependent on the glucose tolerance status and body composition, thus suggesting the importance of other factors in the relationship between menopause and insulin resistance *(24)*. There is no doubt that this topic should be subjected to more intense investigation, taking into consideration different ages, including fertility and menopause. In addition, much more information is needed on the influence of the environmental factors described above.

THE METABOLIC SYNDROME, CARDIOVASCULAR RISK FACTORS, AND CARDIOVASCULAR EVENTS IN WOMEN

In 1988, Reaven proposed that individuals who displayed the cluster of abnormalities associated with insulin resistance and compensatory hyperinsulinemia were at significant risk for CVDs *(10)*. Over the last 15 years, the concept underlying the common aggregation of major abnormalities associated with an insulin-resistant state has emerged as a unique entity, the so-called metabolic syndrome. Although there is a concept that insulin resistance is ontologically different from the metabolic syndrome, for many years these two expressions have nonetheless often been used more or less synonymously. This issue is, however, a matter of great controversy at the present time. One of the reasons is certainly represented by the difficulty of measuring the insulin resistance state and the need for more reliable parameters defining the risk for CVD. The need to simplify the definition of the metabolic syndrome for epidemiological studies contrasts with the complexity of the geographical and cultural differences, ethnicity, and lifestyle habits which influence its phenotypic expression and make it difficult to define the potential etiological roles of these factors across different cohorts and cross-sectional comparisons. Overall, each of these definitions proposes the collection of very simple parameters, mostly based on a clinical approach. Particular attention has been paid to the original National Cholesterol Education Program Expert Panel on Detection, Evaluation and Treatment of High Blood Cholesterol in Adults (NCEP/ATP III) 2001 report *(25)*. Several reports on the prevalence of the metabolic syndrome using the NCEP/ATPIII criteria have been recently reviewed and summarized *(26)*. Based on these studies, the estimate of the prevalence has been reported to range from 4.6 to 29.4%, although an adequate comparison is difficult because of the different definition criteria, demographic variability, and geographical heterogeneity. Results from the National Health and Nutrition Survey III have documented a prevalence rate of the metabolic syndrome of 23% in the adult US population, with peak values of more than 40% in subjects aged 60 years or more, and with significant ethnic differences *(27)*. In other studies, the prevalence rate was found to range from 13 to 55% *(28)*. The main reasons for these large differences were again ethnicity and sex. Comparison of the NCEP/ATP III criteria with those proposed by the World Health Organization (WHO) *(29, 30)* in different studies performed in US populations showed that the prevalence using these two criteria was more or less similar *(31)*. In contrast, a study performed using data from the Framingham Offspring Study and the San Antonio Heart Study *(32)* found that the NCEP/ATP III criteria produced somewhat higher estimates in the former study, with minor differences according to ethnicity, and no difference in men in the latter study. Interestingly, using the NCEP/ATP III criteria, and considering only individuals more than 20 years old, prevalence rates have been estimated to range from 8 to 24% in men and from 7 to 46% in women *(33)*. More recently, a study performed in a nationally representative sample of 15,540 Chinese adults, aged 35–74 years, found that the age-standardized prevalence of the metabolic syndrome (as defined by the NCEP/ATP III criteria) was 9.8% and 17.8% in men and women, respectively, whereas the age-standardized prevalence of overweight or obesity was 26.9% and 31.1%, respectively *(34)*. This partially contrasts with data by the EGIR group, which found that prevalence rates ranged from 10 to 20% for men and 10 to 15% for women *(35)*.

There are few systematic reviews on the impact of the metabolic syndrome according to sex. As reported above, major studies have shown a great difference in prevalence rates in both men and women. In 2004, Cameron and coworkers *(33)* reported an in-depth literature search for publications documenting the prevalence of the metabolic syndrome according to any of the WHO *(29)*, NCEP/ATP-III *(25)*, or EGIR *(35)* criteria. Although the differences in the definition criteria made it difficult to draw general conclusions, the authors evaluated the data separately for men and women, according to each factor. A wide range of prevalence was clearly apparent, regardless of the criteria used. However, it appeared that prevalence increased with increasing age in both groups. They reviewed many large studies using the NCEP/ATP III criteria, and found that women had a tendency to have higher prevalence rates [29.8% (range 7.0–56.1)] than men [22.7% (range 10.0–43.6%)]. However, in the fewer studies using the WHO criteria, they found the opposite [women: 17.9% (range 5.1–33.9); men: 27.4% (range 12.2–44.8)]. It is likely that these discrepancies may be accounted for by some important differences in the definition of the metabolic syndrome according to the WHO and the NCEP/ATP III criteria. In fact, according to the WHO criteria, diabetes or impaired fasting glycemia or impaired glucose tolerance or insulin resistance (under hyperinsulinemic euglycemic conditions) represent a prerequisite for including other criteria, and obesity (BMI > 30) and the waist-to-hip ratio are also included, whereas fasting glucose higher than 110 mg/dL and waist circumference are included in the NCEP/ATP III original definition. Notably, when Cameron and coworkers (33) examined all studies using the EGIR criteria, they found that men [16.0% (range 4.7–24.6)] tended to have higher prevalence rates than women [10.9% (range 1.7–16.0)], although collectively in both sexes rates were lower than in the studies using either the WHO or the NCEP/ATP III criteria. Very few studies are available using the more recent criteria proposed by the International Diabetes Federation (IDF) (36, 37).

Overall, the data support the concept that the prevalence of the metabolic syndrome may differ according to sex, and this may be particularly relevant for women, who physiologically undergo several vulnerable periods during their life, such as menopause. Menopause is in fact a typical physiological event in women, but its occurrence considerably changes their susceptibility to develop metabolic diseases and CVDs. Although the mechanisms responsible for these dramatic events are not completely understood, there is nonetheless evidence that changes in the hormone milieu, other than age, play an important role. Both these factors do in fact have an important regulatory function on metabolism and cardiovascular physiology. The emergence of the metabolic syndrome with menopause has been reviewed recently by Carr (38). In fact, the prevalence of the metabolic syndrome tends to increase with menopause and may partially explain the apparent acceleration in CVD after menopause. The transition from pre- to postmenopause is associated with the emergence of many features of the metabolic syndrome, including increased central body fat, a shift toward a more atherogenic lipid profile, increased low-density lipoprotein and triglyceride levels, reduced high-density lipoprotein, small low-density lipoprotein particles, and increased insulin levels associated with more frequent glucose intolerance (38). Whether this list of abnormalities may be a direct result of ovarian failure or, alternatively, an indirect result of the metabolic consequences of central fat redistribution with estrogen deficiency is a matter of increasing scientific debate (see below). Moreover, it is unclear whether the transition to menopause increases CVD risk in all women or only in those who develop features of the metabolic syndrome.

The role of sex hormones, specifically androgens, in the regulation of insulin secretion and action and in the regulation of major metabolic pathways will be summarized in a further paragraph. On the other hand, many other factors need to be further investigated in relation to sex. They include classic factors such as glucose intolerance, endothelial dysfunction, procoagulant factors, hemodynamic changes, low-grade inflammation, abnormal serum uric acid (39), as well as several hormonal derangements, such as low or high testosterone in men and women, respectively (40), some degree of hyperactivity of the hypothalamic–pituitary–adrenal axis (41), and sex-dependent genetic predisposition (42). Focusing on sex differences among these risk factors will improve our understanding of the impact of the metabolic syndrome on the risk for CVD in women.

HOW THE DEFINITION OF THE METABOLIC SYNDROME OVERLAPS THAT OF INSULIN RESISTANCE

As reported above, the NCEP/ATP III report designated a cluster of related CVD risk factors as a definition of the metabolic syndrome, and stated that "this syndrome is closely linked to insulin resistance" (25). Insulin resistance and/or compensatory hyperinsulinemia are undoubtedly CVD risk factors (10). On the other hand, although insulin resistance is believed to be the basic pathophysiological alteration leading to the metabolic syndrome, neither assessment of insulin resistance nor hyperinsulinemia were among the criteria proposed by the NCEP/ATP III report. This omission was justified by the lack of adequate sensitivity and specificity of the different insulin assays used in clinical practice and other potential limitations. This is of importance, because there are patients with the metabolic syndrome who are unlikely to have insulin resistance and vice versa (35).

There are several other considerations emphasizing why different definitions of the metabolic syndrome and of the insulin resistance may in some way represent different entities and they should not therefore be used synonymously *(37)*. In fact, many studies indicate that relatively new indices related to both insulin resistance and CVD may also be useful predictive tools or useful additions to the definition of the metabolic syndrome. These indices include markers of low-grade inflammation, which is currently suggested to play a major role in atherogenesis development. In fact, recent studies have shown that a relationship exists between inflammatory markers and indices of insulin resistance, both in subjects with the metabolic syndrome and in those with DM2 and obesity [reviewed in *(37)*], as well as in those with PCOS (see paragraph below) *(43)*. It is now well established that there is a strong and consistent inverse association between adiponectin and both insulin resistance and inflammatory markers *(37)*. In addition, adiponectin is also inversely related with other CVD risk factors, such as blood pressure, HDL-cholesterol, and triglycerides, in addition to abdominal fatness, thereby clustering all definitions of the metabolic syndrome. Several other molecular factors (such as fibrinogen, plasminogen activator inhibitor-PAI-1, etc.) have also been found to be closely associated with insulin resistance, metabolic syndrome risk factors, and risks for CVD. The reasons supporting the possibility that the term "insulin resistance" may not adequately describe the hallmark of the metabolic syndrome or vice versa, even though insulin resistance may represent a component or a main pathophysiological factor of the metabolic syndrome itself, have been recently and extensively discussed by Kahn et al. *(37)* in a provocative report which the readers should refer to for further details to understand the fundamental issues of the debate. Therefore, the attempt to define the metabolic syndrome as a result of a simple unifying pathophysiological process is problematic, because there are very few studies which have described the relationship between reliable measurements of insulin resistance and all of the factors used to define the metabolic syndrome. One example of these studies is the report by Cheal et al. *(22)*. These authors investigated a large group of healthy volunteers with different anthropometric and metabolic measurements, and insulin resistance was defined as being in the top tertile of the steady-state plasma glucose during the combined octreotide–insulin–glucose test *(44)*. They found that, although insulin resistance and the presence of the metabolic syndrome were significantly associated ($p < 0.001$), the sensitivity and positive predictive values equaled 46 and 76%. Being overweight with high triglycerides, low HDL-cholesterol or elevated blood pressure were the most common factors included in the diagnosis of the metabolic syndrome itself. No systematic difference, however, was found in relation to sex. When all criteria of the NCEP/APT III definition were considered, approximately more than 90% of women and all men were insulin resistant, and there was still no sex difference when only three criteria were used.

Whatever the truth, it is quite clear that the presence of the metabolic syndrome includes a high proportion of subjects with an insulin resistance state and vice versa. Therefore, with some caution, it could be argued that defining clinical characteristics of the metabolic syndrome may be a justified method of detecting insulin-resistant individuals, although some of them may be lost in the analysis. This is particularly important not only in the general female population and in women with DM2, but also in those with other clinical conditions, such as PCOS.

DIABETES AND CARDIOVASCULAR RISK FACTORS IN WOMEN

There is emerging evidence that DM2 is an important risk factor for the development of CVD, with some difference between women and men. As discussed in more detail in Chap. 3, death rates for coronary heart disease (CHD) are 3–7 times greater among diabetic than nondiabetic women, whereas rates are twice or three times greater in diabetic vs. nondiabetic men *(45)*. Furthermore, evidence suggests that the positive association between adiposity and risk for DM2 is stronger for women compared with men *(46)*, although this association appears to largely depend on the patterns of body fat distribution. Importantly, excess body weight, together with insulin resistance, appears to significantly predict the incidence of DM2 not only in high-risk populations, but also in low-risk groups *(47)*.

In general, estimates of CHD incidence in patients with diabetes vary across studies and countries, mainly because of differences in selection criteria and risk assessment. In a recent study performed in a large cohort of 6,032 women and 5,612 men, sampled from a nationwide network of hospital-based diabetes clinics in Italy and followed up for 4 years, it was reported that the age-standardized rate (per 1,000 person-year) of the first CHD event was 28.0 (95% CL 5–4–32.2) in men and 23.3 (20.2–26.4) in women *(48)*. Major CHDs were less frequent in women than in men, with a sex ratio of 0.5. However, by multivariate Cox analysis, age and diabetes duration were risk factors for both sexes, whereas glycemic control and treated hypertension were additional risk factors for men, and higher triglyceride/low HDL-cholesterol and microvascular complications were independent risk factors for women. These data further indicate that specific risk factors may be different between the sexes, emphasizing the need for additional epidemiological and clinical research in this area. Additionally, these findings raise questions about the possibility that treatment of DM2 should differ in order to prevent CVD according to sex. In fact, the data support the concept that hyperglycemia and hypertension in men, and diabetic dyslipidemia in women should be considered as risk factors amenable to more aggressive treatment. In a recent review by Legato et al. *(49)*, it was found that even when women were included in clinical trials on diabetes, most investigators typically made no attempt to assess the impact of sex difference on the reported results. There is also evidence that DM2 is growing faster in older women, and, most importantly, that women with diabetes appear to have a poorer prognosis after myocardial infarction than men. In addition, Legato et al. *(49)* pointed out that obesity, an important contributor of DM2, is more prevalent in women, and that women with diabetes also have an increased risk for hypertension and hyperlipidemia compared with men. Finally, they found that women are less likely to receive aggressive treatment for CHD and to achieve treatment goals. Disparities in the treatment of diabetes between sexes may therefore be relevant in order to explain the poorer outcomes in women. This could be explained by the heavier burden of other cardiovascular traditional risk factors within the context of the metabolic syndrome, but there is also evidence for a less effective management of these risk factors in women, particularly those with DM2 *(50)*, which suggests the need for better strategies in the treatment of this disorder and in the prevention of CVD in women.

Predictors of DM2 in women include factors that are common in the general population, independent of sex differences. They include insulin resistance and the metabolic syndrome. Recently, particular attention has been paid to chronic subclinical inflammation, which has been suggested as being involved in the pathogenesis of DM2 *(51, 52)*. This hypothesis has recently been supported by several prospective studies showing that subjects who developed DM2 during the follow-up period had elevated levels of markers of inflammation such as C-reactive protein (CRP) or interleukin-6 (IL-6) at baseline compared with subjects who did not develop the disease *(53, 54)*. However, although various studies have examined these associations, few reported sex-specific results *(54–57)*. This lack of data is surprising, since there is strong evidence for sex differences in associations between DM2, obesity, endogenous sex hormones, and inflammation *(58, 59)*. Most of the studies that investigated sex differences concerning inflammatory markers and risk for DM2 were relatively small and yielded contradictory results, especially for CRP. While the Hoorn Study, conducted in the Netherlands, reported a significant association between CRP and incidence of diabetes in men, but not in women *(56)*, the opposite was seen in the Mexico City Diabetes Study *(55)*. Finally, in two studies conducted in subjects of Japanese origin, CRP was significantly associated with incident DM2 in both sexes *(57)*. More recently, however, in a study performed in subjects participating in the population-based MONICA/KORA study between 1984 and 2002, Thorand et al. *(60)* reassessed the sex-related association of CRP and IL-6 with DM2 risk, in 527 cases of DM2 (305 men and 222 women) and 1,698 controls (889 men and 809 women). After adjustment for confounding variables, also including metabolic risk factors, elevated concentrations of CRP and IL-6 were found to present a considerably stronger association with risk of DM2 in women than in men, thus suggesting that inflammatory processes may be of particular importance in the pathogenesis of type DM2, particularly in women.

Obesity is one of the most important risk factors for DM2. In North America as well as in Europe and East Asia, the number of people considered overweight or obese is dramatically increasing (61), involving approximately half the population. Sex differences in weight are clearly influenced by geography and ethnic background. For example, data coming from the United States show that among whites and Mexican Americans, the prevalence is higher among men than among women. However, among black Americans, the prevalence of being overweight or obese is higher in women than in men (62). These figures are more or less similar in Canada (63). In Europe these trends are also similar, although the extent of this epidemic appears to be lower (61). In addition, obesity is also prevalent in many developing countries, with some geographical and ethnic differences. Collectively, prevalence rates appear to be similar for the two sexes, although available data suggest that countries reporting higher levels among women are located in Africa, Latin America, Asia, and Oceania, whereas male obesity appears to be more prevalent in European and North American countries (64). The abdominal obesity phenotype has a dominant importance in whatever definition of the metabolic syndrome is used. Epidemiology of different fat distribution phenotypes is complicated by the need for anthropometric measurements according to body size and ethnicity. This has been clearly recognized by the IDF (36), by defining different cut-off values of waist circumference, according to different populations. With a larger waist circumference, the prevalence of abdominal excess fat, defined as a specific enlargement of visceral fat tissues, tends undoubtedly to increase, although mechanistically a distinction between a large waist due to increases in subcutaneous adipose tissue vs. visceral fat is debated, based on studies using computer tomography or magnetic resonance (39). However, it is widely accepted that abdominal obesity measured by waist circumference or the waist-to-hip ratio confers an independent and additional risk for metabolic (chiefly DM2) diseases and CVDs independent of the degree of obesity (25–30, 65). It should be argued that although abdominal visceral fat has several important differences with respect to subcutaneous abdominal fat, older and recent studies on fat metabolism have shown that abdominal subcutaneous fat has specific and distinct features with respect to subcutaneous fat depots in other areas of the body, particularly gluteofemoral fat (41). This is particularly relevant for women. In fact, while there is evidence that obesity in males is invariably associated with a parallel increase in abdominal and visceral fat, meaning that the central distribution of body fat in the majority of males depends on the actual presence of obesity, by contrast in women a clear dichotomy of fat distribution occurs, with the abdominal phenotype being characterized by an enlargement of both subcutaneous and visceral fat depots and a modest increase of fat in the gluteofemoral areas (66). Women with abdominal obesity have distinct metabolic and hormonal features with respect to those with the subcutaneous peripheral phenotype (2). Metabolic specificities and regulatory factors differentiating visceral fat vs. subcutaneous fat in both sexes have been extensively discussed in recent review articles (2, 66) (see also Chap. 1). Undoubtedly, abdominal obesity is the body fat parameter most closely associated with the metabolic syndrome (11, 67, 68), DM2 (69–71), and cardiovascular risk (72) in women, particularly in postmenopausal women (73). Of particular interest is the association between DM2 and different obesity phenotypes in women with respect to men. Studies performed in the 1990s clearly demonstrated that age-adjusted RR for DM2 increases with increasing BMI in both men (74) and women (75). However, more recent studies performed in Italian cohorts of diabetics have repeatedly shown that the prevalence of abdominal obesity, as defined by a waist circumference greater than 88 cm in women and 102 cm in men, was

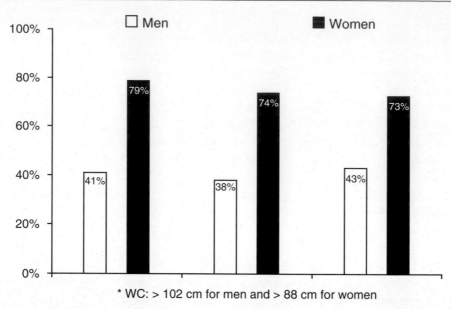

* WC: > 102 cm for men and > 88 cm for women

Fig. 1. Prevalence of abdominal obesity in Italian women with type 2 diabetes mellitus (*bars* on the *left*, *middle* and *right* are obtained from *(78–80)*, respectively).

more than 70% in women compared with approximately 40% in men *(69–71)* (Fig. 1). These data therefore indicate that the association between abdominal obesity and DM2 is stronger in women than in men, reflecting the need for a careful recognition of the abdominal fatness phenotype as a specific target for prevention and possibly for treatment in women, in order to decrease the risk for CVDs.

THE PARADIGM OF PCOS

PCOS is one of the most common causes of ovulatory infertility, affecting 4–7% of women. After the original description by Stein and Leventhal *(76)*, this syndrome has been defined in different ways over the last 15 years. In 1990 the National Institutes of Health (NIH) established very simple new diagnostic criteria, which were based on the presence of hyperandrogenism (either clinical, such as hirsutism, etc., or biochemical) and chronic oligo-anovulation, with the exclusion of other causes of blood androgen excess, such as adult-onset congenital adrenal hyperplasia, Cushing's syndrome, androgen-secreting neoplasms, and others *(77)*. More recently, a consensus conference held in Rotterdam, in 2003 *(78)*, re-examined the 1990 criteria and admitted the appropriateness of including ultrasound morphology of the ovaries among the diagnostic criteria of the syndrome. It was also established that at least two of the proposed diagnostic criteria, i.e., oligo-anovulation, clinical and/or biochemical signs of hyperandrogenism, and polycystic ovaries at ultrasound, were sufficient to make the diagnosis *(2)*. However, debate is still continuing in relation to which criteria should be used to define PCOS. One major concern in the definition of PCOS is related to the fact that insulin resistance and hyperinsulinemia are present in the majority of women with PCOS *(79, 80)*, as is obesity, particularly the abdominal phenotype *(81)*. The presence of these features has important effects in the pathophysiology of PCOS and largely contributes to the changing aspects of this disorder throughout the lifespan. Insulin excess does in fact have a direct responsibility in determining the production of ovarian androgens and increasing their availability in the target tissues through different mechanisms, i.e., a synergistic stimulatory effect with LH on ovarian steroidogenetic enzyme activity, and an inhibition of sex-hormone binging globulin (SHBG) synthesis and secretion from the liver *(80)*. Insulin resistance per se may be responsible for the development of compensatory hyperinsulinemia. It also represents the main pathophysiological event leading to the development of the metabolic syndrome, which is largely prevalent in PCOS women *(82)*, thereby increasing the risk for the development of DM2 and, possibly, CVD in these patients. The presence of obesity could also have a pathophysiological responsibility in the development not only of the insulin-resistant state and associated metabolic abnormalities, but also of hyperandrogenism and associated clinical consequences, such as menstrual disturbances and infertility *(81)*.

Insulin Resistance in PCOS

Insulin resistance in women with PCOS appears even more common than in the general population *(79, 83)*. It should, however, be emphasized that the majority of the studies have simply demonstrated that, in comparison to adequate control groups, insulin resistance, as measured by various techniques or methods, was more common in subjects with PCOS. There are no epidemiological studies focusing on the prevalence of insulin resistance in PCOS. In one study examining the characteristics of more than 1,000 consecutive women with androgen excess, Azziz et al. *(84)* found that 716 of them had PCOS and were characterized, as a group, by hyperinsulinemia and insulin resistance. Interestingly, 60% of them were obese, which indicates that obesity per se may be an amplifier of a cause of this metabolic derangement. Many other studies have in fact reported that insulin resistance is very common in the presence of obesity, particularly the abdominal phenotype *(79–81)*. The common thought is that obesity and PCOS have additive deleterious effects on insulin sensitivity, by mechanisms that have still not been adequately defined and could be partly different *(79, 80, 85)*. Reports on the prevalence of insulin resistance in women with PCOS are not homogeneous, depending on the sensitivity and specificity of the test employed. Due to the lack of epidemiological studies, available data refer to clinical studies performed in different referral centers worldwide and including only PCOS patients attending each institution for medical problems or personal complaints, particularly hirsutism, menses abnormalities, infertility, or obesity.

Both fasting and glucose-stimulated insulin concentrations are usually significantly higher in PCOS women than in non-PCOS controls *(79–81)*. Accordingly, studies examining insulin sensitivity by using different methods, such as the euglycemic hyperinsulinemic clamp technique, the FSIVGTT, or the insulin tolerance test, have demonstrated that PCOS women had significantly lower insulin sensitivity compared with age- and weight-matched controls. In addition, they demonstrated that almost all obese PCOS women have some degree of insulin resistance, whereas this abnormality is present in more than half of their non-obese PCOS counterparts [see extensive reviews in *(79–81)*].

Interestingly, however, some studies found some degree of deficiency in the first phase of insulin secretion in selected groups of PCOS women with obesity investigated in the United States *(8, 86)*, which were not confirmed by other studies performed in Europe *(87, 88)*. A more recent study using the FSIVGTT technique has produced additional data in European PCOS women, showing that in those with normal weight, insulin sensitivity and β-cell function are preserved, whereas glucose effectiveness (which is the insulin-independent glucose uptake) may be decreased *(89)*.

At variance, other relevant studies did not confirm decreased insulin sensitivity in PCOS, particularly in those with normal weight. In addition, these papers raised several questions regarding the opportunity of evaluating potential confounding factors, which, if not considered, can lead to false-positive results. Holte et al. *(90)* reported that some differences in the insulin sensitivity index, defined as the ratio of the glucose disposal rate to the insulin concentrations at the end of a euglycemic hyperinsulinemic clamp, were present only in subjects with high BMI values. While examining insulin sensitivity (measured by the FSIVGTT) in relation to the presence of a heredity risk for DM2,

Ehrmann et al. *(86)* were not able to find any difference in the insulin sensitivity index between obese PCOS and controls in affected women with a negative family history, whereas the difference was present in those with a positive one. Morin Papunen et al. *(91)* found that, compared with adequate control groups, only obese PCOS women were more insulin resistant, without any difference between normal weight PCOS and normal weight controls. More recently, these findings have been confirmed by another study *(92)*. Among potential factors explaining these different findings, dietary factors *(93)*, heredity, or pattern of fat distribution (in both obese and nonobese women) *(81)* should therefore be considered in all studies performed in this field.

Another important aspect in this complex issue is represented by the various methods used to define insulin sensitivity in women with PCOS. In fact, most clinical studies performed in the last two decades used the simple mathematical test cited above rather than the more complex standard tests, such as the clamp technique, the FSIVGTT, or the insulin tolerance test. When HOMA or QUICKI parameters, or an insulin sensitivity parameter derived from the OGTT *(94)*, were used as markers of insulin resistance, it was commonly found that, compared with appropriate age- and weight-matched controls, PCOS women are more insulin resistant *(79–81)*. In addition, in a group of normal-weight and obese PCOS women, some authors *(17)* found that insulin resistance, as measured by the kinetic disappearance rate obtained by the insulin tolerance test, was detectable in approximately 80% of PCOS women and in 95% of those with obesity, and that this index was significantly correlated with both HOMA and QUICKI. These results were not supported by another study which did not show a significant correlation between M value and HOMA or QUICKI in a group of normal-weight, over-weight, and obese PCOS women *(94)*. By contrast, others found that in PCOS patients a highly significant correlation existed between M values and the ratio between basal glucose and insulin values *(79–81)*. These data therefore imply that simple mathematical indices should be applied with some caution in insulin-resistant populations, such as PCOS patients, and should not be considered a priori as equivalent to the clamp technique. More recent data suggest that the evaluation of insulin secretion during an OGTT may provide a reliable and simple way to evaluate insulin sensitivity in vivo *(21)*.

The Metabolic Syndrome in PCOS

Due to the high prevalence of insulin resistance in PCOS, some recent studies used the NCEP/ATP III criteria to assess the prevalence of the metabolic syndrome in PCOS women. Glueck et al. *(95)* studied 138 PCOS patients and found a prevalence rate of 46%, whereas, more recently, Apridonidze et al. *(82)* found a prevalence of 43% by retrospectively reviewing the medical charts of 106 PCOS women attending the Endocrine Clinic of Richmond, Virginia. Both these studies, therefore, described a prevalence of the metabolic syndrome in PCOS women nearly twofold higher than that reported in the general population investigated in the cited NHANES III report *(96)*, matched for age and body weight. Apridonidze et al. *(82)* also described higher free testosterone and lower SHBG levels in those women with the metabolic syndrome compared with those without it, as well as a higher prevalence of acanthosis nigricans and a tendency toward a greater family history for PCOS. These results were in accordance with a cross-sectional population-based study conducted by Korhonen et al. *(97)* who reported different concentrations of some sex hormones between premenopausal women with and without the NCEP/ATP III defined metabolic syndrome. In a recent study *(98)*, we investigated the prevalence of the metabolic syndrome according to the NCEP/ATP III and IDF criteria in 200 Italian women with PCOS (Fig. 2). Among all individuals, 32% were similarly classified under the two defi-nitions. Sixty-one percent were not affected using both classifications. Interestingly, we found that fasting and glucose-stimulated (as AUC) insulin were significantly ($p < 0.01$) higher and QUICKI and the OGTT-derived insulin sensitivity index were significantly ($p < 0.05$) and similarly lower in the

Fig. 2. Prevalence of the metabolic syndrome according to the criteria of the NCEP/ATP III *(25)* and IDF *(36)* in 200 women with PCOS and in 200 controls.

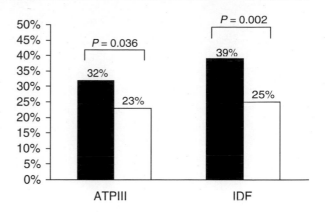

NCEP/ATP III(+)/IDF(+) group with respect to the NCEP/ATP III(−)/IDF(−) group. Additionally, those presenting the metabolic syndrome had significantly higher testosterone levels and selected markers of low-grade inflammation, such as white cells and fibrinogen. These data therefore confirm that the prevalence of the metabolic syndrome is higher than expected in PCOS women and that their insulin-resistant state is worsened as well as their metabolic, hormonal, and inflammatory profile.

In another study, we investigated how many PCOS women with the metabolic syndrome according to the NCEP/ATP III criteria were insulin resistant, in comparison with PCOS women without the metabolic syndrome (therefore with only two or fewer criteria). Collectively, 55% of PCOS women had fasting insulin values 2 SD higher than those observed in the control group, 37% had higher HOMA values, and 49.5% had higher insulin sensitivity index [derived from the OGTT *(99)*], which indicates that approximately 40–50% of PCOS subjects were insulin resistant, therefore confirming previous reports. When PCOS subjects were classified as having or not having the metabolic syndrome, according to the NCEP/ATP III criteria, we found that in the former, higher (i.e., values 2 SD above those found in the controls) fasting insulin was present in 87.3%, higher HOMA in 74.6%, and higher ISI in 79.4% compared with 54.7% ($p < 0.001$), 32.8% ($p < 0.001$), and 56.7% ($p < 0.001$) in those without the metabolic syndrome *(100)*. Notably, BMI was significantly higher in the former. Therefore, these data suggest that insulin resistance is present at least in 70–85% of women with PCOS and that obesity should be considered an additional relevant factor responsible for this metabolic abnormality.

Obesity and the Abdominal Phenotype in PCOS

The prevalence of obesity in PCOS subjects appears to be much greater that that expected in the general population *(81)*. Although the cause of this association remains unknown, a recent comprehensive review by Ehrmann *(83)* reported an estimated prevalence rate of more than 30% of cases and, in some series, a percentage as high as 75%. In the few epidemiological articles cited above, we observed that the prevalence of being overweight or obese among PCOS women ranged from 40 to 66%.

Obesity tends to be abdominal in its distribution in PCOS women, and even lean-affected women may have a fat distribution favoring visceral depots, particularly in the abdomen *(81)*. This is not unexpected, since androgens do in fact have an important role in the regulation of fat metabolism, differentiation, and morphology, through specific receptors whose distribution and characteristics vary according to different fat localization *(101)*. Importantly, stimulation with androgens seems to upregulate the expression of their own receptors *(102)*, but estrogens downregulate the density of these receptors *(103)*. For more details on the effect of androgens on body fat distribution patterns, please see Section "Androgens" in Chap. 1. Interestingly, testosterone in physiological concentrations appears to inhibit catecholamine-induced lipolysis in differentiated preadipocytes from the subcutaneous but not the visceral fat depots. This could be due to a depot-specific inhibition of the expression of hormone-sensitive lipase (HSL) by testosterone and/or to a decrease in the amount of β2 adrenergic receptors. This could also be an important pathophysiological factor behind the insulin-resistant phenotype of the upper-body obesity in men and of the hyperandrogenic PCOS *(104)*.

In humans, it is demonstrated that testosterone increases visceral fat in women. Female-to-male transsexuals treated with testosterone do in fact have an increase in visceral fat only when oophorectomized and thus eliminating the protective effects of estrogens *(105)*. In addition, administration of androgens in postmenopausal women has been documented to increase visceral fat while reducing subcutaneous fat *(106)*. This indicates that an increase in the testosterone to estrogen ratio in women causes accumulation of visceral adipose tissue, consistent with the important role of testosterone in determining the high prevalence of abdominal fat distribution pattern in hyperandrogenized women with PCOS.

Obesity has profound effects on the clinical and hormonal and metabolic features of PCOS, which largely depend on the degree of excess body fat and on the pattern of fat distribution. The recognition of the impact of obesity on PCOS may have some relevance in the pathophysiology of the disorder. In addition, obesity intuitively represents a target for therapeutic strategies, as weight loss produces several benefits on major complaints of women with PCOS, including hormonal and metabolic abnormalities, menses and ovulation, and therefore, fertility *(107)*. Finally, the definition of the obesity phenotype is of great importance for prognosis, since abdominal obesity is not only associated with poorer fertility outcomes *(108)* but also associated with a higher probability of developing the metabolic syndrome, DM2 and, possibly, CVD.

Glucose Intolerance and DM2 in PCOS

Worsening insulin resistance in the long term is an important factor in the development of glucose intolerance states in PCOS *(109, 110)*. Clinical studies have in fact shown that glucose intolerance is present, at the first clinical examination, in as many as 30–40% of obese PCOS women in the United States *(79)*, in Australia *(111)* and, probably, to a lesser extent in those living in Europe *(88)*, while it is uncommon in their normal-weight counterparts *(87, 88)*. In any case, the prevalence rate for impaired glucose tolerance in the population of obese PCOS subjects appears to be higher than that reported in population-based studies on the incidence of glucose intolerance in women of similar ages *(112)*, although cross-sectional or longitudinal epidemiological studies are lacking. Obesity represents the major determinant of glucose tolerance in PCOS *(79, 81)*. Although insulin resistance seems to play a determining role in the development of DM2, the presence of insulin resistance does not immediately imply a concomitant alteration of glucose tolerance. In fact, most obese insulin-resistant PCOS women still have normal glucose tolerance. On the other hand, it has recently been found that PCOS women with impaired glucose tolerance or DM2 are significantly more insulin resistant and hyperinsulinemic than those with normal glucose tolerance, regardless of the presence of obesity *(88)*. It has also been reported that the development of glucose intolerance can be predicted to a certain extent, since there are early markers such as low birth weight in PCOS subjects *(88)*, as in the general population *(113, 114)*. Prospective studies in PCOS women also found that insulin resistance tends to worsen over time together with an increment of insulin and c-peptide response to an oral glucose challenge, and that, in several cases, glucose intolerance develops *(110, 112)*. Taken together, these findings strongly support the role of insulin resistance in the development of altered glucose tolerance states in PCOS women.

Studies in American *(115, 116)*, Asian *(128)*, and Italian *(88)* subjects have also shown that women with PCOS have an increased risk of developing DM2 (Table 1). In addition, all the studies show that

DM2 may appear earlier than expected, often in the second or third decade of life. Prevalence rates range from 10 to 17% in the United States and Asia, while they are around 2–3% in Europe, suggesting that environmental factors may play a dominant role in determining individual susceptibility to metabolic disorders. This is in agreement with recent long-term prospective studies demonstrating that the incidence of DM2 can be dramatically reduced by adequate lifestyle interventions, focusing on dietary habits and increased physical activity *(118, 119)*. As reported above, among other factors, obesity has a profound impact on the susceptibility of PCOS subjects to develop DM2.

Cardiovascular Risk in PCOS Women

PCOS is considered a pathological condition at high risk for CVDs. This is not only due to the presence of androgen excess, insulin resistance, obesity, DM2, and dyslipidemia, but also because of many other risk factors *(120)* (Table 2). These cardiovascular risk factors are often evident at an early age, suggesting that women with PCOS represent a large population at increased risk for developing

Table 1
Prevalence of Impaired Glucose Tolerance (IGT) and Type 2 Diabetes Mellitus (DM2) in Women with PCOS Living in Different Geographical Areas in the World

Reference	Ethnicity	IGT	T2D	Age range (years)
Legro ct al. 1999 *(115)*	Hispanic-American	31.1%	7.5%	14–44
Ehrmann et al. 1999 *(116)*	Hispanic-American	35%	10%	13.5–40
Weerakiet et al. 2001 *(117)*	Asian Thai	22.8%	17.7%	15–40
Gambineri et al. 2004 *(88)*	Italian	15.7%	2.5%	14–37

Table 2
Classic and Newer Risk Factors for Cardiovascular Diseases in PCOS

- Insulin resistance
- Obesity (abdominal)
- Metabolic syndrome (glucose, lipid, ABP disorders)
- Impaired glucose tolerance and type 2 diabetes mellitus
- Decreased cardiac systolic flow velocity and diastolic dysfunction
- Endothelial dysfunction
- Increased vascular stiffness
- Low-grade chronic inflammation
- Increased oxidative stress
- Altered circulating divalent cations
- Altered hemostasis including impaired fibrinolysis
- Increased tissue plasminogen activator antigen
- Homocysteine
- Left ventricular hypertrophy
- Increased endothelin 1
- Impaired arterial viscoelastic properties
- Increased intima media thickness
- Others

early-onset CVD, even if this has not yet been confirmed in prospective studies *(121)*. The risk of CHD and myocardial infarction has been reported to be increased in patients with PCOS compared with regularly cycling women *(122)*, although, to date, no prospective study of cardiovascular mortality in PCOS has been performed *(123)*. On the other hand, several studies reported alterations in intermediate end-points for CVD in this population *(120)*. In fact, endothelial *(124)* and diastolic *(125)* dysfunction have been demonstrated in PCOS subjects and have been associated with both elevated androgen levels and insulin resistance. Elevated homocysteine and left ventricular hypertrophy have recently been shown to be independently associated with an increased risk of CVD *(126)*. Other biochemical, morphological, and functional markers of early CVD have been evaluated to correctly identify the cardiovascular morbidity of this syndrome. One of the early signs of CVD is endothelial injury. Precocious anatomical and functional arterial changes have also been reported in PCOS women *(120, 121)*. In this case too, insulin resistance is likely the major risk factor for the occurrence of CVD in PCOS women and could play a key role in the development of endothelial damage, which is an early sign of atherosclerosis.

Data on endothelial dysfunction in PCOS patients are poor and conflicting. An association between PCOS and early carotid atherosclerosis was demonstrated in several studies *(120, 121)*. Some authors *(127)* reported no difference in flow mediated dilation, which is a measure of reactive vascular hyperemia, between PCOS patients and controls. Conversely, others *(124)* showed markedly diminished endothelium-dependent and insulin-mediated flow responses in the femoral artery of women with PCOS. Furthermore, endothelin-1, a marker of vasculopathy and of endothelial dysfunction, has been reported to be increased in PCOS women *(128)*. In addition, some authors *(129)* have reported impaired carotid viscoelastic properties in PCOS women, providing additional evidence of vascular dysfunction in women with this syndrome.

A recent study *(130)* reported increased vascular stiffness and a functional defect in the vascular action of insulin in PCOS patients. In young, normal weight women with PCOS who had normal lipids and blood pressure, endothelial function was altered and intima media thickness was increased, suggesting early functional and structural preatherosclerotic vascular impairment *(131)*. Furthermore, some studies have shown that a 6-month course of metformin improved endothelial structure and function in these young, normal-weight PCOS women *(132)*, further supporting a role for insulin resistance in the pathogenesis of these abnormalities. Intriguingly, some authors have even hypothesized a cardioprotective effect of androgens on the vascular wall in women with PCOS *(133)*. Impaired fibrinolysis, one of the more important cofactors in the development of fatal ischemic heart disease in women *(134)*, has also been demonstrated in women with PCOS. Specifically, a significant increase in serum PAI-1 activity has been reported. This increase was again positively related to insulin resistance but independent of obesity *(120)*. Recently, several data have demonstrated a correlative and causative relationship between insulin resistance and low-grade inflammation *(135)*, which are both important predictors of CVD. Increased levels of CRP have been demonstrated in PCOS women, as well as an increased leukocyte count, specifically in lymphocytes and monocytes *(136)*. Several studies have also shown increased circulating levels of TNF-α and IL-6 *(137)*, although the direct impact of obesity per se, particularly the abdominal phenotype, has been questioned. Other proinflammatory cytokines, such as IL-18, were reported to be increased in PCOS *(138)*. Collectively, the above findings indicate that low-grade chronic inflammation could be a novel mechanism contributing to the increased risk of CHD in PCOS.

Preliminary studies suggested a slight increase in CVD events in women with PCOS. However, the small size and number of these epidemiological studies have been inadequate for conditions as common as PCOS and CVD in women. Larger prospective trials with long-term follow-up are therefore needed to better define the incidence of CVD in PCOS.

ANDROGENS AND RISK FOR CVD AND DIABETES IN THE FEMALE POPULATION: LESSONS FROM THE PCOS PARADIGM

The androgen balance is profoundly affected in the presence of metabolic disorders, particularly obesity and the metabolic syndrome (2). Androgens have an important impact on both glucose and lipid metabolism, and on fat homeostasis, therefore it is not unlikely that androgen imbalance may play a role in the pathophysiology of the metabolic syndrome. Although the few large prospective studies have not confirmed a significant association, cross-sectional studies have nonetheless provided some evidence for a linkage between low testosterone levels and CHD events, particularly in men (2). One reason for the failure to obtain conclusive information from clinical and epidemiological studies may be partly dependent on the sex-related different behavior of sex hormones in the presence of obesity. On the other hand, this hypothesis has attracted scientific concern since low testosterone in men and a condition of relative hyperandrogenism in women are associated with abdominal obesity, features of the metabolic syndrome, and insulin resistance with compensatory hyperinsulinemia. Accordingly, it has been speculated that altered testosterone concentrations may be a surrogate of the risk represented by the presence of obesity and associated insulin resistance with DM2 and CHD in both women and men, albeit with some differences (40).

In men, there are studies showing that after adjusting for measurement of obesity, fat distribution, and insulin resistance, the correlations of major cardiovascular risk factors with testosterone, but not with visceral fat or insulin, lost their statistical significance (25, 139). Other studies, however, found that, after adjustment for BMI and WHR, the negative correlation of testosterone with insulin and lipid levels remained statistically significant (140). Intriguingly, low testosterone levels in men may therefore be a component of the metabolic syndrome (141). This can also be suspected based on indirect evidence. Hypogonadal men are characterized by enlarged abnormal fat depots and some degree of insulin insensitivity, which is partly dependent on the degree of body fat excess (142). In contrast, suppression of testosterone secretion by long-term administration of a gonadotropin-releasing hormone analog has been found to increase serum leptin and insulin, which are markers of insulin resistance (143). Lowered testosterone blood levels and insulin resistance tend to recover after substantial weight loss and, in addition, long-term treatment with testosterone in obese men with high WHR values has been found to be associated with a selective decrease of visceral fat and a significant improvement of the insulin-resistant state [reviewed in (2)]. There is consistent evidence that in men testosterone reduction may be responsible for excess visceral fat which, in turn, represents a key event in the pathophysiology of insulin resistance, the core abnormality of the metabolic syndrome. In addition, excess insulin accompanying insulin resistance negatively affects SHBG hepatic synthesis; a vicious circle therefore takes place, justifying the strong association between abdominal obesity, insulin resistance, and hyperinsulinemia and hypotestosteronemia in obese men.

Women present the opposite relationships between endogenous androgens and obesity, insulin, DM2, and cardiovascular risk factors (40). As reported above, abdominal obesity in women is a relative hyperandrogenic state, due to increased androgen production rates not adequately compensated by a parallel increase of their metabolic rates. This relative excess of free androgens is also due to the decrease of SHBG concentrations, that generally occurs in abdominally obese women as well as in other conditions of moderate-to-severe insulin resistance (2). Notably, decreased SHBG levels are an independent risk factor for the development of DM2 (144).

In the last few years, several concomitant studies have suggested a role of endogenous androgens in the development of DM2 not only in hyperandrogenic PCOS women but also in the general female population. The potential impact of sex hormones on the susceptibility to develop DM2 has been comprehensively investigated in both men and women in a recent meta-analysis including nine cross-sectional as well as three prospective studies *(58)* (Fig. 2). Cross-sectional studies indicated that testosterone levels were significantly lower than normal in men (−76.6 ng/dL, 95% CI −99.4 to −53.6) and higher than normal in women (6.1 ng/dL, 95% CI 2.3–10.1). Similarly, prospective studies showed that men with higher testosterone levels (RR, 0.58, 95% CI 0.39–0.879) had a 42% lower risk of DM2, while there was suggestion that testosterone increased the risk in women (*p* = 0.06 for sex difference). Conversely, cross-sectional studies found that SHBG was more protective in women than in men, with prospective studies indicating that women with higher SHBG levels (>60 vs. <60 nmol/L) had an 80% lower risk of DM2 (RR, 0.20; 95% CI 0.12–0.30), while men with high SHBG had a 52% lower risk (RR, 0.58; 95% CI 0.33–0.69). In a more recent prospective study, conducted on 6,574 women followed up for an average of 10 years *(145)*, the same authors investigated 359 incident cases of DM2 matched with 359 controls and found that testosterone (and estradiol) levels were strongly and positively associated with the risk of DM2, and that the association remained robust even after accounting for other metabolic syndrome components, HbA1c, BMI, family history, lifestyle, and reproductive variables. These data therefore further suggest a role of sex hormones in the pathogenesis of this complex disease. Obviously, this may have a potential impact on prevention and possibly on treatment of affected women.

By contrast, there are relatively few studies that investigated the relationship between endogenous levels of androgens and CHDs or CVDs in women. In a recent review, Wu and von Eckardstein *(40)* reported only two cross-sectional studies on the relationship between circulating testosterone and CHD in non-PCOS women and found that one was positive whereas the other was negative. In addition, in the prospective Rancho Bernardo Study investigating women with and without a history of heart disease at baseline, and focusing on CVD mortality during the follow up, androgens did not predict death for CVD or CHD during the subsequent 19 years *(146)*. Unfortunately, indirect evidence for the atherogenicity of androgens in women comes in part from clinical observational studies performed in women with PCOS. In the same review, Wu and von Eckardstein *(40)* found that all (*n* = 6) but one cross-sectional study provided consistent evidence for the presence of a strong obesity-independent cluster of CVD risk factors. However, none of the few retrospective studies found a greater incidence of cardiovascular end-points, including stroke as well as myocardial infarction. Therefore the evidence that increased androgenicity in women predisposes to CVDs is still very weak and controversial.

SUMMARY AND CONCLUSIONS

There are many differences between the sexes in the susceptibility and development of chronic metabolic diseases and CVDs. Fundamental differences between males and females primarily involve hormones, which define the secondary sex characteristics at puberty, regulate fertility, metabolism, and behavior, and play an important role in regulating many functions of different nonreproductive tissues. Changes in the androgen balance have been found to be associated with a series of chronic metabolic diseases and CVDs, with different mechanisms according to sex.

Insulin resistance may vary widely in the general population, as well as between sexes. However, data supporting this are still lacking, and this is partly due to the fact that the majority of the studies did not segregate for sex in their analysis, but sex differences were usually taken into consideration by controlling for sex in the statistical approach. In addition, in studies performed in adult populations, simple mathematical models to define insulin resistance have often been used, although they posses intrinsic limitation in this complex pathophysiological area. Nonetheless, available data strongly support the concept that there is some difference in the prevalence of the metabolic syndrome, DM2, and CVD between the sexes, so the hypothesis that insulin resistance and associated hyperinsulinemia may have a sex trait is not arbitrary, although major determinants are not adequately understood. Interestingly, sex-specific genes may therefore have a demonstrable impact on fetal growth and insulin resistance. There is no doubt that this topic should be subjected to a more intense investigation, taking into consideration different stages of women's lives, including the fertility period and menopause. Women, particularly those with the abdominal phenotype of excess body fat, are at risk for the metabolic syndrome, DM2, and, possibly, CVDs. This may be due to their specific hormonal condition, which is characterized by the presence of a relative hyperandrogenic status. Recent meta-analyzes have in fact shown the prevalence of DM2 to be associated with a modest increase of testosterone concentration in the general female population, although whether this also occurs for CVD susceptibility is still controversial.

The paradigm of PCOS is a good example for investigating the relationship between hyperandrogenemia and insulin resistance and metabolic and cardiovascular disorders. In fact, approximately two-thirds of women with PCOS have some degree of insulin resistance, particularly in the presence of obesity. Several studies performed worldwide have also demonstrated that the prevalence of the metabolic syndrome and DM2 is higher in PCOS women than in the general population. PCOS is often associated with the presence of obesity, mostly the abdominal phenotype. On the other hand, there are several differences related to ethnicity and geographical areas, which suggest the possibility that still-undefined environmental (or genetic?) factors may be involved. Importantly, the onset of DM2 tends to develop earlier in women with PCOS than in the general population, which indicates the need for careful early diagnosis and, possibly, preventive intervention, particularly focused on obesity. Although PCOS women are characterized by a higher prevalence of CVD risk factors, whether they are at greater risk for CHD or CVD events is unclear, suggesting the need for careful long-term prospective trials.

REFERENCES

1. Federman DD. The biology of sex differences. N Engl J Med 2006; 354:1507–14.
2. Pasquali R. Obesity and androgens: fact and perspectives. Fertil Steril 2006; 85:1319–40.
3. Beck-Nielsen H, Alford F, Hother-Nielsen O. Insulin resistance in glucose disposal and production in man with specific reference to metabolic syndrome and type 2 diabetes. In Insulin resistance. Kumar S, and O'Railly S, (eds.), Wiley: London. 2000; 155–78.
4. Bergman RN, Finegood DT, Ader M. Assessment of insulin sensitivity in vivo. Endocr Rev 1985; 6:45–86.
5. Weber KM, Martin IK, Best JD, Alford FP, Boston RC. Alternative methods for minimal model analysis of intravenous glucose tolerance data. Am J Physiol 1989; 256:E524–35.
6. Mattews DR, Hosker JP, Rudenski AS, Naylor BA, Treacher DF, Turner RC. Homeostasis model assessment: insulin resistance and B-cell function from fasting plasma glucose and insulin concentrations in man. Diabetologia 1985; 28:412–9.
7. Katz A, Nambi SS, Mater K, Baron AD, Follman DA, Sullivan G, Quon MJ. Quantitative insulin sensitivity check index: a simple, accurate method for assessing insulin sensitivity in humans. J Clin Endocrinol Metab 2000; 85:2402–10.
8. Dunaif A, Finegood DT. β-Cell dysfunction independent of obesity and glucose intolerance in the polycystic ovary syndrome. J Clin Endocrinol Metab 1996; 81:942–7.
9. Yeni-Konshian H, Carantoni M, Abbasi F, Reaven GM. Relationship between several surrogate estimates of insulin resistance and quantification of insulin-mediated glucose disposal in 4090 healthy, nondiabetic volunteers. Diabetes Care 2000; 23:171–5.
10. Reaven GM. Insulin resistance in human disease. Diabetes 1988; 37:1595–607.
11. Regitz-Zagrosek V, Lehmthul E, Weickert MO. Gender differences in the metabolic syndrome and their role for cardiovascular disease. Clin Res Cardiol 2006; 95:136–47.
12. Pollex R, Hegele RA. Genetic determinants of the metabolic syndrome. Nat Clin Pract Cardiovasc Med 2006; 3:482–9.

13. Wilkin TJ, Murphy MJ. The gender insulin hypothesis: why girls are born lighter than boys, and the implications for insulin resistance. Int J Obes (Lond) 2006; 30:1056–61.

14. Baker DJ, Eriksson JG, Forsen T, Osmond C. Fetal origins of adult disease: strength of effects and biological basis. Int J Epidemiol 2002; 31:1235–8.

15. Hofman PL, Regan F, Jackson WE, Jefferies C, Knight DB, Robinson EM, Cutfield WS. Premature birth and later insulin resistance. N Engl J Med 2004; 351:2179–86

16. Shields BM, Knight B, Hopper H, Hill A, Powell RJ, Hattersley AT, Clark PM. Measurement of cord insulin and insulin-related peptides suggests that girls are more insulin resistant than boys at birth. Diabetes Care 2007; 30:2661–6.

17. Murphy MJ, Metcalf BS, Voss LD, Jeffery AN, Kirkby J, Mallam KM, Wilkin TJ; The EarlyBird Study (EarlyBird 6). Girls at five are intrinsically more insulin resistant than boys: the Programming Hypotheses Revisited - The EarlyBird Study (EarlyBird 6). Pediatrics 2004; 113(1 Pt 1):82–6.

18. Travers SH, Jeffers BW, Eckel RH. Insulin resistance during puberty and future fat accumulation. J Clin Endocrinol Metab 2002; 87:3814–8.

19. Moran A, Jacobs DR Jr, Steinberger J, Hong CP, Prineas R, Luepker R, Sinaiko AR. Insulin resistance during puberty: results from clamp studies in 357 children. Diabetes 1999; 48(10):2039–44.

20. Falkner B, Hulman S, Kushner H. Gender differences in insulin stimulated utilization among Afro-Americans. Am J Hypertens 1994; 7:948–52.

21. Ferrannini E, Balkau B, Coppack SW, Dekker JM, Mari A, Nolan J, Walker M, Natali A, Beck-Nielsen H. The EGIR-RISC investigators. Insulin resistance, insulin response, and obesity as indicators of metabolic risk. J Clin Endocrinol Metab 2007; 92:2892–7.

22. Cheal KL, Abbasi F, Lamendola C, McLaughlin T, Reaven GM, Ford ES. Relationship to insulin resistance of the adult treatment panel III diagnostic criteria for identification of the metabolic syndrome. Diabetes 2004; 53:1195–200.

23. Melania M, Giuseppe N, Calvani M, Natali A, Nolan J, Ferrannini E, Mingrone G; On behalf of the European Group for the Study of Insulin Resistance. Menopause, insulin resistance, and risk factors for cardiovascular disease. Menopause 2006; 13:809–17.

24. Piché ME, Lemieux S, Corneau L, Nadeau A, Bergeron J, Weisnagel SJ. Measuring insulin sensitivity in postmenopausal women covering a range of glucose tolerance: comparison of indices derived from the oral glucose tolerance test with the euglycemic-hyperinsulinemic clamp. Metabolism 2007; 56:1159–66.

25. Executive Summary of the Third Report of The National Cholesterol Education Program (NCEP). Expert panel on detection, evaluation, and treatment of high blood cholesterol in adults (Adult Treatment Panel III). JAMA 2001; 285:2486–2497.

26. Ford ES. Prevalence of the metabolic syndrome in US population. Endocrinol Metab Clin North Am 2004; 33:333–50.

27. Resnick HE; Strong Heart Study Investigators. Metabolic syndrome in American Indians. Diabetes Care 2002; 25:1246–7.

28. American College of Endocrinology Task Force on the Insulin Resistance Syndrome. American College of Endocrinology position statement on the insulin resistance syndrome. Endocr Pract 2002; 9:236–252.

29. Alberti K, Zimmet P. Definition, diagnosis and classification of diabetes mellitus and its complications. Part 1: Diagnosis and classification of diabetes mellitus. Report of a WHO consultation. Diabet Med 1998; 15:539–53.

30. World Heath Organization. Definition, diagnosis and classification of diabetes mellitus and its complications. Part 1: Diagnosis and classification of diabetes mellitus. Department of Noncommunicable Disease Surveillance: Geneva (Switzerland); 1999.

31. Ford ES, Giles WH. A comparison of the prevalence of the metabolic syndrome using two proposed definitions. Diabetes Care 2003; 26:575–81.

32. Meigs JB, Wilson PW, Nathan DM, D'Agostino RB Sr, Williams K, Haffner SM. Prevalence and characteristics of the metabolic syndrome in the San Antonio Heart and Framingham Offspring Studies. Diabetes 2003; 52:2160–7.

33. Cameron AJ, Shaw JE, Zimmet PZ. The Metabolic syndrome: prevalence in worldwide populations. Endocrinol Metab Clin North Am 2004; 33:351–75.

34. Gu D, Reynolds K, Wu X, Chen J, Duan X, Reynolds RF, Whelton PK, He J; For the InterASIA Collaborative Group. Prevalence of the metabolic syndrome and overweight among adults in China. Lancet 2005; 365:1398–405.

35. Balkau B, Charles MA. Comment on the provisional report from the WHO consultation. European Group for the Study of Insulin Resistance (EGIR). Diab Med 1999; 16:442–3.

36. International Diabetes Federation: the IDF worldwide definition of the metabolic syndrome. Available from http://www.cdc.gov/nchs/about/major/nhanes/nhanes/99-02.htm. Accessed 18 May 2005.

37. Kahn R, Ferrranini E, Buse J, Stern M. The metabolic syndrome: time for a critical reappraisal. Joint statement from the American Diabetes Association and the European Association for the study of Diabetes. Diabetes Care 2005; 28:2289–304.
38. Carr MC. The emergence of the metabolic syndrome with menopause. J Clin Endocrinol Metab 2003; 88:2404–11.
39. Eckel RH, Grundy SM, Zimmet PZ. The metabolic syndrome. Lancet 2005; 365:1415–28.
40. Wu FC, von Eckardstein A. Androgens and coronary artery disease. Endocr Rev 2003; 24:183–217.
41. Bjorntorp P, Rosmond R. The metabolic syndrome-a neuroendocrine disorder. Br J Nutr 2000; 83(Suppl1):S49–57.
42. Pollex RL, Hegele RA. Genetic determinants of the metabolic syndrome. Nat Clin Pract Cardiovasc Med 2006; 3:482–9.
43. Möhlig M, Spranger J, Osterhoff M, Ristow M, Pfeiffer AF, Schill T, Schlösser HW, Brabant G, Schöfl C. The polycystic ovary syndrome per se is not associated with increased chronic inflammation. Eur J Endocrinol 2004; 150:525–32.
44. Greenfield MS, Doberne L, Kraemer F, Tobey T, Reaven GM. Assessment of insulin resistance with insulin suppression test and the euglycemic clamp. Diabetes 1981; 30:387–92.
45. Hennekens CH. Risk factors for coronary heart disease in women. Cardiol Clin 1998; 16:1–16.
46. Willet WC, Dietz WH, Colditz GA. Guidelines for healthy weight. N Engl J Med 1999; 341:427–34.
47. Bonora E, Kiechl S, Willeit J, Oberhollenzer F, Egger G, Maigs JB, Bonadonna RC, Muggeo M. Population-based incidence and risk factors for type 2 diabetes in white individuals. The Bruneck study. Diabetes 2004; 53:1782–89.
48. Avogaro A, Giorda C, Maggini M, Mannucci E, Raschetti R, Lombardo F, Spila-Alegiani S, Turco S, Velussi M, Ferrannini E. Incidence of coronary heart disease in type 2 diabetic men and women. Impact of microvascular complications, treatment, and geographical location. Diabetes 2007; 30:1241–7.
49. Legato MJ, Geizer A, Goland R, Ebner SA, Rajan S, Villagra V, Kosowski M. Writing group for partnership for gender medicine. Gend Med 2006; 3:131–58.
50. Sarafidis PA, McFarlane SI, Bakris GL. Gender disparity in outcomes of care and management for diabetes and the metabolic syndrome. Curr Diab Rep 2006; 6:219–24.
51. Pickup JC. Inflammation and activated innate immunity in the pathogenesis of type 2 diabetes. Diabetes Care 2004; 27:813–23.
52. Kolb H, Mandrup-Poulsen T. An immune origin of type 2 diabetes. Diabetologia 2005; 48:1038–50.
53. Barzilay JI, Abraham L, Heckbert SR, Cushman M, Kuller LH, Resnick HE, Tracy RP. The relation of markers of inflammation to the development of glucose disorders in the elderly: the Cardiovascular Health Study. Diabetes 2001; 50:2384–9.
54. Nakanishi S, Yamane K, Kamei N, Okubo M, Kohno N. Elevated C-reactive protein is a risk factor for the development of type 2 diabetes in Japanese Americans. Diabetes Care 2003; 26:2754–7.
55. Han TS, Sattar N, Williams K, Gonzalez-Villalpando C, Lean ME, Haffner SM. Prospective study of C-reactive protein in relation to the development of diabetes and metabolic syndrome in the Mexico City Diabetes Study. Diabetes Care 2002; 25:2016–21.
56. Snijder MB, Dekker JM, Visser M, Stehouwer CD, Yudkin JS, Bouter LM, Heine RJ, Nijpels G, Seidell JC. Prospective relation of C-reactive protein with type 2 diabetes: response to Han et al. Diabetes Care 2003; 26:1656–7.
57. Doi Y, Kiyohara Y, Kubo M, Ninomiya T, Wakugawa Y, Yonemoto K, Iwase M, Iida M. Elevated C-reactive protein is a predictor of the development of diabetes in a general Japanese population: the Hisayama Study. Diabetes Care 2005; 28:2497–500.
58. Ding AL, Song Y, Malik V3, Liu 3. Sex differences of endogenous sex hormones and risk of type 2 diabetes. A systematic review and meta-analysis. JAMA 2006; 295:1288–99.
59. Tchernof A, Després JP. Sex steroid hormones, sex hormone-binding globulin, and obesity in men and women. Horm Metab Res 2000; 32:526–36.
60. Thorand B, Baumert J, Kolb H, Meisinger C, Chambless L, Koenig W, Herder C. Sex differences in the prediction of type 2 diabetes by inflammatory markers: results from the MONICA/KORA Augsburg case-cohort study, 1984–2002. Diabetes Care 2007; 30:854–60.
61. James WPT, Rigby N, Leach R. The obesity epidemic, metabolic syndrome and future preventive strategies. Eur J Cardiovasc Prev Rehabil 2004; 11:3–8.
62. National Health and Nutrition Examination Survey: Healthy weight, overweight, and obesity among U.S. adults (Web site of the Centers for Disease Control and Prevention). Available www. Cdc.gov/nchs/data/nhanes/databrief/adult-weight.pdf (accessed 2006 Dec 19).
63. Tremblay MS, Pérez CE, Ardern CI, Bryan SN, Katzmarzyk PT. Obesity, overweight and ethnicity. Health Rep 2005; 16:23–34.

64. Pilote L, Dasgupta K, Guru V, Humphries KH, McGrath J, Norris C, Rabi D, Tremblay J, Arsham A, Barnett T, Cox J, Ghali WA, Grace S, Hamet P, Ho T, Kirkland S, Lambert M, Libersan D, O'Loughlin J, Paradis M, Tagalakis V. A comprehensive review of sex specific issues related to cardiovascular disease. CMAJ 2007; 176(6):S1–S44.

65. Despres JP. Abdominal obesity as important component of insulin resistance syndrome. Nutrition 1993; 9:452–9.

66. Wajchenberg BL. Subcutaneous and visceral adipose tissue: their relation to the metabolic syndrome. Endocr Rev 2000; 21:697–738.

67. National Cholesterol Education Program (NCEP). Expert Panel on Detection, Evaluation, and Treatment of High Blood Cholesterol in Adults (Adult Treatment Panel III). Third Report of the National Cholesterol Education Program (NCEP) Expert Panel on Detection, Evaluation, and Treatment of High Blood Cholesterol in Adults (Adult Treatment Panel III) final report. Circulation 2002; 106:3143–421.

68. Carr DB, Utzschneider KM, Hull RL, Kodama K, Retzlaff BM, Brunzell JD, Shofer JB, Fish BE, Knopp RH, Kahn SE. Intra-abdominal fat is a major determinant of the National Cholesterol Education Program Adult Treatment Panel III criteria for the metabolic syndrome. Diabetes 2004; 53:2087–94.

69. Comaschi M, Coscelli C, Cucinotta D, Malini P, Manzato E, Nicolucci A; SFIDA Study Group – Italian Association of Diabetologists (AMD). Cardiovascular risk factors and metabolic control in type 2 diabetic subjects attending outpatient clinics in Italy: the SFIDA (survey of risk factors in Italian diabetic subjects by AMD) study. Nutr Metab Cardiovasc Dis 2005; 15:204–11.

70. Mannucci E, Alegiani SS, Monami M, Sarli E, Avogaro A; DAI (Diabetes and Informatics) Study Group. Indexes of abdominal adiposity in patients with type 2 diabetes. J Endocrinol Invest 2004; 27:535–40.

71. Marchesini G, Forlani G, Cerrelli F, Manini R, Natale S, Baraldi L, Ermini G, Savorani G, Zocchi D, Melchionda N. WHO and ATPIII proposals for the definition of the metabolic syndrome in patients with Type 2 diabetes. Diabet Med 2004; 21:383–7.

72. Sundstrom J, Riserus U, Byberg L, Zethelius B, Lithell H, Lind L. Clinical values of the metabolic syndrome for long term prediction of total and cardiovascular mortality: prospective, population based cohort study. BMJ 2006; 332:878–82.

73. Kanaya AM, Vittinghoff E, Shlipack MG, Rosnick HE, Visser M, Grady D, Barrett-Connor E. Association of central obesity with mortality in postmenopausal women with coronary artery disease. Am J Epidemiol 2003; 158:1161–70.

74. Chan JM, Rimm EB, Colditz GA, Stampfer MJ, Willett WC. Obesity, fat distribution, and weight gain as risk factors for clinical diabetes in men. Diabetes Care 1994; 17(9):961–9.

75. Colditz GA, Willett WC, Rotnitzky A, Manson JE. Weight gain as a risk factor for clinical diabetes mellitus in women. Ann Intern Med 1995; 122:481–6.

76. Stein IF, Leventhal ML. Amenorrhea associated with bilateral polycystic ovaries. Am J Obstet Gynecol 1935; 29:181–91.

77. Zawadzki JK, Dunaif A. Diagnostic criteria for polycystic ovary syndrome: towards a rationale approach. In Polycystic ovary syndrome. Dunaif A, Givens JR, Haseltine FP, and Merriam GR, (eds.), Blackwell: Boston, MA. 1992; 377–84.

78. The Rotterdam ESHRE/ASRM-Sponsored PCOS consensus workshop group. Revised 2003 consensus on diagnostic criteria and long-term health risks related to polycystic ovary syndrome (PCOS). Hum Reprod 2004; 19:41–7.

79. Dunaif A. Insulin resistance and the polycystic ovary syndrome: mechanisms and implications for pathogenesis. Endocr Rev 1997; 18:774–800.

80. Poretsky L, Cataldo NA, Rosenwaks Z, Giudice LC. The insulin-related ovarian regulatory system in health and disease. Endocr Rev 1999; 20:535–82.

81. Gambineri A, Pelusi C, Vicennati, Pagotto U, Pasquali R. Obesity and the polycystic ovary syndrome. Int J Obes Relat Metab Dis 2002; 26:883–96.

82. Apridonidze T, Essah P, Iourno MJ, Nestler JE. Prevalence and characteristics of the metabolic syndrome in women with PCOS. J Clin Endocrinol Metab 2005; 90:1929–35.

83. Ehrmann DA. Polycystic ovary syndrome. N Engl J Med 2005; 352:1223–36.

84. Azziz JR, Sanchez LA, Knochenhauer ES, Moran C, Lazenby J, Stephens KC, Taylor A, Boots LR. Androgen excess in women: experience with over 1000 consecutive patients. J Clin Endocrinol Metab 2004; 89:453–62.

85. Cibula D. Is insulin resistance an essential component of PCOS? Hum Reprod 2004; 19:757–9.

86. Ehrmann DA, Sturis J, Byrne MM, Karrison T, Rosenfield RL, Polonsky KS. Insulin secretory defects in polycystic ovary syndrome. Relationship to insulin sensitivity and family history of non-insulin-dependent diabetes mellitus. J Clin Invest 1995; 96:520–7.

87. Holte J, Bergh T, Berne C, et al. Restored insulin sensitivity but persistently increased early insulin secretion after weight loss in obese women with polycystic ovary syndrome. J Clin Endocrinol Metab 1995; 80:2586–93.

88. Gambineri A, Pelusi C, Manicardi E, Vicennati V, Cacciari M, Morselli-Labate AM, Pagotto U, Pasquali R. Glucose intolerance in a large cohort of Mediterranean women with polycystic ovary syndrome: phenotype and associated factors. Diabetes 2004; 53:2353–8.

89. Gennarelli G, Roveri RNovi F, Holte J, Bongiovanni F, Revelli A, Pacini A, Cavallo-Perin P, Massobrio P. Preserved insulin sensitivity and b-cell activity, but decreased glucose effectiveness in normal weight women with polycystic ovary syndrome. J Clin Endocrinol Metab 2005; 90:3381–6.

90. Holte J, Bergh Ch, Berglund L, Litthell H. Enhanced early phase insulin response to glucose in relation to insulin resistance in women with polycystic ovary syndrome. J Clin Endocrinol Metab 1994; 78:1052–8.

91. Morin Papunen LC, Vahkonen I, Koivunen RM, Ruokonen A, Tapanainen JS. Insulin sensitivity, insulin secretion and metabolic and hormonal parameters in healthy women and women with polycystic ovary syndrome. Hum Reprod 2004; 15:1266–74.

92. Vrbikova J, Cibula D, Dvorakova K, Stanicka S, Sindelka G, Hill M, Fanta M, Vondra K, Skrha J. Insulin sensitivity in women with polycystic ovary syndrome. J Clin Endocrinol Metab 2004; 89:2942–5.

93. Wijeyartne CN, Balen AH, Barth JH, Belchetz PE. Clinical manifestation and insulin resistance (IR) in polycystic ovary syndrome (PCOS) among South Asians and Caucasians: is there a difference? Clin Endocrinol (Oxf) 2002; 57:343–50.

94. Pasquali R, Gambineri A. Insulin resistance. Definition and epidemiology in normal women and polycystic ovary syndrome. Diamanti-Kandarakis E, Nestler JE, Panidis D, and Pasquali R, (eds.), Humana Press Inc.: Totowa, NJ, 2007; 13–31.

95. Glueck CJ, Papanna R, Wang P, Goldemberg N, Sieve-Smith L. Incidence and treatment of metabolic syndrome in newly referred women with confirmed polycystic ovarian syndrome. Metabolism 2003; 52:908–15.

96. U.S. Department of Health and Human Services (DHHS). National Center for Health Statistics. Third National Health and Nutrition Examination Survey, 1988–1994, NHANES III. 1996. Hyattsville, MD, Center for Disease Control and Prevention. Ref type: Data File.

97. Kohronen S, Hippelainen M, Vanhala M, Heinonen S, Niskanen L. The androgenic sex hormone profile is an essential feature of metabolic syndrome in premenopausal women: a controlled community-based study. Fertil Steril 2003; 79:1327–34.

98. Patton L, Gambineri A, Repaci A, Forlani G, Fagotto U, Pasquali R. Prevalence of metabolic syndrome in a cohort of young Mediterranean women with polycystic ovary syndrome and association with clinical and biochemical parameters. Endocrine Abstract. 9th European Congress of Endocrinology, Budapest 1007. Endocrine abstracts 2007; 14:P259.

99. Matusda M, De Fronzo RA. Insulin sensitivity indices obtained from oral glucose tolerance testing. Diabetes Care 1999; 22:1462–70.

100. Pasquali R, Gambineri A, Pagotto U. The impact of obesity on reproduction in women with polycystic ovary syndrome. BJOG 2006; 113:1148–59.

101. Pasquali R, Vicennati V, Pagotto U. Endocrine determinants of fat distribution. In Handbook of obesity. Bray GA, and Bouchard C, (eds.), Marcel Dekker: New York, NY, 2003; 671–92.

102. De Pergola G, Xu XF, Yang SM, Giorgino R, Bjorntorp P. Up-regulation of androgen receptor binding in male rat fat pad adipose precursor cells exposed to testosterone: study in a whole cell assay system. J Steroid Biochem Mol Biol 1990; 37:553–8.

103. Bjorntorp P. The regulation of adipose tissue distribution in humans. Int J Obes 1996; 20:291–302.

104. Dicker A, Ryden M, Naslund E, Muchlen IE, Wiren M, Lafontan M, Arner P. Effect of testosterone on lipolysis in human pre-adipocytes from different fat depots. Diabetologia 2004; 47:420–8.

105. Elbers JMH, Asscheman H, Seidel JC, Megens JA, Gooren LJG. Long-term testosterone administration increases visceral fat in female to male transsexuals J Clin Endocrinol Metab 1997; 79:265–71.

106. Lovejoy JC, Bray GA, Bourgeois MO, Macchiavelli R, Rood JC, Greeson C, Partington C. Exogenous androgens influence body composition and regional body fat distribution in obese postmenopausal women-A clinical research center study. J Clin Endocrinol Metab 1996; 81:2198–203.

107. Pasquali R, Patton L, Diamanti-Kandarakis E, Gambineri A. Role of obesity and adiposity in PCOS. In The polycystic ovary syndrome. Current concepts on pathogenesis and clinical care. Azziz R, (ed.), Endocrine Updates, Melmed S, series editor, Springer: New York, NY, 2007; 85–98.

108. Zaadstra BM, Seidell JC, Van Noord PA, Te Velde ER, Habbema JD, Vrieswijk B, Karbaat J. Fat and female fecundity: prospective study of effect of body fat distribution on conception rates. Br Med J 1993; 306:484–7.

109. Pasquali R, Patton L, Pagotto U, Gambineri A. Metabolic alterations and cardiovascular risk factors in the polycystic ovary syndrome. Minerva Ginecol 2005; 57:79–85.

110. Pasquali R, Gambineri A, Anconetani B, Vicennati V, Colitta D, Caramelli E, Casimirri F, Morselli-Labate AM. The natural history of the metabolic syndrome in young women with the polycystic ovary syndrome and the long-term effect of oestrogen-progestogen treatment. Clin Endocrinol (Oxf) 1999, 50:517–27.

111. Norman RJ, Masters L, Milner CR, Wang JX, Davies MJ. Relative risk of conversion from normoglycaemia to impaired glucose tolerance or non-insulin dependent diabetes mellitus in polycystic ovarian syndrome. Hum Reprod 2001; 16:1995–8.

112. Legro RS, Gnatuk CL, Kunselman AR, Dunaif A. Changes in glucose tolerance over time in women with polycystic ovary syndrome: a controlled study. J Clin Endocrinol Metab 2005; 90:3236–42.

113. Harris MI, Hadden WC, Knowler WC. Prevalence of diabetes and impaired glucose tolerance and plasma glucose levels in the US population aged 20–74. Diabetes 1987; 36:523–34.

114. Hofman PL, Cutfiled WS, Robinson EM, Bergman RN, Menon RK, Sperling MA, Gluckman PD. Insulin resistance in short children with intrauterine growth retardation. J Clin Endocrinol Metab 1997; 82:402–6.

115. Legro RS, Kunselman AR, Dodson WC, Dunaif A. Prevalence and predictions of the risk of type 2 diabetes mellitus and impaired glucose tolerance in polycystic ovary syndrome: a prospective, controlled study in 254 affected women. J Clin Endocrinol Metab 1999; 84:165–9.

116. Ehrmann DA, Barnes RB, Rosenfield RL, Cavaghan MK, Imperial J. Prevalence of impaired glucose tolerance and diabetes in women with polycystic ovary syndrome. Diabetes Care 1999; 22:141–6.

117. Weerakiet S, Srisombut C, Bunnag P, Sangtong S, Chuangsoongnoen N, Rojanasakul A. Prevalence of type 2 diabetes mellitus and impaired glucose tolerance in Asian women with polycystic ovary syndrome. Int J Gynaecol Obstet 2001; 75:177–84.

118. Norris SL, Zhang X, Avenell A, Gregg E, Bowman B, Serdula M, Brown TJ, Schmid CH, Lau J. Long-term effectiveness of lifestyle and behavioral weight loss interventions in adults with type 2 diabetes: a meta-analysis. Am J Med 2004; 117:762–74.

119. Kanaya AM, Narayan KM. Prevention of type 2 diabetes: data from recent trials. Prim Care 2003; 30:511–26.

120. Orio D, Diamanti-Kandarakis E, Palomba S. Cardiovascular disease and inflammation. In Contemporary endocrinology: insulin resistance and polycystic ovary syndrome: Pathogenesis, evaluation, and treatment. Diamanti-Kandarakis E, Nestler JE, Panidis D, and Pasquali R, (eds.), Humana: Totowa, NJ, 2007; 259–6.

121. Legro RS. Polycystic ovary syndrome and cardiovascular disease: a premature association? Endocr Rev 2003; 24:302–12.

122. Dahlgren E, Janson PO, Johansson S, Lapidus L, Oden A. Polycystic ovary syndrome and risk for myocardial infarction. Evaluated from a risk factor model based on a prospective population study of women. Acta Obstet Gynecol Scand 1992; 71:599–604.

123. Pierpoint T, McKeigue PM, Isaacs AJ, Wild SH, Jacobs HS. Mortality of women with polycystic ovary syndrome at long-term follow-up. J Clin Epidemiol 1998; 51:581–6.

124. Paradisi G, Steinberg HO, Hempfling A, Cronin J, Hook G, Shepard MK, Baron AD. Polycystic ovary syndrome is associated with endothelial dysfunction. Circulation 2001; 103:1410–5.

125. Yarali H, Yildirir A, Aybar F, Kabakci G, Bukulmez O, Akgul E, Oto A. Diastolic dysfunction and increased serum homocysteine concentrations may contribute to increased cardiovascular risk in patients with polycystic ovary syndrome. Fertil Steril 2001; 76:511–6.

126. Kishore J, Harjai MBBS. Potential new cardiovascular risk factors: left ventricular hypertrophy, homocysteine, lipoprotein(a), triglycerides, oxidative stress, and fibrinogen. Ann Intern Med 1999; 131:376–86.

127. Mather KJ, Verma S, Corenblum B, Anderson T. Normal endothelial function despite insulin resistance in healthy women with the polycystic ovary syndrome. J Clin Endocrinol Metab 2000; 85:1851–6.

128. Diamanti-Kandarakis E, Spina G, Kouli C, Migdalis I. Increased endothelin-1 levels in women with polycystic ovary syndrome and the beneficial effect of metformin therapy. J Clin Endocrinol Metab 2001; 86:4666–73.

129. Lakhani K, Seifalian AM, Hardiman P. Impaired carotid viscoelastic properties in women with polycystic ovaries. Circulation 2002; 106:81–5.

130. Kelly CJG, Speirs A, Gould GW, Petrie JR, Lyall H, Connell JMC. Altered vascular function in young women with polycystic ovary syndrome. J Clin Endocrinol Metab 2002; 87:742–6.

131. Orio F Jr, Palomba S, Cascella T, De Simone B, Di Biase S, Russo T, Labella D, Zullo F, Lombardi G, Colao A. Early impairment of endothelial structure and function in young normal-weight women with polycystic ovary syndrome. J Clin Endocrinol Metab 2004; 89:4588–93.

132. Diamanti-Kandarakis E, Alexandraki K, Protogerou A, Piperi C, Papamichael C, Aessopos A, Lekakis J, Mavrikakis M. Metformin administration improves endothelial function in women with polycystic ovary syndrome. Eur J Endocrinol 2005; 152:749–56.

133. Meyer C, McGrath BP, Cameron J, Kotsopoulos D, Teede HJ. Vascular dysfunction and metabolic parameters in polycystic ovary syndrome. J Clin Endocrinol Metab 2005; 90:4630–5.

134. Levy D, Garrison RH, Savage DD, Kannell WB, Castelli WP. Prognostic implication of echocardiographically determined left ventricular mass in the Framingham Heart Study. N Engl J Med 1991; 322:1561–6.

135. Bloomgarden ZT. Inflammation and insulin resistance. Diabetes Care 2003; 26:1922–6.

136. Orio F, Jr., Palomba S, Cascella T, Di Biase S, Manguso F, Tauchmanova L, Nardo LG, Labella D, Savastano S, Russo T, Zullo F, Colao A, Lombardi G. The increase of leukocytes as a new putative marker of low-grade chronic inflammation and early cardiovascular risk in polycystic ovary syndrome. J Clin Endocrinol Metab 2005; 90:2–5.

137. Kelly CC, Lyall H, Petrie JR, Gould GW, Connell JM, Sattar N. Low grade chronic inflammation in women with polycystic ovarian syndrome. J Clin Endocrinol Metab 2001; 86:2453–5.

138. Escobar-Morreale HF, Botella-Carretero JI, Villuendas G, Sancho J, San Millan JL. Serum interleukin-18 concentrations are increased in the polycystic ovary syndrome: relationship to insulin resistance and to obesity. J Clin Endocrinol Metab 2004; 89:806–11.

139. Tsai EC, Boyko EJ, Leonetti DL, Fujimoto WY. Low serum testosterone levels as a predictor of increased visceral fat in Japanese-American men. Int J Obes Relat Metab Disord 1996; 24:485–91.

140. Simon D, Charles MA, Nahoul K, Orssaud G, Kremski J, Hully V, et al. Association between plasma total testosterone and cardiovascular risk factors in healthy adult men: the TELECOM study. J Clin Endocrinol Metab 1997; 82:682–5.

141. Malkin CJ, Pugh PJ, Jones TH, Channer KS. Testosterone for secondary prevention in men with ischaemic heart disease. Q J Med 2003; 96:521–9.

142. Wang C, Swerdloff RS, Iranmanesh A, Dobs A, Snyder PJ, Cunningham G, et al. Transdermal testosterone gel improves sexual function, mood, muscle strength, and body composition parameters in hypogonadal men. Testosterone gel study group. J Clin Endocrinol Metab 2000; 85:2839–53.

143. Buchter D, Behere HM, Kliesch S, Chirazi A, Nieschlag E, Assmann G, et al. Effect of testosterone suppression in young men by the gonadotropin releasing hormone antagonist cetrorelix on plasma lipids, lipolytic enzymes, lipid transfer proteins, insulin, and leptin. Exp Clin Endocrinol Diabetes 1999; 107:522–9.

144. Lindstedt G, Lundberg P, Lapidus L, Lundgren H, Bengtsson C, Bjorntorp P. Low sex hormone binding globulin concentration as an independent risk factor for development of NIDDM: 12 yr follow-up of population study of women in Goteborg. Diabetes 1991; 40:123–8.

145. Ding AL, Song Y, Manson JE, Rifai N, Buring JE, Liu S. Plasma sex steroid hormones and risk of developing type 2 diabetes in women: a prospective study. Diabetologia 2007; 50:2076–84.

146. Barrett-Connor EL, Goodman-Gruen D. Prospective study of endogenous sex hormones and fatal cardiovascular disease in port-menopausal women. Br Med J 1995; 311:1193–6.

5

Developmental Programming of Polycystic Ovary Syndrome: Role of Prenatal Androgen Excess

Agathocles Tsatsoulis

CONTENTS

ABSTRACT

Polycystic ovary syndrome (PCOS) is a common endocrine/metabolic disorder in women, characterized by hyperandrogenism, chronic anovulation, and/or polycystic ovaries in association with android fat distribution and insulin resistance/hyperinsulinism. The etiology of PCOS remains elusive but there is increasing evidence that the phenotypic traits of the syndrome may be programmed in utero by androgen excess.

Thus, female primates, exposed to androgen excess during fetal life, exhibit the reproductive and metabolic features of PCOS in adulthood. Women with congenital 21-hydroxylase deficiency and congenital adrenal virilizing tumors develop features characteristic of PCOS during adult life, despite the normalization of androgen excess after birth. Rare cases of women with congenital sex hormone-binding globulin (SHBG) and P450 aromatase deficiency may also develop some of the features of PCOS in adulthood.

The potential sources of gestational hyperandrogenism to account for the developmental programming of PCOS in humans are not clearly understood. However, maternal and/or fetal hyperandrogenism, in association with reduced placental SHBG and/or aromatase activity, can provide a plausible mechanism and this, in part, may be genetically determined. Indeed, genetic association studies have indicated that common variants of genes determining androgen activity or genes that influence the availability of androgens to target tissues are associated with PCOS and increased androgen levels. These genetic variants may provide the genetic link to prenatal androgenization in human PCOS.

From: *Diabetes in Women: Pathophysiology and Therapy*
Edited by: A. Tsatsoulis et al. (eds.), DOI 10.1007/978-1-60327-250-6_5
© Humana Press, a part of Springer Science+Business Media, LLC 2009

It appears, therefore, that prenatal androgenization of the female fetus, induced by genetic factors and environmental signals, or by the interaction of both, may program the differentiating target tissues toward the development of PCOS in adult life.

Key words: Polycystic ovary syndrome; Hyperandrogenism; Developmental programming; Genetic polymorphisms; Prenatal androgenization.

INTRODUCTION

The prenatal and early postnatal period is a time of rapid cellular proliferation and differentiation as well as functional maturation of the various organ systems. These processes are very sensitive to changes in the intrauterine and early postnatal environment.

Epidemiological studies have shown that impaired fetal growth is associated with an increased risk of cardiometabolic disease in adult life. In particular, low birth weight (LBW) has been linked to cardiometabolic risk factors including obesity, hypertension, dyslipidemia, and type 2 diabetes in adulthood *(1, 2)*. Importantly, LBW has also been associated with early pubertal development in girls, followed by functional hyperandrogenism in adolescence *(3)*.

These observations have led to the concept of developmental origins of adult disease, suggesting that adult diseases may originate in utero as a result of changes in the intrauterine environment *(4)*. The process whereby a stimulus or insult, acting at a sensitive or critical period of development, leads to permanent changes in structure or function is known as developmental programming *(5)*. Of course, different tissues are sensitive at different times, so the impact of intrauterine challenges may have distinct effects depending not only on the stimulus but also upon its timing.

Two major processes are believed to affect intrauterine programming and produce alterations in both fetal growth and adult pathophysiology; maternal/fetal nutrition and hormonal programming. Suboptimal intrauterine conditions such as reduced nutrient or oxygen supply that alter the balance between anabolic and catabolic pathways and the partitioning of fuel may exert programming effects on the development of metabolic and cardiovascular diseases in adult life *(6)*. Fetal exposure to glucocorticoid excess may also program the same adult traits induced by maternal/fetal suboptimal nutrition, and has been proposed as the common physiological mechanism translating adverse intrauterine environment into impaired fetal growth and programming of cardiometabolic disease in later life *(7)*.

A well-characterized hormonal programming is the phenomenon of perinatal programming by sex steroids. Specifically, the surge of sex steroid secretion in early neonatal life has been linked to neuroanatomical and functional changes in the forebrain and associated sexual behavior and changes in the expression of steroid-metabolizing enzymes in the liver *(8, 9)*.

In this context, evidence has accumulated in support of the developmental origins hypothesis for polycystic ovary syndrome (PCOS). According to this hypothesis, the development of PCOS is a linear process with its origins in intrauterine life, induced by androgen excess, and expressed during adolescence and adulthood *(10)*.

In this chapter, the evidence from clinical and experimental animal research supporting the developmental programming of PCOS by androgen excess is analyzed. The potential environmental and genetic factors that may be linked to prenatal androgen excess are also discussed. This is preceded by a brief review of the clinical and molecular phenotype of PCOS.

THE CLINICAL AND MOLECULAR PHENOTYPE OF PCOS

PCOS is a common endocrine-metabolic disorder affecting 6–8% of women during their reproductive age. The endocrine abnormalities include hyperandrogenism of ovarian and/or adrenal origin, with variable clinical expression, and arrested follicular development leading to oligo- or anovulation and manifesting with oligo- or amenorrhea. Often women with PCOS have augmented luteinizing hormone (LH) secretion that contributes to hyperandrogenemia (11, 12). The metabolic trait of PCOS is characterized by central adiposity with associated insulin resistance and hyperinsulinemia, which further exacerbates the hyperandrogenism and ovulatory dysfunction. These, together with other features of the metabolic syndrome, impose an increased risk for type 2 diabetes and cardiovascular disease (13, 14). A common feature of PCOS resulting from aberrant folliculogenesis is the accumulation of small follicles in the periphery of a thickened ovarian stroma, yielding the characteristic polycystic ovarian (PCO) morphology on ultrasound (15).

The spectrum of the endocrine and metabolic abnormalities of PCOS and their clinical expression may vary among affected women, creating a heterogeneous biochemical and clinical phenotype and precluding a precise diagnosis of the syndrome. Recently, an international consensus group proposed that PCOS can be diagnosed if two of the following three criteria are present: oligo- or amenorrhea, biochemical or clinical signs of hyperandrogenism, or PCO as defined by ultrasound examination (16). This consensus broadened the previous definition of the 1990 National Institutes of Health Conference (17) by also including the ovarian morphology. Both definitions require that other causes of menstrual irregularity and hyperandrogenism are excluded. Although central adiposity, insulin resistance, and hyperinsulinemia are common, neither is included in the diagnostic criteria.

The fundamental manifestation of PCOS is excess in androgen secretion by the theca cells of the ovary and/or the zona reticularis of the adrenal cortex (18). Theca cells obtained from women with PCOS have an inherent tendency to synthesize and secrete excessive amounts of androgen. This phenotype persists despite many passages in cell culture, indicating that it is an intrinsic property of PCOS theca cells (19). A number of molecular studies suggest that increased functional activity of cytochrome P450 17-alpha hydroxylase (CYP17), cholesterol side chain cleavage P450 (CYP11A), and 3-beta hydroxysteroid dehydrogenase (HSD3B2) contribute to the molecular phenotype of PCOS theca cells (20). Furthermore, recent studies using DNA microarrays in cultured theca cells from women with PCOS reported increased expression of the genes encoding aldehyde dehydrogenase-6 and retinol dehydrogenase-2. These factors play a role in all-*trans*-retinoic acid synthesis and the transcription factor GATA6 that, in turn, increases the expression of CYP17, a functional characteristic of PCOS theca cells (21, 22).

These findings support the notion that PCOS theca cells have a hyperandrogenic phenotype suggestive of a genetic alteration or an epigenetic effect. In this regard, a recent molecular analysis, that compared gene expression profiles in ovaries from PCOS patients and female-to-male transexuals receiving long-term androgen therapy, reported a considerable overlap in gene expression profiles in both groups, indicating that androgens may influence the functional phenotype of ovarian theca cells that become more hyperandrogenic (23).

In summary, hyperandrogenism appears to be the fundamental manifestation of PCOS, probably driven by an inherent hyperandrogenic activity of the ovarian theca cells and/or the androgen producing adrenocortical cells. This is associated with the metabolic trait of central adiposity and features of the metabolic syndrome, including insulin resistance and hyperinsulinemia which further exaggerates the hyperandrogenic phenotype. Both abnormalities contribute to aberrant follicular development manifesting with oligo- or anovulation and the characteristic ovarian morphology. A third abnormality, present in many but not all women with PCOS, is an altered hypothalamic gonadotropic releasing hormone (GnRH) pulsatility associated with augmented LH secretion that also contributes to an ovarian androgen production (Fig. 1). In the following sections, evidence is presented supporting the hypothesis that the endocrine and metabolic traits of PCOS may be programmed in utero by androgen excess.

Fig. 1. The cardinal features of polycystic ovary syndrome (PCOS) and the feet-forward vicious cycle.

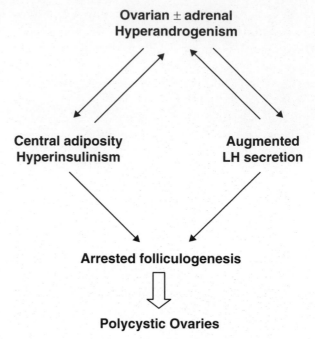

EVIDENCE FOR THE DEVELOPMENTAL ORIGINS OF PCOS

Two sources of evidence in human beings and animals suggest that PCOS may originate in intrauterine life. The first is evidence from clinical observations and experimental animal research suggesting that fetal exposure to androgen excess may program in utero, the development of PCOS traits that are expressed in adulthood *(24)*. Further evidence comes from longitudinal observations of girls with LBW that follow a path through postnatal catch-up weight gain, amplified adrenarche, and ovarian hyperandrogenism in adolescence *(3)*. This pathway is strongly related to central adiposity and insulin resistance, and has been thought of as the hyperinsulinemic pathway to PCOS as opposed to the hyperandrogenic pathway suggested above. It is likely, however, that both pathways have a common origin in intrauterine life as discussed below.

Prenatal Androgenization and PCOS

CLINICAL OBSERVATIONS

The developmental origins hypothesis of PCOS emerged following astute clinical observations in women with congenital virilizing disorders and was further substantiated by experimental animal research. Examples of prenatally androgenized humans are women with classical congenital adrenal hyperplasia from 21-hydroxylase deficiency and rare cases of women with congenital adrenal virilizing tumors*(25, 26)*. These women are exposed to excess adrenal androgens during intrauterine life and, despite the normalization of androgen excess with treatment, manifest a PCOS-like syndrome in adult life, including functional ovarian hyperandrogenism, LH hypersecretion, anovulatory cycles, and polycystic ovarian morphology as well as central adiposity and insulin resistance *(25, 26)*. Similar PCOS traits have also been reported recently for girls with congenital P450 oxidoreductase deficiency who are exposed to excess adrenal androgens in prenatal life but not after birth *(27)*.

Additional experiments of nature associated with prenatal androgenization in humans are women with rare loss-of-function mutations of P450 aromatase (*CYP19*) gene or the sex hormone-binding globulin (*SHBG*) gene. Such patients are reported to develop features of PCOS in adult life *(28, 29)*. These clinical observations suggest that androgen excess during early life might provide a crucial hormonal insult that is necessary for the developmental programming of PCOS.

PRENATALLY ANDROGENIZED ANIMAL MODELS

An appropriate animal model to study the reproductive and metabolic outcomes of fetal programming by androgen excess is the prenatally androgenized female rhesus monkey. This primate shares similar chronological patterns of reproductive function and growth with humans *(30)*.

Studies using this animal model have convincingly shown that a PCOS-like phenotype can be produced by injecting pregnant rhesus monkeys, carrying female fetuses, with 10–15 mg of testosterone propionate for 15–35 days, starting on gestational days 40–60 (early gestation) or days 100–115 (late gestation). Such treatment achieves circulating testosterone levels in female fetuses similar to those normally seen in male fetuses *(31)*. This prenatally androgenized animal model manifests, in adult life, the reproductive and metabolic traits of human PCOS, as described below. Similar outcomes, albeit with some differences, have been reported with other animal models such as prenatally androgenized sheep and rats.

Prenatally treated adult female monkeys exhibit basal hyperandrogenemia with exaggerated androgen responses to hCG stimulation as well as ACTH-stimulated adrenal androgen secretion *(32, 33)*. These findings indicate the development of functional ovarian and adrenal hyperandrogenism, respectively. In addition, prenatally testosterone-treated female monkeys demonstrate ovulatory dysfunction resulting in about 40–50% fewer menstrual cycles than normal females *(34)*. Moreover, a high proportion of prenatally androgenized female monkeys have enlarged polyfollicular ovaries resembling the morphology of polycystic ovaries seen in PCOS women *(30)*. A similar PCOS-like reproductive outcome has been reported in the prenatally androgenized sheep *(35)*.

A neuroendocrine hallmark of PCOS is an enhanced LH secretion from enhanced GnRH pulsatility. Prenatally androgenized female monkeys exhibit abnormal neuroendocrine function, such as increased LH concentrations and LH pulse frequency during subsequent maturation *(36)*. Similar to women with PCOS, prenatally androgenized sheep demonstrate decreased sensitivity to progesterone suppression of LH secretion *(37)*. Interestingly, this neuroendocrine dysfunction is manifested only in animals treated in early gestation but not in late gestation, indicating that the timing of fetal androgen excess may be important for the expression of this PCOS phenotype *(36, 38)*.

Collectively, these findings provide strong evidence that reduced hypothalamic sensitivity to steroid negative feedback, entrained by exposing the developing female hypothalamic-hypophyseal unit to prenatal androgens may cause LH hypersecretion after birth.

In addition to its impact on the reproductive endocrine axis, prenatal androgenization of female rhesus monkeys may also induce metabolic defects that resemble those of PCOS. Like humans, rhesus monkeys are susceptible to obesity and its glucoregulatory effects. Prenatally androgenized female monkeys tend to deposit fat in the visceral area and exhibit impaired insulin secretion or action, depending on the timing of androgen exposure during gestation. Thus, studies of body composition using CT combined with dual X-ray absorptiometry revealed that females treated early in gestation have increased visceral fat compared with controls, even when corrected for BMI and total body fat *(40)*. On the other hand, monkeys treated late in gestation have increased total body fat and nonvisceral abdominal fat compared with control females *(40)*. However, both groups of testosterone-treated females preferentially accumulate visceral fat with increasing BMI, while normal females preferentially accumulate nonvisceral fat *(40)*. Further metabolic studies showed that females treated with testosterone early in gestation liberate more fatty acids than controls and have reduced insulin secretion, whereas those treated late in gestation show reduced insulin sensitivity with increasing adiposity and preservation of insulin secretory function (41). As is the case with women who have PCOS, the altered body composition and resulting metabolic abnormalities in prenatally androgenized female monkeys contribute to an increased risk of diabetes mellitus (38). Similarly, prenatally androgenized sheep develop reduced insulin sensitivity in postnatal life, together with hypertension and hypercholesterolemia after puberty as additional components of the metabolic syndrome as seen in patients with PCOS (42, 43). Interestingly, adult male monkeys exposed to excess androgens in utero may also develop defects in insulin secretion and action in a similar way to female counterparts (44).

Such parallels of metabolic traits between PCOS patients and prenatally androgenized female monkeys, as well as sheep provide convincing evidence that fetal androgen excess programs both the metabolic as well as the reproductive-endocrine phenotypes of PCOS.

Prenatal Growth Restraint and PCOS

A putative developmental program linking LBW and precocious pubarche (PP) with functional ovarian hyperandrogenism in adolescence has been suggested by Ibanez et al., following a series of studies in a Spanish population of girls (45). Girls with PP associated with elevated dihydroepiandrosterone sulfate (DHEAS) or androstenedione levels were more likely to be small for gestational age (SGA). Thus, birth weight SD scores (mean ± SEM) of PP girls (-0.81 ± 0.13; $n = 102$) were lower ($p < 0.0001$) than those in control girls (0.38 ± 0.08; $n = 83$) (46). One French study also reported that birth weight in unselected girls with PP was lower than expected (47). However, no association between SGA and PP was found in another smaller Parisian cohort (48).

In addition, postmenarcheal Spanish girls without PP who were born SGA had DHEAS levels higher than those with normal birth weight (49). In a smaller study, Italian girls who were SGA examined at 6.0–7.5 years of age were found to have 30% higher DHEAS levels than matched controls, although pubarche had not occurred (50). However, when this SGA cohort was evaluated at 17.5–18.5 years, they showed no significant DHEAS elevation or clinical evidence of PCOS. A Dutch study showed significantly increased DHEAS levels in SGA children before puberty but loss of significance after puberty (51). A study from the UK revealed an inverse relationship between the birth weight at term and mid-childhood DHEAS levels (52). Collectively, these findings confirm an association between early adrenarche and SGA but indicate that this may be symptomatic or a harbinger of persistent adrenal hyperandrogenism in some but not all populations.

Further studies by Ibanez et al., in their Spanish cohort, identified additional markers along the pathway of LBW, PP, and PCOS: PP was preceded by central adiposity accompanied by hyperinsulinism, low SHBG, low grade inflammation, and hypoadiponectinemia (53). PP was also found to be followed by early menarche and anovulation.

Postmenarcheal follow-up of the same population with exaggerated adrenarche at an average age of 28 years revealed that 52% were not hyperandrogenic, whereas 25% had the PCOS type of functional ovarian hyperandrogenism without hyperinsulinemia and 23% had both hyperandrogenism and hyperinsulinemia (54). The birth weight of these successive groups was on average 0.25, 1.0, and 2.0 SD below average. Thus, increasing degrees of intrauterine growth restriction appeared to be associated with successively increasing risk for PP, PCOS, and hyperinsulinemia. Interestingly, SGA appeared to protect those who developed PCOS from developing polycystic ovaries.

The above data were interpreted as consistent with the hypothesis that intrauterine growth restraint predisposes to postnatal insulin resistance, an association that is well established (55). In addition, the investigators postulated that PP and PCOS were likewise consequences of LBW-related insulin resistance and hyperinsulinism.

However, studies of birth cohorts in other populations have found no relationship between LBW and PCOS. A large British group followed for an average age of 27 years showed no relationship of SGA to PCOS but large for gestational age (LGA) babies from overweight mothers developed the PCOS phenotype (56). A Finnish study showed no relationship between LBW and PCOS phenotype (57). The above-mentioned Parisian study that found no relationship of SGA to PP also found that young adult women born SGA did not have an increased prevalence of menstrual irregularity or higher androgen levels, although they did have insulin resistance and hyperinsulinemia (48). Thus, although LBW predisposes to insulin resistance, it appears to pose a risk for PP and PCOS in some but not all the populations studied to date. On the other hand, high birth weight may also predipose to the development of PCOS (58).

POTENTIAL ORIGIN OF PRENATAL ANDROGEN EXCESS IN HUMANS

The Placental Barrier to Excess Androgens

The experimental animal research and the clinical observations cited above suggest a common prenatal etiology for the postnatal endocrine/metabolic manifestations of PCOS. The potential sources of excess androgens during intrauterine life to account for fetal programming of PCOS in humans, however, are not clearly known and remain an issue for further research. Normally, the female fetus is protected from the effect of maternal or fetal adrenal androgens by a combination of high SHBG that binds androgens and a high level of placental aromatase activity that converts androgens to estrogens. In a similar way, the fetus is also protected from excess maternal glucocorticoids by the feto-placental 11β-hydroxysteroid dexydrogenase type 2 (11β-HSD2), which catalyzes the metabolism of active cortisol to inactive cortisone (59). Thus, the primary function of placental SHBG and aromatase is to maintain the androgen to estrogen balance and protect the female fetus from the high concentration of endogenous maternal and/ or fetal adrenal androgens. However, this buffering capacity may be overcome if the production of SHBG or the aromatase activity is suboptimal. Theoretically, therefore, exposure of the female fetus to gestational hyperandrogenism may occur due to increased maternal or endogenous fetal androgen production, and decreased placental SHBG or aromatase activity. These possibilities are discussed below.

Gestational Hyperandrogenism of Maternal Origin

The possible role of PCOS itself as a cause for gestational hyperandrogenism was evaluated in a recent study by Sir-Petermann et al. (60). Pregnant PCOS women were found to have higher concentrations of androgens than normal pregnant women, thus potentially exposing their unborn daughters to elevated androgen levels in utero.

The origin of the androgen excess during pregnancy in women with PCOS women is uncertain but it could be due to increase in androgen production by the maternal theca interstitial cells stimulated by hCG. In this respect, the same investigators also reported that after delivery, androstenedione levels and ovarian volume of patients with PCOS were increased, suggesting that their ovaries were persistently stimulated during pregnancy (61). In addition, while the human placenta lacks 17β-hydroxylase and 17, 20-lyase, it does express 17β-hydroxysteroid dehydrogenase (17 β-HSD) and aromatase as well as 3β-hydroxysteroid dexydrogenase (3β-HSD) (62). It can therefore synthesize androstenedione from adrenal or ovarian DHEAS, and can continue with the synthesis of both testosterone and estradiol.

As mentioned above, normally androgens from maternal origin, or those synthesized by the placenta, are rapidly converted to estrogens due to activity of the placental aromatase and therefore, they probably contribute only slightly to gestational hyperandrogenism. However, when the enzyme capacity of the placental aromatase is suboptimal, androgens of maternal or placental origin could increase. In this respect, insulin has been shown to reduce aromatase and stimulate 3 β-HSD activity in human cytotrophoblasts (63, 64). Therefore, in women with PCOS in whom insulin levels are high, this could be a mechanism to explain, in part, the high androgen levels observed in these patients during gestation. In addition, hyperinsulinemia is also known to reduce SHBG production (65). Therefore, in pregnant women with PCOS with hyperinsulinemia, the combination of excess androgen production and the associated low aromatase activity and SHBG production could conceivably contribute to excess androgen exposure in their female offspring.

Studies on mothers of women with PCOS have reported increased androgen levels, insulin resistance, and an increased prevalence of glucose intolerance, suggesting that these abnormalities are heritable (66). In the light of the above observations, this "heritability" may not be genetic in nature but may result from gestational hyperandrogenism that programs in utero the PCOS phenotype. Recent studies on daughters of women with PCOS also support this notion. Thus, prepubertal daughters of mothers with PCOS exhibit early metabolic derangements similar to those in PCOS and increased anti-Mullerian hormone levels, a marker of early follicular development that also characterizes the syndrome (67, 68).

An interesting observation made by Sir-Petermann et al. was the high prevalence of SGA births in mothers with PCOS compared with control pregnancies (12.8% vs. 2.8%), while the prevalence of large for gestational age births were the same in both groups (69). Other studies, however, did not find a sex-specific decrease in birth weight in offsprings of PCOS women (70, 71). A study based on a random selection of pregnant women reported that endogenous maternal circulating androgen levels were negatively associated with birth size of the offspring (72). This inverse association remained unchanged after correction of several known factors associated with intrauterine growth. At gestational week 17, an increase in the circulating maternal testosterone levels from the 25th to the 75th percentile corresponded to decrease in birth weight of 160 g. These findings are in accordance with animal data. For instance, in sheep, testosterone treatment of the mother during early to mid pregnancy reduced birth weight in the offspring of either gender (73). This, however, was not observed in the prenatally androgenized female monkey model (34).

These data support the concept that fetal growth restriction, an early marker of adult disease, is somehow related to prenatal exposure to excess androgens. Interestingly, a recent study suggested that, unlike the norm in the adult, where testosterone production is often inhibited by cortisol, in the fetus, there is a positive link between the two (74). Thus, fetal testosterone correlated positively with both fetal cortisol and maternal testosterone concentrations.

These findings suggest that some of the factors that cause raised cortisol levels during fetal life, for example fetal stress, may also cause an increase in testosterone. This, in turn, may influence fetal growth and development in ways associated with fetal growth restraint and a more androgenic profile expressed with LBW, premature adrenarche, and PCOS in postnatal life (Fig. 2).

Environmental Influences on Prenatal Androgenization

As mentioned above, alterations in placental function with regard to aromatase activity or SHBG production may contribute to prenatal androgenization. Evidence is emerging that nutritional factors or factors associated with oxygen supply may also influence placental function and alter the intrauterine milieu.

In the pregnancy-associated disease preeclampsia, in which the placenta is relatively hypoxic, cytotrophoblast proliferation is increased and differentiation into invasive cells is reduced. Thus, oxygen

Fig. 2. Fetal stress as a potential cause of fetal growth restraint and prenatal androgenization leading to postnatal development of premature adrenarche and polycystic ovary syndrome (PCOS).

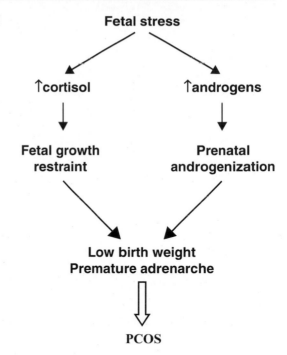

availability to the hormone-producing syncytiotrophoblasts is reduced *(75, 76)*. Such pregnancies are frequently associated with increased synthesis of progesterone and reduced synthesis of estradiol and insulin growth factor I (IGF-1) as well as fetal growth restriction *(77)*. Interestingly, in this regard, experimental evidence suggests that hypoxia prevents induction of aromatase expression in human trophoblast cells in culture *(78)*.

On the other hand, low SHBG levels are a biomarker of the metabolic syndrome and a harbinger of its associated pathologies *(79)*. In insulin-resistant individuals, elevated insulin levels have been linked to low plasma SHBG levels, but hyperglycemia in conjunction with hypertriglyceridemia is also present *(80)*. The reason why plasma SHBG levels are low in obese individuals with metabolic syndrome is not clearly known. The widely held explanation is that elevated insulin in obese and insulin-resistant individuals act in the liver to decrease hepatic SHBG production *(65, 81)*.

A recent study, however, conducted in both transgenic mice and HepG2 hepatoblastoma cells showed that monosaccharide (glucose and fructose)-induced lipogenesis reduced hepatic HNF-4α levels which, in turn, attenuated SHBG expression *(82)*. This may provide an additional biological explanation for why SHBG is low in conditions associated with increased dietary energy consumption. Whether placental SHBG production is also affected in a similar way by nutritional factors remains a speculation. This, in turn, may explain the observation that heavy babies from overweight mothers may also develop PCOS in adult life *(57)*.

An additional consideration is whether environmental chemicals with hormone-like activity, collectively known as endocrine disruptors, might also cause androgenization in utero and exert fetal programming effects. Theoretically, this would occur if such compounds have androgenic or antiestrogenic effects, or effects on *P450* aromatase activity, thus altering the ratio of androgens to estrogens in target tissues.

There has been a flurry of interest in recent years on xenobiotic compounds and dietary substances that can disrupt endocrine signaling, particularly of steroid receptors, during perinatal differentiation, with consequences of this disruption appearing in later life *(83)*.

In this respect, there is a potential fetal programming link between in utero estrogen and androgen excess: exposure of fetal rats to diethylstilbestrol (DES), a synthetic estrogen or to environmental toxicants with estrogenic activity, such as bisphenol A, increases binding activity at the androgen receptor *(84)*. In female mice exposed to DES during fetal life, adult ovarian size is diminished, follicle numbers are reduced, there is relative hyperplasia of ovarian stroma, and cultured ovarian tissue is hyperandrogenic *(85)*. In women, such fetal estrogen excess induces moderate hyperandrogenism, intermittent or absent menstrual cycles, and reduced fertility *(86, 87)* Furthermore, studies on an animal model of developmental exposure to DES indicated that prenatal exposure to environmental estrogen may also program the development of obesity through alteration of adipogenic mechanisms *(88)*.

Another interesting class of widespread persistent organic pollutants with endocrine-disrupting properties is the diverse group of organotins. Tributiltin (TBT) and bis(triphenyltin) oxide (TPTO) in this group have pleiotropic adverse effects on the endocrine system. Thus, exposure to TBT or to TPTO results in imposex, the abnormal induction of male sex characteristics in female gastropod mollusks *(89)*. Bioaccumulation of organotins decreases aromatase activity leading to a rise in testosterone levels that promotes development of male characteristics *(89)*. However, TBT is reported to have modest adverse effects on mammalian male and female reproductive tracts and does not alter sex ratios *(90)*.

Recent work has shown that aromatase mRNA levels can be downregulated in human ovarian granulosa cells by treatment with organotins, similar to the effect of ligands for the nuclear hormone receptors, retinoid X receptors (RXRs), or peroxisome proliferator-activated receptor γ (PPAR γ) *(91, 92)*. New data indicate that organotins are potent agonist ligands of RXRs and PPAR γ nuclear receptors and can induce differentiation of adipocytes in vitro, and increase adipose mass in vivo (93). In utero exposure to organotins leads to elevated lipid accumulation in adipose depots, liver, and testis of neonate mice and results in increased adipose tissue in adults *(93)*. These data suggest that developmental or chronic exposure to organotins may act as a chemical stressor for obesity and related disorders *(94)*. This opens an important new area of research into potential environmental influences on the developmental origins of health and disease. Whether organotins acting through RXR/PPARγ nuclear receptors and affecting aromatase activity and adipogenesis can also program in utero the reproductive and metabolic traits of PCOS in humans is an intriguing hypothesis that needs further investigation.

Thus, environmental factors acting during pregnancy may influence placental function in ways associated with reduced P450 aromatase activity or decreased SHBG production, and this may influence androgen availability to target fetal tissues. In addition, genetic factors may also influence SHBG levels or aromatase activity, and these may also contribute to prenatal androgenization as will be discussed in the following section (Table 1).

Plausible Genetic Contribution to Prenatal Androgenization

Evidence is accumulating that genetic modifiers of placental barrier to androgens, such as polymorphisms of the *SHBG* and P450 aromatase (*CYP19*) genes, or genetic variants associated with increased androgen receptor (AR) sensitivity may also contribute to fetal programming of PCOS by androgen excess.

GENETIC CONTRIBUTION TO PLACENTAL BARRIER FUNCTION

Human SHBG is a homodimeric glycoprotein produced in the liver as well as the placenta and gonadal tissues, and is encoded by a 4-kb gene spanning eight exons on the short arm of chromosome 17 *(95)*. The hepatic synthesis of SHBG is upregulated by estrogens and thyroid hormones and downregulated by androgens as well as insulin and nutritional factors, and plays an important role in the control of sex steroid bioavailability to target tissues, as already mentioned *(96)*.

Table 1

Potential Causes of Prenatal Androgenization

1. Maternal factors (PCOS)
   - Hyperandrogenemia
   - Hyperinsulinemia
2. ↓ Fetoplacental barrier to androgens
   Environmental influences
   - Hypoxia
   - Hyperinsulinemia
   - Over/undernutrition
   - Endocrine disruptors
   Genetic polymorphisms
   - *SHBG* (TAAAA)n
   - *CYP19* (TTTA)n
3. Hyperandrogenic fetal ovaries
   Environmental influences
   - ↑ hCG/insulin
   Genetic polymorphisms
   - *AR* (CAG)n

SHBG levels are often low in women with PCOS as well as in subjects with abdominal obesity and features of the metabolic syndrome *(65, 79)*. Although this is thought to be the result of hyperinsulinemia and hyperandrogenemia or other nutritional factors, there is also evidence that SHBG production may be genetically determined *(29, 97)*.

In this regard, a (TAAAA)n pentanucleotide repeat polymorphism at the 5′ boundary of the human *SHBG* promoter has been described and reported to influence its transcriptional activity in vitro *(98)*. It has been suggested that this functional polymorphism could contribute to the individual differences in plasma SHBG levels and thereby influence the access of free androgens to target tissues. Notably, rare mutations of the *SHBG* gene are associated with very low SHBG levels and a prominent hyperandrogenic phenotype in affected women *(29, 98)*.

We have recently shown, in a case–control study, an association between the (TAAAA)n polymorphism of the *SHBG* gene and PCOS among Greek women *(99)*. In particular, women with PCOS were more frequently carriers of longer (TAAAA)n alleles, compared with control women. Furthermore, carriers of the longer allele genotypes had lower SHBG levels and higher free androgen index (FAI) than those with shorter alleles (Fig. 3). Similar findings were reported among French women with hirsutism and hyperandrogenism *(100)* and, in a more recent study, among Slovenian women *(101)*. In the latter study, however, the distribution of the *SHBG* alleles or genotypes was not different between patients and controls, but SHBG levels were strongly influenced by the (TAAAA)n polymorphism, in both the PCOS and the control women *(101)*. These studies suggest that there may be a genetic contribution to decreased SHBG levels in women with PCOS. Those individuals with genetically determined low SHBG levels may be exposed to higher than normal free androgens during their reproductive life but, more importantly, in intrauterine and early postnatal life, when programming of sexually dimorphic traits takes place.

In a similar way to SHBG variation, genetic variations in the aromatase (*CYP19*) gene may also contribute to increased prenatal androgenization in humans *(102)*. Indeed, women with congenital aromatase deficiency, caused by loss-of-function mutations of *CYP19* gene, develop phenotypic features of PCOS *(28)*. Although earlier linkage and association studies failed to find an association between

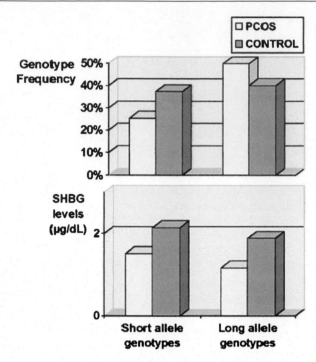

Fig. 3. *Upper panel*: Frequency of genotypes, grouped in short and long genotypes, show significant differences between polycystic ovary syndrome (PCOS) and controls (*p* = 0.009). *Lower panel*: Correlation of (TAAAA)n genotypes with sex hormone-binding globulin (SHBG) levels. PCOS women with short allele genotypes had higher SHGB levels compared to women with long allele genotypes (*p* = 0.02). With permission from the Endocrine Society.

CYP19 and PCOS, probably due to low statistical power *(103–105)*, a recent population study found a strong association between a common genetic variant [the single nucleotide polymorphism (SNP 50)] in *CYP19* and androgen excess in girls with PP and functional hyperandrogenism *(106)*. Furthermore, another study indicated that a short microsatellite (TTTA)n repeat allele in the fourth intron of the *CYP19* gene is associated with elevated androgens, perturbed regulation of the hypothalamic–pituitary–adrenal axis, and abdominal obesity among premenopausal women from the general population *(107)*.

We examined the distribution of the *CYP19* (TTTA)n polymorphism and its association with androgen levels in our cohort of 180 PCOS women and 160 controls. We identified seven *CYP19* (TTTA)n alleles in both patients and controls with 7–12 repeats. Comparing the frequency of (TTTA)n alleles between the two groups, we found that women with PCOS tended to have shorter *CYP19* alleles (≤9 repeats) than controls, although the difference did not reach significance (33.1% vs. 29.5%). However, in PCOS patients, homozygous for short (TTTA)n genotypes had the highest testosterone/estradiol (T/E2) ratios compared with homozygous for long allele genotypes, and those heterozygous for short and long alleles had intermediate values (Fig. 4). In addition, women homozygous for short *CYP19* alleles had higher levels of testosterone and LH/follicle stimulating hormone (FSH) ratios (*p* = 0.05) compared with patients with longer alleles (unpublished data). These findings indicate that, although *CYP19* may not be a major determinant for the development of PCOS, it may be a genetic modifier of the hyperandrogenic phenotype of PCOS.

We further sought to examine whether the *SHBG* and *CYP19* genes may exert a synergistic effect on the development of PCOS *(108)*. By subdividing the study population into subgroups according to the number of repeats of both *SHBG* and *CYP19* polymorphisms, we found that women with PCOS had the combination of long *SHBG* (TAAAA)n and short *CYP19* (TTTA)n alleles more frequently,

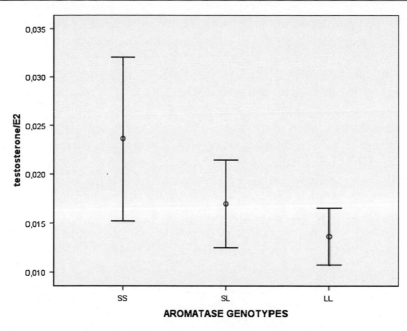

Fig. 4. Differences in testosterone/estradiol (E2) ratio between patients homozygous (SS) for short *CYP19* (TTTA)n alleles (≤9 repeats) and patients being either heterozygous (SL) or homozygous (LL) for long *CYTP19* (TTTA)n alleles (>9 repeats).

compared with control women although this did not reach statistical significance ($p = 0.07$). More importantly, PCOS women who were carriers of the above genotype combination had a higher androgenic profile (including total testosterone, FAI, and testosterone/estradiol ratio) compared to patients with other genotype combinations *(108)*. These findings support the hypothesis that *SHBG* and *CYP19* gene variants may play a synergistic role in the phenotypic expression of PCOS.

GENETIC CONTRIBUTION TO HYPERANDROGENIC FETAL OVARIES

In considering the potential causes of prenatal androgenization in humans to account for fetal programming of PCOS, we discussed above plausible maternal sources in conjunction with environmental and genetic factors altering placental barrier function. Another potential source of prenatal androgenization could be a hyperandrogenic fetal ovary. Ovarian hyperandrogenism is considered the fundamental abnormality and a heritable PCOS trait. Indeed, increased functional activity of all steroidogenic enzymes involved in ovarian theca cell steroidogenesis appears to constitute the molecular phenotype of PCOS theca cells *(21)*. These observations prompted the consideration of genes encoding steroidogenic enzymes as potential candidate genes for the etiology of ovarian hyperandrogenism in PCOS. However, almost all initial candidate genes regulating theca cell steroidogenesis including *CYP17* and *CYP11A*, encoding the P450 17α and P450scc enzymes, respectively, have failed to show association or linkage to PCOS phenotype *(103–109)*.

On the other hand, ovarian theca cells have been shown to express androgen receptors (AR) that may act as transcriptional factors in molecular pathways involved in cellular differentiation and function *(110)*. In this regard, ovarian hyperandrogenism might relate to genetic variation in *AR* sensitivity. Indeed, a CAG repeat polymorphism in exon 1 of the *AR* gene on chromosome X appears to influence the function of the receptor as a transcription factor, so that relatively long fragments are associated with a low level of receptor function *(111)*. A study on premenopausal women in the general population showed that those women with relatively shorter CAG repeats in the *AR* gene, resulting in higher transcriptional activity of the receptor, exhibited higher androgen levels, than women with longer repeat alleles *(112)*. It is possible therefore, that variation in the length of the *AR* (CAG)*n* repeat may also contribute to the hyperandrogenic phenotype of PCOS.

In this context, a recent study by Ibanez et al. *(113)* showed that genetically determined higher AR sensitivity, as indicated by shorter *AR* (CAG) repeat alleles, is a risk factor for the development of ovarian hyperandrogenism among Spanish adolescent girls. This study demonstrated that clinical hyperandrogenism and androgen levels were increased in those girls with shorter *AR* (CAG) repeat alleles, indicating that higher *AR* sensitivity is associated, through a positive feedback mechanism, with increased ovarian androgen production *(113)*. The same study also showed that both LBW and shorter CAG repeats are independently related to ovarian hyperandrogenism and hyperinsulinemia and their effects appear to be additive.

Although, the association of genomic variants of *AR* with PCOS has been confirmed in some case–control studies, other population studies have reported no linkage or association of PCOS with *AR* locus *(112–118)*. These discrepant findings may be due to the reported wide population differences in *AR* CAG repeat distribution and could relate to ethnic differences in body habitus and PCOS phenotype *(119)*.

In our cohort of women with PCOS and controls, described above, we investigated the possible interaction of *SHBG* and *AR* genes on the phenotypic expression of PCOS. In particular, we examined the combined effect of the two functional polymorphisms, the *SHBG*(TAAAA)*n* and the *AR*(CAG)*n* repeat polymorphisms on the hyperandrogenic phenotype of PCOS *(120)*.

As mentioned earlier, women with PCOS were more frequent carriers of longer TAAAA repeat alleles than normal women, and these alleles were associated with lower SHBG levels *(99)*. Regarding the *AR* gene, patients tended to have in higher frequency shorter *AR* (CAG)*n* repeat alleles than controls, although the difference was not statistically significant. Focusing on the distribution of the combined polymorphic variants of the two genes, women with PCOS tended more frequently to have the combination of long *SHBG*(TAAAA)*n* and short *AR*(CAG)*n* alleles compared with healthy controls. The novel finding, in this study however, was the synergistic effect of the combined genotypes on the hyperandrogenic phenotype of PCOS. PCOS women with the combination of long *SHBG*(TAAAA)*n* and short *AR*(CAG)*n* alleles had the lowest *SHBG* and the highest androgen levels compared with other patient subgroups. A similar, but not significant trend was also seen among the healthy women. Conversely, women with short *SHBG* (TAAAA)*n* and long *AR* (CAG)*n* alleles were found to have the lesser androgenic profile *(120)*. Taken together, these findings indicate that PCOS women tend to have more frequently the combination of SHBG and AR polymorphic variants, that is associated with increased "androgenic" activity and less frequently the "protective" genotype combination than normal women. Thus, the combination of long *SHBG* (TAAAA)*n* alleles and short *AR* (CAG) alleles may contribute to a more severe hyperandrogenic state in PCOS women.

In summary, genetic variation in androgen availability, as exemplified by *SHBG* (TAAAA)*n* and *CYP19*(TTTA)*n* polymorphic variants as well as androgen receptor sensitivity determined by *AR* (CAG)*n* repeat alleles, may, in isolation or more importantly in combination, contribute to prenatal androgenization. These genetic variants may provide the genetic link to the developmental programming of PCOS.

PLAUSIBLE BIOLOGICAL MECHANISMS

Fetal programming of PCOS by androgen excess may be related to the phenomenon of sexually dimorphic programming of tissues. Normally, sexually dimorphic traits are programmed during the early neonatal period by the burst of gonadotropin and sex-steroid secretion in both sexes *(8)*. Such developmental programming in the female may occur in prenatal life, under the influence of

Fig. 5. Fetal programming of neuroendocrine, reproductive and metabolic traits of polycystic ovary syndrome (PCOS) by androgen excess.

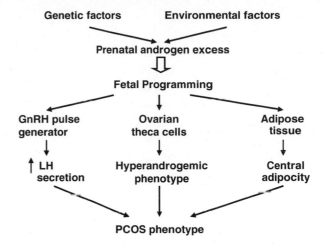

androgen excess, and be directed toward a more masculine phenotype with regard to reproductive, neuroendocrine, and metabolic traits in the female (Fig. 5).

In the reproductive context, a key trait of PCOS is the hyperandrogenic phenotype of the ovarian theca cells, as mentioned earlier in this chapter. It is likely, that the structural and functional phenotype of PCOS theca cells is programmed during differentiation in prenatal life by the altered sex-steroid milieu. This notion is supported by reports on the phenotype of the aromatase knockout female mice in which the androgen to estrogen ratio is altered in favor of androgen excess. The ovaries of these mice exhibit an increased interstitium with the presence of theca cells morphologically resembling Leydig cells *(121)*. It is likely, therefore, that alteration in the androgen to estrogen balance may influence the differentiation of the ovarian theca cells toward a male-type phenotype.

Another sexually dimorphic trait in humans and in animals is neuroendocrine development. The pattern of hypothalamic GnRH pulsatility is different between the sexes, being more frequent in the male (and women with PCOS) and resulting in LH hypersecretion relative to FSH *(12)*. This functional neuroendocrine dimorphism is partly related to androgen-dependent decrease in GnRH pulse generator sensitivity to the negative feedback action of sex steroids *(35)*. Thus, it is possible that androgen excess during fetal life may program a male-type pattern of GnRH secretion *(122)*. Of course, the resulting abnormality in gonadotropin secretion (increase in the LH to FSH ratio) would further contribute to ovarian hyperandrogenism, establishing a vicious cycle that promotes the progress towards the adult PCOS phenotype.

On the other side, an important metabolic trait of PCOS is visceral adiposity associated with insulin resistance and hyperinsulinism *(38, 123)*. Since body fat distribution in humans is sexually dimorphic, the central adiposity in PCOS, in part, reflects an android pattern of fat distribution programmed in utero at a time of tissue differentiation.

The molecular mechanisms underlying the programming of the above endocrine and metabolic traits of PCOS by androgens are not known. Androgens produced during differentiation may act as potent gene transcription factors and induce other critical transcription factors that may permanently alter gene expression *(124)*. It has been suggested that epigenetic change in gene expression, through DNA methylation or histone modification, may be the underlying mechanism in the fetal programming of the metabolic syndrome by maternal nutrition *(125)*. Whether epigenetic modification of gene expression is also implicated in the fetal programming by androgen excess is an interesting hypothesis that needs verification *(126, 127)*. Epigenetic changes in gene expression can occur at any point during development but are more likely to occur during formation of cell lineages and when cells are differentiating during gestation, and have long-term consequences *(127)*.

In a number of diseases with fetal origin, besides epigenetic abnormalities in the offspring, there is also evidence for epigenetic inheritance, that is, nongenomic transmission of environmentally induced abnormalities across several generations *(128)*. Whether epigenetic inheritance with its intergenerational effect is also implicated for the familial clustering of PCOS is another point that needs further investigation.

Developmental programming of the metabolic syndrome due to fetal undernutrition is related to adaptive homeostatic processes that confer a survival advantage *(4)*. Whether such predictive adaptive mechanisms are also involved in the programing of PCOS remain a matter of speculation. Shorter *AR* (CAG) repeat alleles, longer SHBG (TAAAA)*n* alleles, and shorter *CYP 19* (TTTA) repeat alleles could represent thrifty genotypes, since increased androgenic activity and central fat accumulation may confer a survival advantage during periods of limited nutritional resources. In our modern environment, these thrifty genes may be disadvantageous *(129)*.

In summary, fetal programming of PCOS by androgen excess may be related to sexually dimorphic programming of tissues during intrauterine life, but the underlying molecular mechanisms implicated in this process remain to be elucidated by further research.

CONCLUSIONS AND FUTURE IMPLICATIONS

Both experimental animal research and clinical observations have strongly indicated that fetal exposure to androgen excess may program the reproductive and metabolic manifestations of PCOS in adult women. Environmental and/or genetic factors influencing the functional capacity of the fetoplacental barrier, that normally protects the female fetus from androgen excess, are likely to contribute to prenatal androgenization in humans. It is hypothesized that androgens acting on the differentiating tissues of the female fetus may program the ontogenic development and phenotypic expression of sexually dimorphic traits toward a more masculine phenotype in adult life.

The molecular mechanisms underlying the developmental programming of PCOS by androgen excess are not known but may be related to epigenetic changes in gene expression induced by androgens during fetal development. In addition, such epigenetic modifications may also promote the transgenerational transmission of the PCOS phenotype. This, however, remains a hypothesis that requires further substantiation. In the future, carefully planed clinical studies are needed to define the role of prenatal androgenization in the etiology of PCOS in human beings. Further studies using animal models that mimic fetal exposure to androgen excess are also necessary to provide a better insight into the molecular mechanisms that underline the developmental programming of PCOS and its inheritance pattern. Hopefully, such studies will provide a more clear evidence for the developmental origin hypothesis of PCOS. If verified, this hypothesis will open new avenues for the possible intervention at the critical period of prenatal life to prevent PCOS occurrence. Moreover, identification of possible epigenetic changes will help develop new tools for monitoring fetal health state in a hyperandrogenic intrauterine environment.

REFERENCES

1. Barker DJP, Gluckman PD, Godfrey KM, Harding JE, Owens JA, Robinson JS. Fetal nutrition and cardiovascular disease in adult life. Lancet 1993;345:938–941
2. Barker DJP, Hales CN, Fall CH, Osmond C, Phipps K, Clark PMS. Type 2 (non-insulin dependent) diabetes mellitus, hypertension and hyperlipidaemia (syndrome x): relation to reduced fetal growth. Diabetologia 1993;36:62–67

3. Ibanez L, Potau N, Francois I, De Zegher F. Precocious pubarche, hyperinsulinism, and ovarian hyperandrogenism in girls: relation to reduced fetal growth. J Clin Endocrinol Metab 1998;83:3558–3562

4. Gluckman PD, Hanson MA. The developmental origins of the metabolic syndrome. Trends Endocrinol Metab 2004;15:183–187

5. Lucas A. Programming by early nutrition in man. Ciba Found Symp 1991;156:38–50

6. Fowden AL, Giussani DA, Forhead AJ. Intrauterine programming of physiological systems: causes and consequences. Physiology 2005;21:29–37

7. Seckl JR. Glucocorticoid programming of the fetus; adult phenotypes and molecular mechanisms. Mol Cell Endocrinol 2000;185:61–71

8. Arai Y, Gorski RA. Critical exposure time for androgenization of the developing hypothalamus in the female rat. Endocrinology 1968;82:1010–1014

9. Gustafsson J-A, Mode A, Norstedt G, Skett P. Sex steroid induced changes in hepatic enzymes. Annu Rev Physiol 1983;45:51–60

10. Abbott DH, Dumesic DA, Franks S. Developmental origin of polycystic ovary syndrome – a hypothesis. J Endocrinol 2002;174:1–5

11. Azziz R, Woods KS, Reyna R, Key TJ, Knochenhauer ES, Yildiz BO. The prevalence and features of the polycystic ovary syndrome in an unselected population. J Clin Endocrinol Metab 2004;89:2745–2749

12. Ehrmann DA. Polycystic ovary syndrome. N Engl J Med 2005;352:1223–1236

13. Ehrmann DA, Liljenquist DR, Kasra K et al. Prevalence and predictors of the metabolic syndrome in women with polycystic ovary syndrome. J Clin Endocrinol Metab 2006;91:48–53

14. Kravariti M, Naka KK, Kalantaridou SN et al. Predictors of endothelial dysfunction in young women with polycystic ovary syndrome. J Clin Endocrinol Metab 2005;90:5088–5095

15. Franks S. Polycystic ovary syndrome. N Engl J Med 1995;333:853–861

16. Rotterdam ESHRE/ASRM-Sponsored PCOS Consensus Workshop Group. Revised 2003 consensus on diagnostic criteria and long-term health risks related to polycystic ovary syndrome. Fertil Steril 2004;81:19–25

17. Zawadski JK, Dunaif A. Diagnostic criteria for polycystic ovary syndrome: towards a national approach. In: Dunaif A, Givens JR, Haseltine FP (eds). Polycystic Ovary Syndrome. Current Issues in Endocrinology and Metabolism. Boston, MA: Blackwell, 1992, pp. 337–384

18. Azziz R, Carmina E, Dewailly B, et al. Position statement: criteria for defining polycystic ovary syndrome as a predominantly hyperandrogenic syndrome: an Androgen Excess Society guideline. J Clin Endocrinol Metab 2006;91:4237–4245.

19. Nelson VL, Legro RS, Strauss JF, McAllister JM. Augmented androgen production is a stable steroidogenic phenotype of propagated theca cells from polycystic ovaries. Mol Endocrinol 1999;13:946–957

20. Wickenheisser JK, Nelson-De Grave VL, McAllister JM. Human ovarian theca cells in culture. Trends Endocrinol Metab 2006;17:63–69

21. Wood JR, Nelson VL, Ho C, et al. The molecular phenotype of polycystic ovary syndrome (PCOS) theca cells and new candidate PCOS genes defined by microarray analysis. J Biol Chem 2003;278:26380–26390

22. Wood JR, Ho CK, Nelson-De Grave VL, McAllister JM, Strauss JF III. The molecular signature of polycystic ovary syndrome (PCOS) theca cells defined by gene expression profiling. J Reprod Immunol 2004;63:51–60

23. Jansen E, Laven JSE, Dommerhot HBR, et al. Abnormal gene expression profiles in human ovaries from polycystic ovary syndrome patients. Mol Endocrinol 2004;18:3050–3063

24. Xita N, Tsatsoulis A. Fetal programming of polycystic ovary syndrome by androgen excess: evidence from experimental, clinical, and genetic association studies. J Clin Endocrinol Metab 2006;91:1660–1666

25. Haque WM, Adams J, Rodda C, et al. The prevalence of polycystic ovaries in patients with congenital adrenal hyperplasia and their close relatives. Clin Endocrinol (Oxf) 1990;33:501–510

26. Barnes RB, Rosenfield RC, Ehrmann DA et al. Ovarian hyperandrogenism as a result of congenital adrenal virilizing disorders: evidence for perinatal masculinization of neuroendocrine function in women. J Clin Endocrinol Metab 1994;79:1328–1333

27. Miller WL. P450 oxidoreductase deficiency: a new disorder of steroidogenesis with multiple clinical manifestations. Trends Endocrinol Metab 2004;15:311–315

28. Morishima A, Grumbach MM, Simpson ER, Fisher C, Kenan Q. Aromatase deficiency in male and female siblings caused by a novel mutation and the physiological role of estrogens. J Clin Endocrinol Metab 1995;80:3689–3698

29. Hogeveen KN, Cousin P, Pugeat M, Dewailly D, Soudan B, Hammond GL. Human sex-hormone-binding globulin variants associated with hyperandrogenism and ovarian dysfunction. J Clin Invest 2002;109:973–981

30. Abbott DH, Dumesic DA, Eisner JR, Kemnitz JW, Goy RW. The prenatally androgenized female rhesus monkey as a model for polycystic ovarian syndrome. In: Azziz R, Nestler JE, Dewailly D (eds). Androgen Excess Disorders in Women. Philadelphia, PA: Lippincott-Raven, 1997, pp. 369–382

31. Resko JA, Buhl AE, Phoenix CH. Treatment of pregnant rhesus macaques with testosterone propionate: observations on its fate in the fetus. Biol Reprod 1987;37:1185–1191

32. Eisner JR, Barnett MA, Dumesic DA, Abbott DH. Ovarian hyperandrogenism in adult female rhesus monkeys exposed to prenatal androgen excess. Fertil Steril 2002;77:167–172

33. Zhou R, Bird IM, Dumesic DA, Abbott DH. Adrenal hyperandrogenism is induced by fetal androgen excess in a rhesus monkey model of polycystic ovary syndrome. J Clin Endocrinol Metab 2005;90:6630–6637

34. Abbott DH, Dumesic DA, Eisner JR, Colman RJ, Kemnitz JW. Insights into the development of PCOS from studies of prenatally androgenized female rhesus monkeys. Trends Endocrinol Metab 1998;9:62–67

35. Padmanabhan V, Evans N, Taylor JA, Robinson JE. Prenatal exposure to androgens leads to the development of cystic ovaries in the sheep. Biol Reprod 1998;56(Suppl 1):194

36. Dumesic DA, Abbott DH, Eisner JR, Goy RW. Prenatal exposure of female rhesus monkeys to testosterone propionate increases serum luteinizing hormone levels in adulthood. Fertil Steril 1997;67:155–163

37. Robinson JE, Forsdike RA, Taylor JA. In utero exposure of female lambs to testosterone reduces the sensitivity of the gonadotropin-releasing hormone neuronal network to inhibition by progesterone. Endocrinology 1999;140:5797–5805

38. Abbott DH, Barnett DK, Bruns CM, Dumesic DA. Androgen excess fetal programming of female reproduction: a developmental aetiology for polycystic ovary syndrome. Hum Reprod Update 2005;11:357–374

39. Eisnher JR, Dumesic DA, Kemnitz JW, Colman RJ, Abbott DH. Increased adiposity in female rhesus monkeys exposed to androgen excess during early gestation. Obes Res 2003;11:279–286

40. Bruns CM, Baum ST, Colman RJ, et al. Prenatal androgen excess negatively impacts body fat distribution in a nonhuman primate model of polycystic ovary syndrome (PCOS). Int J Obes 2007;31:1579–1585

41. Eisner JR, Dumesic DA, Kemnitz JW, Abbott DH. Timing of prenatal androgen excess determines differential impairment in insulin secretion and action in adult female rhesus monkeys. J Clin Endocrinol Metab 2000;85:1206–1210

42. Recabarren SE, Padmanabhan V, Codner E, et al. Postnatal developmental consequences of altered insulin sensitivity in female sheep treated prenatally with testosterone. Am J Physiol 2005;289:E801–E806

43. King AJ, Olivier NB, Mohankumar PS, Lee JS, Padmanabham V, Fink GD. Hypertension caused by prenatal testosterone excess in female sheep. Am J Physiol Endocrinol Metab, 2007;292:E1837–E1841

44. Bruns CM, Baum ST, Colman RJ, et al. Insulin resistance and impaired insulin secretion in prenatally androgenized male rhesus monkeys. J Clin Endocrinol Metab 2004;89:6218–6223

45. Ibanez L, Dimartino-Nardi J, Potan N, Saenger P. Premature adrenarche-normal variant or forerunner of adult disease? Endocr Rev 2000;21:671–696

46. Ibanez L, Potau N, deZegher FI. Precocious pubarche, hyperinsulinism, and ovarian hyperandrogenism in girls: relation to reduced fetal growth. J Clin Endocrinol Metab 1998;83:3558–3562

47. Charkaluk ML, Trivin C, Brauner R. Premature pubarche as an indicator of how body weight influences the onset of adrenarche. Eur J Pediatr 2004;163:89–93

48. Meas T, Chevenne D, Thibaud E, et al. Endocrine consequences of premature pubarche in postpubertal caucasian girls. Clin Endocrinol (Oxf) 2002;57:101–106

49. Ibanez L, Potau N, Marcos MV, de Zegher F. Exaggerated adrenarche and hyperinsulinism in adolescent girls born small for gestational age. J Clin Endocrinol Metab 1999;84:4739–4741

50. Ghirri P, Bernardini M, Vuerich M, et al. Adrenarche, pubertal development, age at menarche and final height of full-term, born small for gestational age (SGA) girls. Gynecol Endocrinol 2001;15:91–97

51. Veening MA, van Weissenbruch MM, Roord JJ, de Delamarre-van Waal HA. Pubertal development in children born small for gestational age. J Pediatr Endocrinol Metab 2004;17:1497–1506

52. Ong KK, Potau N, Petry CJ, et al. Opposing influences of prenatal and postnatal weight gain on adrenarche in normal boys and girls. J Clin Endocrinol Metab 2004;89:2647–2651

53. De Zegher F, Ibanez L. Prenatal growth restraint followed by catch-up of weight: a hyperinsulinemic pathway to polycystic ovary syndrome. Fertil Steril 2006;86:S4-S5

54. Ibanez L, Jaramillo A, Enriquez G, et al. Polycystic ovaries after precocious pubarche: relation to prenatal growth. Hum Reprod 2007;22:395–400

55. Barker DJ, Eriksson TG, Forsen T, Osmond C. Fetal origins of adult disease: strength of effects and biological basis. Int Epidemiol 2002;31:1235–1239

56. Cresswell JL, Barker DJ, Osmond C, Egger P, Phillips DI, Fraser RB. Fetal growth, length of gestation, and polycystic ovaries in adult life. Lancet 1997;350:1131–1135

57. Laitinen J, Taponen S, Martikainen H, et al. Body size from birth to adulthood as a predictor of self-reported polycystic ovary syndrome symptoms. Int J Obes Relat Metab Disord 2003;27:710–715

58. Michelmore K, Ong K, Mason S, et al. Clinical features of women with polycystic ovaries: relationships to insulin sensitivity, insulin gene VNTR and birth weight. Clin Endocrinol (Oxf) 2001;55:439–446

59. Benediktsson R, Calder AA, Edwards CR, Seckl JR. Placental 11β-hydroxysteroid dehydrogenase: a key regulator of fetal glucocorticoid exposure. Clin Endocrinol (Oxf) 1997;46:161–166

60. Sir-Petermann T, Maliqueo M, Angel B, Lara HE, Perez-Bravo F, Recabarren SE. Maternal serum androgens in pregnant women with polycystic ovarian syndrome: possible implications in prenatal androgenization. Hum Reprod 2002;17:2573–2579

61. Sir-Petermann T, Devoto L, Maliqueo M, Peirano P, Recabarren SE, Wildt L. Resumption of ovarian function during lactational amenorrhoea in breastfeeding women with polycystic ovarian syndrome: endocrine aspects. Hum Reprod 2001;16:1603–1610

62. Mason JI, Vshijima K, Doody KM, et al. Regulation of expression of the 3β-hydroxysteroid dehydrogenase of human placenta and fetal adrenal. J Steroid Biochem Mol Biol 1993;47:151–159

63. Nestler JE. Modulation of aromatase and P450 cholesterol side-chain cleavage enzyme activities of human placental cytotrophoblasts by insulin and insulin-like growth factor-1. Endocrinology 1987;121:1845–1852

64. Nestler JE. Insulin and insulin-like growth factor-1 stimulate the 3β-hydroxysteroid dehydrogenase activity of human placental cytotrophoblasts. Endocrinology 1989;125:2127–2133

65. Nestler JE, Powers LP, Matt DW et al. A direct effect of hyperinsulinemia on serum sex hormone-binding globulin levels in obese women with the polycystic ovary syndrome. J Clin Endocrinol Metab 1991;72:83–89

66. Sam S, Legro RS, Essah P, Apridonidze T, Dunaif A. Evidence for metabolic and reproductive phenotypes in mothers of women with polycystic ovary syndrome. Proc Natl Acad Sci U S A 2006;103:7030–7035

67. Sir-Petermann T, Maliqueo M, Codner E et al. Early metabolic derangements in daughters of women with polycystic ovary syndrome. J Clin Endocrinol Metab 2007;92:4637–4642

68. Sir-Petermann T, Codner E, Maliqueo M, et al. Increased anti-mullerian hormone serum concentrations in prepubertal daughters of women with polycystic ovary syndrome. J Clin Endocrinol Metab 2006;91:3105–3109

69. Sir-Petermann T, Hitchsfeld C, Maliqueo M, et al. Birth weight in offspring of mothers with polycystic ovarian syndrome. Hum Reprod 2005;20:2122–2126

70. Turhan NO, Seckin NC, Rybar F, Inegol I. Assessment of glucose tolerance and pregnancy outcome of polycystic ovary patients. Int J Gynecol Obstet 2003;81:163–168

71. Glueck CJ, Goldenberg N, Pranikoff J, Loftspring M, Sieve L, Wang P. Height, weight and motor-social development during the first 18 months of life in 126 infants born to 109 mothers with polycystic ovary syndrome who conceived on and continued metformin through pregnancy. Hum Reprod 2004;19:1323–1330

72. Gartsen SM, Jacobsen G, Romundstad P. Maternal testosterone levels during pregnancy are associated with offspring size at birth. Eur J Endocrinol 2006;155:365–370

73. Steckler T, Wang T, Bartol FF, Roy SK, Padmanabhan V. Fetal programming: prenatal testosterone treatment causes intrauterine growth retardation, reduces ovarian reserve and increases ovarian follicular recruitment. Endocrinology 2005;146:3185–3193

74. Gitau R, Adams D, Fisk NM, Glover V. Fetal plasma testosterone correlates positively with cortisol. Arch Dis Child Fetal Neonatal Ed 2005;90:F166-F169

75. Genbacev O, Zhou Y, Ludlow JW, Fisher SJ. Regulation of human placental development by oxygen tension. Science 1997;277:1669–1672

76. Zhou Y, Genbacer O, Damsky CH, Fisher SJ. Oxygen regulates human cytotrophoblast differentiation and invasion: implications for endovascular invasion in normal pregnancy and pre-eclampsia. J Reprod Immunol 1998;39:197–213

77. Zamudio S, Leslie KK, White M, Hagerman DD, Moore LG. Low serum estradiol and high serum progesterone concentrations characterize hypertensive pregnancies at high altitude. J Soc Gynecol Investig 1994;1:197–205

78. Jiang B, Kamat A, Mendelson CR. Hypoxia prevents induction of aromatase expression in human trophoblast cells in culture: potential inhibitory role of the hypoxia-inducible transcription factor Mash-2 (Mammalien Achaete-Scute Homologous Protein2). Mol Endocrinol 2000;14:1661–1673

79. Tchernof A, Toth MJ, Poehlanan ET. Sex hormone-binding globulin levels in middle-aged premenopausal women. Association with visceral obesity and metabolic profile. Diabetes Care 1999;22:1875–1881

80. Haffner SM, Katz MS, Stern MP, Dunn JF. The relationship of sex hormones to hyperinsulinemia and hyperglycemia. Metabolism 1988;67:460–464

81. Plymate SR, Matej LA, Jones RE, Friedl KE. Inhibition of sex hormone-binding globulin production in the human hepatoma (HepG2) cell line by insulin and prolactin. J Clin Endocrinol Metab 1998;67:460–464

82. Selvo DM, Hogerveen KN, Innis SM, Hammond GL. Monosaccharide-induced lipogenesis regulates the human hepatic sex hormone-binding globulin gene. J Clin Invest 2007;117:3979–3987

83. Dickenson SM, Gore AC. Estrogenic environmental endocrine-disrupting chemical effects on reproductive neuroendocrine function and dysfunction across the life cycle. Rev Endocr Metab Disord 2007;8:143–159

84. Gupta C. Reproductive malformation of the male offspring following maternal exposure to estrogenic chemicals. Proc Soc Exp Biol Med 2000;224:61–68

85. Haney AF, Newbold RR, McLachlan JA. Prenatal diethylstilbestrol exposure in the mouse: effects on ovarian histology and steroidogenesis in vitro. Biol Reprod 1984;30:471–478

86. Wu CH, Mangan CE, Burtnett MM, Michail G. Plasma hormones in DES-exposed females. Obstet Gynecol 1980;55: 157–162

87. Bibbo M, Gill WB, Azizi F, et al. Follow-up study of male and female offspring of DES-exposed mothers. Obstet Gynecol 1977;49:1–8

88. Newbold RR, Padilla-Banks E, Snydrer RJ, Jefferson WN. Perinatal exposure to environmental estrogens and the development of obesity. Mol Nutr Food Res 2007;51:912–917

89. Matthiessen P, Gibbs P. Critical appraisal of the evidence for tributyltin-mediated endocrine disruption in mollusks. Environ Toxicol Chem 1998;17:37–43

90. Ogata R, Omara M, Shimasaki Y, et al. Two-generation reproductive toxicity study of tributyltin chloride in female rats. J Toxicol Environ Health 2001;63:127–144

91. Cooke GM. Effect of organotins on human aromatase activity in vitro. Toxicol Lett 2002;126:121–130

92. Mu YM, Yanase T, Nishi Y, Takayanagi R, Goto K, Nawata H. Combined treatment with specific ligands for PPARγ: RXR nuclear receptor system markedly inhibits the expression of cytochrome P450 arom in human granulosa cancer cells. Mol Cell Endocrinol 2001;181:239–248

93. Grun F, Watanabe H, Zamanian Z, et al. Endocrine-disrupting organotin compounds are potent inducers of adipogenesis in vertebrates. Mol Endocrinol 2006;20:2141–2155

94. Grun F, Blumberg B. Environmental obesogens: organotins and endocrine disruption via nuclear receptor signalling. Endocrinology 2006;147:550–555

95. Berube D, Sevalini GE, Gagne R, Hammond GL. Localization of human sex hormone-binding gene (SHBG) to the short arm of chromosome 17(17p12-p13). Cytogenet Cell Genet 1990;54:65–67

96. Toscano V, Balducci R, Bianchi P, Guglielmi R, Mangiantini A, Sciara F. Steroidal and non-steroidal factors in plasma sex hormone binding globulin regulation. J Steroid Biochem Mol Biol 1992;43:431–437

97. Ahrentsen OD, Jensen HK, Johnsen SG. Sex hormone-binding globulin deficiency 1982;2:377–378

98. Hogeveen KN, Talikka M, Hammond GL. Human sex hormone-binding globulin promoter activity is influenced by a (TAAAA)n repeat element within an Alu sequence. J Biol Chem 2001;276:36383–36390

99. Xita N, Tsatsoulis A, Chatzikyriakidou A, Georgiou I. Association of the (TAAAA)n repeat polymorphism in the sex hormone-binding globulin (SHBG)gene with polycystic ovary syndrome and relation to SHBG serum levels. J Clin Endocrinol Metab 2003;88:5976–5980

100. Cousin P, Calemard-Michel L, Lejeune H, et al. Influence of SHBG gene pentanucleotide TAAAA repeat and D 327 N polymorphism on serum sex hormone-binding globulin concentrations in hirsuit women. J Clin Endocrinol Metab 2004;89:917–924

101. Polonca F, Teran N, Gersak K. The (TAAAA)n microsatellite polymorphism in the SHBG gene influences serum SHBG levels in women with polycystic ovary syndrome. Hum Reprod 2007;22:1031–1036

102. Bulun SE. Aromatase deficiency in women and men: would you have predicted the phenotype? J Clin Endocrinol Metab 1996;81:867–871

103. Urbanek M, Legro RS, Driscoll DA et al. Thirty-seven candidate genes for polycystic ovary syndrome: strongest evidence for linkage is with follistatin. Proc Natl Acad Sci U S A 1999;69:8573–8578

104. Söderlund D, Canto P, Carranza-Lira S, Méndez JP. No evidence of mutations in the P450 aromatase gene in patients with polycystic ovary syndrome. Hum Reprod 2005;20:965–969

105. Gharani N, Waterworth BW, Batty S, et al. Association of the steroid synthesis gene CYP11a with polycystic ovary syndrome and hyperandrogenism. Hum Mol Genet 1997;6:397–402

106. Petry CJ, Ong KK, Michelmore KF, et al. Association of aromatase (CYP19) gene variation with features of hyperandrogenism in two populations of young women. Hum Reprod 2005;20:1837–1843

107. Baghaei F, Rosmond R, Westberg L, et al. The CYP19 gene and associations with androgens and abdominal obesity in premenopausal women. Obes Res 2003;11:578–585

108. Xita N, Georgiou I, Lazaros L, Psofaki V, Kolios G, Tsatsoulis A. The synergistic effect of sex hormone-binding globulin and aromatase genes on polycystic ovary syndrome phenotype. Eur J Endocrinol 2008;158:861–865

109. Gaasenbeek M, Powell BL, Sovio U et al. Large-scale analysis of the relationship between CYP11A promoter variation, polycystic ovarian syndrome, and serum testosterone. J Clin Endocrinol Metab 2004;89:2403–2413

110. Kimura S, Matsumoto T, Matsuyama K et al. Androgen receptor function in folliculogenesis and its clinical implication in premature ovarian failure. Trends Endocrinol Metab 2007;18:181–189

111. Chamberlain NL, Driver ED, Miesfeld RL. The length and location of CAG trinucleotide repeats in the androgen receptor N-terminal domain affect transactivation function. Nucleic Acids Res 1994;22:3181–3186

112. Westberg L, Baghaei F, Rosmond R, et al. Polymorphisms of the androgen receptor gene and the estrogen receptor β gene are associated with androgen levels in women. J Clin Endocrinol Mctab 2001;86:2562–2568

113. Ibanez L, Ong KK, Mongan N, et al. Androgen receptor gene CAG repeat polymorphism in development of ovarian hyperandrogenism. J Clin Endocrinol Metab 2003;88:3333–3338

114. Legro RS, Shahbahrami B, Lobo PA, Kovacs BW. Size polymorphisms of the androgen receptor among female Hispanics and correlation with androgenic characteristics. Obstet Gynecol 1994;83:701–706

115. Misfud A, Ramirez S, Yong EL. Androgen receptor gene CAG trinucleotide repeats in anovulatory infertility and polycystic ovaries. J Clin Endocrinol Metab 2000;85:3484–3488

116. Hickey T, Chandy A, Norman RJ. The androgen receptor CAG repeat polymorphism and X-chromosome inactivation in Australian Caucasian women with infertility related to polycystic ovary syndrome. J Clin Endocrinol Metab 2002;87:161–165

117. Calvo RM, Asuncion M, Saucho J, San Millan JL, Escobar-Morreale HF. The role of the CAG repeat polymorphism in the androgen receptor gene and of skewed X-chromosome inactivation in the pathogenesis of hirsutism. J Clin Endocrinol Metab 2000;85:1735–1740

118. Jaaskelainen J, Korhonen S, Voutilainen R, Hippelainen M, Heinonen S. Androgen receptor gene CAG length polymorphism in women with polycystic ovary syndrome. Fertil Steril 2005;83:1724–1728

119. Edwarls A, Hammond HA, Jin L, Caskey CT, Chakraborty R. Genetic variations at five trimeric and tetrameric tandem repeat loci in four human population groups. Genomics 1992; 241–253

120. Xita N, Georgiou I, Lazaros L, Psofaki V, Kolios G, Tsatsoulis A. The role of sex hormone-binding globulin and androgen reception gene variants in the development of polycystic ovary syndrome. Hum Reprod 2008;23:693–698

121. Britt KL, Findlay JK. Estrogen actions in the ovary revisited. J Endocrinol 2002; 175:269–276

122. Robinson J. Prenatal programming at the female reproductive neuroendocrine system by androgens. Reproduction 2006; 132:539–547

123. Escobar-Morreale HF, Sam Millan JL. Abdominal adiposity and the polycystic ovary syndrome. Trends Endocrinol Metab 2007;18:266–272

124. Auger AP, Hexter DP, McCarthy MM. Sex differences in the phosphorylations of cAMP response element binding protein (CREB) in neonatal fat brain. Brain Res 2001; 890:110–117

125. Waterland RA, Jirtle RL. Early nutrition, epigenetic changes at transposons and imprinted genes, and enhanced susceptibility to adult chronic disease. Nutrition 2004; 20:63–68

126. Li Z, Huang H. Epigenetic abnormality: a possible mechanism underlying the fetal origin of polycystic ovary syndrome. Med Hypotheses 2008; 70:638–642

127. Lavoie HA. Epigenetic control of ovarian function: the emerging role of histone modification. Mol Cell Endocrinol 2005; 243:12–18

128. Drake AJ, Walker BR. The intergenerational effects of fetal programming: non-genomic mechanisms for the inheritance of low birth weight and cardiovascular risk. J Endocrinol 2004; 180:1–16

129. Escobar-Morreale HF, Luque-Ramirez M, San Millan JL. The molecular-genetic basis of functional hyperandrogenism and the polycystic ovary syndrome. Endocr Rev 2005; 26:251–282

6   An Anthropological View of the Impact of Poverty and Globalization on the Emerging Epidemic of Obesity

Patricia Aguirre

CONTENTS

ABSTRACT

This chapter explores how social relations have contributed to the emerging obesity epidemic, both in developed and developing countries. It poses that the most important factor in the global increase of obesity at the world level lies in the integrated agroindustry, which produces and distributes cheap energy and expensive micronutrients. This industry has homogenized world tastes and is pursuing ever more distant and specific market niches (i.e., low-income populations, women, teenagers, or children). If the only value dominating present-day nutrition is profit, it is understandable that production should stand on the edge of a sustainability crisis, that distribution should be facing an equity crisis, and that consumption is confronting a commensality crisis.

The economic principles ruling current eating habits are at odds with human needs and health, generating both hunger and obesity.

Key words. Obesity, Poverty, Food, Globalization; AgroIndustry.

The rapid changes in dietary habits and lifestyle as a result of industrialization, town planning, economic development, and market globalization over the last century have made a serious impact on people's health and nutrition. This economic transition ensuing industrialization was accompanied by demographic, epidemiological, and nutritional transitions, which have contributed to define political developments in the twentieth century. The demographic transition may be briefly summarized as an

From: *Diabetes in Women: Pathophysiology and Therapy*
Edited by: A. Tsatsoulis et al. (eds.), DOI 10.1007/978-1-60327-250-6_6
© Humana Press, a part of Springer Science+Business Media, LLC 2009

increase in urban population at the expense of the rural areas, along with lower fertility and mortality rates which, in the long term, will result in an aging population. The epidemiological transition is associated with a significant decrease in the prevalence of infectious/contagious diseases, which have been gradually replaced by noncontagious chronic diseases such as diabetes, hypertension, cardiovascular disease, and some types of cancer among others.

The nutritional transition has varied between regions, even within one and the same society, but the trend globally has been that traditional nutrition patterns have been abandoned for diets dependent on out-of-season, imported foods rich in saturated fats, sugar, and other refined carbohydrates while low in fibers and polyunsaturated fats. At nearly the same time, the level of physical activity has declined.

In the 1990s, American epidemiologists (1) first characterized obesity, a noncontagious disease, as an epidemic. By calling it "global," they raised it to the category of a pandemic disease. Nowadays, type 2 diabetes (DM2) has reached the same status. While the prevalence of obesity varies greatly from country to country, all countries share common characteristics: the condition has continued to spread, and even countries with low-obesity prevalence rates at baseline have demonstrated an increase in prevalence with time. It should be noted that the increase in obesity has been exceedingly fast and reached all social classes, sexes, and age groups. In other words, it is a truly global issue, since it reaches across geographic, cultural, economic, gender, and age barriers.

In Europe, concern about the problem was translated into political action by the 53 member states following the Istanbul Encounter (2). On the other hand, Latin American countries, where public policies are as poor as the population, have not addressed this disorder.

According to the ENNYS 2004, in Argentina, 2.3% of children under 5 years of age are underweight (3) and 9.8% are overweight as defined by international standards (4). In Chile, 27% of the population is obese; the risk of being overweight increases with age and is inversely proportional to income (5). In Brazil, the body mass index (BMI) over a 15-year period survey indicated a remarkable reduction in the prevalence of underweight and an increase in the prevalence of overweight (6). This represents a shift from the traditional pattern where, until the second half of the twentieth century, being overweight was a consequence of affluence. Obesity has now been displaced toward low-income population groups, which includes the majority of women and children below the poverty line (7).

Latin America experienced nutritional transformation later than other regions, triggered by the economic and social transformations (8). In their survey of epidemiological studies of 36 developing countries, Menendez and Popkin showed that in more than half of these countries, obesity proved more frequent than malnutrition. Malnutrition, obesity, infectious/contagious diseases, and noncontagious diseases are not found at the extremes of the socioeconomic range but rather tend to converge in poverty, even within the same family. This picture, known as the "nutritional paradox," has been observed in developing countries undergoing nutritional transition. In such countries, about 60% of the families with an underweight member – usually a child – also have an overweight member – generally the mother – a fact that imposes a "dual burden" on these families (9).

In countries defined as "middle income" by the World Bank, overweight appears in fifth place among the first ten causes of disease, just as it does in the developed world, but from the anthropometric standpoint, the most serious public health problem to be tackled is inadequate body size. This is related to poverty, in so far as it results from adverse social and environmental conditions, insufficient nutrition in utero and in the first few years of life (for linear growth is more demanding in terms of diet quality), and frequent infections. This stunted linear growth will later be found associated with obesity, type 2 diabetes, and other disorders. The obese poor often begin their path toward obesity in the womb as undernourished fetuses. After birth, they are often undernourished children who are fed cheap high-carbohydrate food, which is low in protein and micronutrients. Later on, particularly in the case of women whose activity is restricted to the household, the accumulation of fat will ensure their joining the ranks of the obese with the subsequent social stigmatization. This is due to the fact that obese poor are pointed at by society as the perfect example of what one "should not be" in a modern, stratified society *(10)* responding to the beauty paradigms of the global world.

THE BIG THREE

The Homo sapiens Genotype

Bearing in mind the difficulties of inquiring into the causes of the epidemic spread of a noncontagious disease - that is, a disease without an external agent – it is frequent for medical literature, particularly in the USA, to speak of "The Big Two": (1) an increase in food availability and (2) a forced sedentary lifestyle. No doubt these factors play a decisive role in precipitating the phenomenon, but not without a third factor shared by mankind as a whole: the "thrifty" genotype of *Homo sapiens*. This exerts its influence when the social conditions in which it operates experience a change.

The obesity epidemic afflicting the globe is closely related to the fact that our still Paleolithic body is operating in a postindustrial social environment. Our bodies, metabolism, and genes are the result of a time-out-of-mind adaptation to living conditions that have suffered such radical changes that what used to be an advantage has become a handicap.

It would be wise to bear in mind that for millions of years, we lived as hunters-gatherers. We were agriculturists for no longer than 10,000 years, and barely 150 years have passed since we began to industrialize food production. Thus, our genomic baggage was shaped by those distant adaptation contexts. It is interesting to examine our ancestors' ways of life and eating habits in order to have an insight into the adaptive restrictions that modeled our bodies and to compare our characteristics of yore to our present shape. Not long ago, anthropologists restrained both catastrophic and state-of-bliss views (that is to say, a short, starved, brutal life vs. the affluent primitive society) and agreed that the model that best reflected reality was one of alternate *periods of plenty and dearth*, none of which proved determinant. Plenty did not amount to obesity, nor did dearth amount to starvation.

It would be a mistake to envisage a single mode of life in the Paleolithic era, evenly developed throughout time in every geography. It stands to reason that there must have been great diversity in the creative solutions that the hunter-gatherer lifestyle gave to problems rising from the need to colonize the various continents, to overcome dramatic climatic changes such as the forward and backward movement of glaciers, and to interact with other human groups over the full length of the era. To achieve our physical and social reproduction, we humans devised mainly cultural strategies, including the ability to draw on particular experiences so as to transmit them to others, to organize the group, to divide labor, to improve techniques for the protection of the weak, to intensify production, and to implement changes at the same speed as new problems arose. In fact, cultural change occurs almost as quickly as problems arise to challenge a culture, whereas biological changes occur slowly. Still, regardless of man's will, there was enough time to fixate such biological traits as the capacity to accumulate caloric reserves in order to survive the plenty–dearth oscillation periods.

Beginning in 1985 *(11)* we anthropologists devised various *models* of Paleolithic diets, each of them resulting from adaptation to different habitats in which the available technology varied, as did the social and symbolic organization. The latter determined what could and could not be eaten depending on gender, age, and social status, at the same time legitimizing the distribution bias and the very conception of what was conceived of as "food." Although in different Paleolithic groups we found ecological and cultural restraints that "specialized" the diet, encouraging consumption of very large quantities of either meat or vegetables, we also found nonspecific diets in which both these food varieties were consumed, at varying percentages. Thanks to our flexible eating habits – we have succeeded in adapting to every new situation, including arctic climates in which meat abounds but vegetables are in poor supply or to sylvan environments with an abundance of crisp vegetables and a lack of animal proteins.

One common theme seems to be that fats and sugars were generally scarce. Even though protein intake was high, the intake of fats was remarkably lower than anticipated. Game tends to be leaner than farmed animals on account of the animals' diets and yields a more favorable polyunsaturated/saturated (P/S) ratio. Although the total cholesterol contained in such diets has been estimated to be higher than present-day ideal levels, it is quite likely that cholesterol levels in blood proved low – thanks to the combination of the polyunsaturated fatty acids mentioned and the exertion of physical activity, which amply exceeded present levels *(12)*. Ross *(13)* points out that the limitations set by energy led hunters to opt for species rich in fats. Perhaps that explains the high protein intake as a way to obtain enough calories.

Nonrefined sugars must have been seasonably available as a "safe" and immediate source of energy (most poisonous substances are bitter). Judging from present-day parameters, the intake of fibers may have been excessive, while that of iron, calcium, and ascorbic acid may have been optimal. Carbohydrates were surely lower than is now recommended. Although nutritionally adequate based on the presence of trace mineral elements and the absence of growth stop signals in our ancestors' bones, their food must have been heavily dependent on the cyclical alternation of the ecosystem, for they could not rely on conservation. All ecosystems are subject to larger and smaller variations. They may be periodic and short-lasting (as is the case with seasonal changes), medium term (like the 8-year drought 2-year flood alternation in the Argentine *pampas*), or long-lasting (as happens during glaciation). Hence, societies that did not implement accumulation practices were forced to devise cultural strategies such as gathering together in large hunting parties and holding binge feasts in order to consume as much as possible during periods of plenty while splitting into small groups to spend the accumulated reserves in times of scarcity.

In the plenty–dearth alternation context, suitable physiological mechanisms to store calories in the form of fat reserves must have been crucial. In 1962, Neel *(14)* pointed to the possible existence of a thrifty gene, an efficient mechanism that quickly and massively released insulin after a copious meal. This minimized hyperglycemia and glycosuria, allowing for a larger energy reservoir. Those who succeeded in storing the most energy were better suited to survive the inevitable period of scarcity that was bound to follow the times of plenty. In other words, they enjoyed selective advantages that were translated into reproductive advantages within the adaptation context, and their offspring inherited these genes. Should this be true, alleles related to current chronic metabolic diseases, such as obesity, arteriosclerosis, and diabetes, are, in fact, part of *the species' normal genotype* and are the result of a process of positive selection that occurred in adaptive contexts, which, in our days, have come to be a handicap and labeled as disease-predisposing alleles.

Nevertheless, if we view nutrition as a social fact, something other than thrifty genes was needed to create Palaeolithic eating habits. Cultural regulations, in the form of prescriptions, habits, customs, and taboos must have reenforced certain behaviors, endowing with meaning the fact of eating as much as possible whenever it was possible, so as to store energy for the hard times to come. In other words, *the thrifty biological process was overlaid with a regulatory culture*, which aided individual adjustment to changing local conditions: possibility of production, manner of distribution, and ways of food consumption. Such adjustments must be quick and cannot be subject to the slow pace of biological evolution. Since those days, it has been culture rather than nature that has dictated what to eat, how to eat, how much to eat, and who to eat with. This is why we had better speak of human bodies rather than of genes. In hunting-and-gathering based cultures, the thrifty genome gave rise to the tall, lean bodies depicted in cave paintings and archaeological findings. In preindustrial, cereal-growing societies that exercised differential appropriation of the surplus, the very same genotype gave rise to differentiated cuisines (high and low) and to class-differentiated bodies: *the fat rich and the skinny poor*. In the last phase of industrial society, with the same genome deployed in market societies in which access to food is strongly determined by prices, we are witnessing a reversal in this pattern, as we are more likely to find *rich slim people and fat poor people* rather than the other way about *(15)*. Summing up, we have kept the same biological genotype that proved effective 100,000 years ago, but our present environment is no longer an alternation between plenty and scarcity, for we enjoy permanent availability and abundance. These same forces that ensure availability have created an unprecedented crisis in health and nutrition.

Activity

Although in the Palaeolithic era hunting and gathering must have been approached at a physiologically bearable pace, Hayes et al. *(16)* have suggested that they had a very high physical activity level (PAL). The PAL is the total daily energy expenditure divided by basal metabolic rate. The PAL in Palaeolithic times was estimated to be 3.2, a value no contemporary population can aspire to. Present foraging groups have much lower PALs ranging from 2.1 to 1.4 while simple agriculturist societies have PALs that range from 2.3 to 1.5 *(17)*. This compares with PAL values ranging between 2.2 and 1.2 among urban populations in industrialized societies. These and many other observations support the idea that low energy expenditure by contemporary adult dwellers of industrially advanced urban locations contributes to the epidemic prevalence of obesity.

Bipedalism was instrumental to the evolutionary pathway that culminated in the *Homo sapiens*. It was our means of transportation for millions of years, even after the invention of the wheel about 5,000 years ago and even after the invention of the steam engine. In the early nineteenth century, Napoleon's army trudged its way into Russia and returned (those who did return, that is) on their own feet. It was the early twentieth century that saw the advent of the first automobiles, which began to encourage the sedentary urban lifestyle. However, although automobiles certainly decreased the amount of walking, they did not entirely delegitimize movement or the pleasures of physical activity. This was done by television, which succeeded in installing immobility as the primary leisure–rest–pleasure pursuit, exchanging enjoyment of "physical activity" for the vicarious "watching of movement" from early childhood. In a 5-year longitudinal study, it was found that the number of hours that 6–11-year olds spent in front of the TV set were the best predictor of obesity *(18)*. At present, more than 60% of the world population engages in less than 30 min of physical activity per day *(19)*. For the average American of our times, the total energy expenditure per kilo of body mass amounts to 65% of that of a Palaeolithic man, which means that an adult city dweller weighing 70 kg should walk 19 km a day to reach a level of activity equivalent to that mentioned by Haynes *(20)*.

Nowadays, as the planet is quickly developing, the activity rate in cities is lower than in rural areas. Agriculture, especially in poorer areas, still demands intensive labor. In cities and developed rural areas, technology has replaced intensive physical labor except in the poorest sectors of society. City culture favors spatial body control, discouraging movement, even if spontaneously prompted. Little movements in everyday life have been reduced to a minimum: we prefer lifts to stairs; we press a button on the remote control to change TV channels and so forth. City distances and strict timetables induce automotive transportation and discourage walking. Such reduction of movement has been occurring progressively over the last 40 years *(21)*. Although high- and middle-income sectors can afford to participate in voluntary physical activities such as aerobics, team sports, and dancing, it is not clear that this activity compensates for lack of movement throughout the day.

In urban industrial societies, activity has dwindled into forced sedentarism. This has imposed a heavy toll on human health: one in four elderly women suffer a hip fracture, which could be in part prevented as brisk walking increases bone density. While "a 30-min walk a day" may sound unimportant in terms of calorie expenditure, walking involves the movement of a large number of muscles, which improves glucose homeostasis by increasing insulin sensitivity through insulin-independent glucose uptake. This in turn improves metabolic activity, causes vasodilatation, and can help to prevent diabetes and dyslipidemias *(19)*. So as we are the product of an active past and are now subjecting our Paleolithic bodies to forced inactivity, we are changing what used to be adaptive advantages into risk factors for present metabolic diseases.

In different societies, the activity rate varies by income, sex, and age. In Argentina, a study of the roles assigned to poor men shows that they perform labor-intensive tasks with high energy expenditure until they turn approximately 30 years old. At this age, their physical deterioration forces them to do more passive jobs. In poor urban Argentine women, the household chores done by some demand high energy expenditure, since they do not have access to technology or to utilities. For example, these women have to carry 10-L containers of water several times a day, hand-wash bed sheets, clean without the aid of laborsaving devices, build their own dwelling, etc. Such activities demand a greater consumption of energy even if they are performed at a physiologically tolerable pace (i.e., on days when washing is scheduled, no other heavy job is done). Poor women who live in violent and unsafe neighborhoods are forced to confine themselves to their homes. So, their appropriation of the urban space is extremely limited as they only go out to take their children to school, do the shopping, or call on relatives. As their daughters grow up, they "help," taking upon themselves the heavier household chores and freeing their mothers so that they can enter the job market. Even those women who become employed as household help will spend less physical energy at their employers' home than at their own, since they work for sectors that have access to laborsaving devices. It should be noted that the replacement of mothers by daughters will inevitably repeat the cycle. Therefore, obesity in poverty is associated with women over 25 and men over 30 years of age *(22)*. At the top of the income pyramid, women in nonpoor sectors not only practice planned physical activity such as sports, gym, and dancing, but also can freely move about the streets, parks, and safe areas of the city. These two different ways of the appropriation of the urban space condition the activity rate of women in the two income layers described.

Growing Availability

The time has come to approach the third – and, in my view, the most important – factor in the obesity epidemic: dietary changes with an exponential increase of energy availability. Food and Agricultural Organization (FAO) estimates that the worldwide average calorie availability was 2,358 kcal/person/day in 1964, 2,655 in 1981, 2,830 in 1997, with a projection of 2,940 for 2015, and 3,950 for 2030 *(23)*, a much higher amount than is needed by the average human. Regarding the composition of the figure, 70% of our present energy comes from carbohydrates, refined sugars, dairy products, and fats, which, in the origins of our biology, either did not exist (milk derivatives are barely 10,000 years old) or were not frequently consumed, as was the case with fats. The consumption of fruit and vegetables, as well as lean meats, has been put aside. Wild fruits were richer in fibers and poorer in sugars, while the choice of animals for taming and breeding purposes was ruled by their mild dispositions and body fat. Bearing this in mind, Swinburn et al. coined the expression "obesogenic environment," arguing that the physical, economic, social, and cultural environments of the majority of industrialized nations encourage a positive energy balance in their populations *(24)*.

Urban industrial societies began to gain weight when they achieved a continuous, guaranteed supply of foodstuffs. It is, therefore, necessary to ponder over the problem of available energy from a more complex stance than mere intake, and this is what the rest of this chapter will be devoted to.

We shall approach the subject as an issue of food security, understood as the *right* to safe, nutritious, and culturally suitable food that may enable people to lead a healthy, active life *(25)*.

Although from a global standpoint current levels of food production are statistically sufficient to feed each and every inhabitant of the planet on a diet that is nutritionally suited to average human needs, inequality of access results in the coexistence and overlap of malnutrition and obesity problems. The 850 million malnourished people recorded by the FAO are not a consequence of unavailability but of inequality – inequality between countries and inequality between different groups within countries. Were there equal access to *distribution*, it would not be necessary to increase current production to feed the 10,000 million people expected by 2050. Of course, such a conclusion would require a context in which the global economy would concern itself with *equity of consumption* and with offering everyone adequate and healthy diets. On the other hand, it would be impossible to feed the present 7,000 million people if the rule were to be guided by the American per capita average food supply, about 40% of which is wasted *(26)*.

If we assume that we have a *production* problem, then it does not lie with underproduction but with overproduction of certain foods, directly related to the organizing criteria of the current global market. The logic of profit drives both the poor and the rich to damage the environment and the diet. If we wish to discuss a long-term nutritional policy, we should remember that all consumption patterns must change, and by "all" I mean those of the ones who have little or nothing as well as the ones who have too much.

THE FOOD PRODUCTION

There is strong integration between industry and agriculture to the extent that we could speak of them as agroindustry. Some authors point out that industry and agriculture behave differently toward globalization. Only industry has become globalized. This can be seen from the free flow of capital and trade, labor decentralization, flexibility, and applied knowledge. However, by differentiating between production and distribution, we realize that, despite agroindustry's unique traits, only industry has become globalized and has exported its consumption model to the whole planet. Agriculture has remained in the field of comparative advantages, since just when it was on the verge of becoming independent of its physical and territorial limitations (i.e., beginning to produce stable molecules, resembling mass production in an assembly line), it was put to question by consumers, who still wish their food natural and territorial. The growing merger between the food industry and the chemical and pharmaceutical industries casts doubts on the possibility that their wish will survive into the future.

In view of the deterritorializing bias of globalization, food companies still need to devise a vertical integration strategy to connect the various links in the production chain [both in Europe *(27)* and the USA, the food industry uses 82% of domestic agricultural raw materials *(28)*] and to establish branches near the places where the raw materials are produced. Now, based on organizational rules established by global production, the branches of the large multinational companies are fairly independent from their headquarters. Adopting a regional profile, they have succeeded in outdoing the central company. According to the United States Department of Agriculture (1998), sales by branches quadrupled (100,000 million dollars) the value exported by US-based companies (25,000 million dollars). Headquarters and branches' main markets are composed of consumers who reside in the region where the companies operate. Of the 300 hundred tons of grain harvested in the USA, two-thirds are consumed by the domestic market, and still the country remains the largest grain exporter worldwide. The exception to the rule is branches exploiting crops in Southern countries and producing against the season when their headquarters cannot produce.

While the industry has been taking dramatic steps toward the world's nutritional homogenization (and doing so unawares, for its sole purpose lies in boosting sales), agricultural trade has survived in a limited manner, since agriculture is still very much protected and subsidized in most developed countries. In fact, tariff barriers to the exchange of agricultural products currently amount to 60% of their value *(29, 30)*, to which we should add the cost of para-tariff barriers, such as those imposed on health issues, for example, which are not easily quantified and which increase the constraints on this kind of trade.

SUBSIDIES

The General Agreement on Tariffs and Trade (GATT) 1947–1995 and Word Trade Organization (WTO) 1995–2001 meetings are seeking to modify a system that has survived since the second post-war period, when the developed countries estimated that the right strategy for them consisted in achieving nutritional adequacy and autonomy.

These goals prompted improved agricultural technology through state subsidies that acted as powerful incentives for producers with a potential to achieve productivity and profitability. Together with frontier protection aimed at avoiding the import of products that might pose a threat on local production, the said subsidies stood out as the main signs of policies seeking ample availability of food. According to FAO, food availability is composed of various items: *sufficiency* regarding food supply, *stability* and continuity in the said food supply, *autonomy* from imported food supplies, and *sustainability* to ensure future food supplies *(31)*. It was also necessary to preserve social order by preventing producers' bankruptcy during market fluctuations. Thus, agricultural trade took on a *complementary* rather than a *competitive* form to suit each country's requirement for autonomy first, and this is why it is not viewed by some as globalized. In other words, even surplus-producing countries export the surplus once they have satisfied domestic needs. The Neo-liberal reforms of the 1980s attempted to change the paradigm by turning it competitive but it was only through the E.U. 1992 and 2003 reforms and the 1996 reforms in the USA that the subsidy-and-protectionism system experienced some *slight* changes. The system persists in the developed world, not only because of the surplus it generates or for fear of future dire times but also because of fear of the effects of open agriculture. Removing this system would bring about the collapse of the agricultural systems of the developed world, since these systems lack the capacity to compete with better quality, more conveniently priced products. If subsidies were cancelled, cereals, legumes, and fruit grown in developing countries where soils and climates are favorable and labor is cheap would have better chances of competing in the markets of developed countries. This would in turn lead to serious social and economic unrest, and no country is willing to deal with such a situation. Perhaps this fear influenced the industry's decision to abandon the decentralized factory structure typical of globalization and to adopt a vertical, geographic concentration. This is not necessarily due to the perishable nature of food since grains, for example, may be transported over long distances. However, as the most severe protection and distortion is exerted on grains, hindering their commercial flow, it is easier for semiprocessed and manufactured foodstuffs to evade protectionism. Nowadays the flow of the latter, regarding both volume and value, has amply exceeded that of natural foodstuffs such as cereals, oilseeds, and horticultural products *(30)*.

Developed countries' subsidies and protectionism have more than fulfilled their commitment to achieve a dynamic agriculture yielding nutritional adequacy, for the current issue happens to be overproduction *(32)*, with its multiple negative effects inside and outside the country.

Overproduction endangers the environment because monoculture agriculture requires ever increasing inputs of water and agrochemicals. In the case of water, the main consumer on the planet is extensive monoculture agriculture rather than human beings. In the case of agrochemicals, it should be taken into account that they are dependent on oil, entailing the risks of reaching beyond the environment's self-purging capacity and thus leading to its local degradation and the contamination of distant ecosystems.

For example, the influence of plain crops is felt many kilometers away at sea. While this production model increased profitability, it is not sustainable and this concern extends to predatory fishing and hormone-based cattle-breeding schemes as well.

The number of resources invested in agricultural subsidies is stunning. Total transfers to agriculture in countries in the Organisation for Economic Cooperation and Development for 2003 amounted to $350 billion (€288 billion), half of which comes from taxpayers and half from consumers. Eliminating all agricultural policy distortions could produce global annual welfare gains up to $165 billion according to FAO because production would move to poor countries with comparative advantages (33). For example, in Argentina the expanse of the plains, the temperate climate, qualified, cheap labor, and low population density satisfy the demands of the domestic market and provide a huge surplus of exportable foodstuff.

As an example, the European Union spends about two billion euros a year to keep milk production 20% above domestic demand, at prices that double those of the world market (34). Were there no subsidies, production would quickly adapt to the levels of demand. Yet, historical and cultural reasons and a powerful industry lobby fiercely protect dairy production in the E.U. creating a surplus of butter and powdered milk. Still, to maintain a surplus of dairy products whose subsidies depend on consumers' taxes is both expensive and unpopular, so they are placed in the market for domestic consumption, subsidized exports, or as nutritional assistance to poor countries. Subsidized dairy exports undermine the traditional gastronomic heritages of the countries it reaches and the local dairy industry of countries such as the Dominican Republic, Kenya, India, and Jamaica among others (35). These local industries are not able to compete with the artificially low prices with which these products penetrate their markets.

For developing countries, subsidized production and barriers to agricultural imports implemented by developed countries constitute a serious obstacle to agricultural growth. It is a known fact that FAO ascribes great importance to local agricultural growth in order to fight poverty and malnutrition. For example, in regions that depend heavily on primary production, the growth of agriculture not only pours more food into local markets, reducing the costs of nutrition for poor consumers, but also creates employment for unskilled workers, distributes income in a progressive manner, and strengthens rural economy, all of which makes an impact on national growth (36).

Besides damaging the poor countries' economies and causing poverty and malnutrition in rural areas, exports of subsidized grains fatten the urban poor. These products, imported at low prices, replace local, traditional, and fresh foodstuffs, so that the poor end up eating subsidized cereals only.

The oversupply fostered by subsidies also makes an impact on the domestic consumption of the subsidizing countries by stimulating an excessive offer of the cheap foodstuffs that lie at the base of the obesity epidemic. For example, the E.U. subsidizes domestic consumption of one-third of the total butter production, at a yearly cost of 500 million euros amounting to 1.5 kg of butter per citizen. The industry uses this cheap butter to make ice-cream and desserts, which increase the average European's calorie intake.

Full-fat milk, subsidized and distributed in schools, is another outlet for the dairy oversupply. The Swedes have come to the conclusion that this is the source of 1.5 kg/year of extra saturated fat in school children, who should be drinking the healthier skimmed variety (37).

In short, rather than encourage a decrease in prices, overproduction has contributed to increase the food offered in developed countries, but we are not talking of just any food, but of cereals, oils, fats, and sugars, all of which contribute to the problem of an overweight society. Should the same amounts of money have been invested to further horticultural production, we would be looking at a quite different outcome.

In 2003, the common European agricultural policy underwent a reform whose main objective consisted in aligning agricultural production and demand and partially reducing subsidies. Judging from the results, the reform *proved to be a failure, since it resulted in*:

1. *Only a 1% decrease* in the production of commodities such as wheat, coarse grains, oilseeds, beef, pork, and poultry.
2. A continued increase in the production of dairy products until 2015.
3. Only rice production is expected to decrease significantly.

Still, this will be accompanied by a reduction in subsidized exports (4% for wheat, 6% for cheese, 8% for skimmed milk powder, and 17% for butter), so it is expected that domestic prices will drop and that consumption will grow. In other words, the project seems to aim at solving the problems rising from communal agriculture by enticing people to eat more. This manner of agricultural policy does not aid the prevention of obesity. Unless the health sector begins to play an active role in agricultural policies, the prospects for obesity prevention look bleak. It is not enough to issue sanitary regulations or to control agrochemicals: it is absolutely necessary to operate directly on the regulations, subsidies, support prices for domestic products, and foreign trade, which have a direct impact on consumption.

It is to be noted, however, that when the subsidy system was strongly put to question, dietary changes associated with the economic growth-related increase in the average income of India and China triggered a huge demand for grain, which resulted in higher international prices. For example, China, with its 1,300 million inhabitants, raised its per capita yearly meat consumption from 20 kg in 1985 to more than 50 kg in 2005. The country increased cattle raising and slaughtering to meet the new demand, but this required importing grain as balanced feed, since 1 kg of beef requires the bovine to consume 8 kg of feed; 1 kg of pork implies a 3-kg feed consumption by the pig; 1 kg of chicken is obtained from 2.5 kg of feed consumption, and 1 kg of fish requires 1.8 kg of feed. Grain prices rose by 75% above inflation between 2005 and 2008, originating the neologism "agflation": inflation in agricultural prices. Rather than stimulate developed countries to lift their subsidies, these prices encourage them to increase these subsidies to increase the production. Thus, if we include biofuel demand in the picture, we may well expect food prices to keep soaring. The British weekly, *The Economist*, which began recording a world price index in 1845, has declared current food prices to have reached a historical high since they first published the indices.

The demand of soy oil and maize ethanol biodiesel (which is already taking up one-third of the American maize harvest) makes a direct impact on the prices of these products and puts indirect upward pressure on displaced crops, as more maize means less of something else. The land has limits; it is a long time since agrarian frontiers have become relatively stable. Very few countries can afford to dedicate more land to agriculture, and when they do so, it is at the expense of woods and forests. Thus, such grains as will be turned into biofuels exit the food circuit and steadily increase their prices until they reach the consumer. A similar substitution and ever-higher prices situation happened in Central America when the countries of the region exported a part of their harvests to the USA for the manufacture of ethanol. When maize was withdrawn from the domestic market, its price went up by 300% in 6 months. As maize is a primary product for 85% of the population, its price was directly relative to the increase in poverty.

EXPORT TAXES (OR "SLIDING SCALE DUTIES" OR "RETENTIONS")

Approximately 50 world economies, mostly those of countries that specialize in exports of primary products, tax their exports on a sliding scale basis in order to recapture a part of the income derived from their natural resources. Examples of this are coffee in Colombia, grains in Argentina, or uncut diamonds in South Africa. In the absence of state-run companies for trade of grains, like the Australian and Canadian Wheat Boards (AWB and CWB), sliding scale duties are a source for the State to benefit from soil-generated income. This type of taxation arises from classic economics *(38)* (after all, nature is unique – it is impossible to duplicate the Argentinean pampas or the Nile's slime) - so extra profit from a unique agricultural source can be equated to the income yielded by a monopoly. If this is so, the export duties do not tax the producer's profit, which remain at an average level, but the land-generated income based on the extraordinary agro-ecological conditions of the soil that allow grain cultivation (Argentina), dry fruit cultivation (Turkey), or diamond extraction (South Africa). According to the WTO, this is a legal instrument, and one-third of the member countries make use of it *(39)*.

Argentina, 76% of whose GNP is dependent on the export of primary products, taxes 35% on soy exports, 28% on corn exports, and 25% on maize exports. This scheme, which had been abandoned in 1992, was reinstated following the 285% depreciation of the currency after the 2002 crisis. It was a fiscal instrument to lay hands on the extraordinary profits that devaluation allowed the 80 exporting business groups. Its additional function consists in differentiating the prices of products sold in foreign markets from those in the domestic market, which is specially important, when exportable goods are either a part of the food basket or constitute important supplies within the production process. It should be noted that these high taxes apply only to 80 companies that control 70% of the total exports of the country, for if thousands of companies composed the export sector, depreciation would have had a serious trickle-down effect.

Although the export taxes were supposed to be temporary, 6 years have passed and they are still in force. They support social aid programs for the unemployed and subsidize several aspects of agribusiness, such as livestock feeds, so as to avoid price increases in the domestic market. In an indirect way, the high exchange rate fosters the substitution of imports so as to encourage national productive activity, a key element for the reindustrialization strategy in the country. Argentina's agricultural potential, added to the expectation of sustained high prices that will grant great profitability to primary activities, enables the State to seize a part of the agribusiness profits through high taxes or "retentions."

GLOBALIZED INDUSTRY

While agroindustry is relatively modern, its origins date back to the sixteenth century, when the seeds for "scientific" agricultural exploitation were sown *(40)*. This simply meant the application of knowledge to intensified profitability, amid a struggle "against" nature perceived as a wild element. The same criteria still rule food production. The international division of labor *(41)*, a salient characteristic of food production in the industrial era, resulted in the delocalization of diets. Ever since the nineteenth century, whenever local supplies have not sufficed to feed the population gathered in the urban and industrial belts, countries have depended on imports and on commercial and political dealings with other regions and nations. The twofold pressure of having to secure social and economic stability by controlling prices and food flows into the cities added to a profitable diversification of financial capital, driving developed countries to seek sources of food farther and farther away from their own territory. Here lies the significance of the role of the state as the protector of economic agents. In developed countries, increases in average income stimulate consumption, and the delocalization of diets causes a corresponding increase in the number and variety of foodstuffs. The seasonal cycles whose alternation used to determine human nutrition are gone for good – today, only Japan values and maintains seasonality of consumption, even though the country's industry possesses the means to end it.

In the industrial era, having food - and cheap food at that – is not enough: food must take on a *different format* if it is to satisfy the needs of urban supply. Foodstuffs are no longer fresh but processed, undergoing transformations in six areas. *Preservation* of food has become extremely complex (canning, dehydration, freezing, sterilization, etc.), so that it can be safely *transported* over long distances. *Mechanized* production ensures stability, promptness, and hygiene. *Wholesale–retail chains* distribute it in the remotest corners of the planet where such foodstuffs can be afforded, and this entails a national and international corpus of *sanitary regulations* that ensure quality. *Brands* identify and point to manufacturer's responsibility toward consumers, and States guarantee that there is no adulteration and control compliance with health regulations (the *expert systems* of modernity) *(42)*. These transformations achieved stability of supply and worldwide coverage: food will reach every place where people can pay for it. However, side by side with this paradise of stability, hygiene, and diversity, the modern urban-industrial consumer perceives the disadvantages of this kind of food. Flavors are lost. Intraspecies diversity is gone (of the 400 potato varieties we used to have, only five are still grown). Consumers have lost control of what they are eating: they no longer know if apples contain apple genes or if "others" have been added. They cannot be sure that agrochemicals are safe and that additives and preservatives involved in food processing are not carcinogenic. Moreover, they do not know if what they eat contains "undetectable" salt or sugar, if fats are hydrogenated, if transportation has been safe (the cold chain in frozen foods may have been broken), or even if the packaging is right (does the three-laminated structure really consist of three layers?). In brief, consumers have no control of what makes their food edible. This is a unique situation in human food culture. Nowadays, we do not know what exactly we are eating, as we delegate knowledge and care to the expert systems of modernity. Cooking mothers and grandmothers have been replaced by industry. With preprocessed and preprepared foodstuffs ("service food"), the factory trespasses into the kitchen, and the culinary knowledge of mothers loses value when confronted with a brand. As women withdraw from their reproductive role to join the labor force, both "service food" and meals eaten out – without any possibility of supervising either the products or the preparation – impinge upon family food intake.

Over the past decade, laboratories have displaced factories and replaced cooking mothers. Genetically modified food and functional food (the ones treated with substances that improve their bioavailability and/or prevent disease), which includes pre and probiotic food (which have a direct effect on the intestinal bacteria), no longer depend on manufacturing but on scientific creativity. While factories chopped and/or cooked, using the same elements as kitchens, though in a different scale, food was still recognizable from the packaging. On the other hand, "created" foodstuffs start from the expert's knowledge about the iron or calcium intake that humans need, which pushes food closer and closer to medicine. Although the industry insists that it responds to the market's demand, experience tells us that it creates artificial needs so that it can shape the demand to suit the offer. In addition, there is technical and scientific knowledge (e.g., molecular biology) that proves unattainable to the majority of people and that "creates" foodstuffs to "outdo" natural products, following the old cultural representations of the Enlightenment, acting against or upon nature. These "created" foods are incomprehensible to simple cooking mothers for nature offers nothing similar. These foods highlight the role of the mass media to devise stories that entice people to buy and consume these foods and generate new symbolic constructions to replace those that used to regulate our thrifty biology.

The food cultures of our past were collective creations that were built on a knowledge resulting from the experience accumulated by numberless generations. This collective creation, maintained and transformed for centuries, guaranteed a degree of rationality that has now been replaced by the mass media and the power of the food industry with its logic of profit. They are the main creators of meaning – that is, of culture – in the eating habits of the industrial world. Not having gone through the "fires" of time or experience, our food lacks a history.

Good to Sell

One of the most important consequences of the growing intensification of the industrial production of food is that it has ceased to target the production of food to focus on profit. When production grows at the expense of investment technology or fossil energy, with new formats raising added value, there is always a concomitant increase in costs. The need for investment causes the search for profit to precede product quality and, in turn, this casts aside the issue of availability by restricting access to those who can afford it. If food is regarded as such insofar as it is saleable, the logic of the market concludes that only those who can afford it will eat.

The dietary repercussions of the evolution of industrial capitalism erased the borders dividing food production and the production of other goods. *Food is merchandise rather than nutrients.* Diversified companies and holdings characterized by highly concentrated capital determine the industrial diet. One-third of the overall world food production is in the hands of 200 companies based in developed countries, mainly in the USA, England, and Japan. In fact, only 5% of these companies lie outside these countries *(43)*. We, therefore, do not eat what we want, but what manufacturers decide to sell us. They do not sell us nourishing food, but food that yields good profit. "What is good to eat turns out to be what is good to sell" *(44)*, regardless of its nutritional value.

Naturally, no food company intends to poison buyers. Still, as is the case with tobacco, if the buyer's health deteriorates in the long term, there is no reason to go out of business. Besides, in the case of food, the dietary diversity would prevent a direct correlation with illness. However, some alarming examples, such as the huge amount of packaged, sugary, colored, inflated, flavored stuff called "junk food," which is sold round the planet, show that industrial food is divorced from nutrition and health.

Industrial consumption has reduced us to mere buyers of eatable goods, which we can neither fathom nor control. This is related not only to the quantity and quality of the food we eat but also to commensality or modes of eating.

While quantity and quality have been extensively discussed in the literature, we are just beginning to grasp the importance of commensality, a key point in the regulating culture and the obesity epidemic. Human modes of eating structure products, concoctions, and dishes following combinations that reflect social, gender, and age categories. Such social categories become "obscured" when they are "naturalized" as if they pertained to the food eaten rather than to the eaters' society. Every culture organizes its own rules of combination into "a knowledge about the art of fine dining," or into a gastronomy. Nowadays, industrialized societies have dropped the rules that endow commensality with meaning and, as Fischler *(45)* says, there is gastro-anomie: lonely eaters who have given up eating patterns and peck at their food whenever they feel like it; people who no longer sit at table but munch away in the streets, in food stores, or standing by the refrigerator. The paradox lies in the fact that present-day eaters lack rules about "the art of fine dining" precisely because of an excess of rules. Chefs, nutritionists, administrators, and advertisers give advice on how to eat tasty, wholesome, inexpensive, or trendy food. Faced with such a lot of simultaneous advice, the eater has to choose without the aid of the culture that used to organize his intake of food. The agroindustry takes good advantage of this unique situation in history – a solitary eater making a food choice. Through the mass media, it directs him to what it needs to sell. In our times, the mass media provides meaning to urban eaters.

In places with sufficient income to buy agroindustrial products – whether in developed countries or in rich areas of poor countries – agroindustries need to keep maximizing profits in a market so saturated with food goods [in 2003, 13,900 new products were launched in the USA *(46)*] that they cannot but resort to ever more aggressive marketing strategies. They insist that we should eat more, moreover, that we should eat more calorie-dense food, and they do so through relentless advertising aimed at ever more specialized market niches: children, teenagers, dancers, athletes, the constipated, the obese, the diabetics, etc. They also reach for markets that have been long neglected, such as developing countries with exceedingly low per capita income. They find strategic locations for their outlets, increase the content in the package, and lower their prices as a manner of rewarding those who consume the most. They cut their costs [by substituting chemical margarine for natural butter *(47)*, for example], even when the cheaper products prove dangerous for health.

I suggest keeping an eye on the number of calories produced by global agroindustry in order to predict obesity indices in the world, since if it produces 4,500 kcal/person/day, it will surely want to sell them; in other words, it will make use of the full power of the media until someone buys them and eats them in some corner of the planet.

It is a great concern that the food industry targets children as a favorite market niche aggressively advertising food that is good to sell and bad to eat. Thirty percent of the calories involved in consumption are sweets, soft drinks, salty snacks, and fast food. It is not unusual for overweight children to consume 1,200 or 2,000 calories a day from soft drinks alone *(48)*. Since 1970, obesity rates have more than doubled among children 6–11 years of age and more than tripled among those 12–19 years of age. As a consequence of this, type 2 diabetes mellitus is no longer rare in pediatric practice *(48)*. Marketing strategies to sell junk food to children is nearly Orwellian, using psychological tests, focus groups, ethnographic studies, profiling, and archetypes to inform them. It has proved effective, though. American children spend 30 billion of their own money on junk food and influence adults to buy them more. In 2004, McDonald's spent 528 million dollars on publicity addressed to children and sold them 24.4 billion dollars worth of products *(49)*.

Although our data come from developed countries, it is known that sister companies apply the very same sales strategies in developing countries in an attempt to attract high- and middle-income sectors, where these products enjoy the prestige of the exotic, modern, exclusive world unknown to most of the people targeted. Once the products have been accessed by this income tier, the "demonstration effect" introduces them into the low-income sector. In spite of their price - or perhaps because of their price – this sector adopts them as prestige food and they become deceptive substitutes for modern, sumptuary forms of consumption. A poor parent cannot buy an electronic toy, but finds affordable "junk food."

In the past, parents used to feed and raise their children. Now, as can be seen from advertisements and commercials, companies do their best to persuade children that they should decide by themselves what to eat and that parents should indulge them. Urgent political action must be taken against this avoidable source of child obesity. It generates private gains and social losses, since families and states will have to cope with obese children, their treatment, and the comorbilities and disabilities to which consumption of such foods exposes them at a very early age.

Some countries (Australia, the Netherlands, Sweden) ban food advertisements and commercials targeting children under 14 years of age *(50)*, or else they regulate the duration of the latter (12 min/h in the USA). Still, rather than subjecting themselves to restrictions, the food companies have adopted "healthy" disguises, funding health campaigns, "enhancing" their products with vitamins, iron, or calcium, or reducing the amounts of salt and trans fats. The inclusion of a "healthy line of products" enables them to keep on selling unwholesome products while rejecting responsibility for consumers' "wrong" choices. A case in point is a multinational soft drinks company that is currently promoting itself as an advocate of "human hydration." The Institute of Medicine (IOM) has launched a warning that unless the industry changes its practices voluntarily "the Congress should enact legislation mandating the shift" *(51)*. Strong words to deal with a serious issue. The Lancet has adopted a militant approach to the junk food industry, declaring that "desperate moments require desperate measures" against the industry's freedom of action *(52)*.

However, as this is a worldwide epidemic, so should be the corresponding regulations; WTO, WHO, FAO, and other international organizations should play an active part in solving the problem. Otherwise, it might just happen that countries with the means to implement effective controls will have healthy food, while developing countries with limited control mechanisms will be flooded with the junk food that cannot be sold elsewhere. This is similar to what occurred when developed countries issued restrictions on tobacco consumption, and tobacco companies increased their penetration in the rest of the world with China becoming the country with the largest smoking population *(53)*.

The Logic of Market Society: Slim Rich and Fat Poor

For thousands of years, different hunter-gatherer societies, whether village-based or in a preindustrial state stage, based their nutrition on the alternation between plenty and scarcity. Intake was regulated by culture, which encouraged the majority groups of the population to eat, so that they could survive through scarcity. At the same time, the privileged minority that enjoyed abundance was encouraged, in all preindustrial cultures, to eat frugally, making the most of table manners, whose function was to replace quality for quantity. Over the last 50 years, there have been radical global changes, and substantial investment has led us to the end of scarcity: now there is food for everybody. Nevertheless, 2,000 million people survive on less than $1 a day, and 850 million suffer from malnutrition because they cannot access the food that is available *(54)*. In our times, hunger exists because we do nothing about it. There are no valid excuses: we cannot blame natural disasters, or the gods, or fate. In a world of abundance, there is no doubt that hunger is a human creation, stemming from human society, from the social relations that legitimize who is entitled to eat and who is not. Present-day values encourage overproduction and overconsumption in some parts of the world and condemn other parts of the world to subproduction and underconsumption. In the global village, malnutrition and obesity are strongly related. Some of the same factors that result in obese individuals also produce malnourished individuals, and among the urban poor in poor countries one same individual may swing from one condition to the other at different stages of his life, as a malnourished fetus and an obese adult *(55)*.

The social consequences and economic cost of these policies cannot be measured, since they create and promote immeasurable human suffering, armed conflict, humanitarian emergency, international crime, terrorism, clandestine migration, and, needless to say, low quality of life followed by premature death for the victims of these scourges. In contrast, the cost of feeding the 850 million malnourished people recorded by FAO amounts to 10.4 billion dollars a year, while the annual cost for ensuring sound nutrition and health in developing countries is estimated to be $70–$80 billion in addition to the $136 billion currently spent by FAO. The official aid needs for achievement of the millennium development goals have been estimated to be $135 billion rising to $195 billion in 2015 *(56)*.

The logic of profit underlying integrated agroindustry planet-wide has turned food into goods just like any others. If food is good to sell, the logic of profit concludes that only those who can afford food will eat, in an equation ruled by budget rather than by need. There is a direct relation between the creation of profit and the creation of nutrition pathologies. In no way can small local producers compete with the world's agroindustry; as a consequence, products manufactured in developed countries reach the farthest corners of the planet, on the basis of price, prestige, and biological security, homogenizing the taste for certain foods and decreasing the diversity of foods. Such nutritional invasion does not promote health but instead profit. In the global culture "the market" that historically was used to organize the interchange has become the legitimizing factor of society: "the market society" that endows nutritional culture with one single meaning: profit. Then, those who eat are the ones who can afford to pay what the market offers. As the market produces cheap energy foods and expensive foods rich in micronutrients, the relationship of socioeconomic status to obesity has changed. In the past, scarcity had dictated that higher socioeconomic status and obesity have been positively related. In industrialized societies, the relationship is inverted. The latter has been linked to dietary energy density and energy-dense foods *(57, 58)*. In the USA, diets that are more energy-dense cost less *(59)*. In recent years the prices of fresh fruit and vegetables have increased as proportions of disposable income, while those of refined grains, sugars, and fats have declined *(60)*. The same can be said wherever the market is dominated by concentrated agroindustry *(61)*. Argentina's Household Expenditure Surveys have accurately recorded that, as the household average income goes down and prices go up, there is also a reduction in the consumption of fruit, vegetables, dairy products, and meat. Nutrition education has been the same. Mothers responding to the first survey held in 1965 were grandmothers in 1996, when the latest survey was conducted. Over a 30-year span, they replaced fruit, vegetables, and high-quality sources of protein with bread, noodles, sugar, and potatoes, ensuring quantity rather than quality in the family consumption basket. As income increased in high- and middle-income sectors, they diversified their consumption of fruit, vegetables, white meats, and dairy products (mostly cheese), though at the top of the price structure *(62)*. Similar patterns have been observed in Chile and Brazil.

The poor do not adopt poor nutritional strategies simply through ignorance; they know that they should eat meat, vegetables, and dairy products, but they choose that poor diet, in part for financial reasons. Because, if they did not, their income would run out on day 12 of the month. Healthier foods cost more. Costs, other than direct food costs, should also be borne in mind. In developing countries, where utilities such as potable water and gas are not available to the total population, the price of fruit and vegetables includes the time taken up by washing them properly with water that must be carried from far away and the time demanded by cooking techniques. As if this were not discouraging enough, fruit and vegetables do not prove satiating, which makes them even more expensive. Replacing them with carbohydrates and fat is a cost-effective "rational" choice aimed at maximizing income, time, and satiety, independently of nutritional education *(63)*. Similar patterns have been observed in the UK *(64)*. In the USA, Drewnowsky has calculated that it would take about 20 h a week to cook the healthy food recipes recommended in the USA, while a poor working woman cannot devote more than 5 h a week to cooking *(65)*. It does not seem realistic to suggest options that rule out either eating or working, particularly in the case of poor women. As more and more poor women become the heads of household, it is obvious that their families depend on these women's incomes.

In some cases, the same economic constraints that dominate food choices generate physical body aspirations that justify preferences for foods rich in carbohydrates, fats, and sugars. Such cultural representations are "food inclusion principles," involving the ideal body image, food itself, and commensality *(48)*. In low-income Argentine households, an ideal body is supposed to be *strong* to perform intensive labor work, be active, resistant to disease, and exhibit the large size that the sector deems beautiful. Sexist societies apply these characteristics to women rather than to men. To feed a strong body, the chosen food must be *"high performance,"* which means that it should be *tasty* (such as sugars), *cheap* (such as carbohydrates), *satiating* (like fats), and lend itself to *shared commensality*, that is to say, apt for group preparation and consumption (as is the case with soups and stews) on the grounds that food should be enjoyed as long as it is available, since there is no telling what can happen in the future. The "strong body" ideal explains that the consumption of "high-performance" food serves as a justification for the inevitable fate of the poor becoming overweight.

Unlike the malnourished and starving whose circumstance evokes social outrage and encourages political vindication, the obesity of scarcity is *functional to society* as a whole and aids the *reproduction* of poverty in the coming generation. By reducing the obesity of scarcity to the level of an individual problem, it is possible to *avoid political vindication* for the poor's right to nourishment, a right that is not questioned as illegitimate when it is claimed by the malnourished or the starving. Victims of the obesity of scarcity serve a purpose to the market, since they are *consumers* in a cheap "junk food" market made to measure for them. In spite of their lack of micronutrients (in Argentina 30% of the population is mildly lacking in iron) these people *are not incapacitated for work*, but they are discriminated against in the formal labor market because of their obesity. So they join the informal market accounting for 30% of the economy, with high production levels and low salaries. These workers receive governmental *social assistance* programs that provide the same *cheap* agroindustry-generated foodstuffs that are more easily distributed than fresh foods, and *will not be rejected*, for it is exactly the same as the poor already consume in excess. In addition, they receive government aid for medical and pharmacological treatment, which boosts private profit and public losses *(62)*.

In high-income households, with access to both quantity and quality of food, there is awareness of beauty and health market values. Inclusion principles are related to an ideal that celebrates a *healthy slim* body, *light* food (no fat or sugar), and *individual commensality*, in which everyone is responsible for their choices with a view to a healthy, pleasant future.

Income levels, education, and power make this sector hegemonic, which implies that it decides what is legitimate regarding ways of eating – and of living – in society. Seen from this class standpoint, the obesity of scarcity is incomprehensible, since it would suffice to abstain from eating poor quality foods by choosing wisely. Those who ignore economic and cultural determining factors (i.e., the ways in which income level constructs the principles that legitimize the foods characteristic of each level's consumption) tend to view obesity in individual terms. They condemn the obesity of scarcity as they suggest that a suitable education would change present choices, as if the poor enjoyed infinite options. Their options are not between noodles and fruit, but rather between noodles and potatoes, which are essentially varieties of one and the same thing. The options of the poor are structurally limited by the economy, and this is the dominant view in related policies: obesity is a low-income problem yet we offer middle-class solutions *(66)*.

FINAL WORDS

Although recent work *(67)* has gathered many other causes involved in the origin of the epidemic [insufficient sleeping hours, endocrine disrupters, longer life spans in thermoneutrality, reduction of tobacco consumption, pharmacological iatrogenesis, factors related to ethnicity, gender, and age, longer reproductive years, intrauterine malnutrition, and even social networks *(68)*], it should be noted that many result from lifestyle, that is to say, from the social relations we enter in our daily lives. While they may be modifiable, these modifications do not depend on only individual action but also on social action.

To summarize, the global obesity epidemic is caused by the *thrifty genome together with the regulating culture*, spreading across a social environment modified by *market* values that have transformed food and health by providing excessive cheap energy and limited expensive micronutrients while impeding movement. The agroindustry market, supported by subsides, has expanded globally, homogenizing production and consumption and undermining the economies of developing nations after decades of globalization in which inequalities grew deeper *(69)*. Thus, obesity may well result from living in ever more *unequal* societies, as has been stated in an ecological study of obesity in 21 developed nations *(70)*.

Perhaps the fact that the medical model prefers individual solutions, most of its proposals have focused on diet and exercise, as if the problems stemmed from *the patients' "errors."* Pharmacological and surgical solutions pivot around identical concepts: the individual must change his eating habits, whether by chemically reducing his appetite or surgically reducing his stomach, thus supporting billion dollar businesses involving diet foods, medical treatments, nutrition counseling, psychological therapy, surgical treatments, self-help groups, gymnasiums, books, videos, and medication of all kinds. Some of these interventions are useful, but they are not cost-effective methods for treating this global problem.

Attempts at changing individual behavior through education have systematically failed, for they do not take into account the social environment. To justify the fact that they address the effects rather than the causes, these approaches blame the patients for adopting irrational conducts and having addictive personalities. However, future health is just one of the many variables that influence a course of action and it is not the one that looks the most attractive. For decades, the mass media have conveyed to us the messages sent by the industry, urging us to indulge here and now in a soft drink, some chocolate, a hamburger rather than in healthy food. Their success lies in that they do not appeal to health but to pleasure. People do not care exclusively about health, and even when they are aware of the risks, they do not do only what is healthy: they work 14 h a day, smoke, climb mountains, stay up with friends until dawn, among other things. The theory of rational choice establishes that people are rational beings who try to attain the maximum happiness within the constraints of their circumstances such as their income, available time, and other resources. If you want to change behavior, change the costs (measured in dollars, time, or opportunity). Just telling people to stop buying cigarettes will not have much impact, but raising the price of smoking by taxing cigarettes and making smoking inconvenient by banning it from workplaces, restaurants and pubs will (71).

In a profit-driven market society, public health planning should pay much more attention to the economic factors of the world obesity epidemic. The purchasing capacity, the prices of healthy food, and people's economic capacity to afford them have greatest influence. Satiation and preparation time are factors as well.

There is negative advertising that insists that healthy food is tasteless, boring, and difficult to prepare while agroindustry promises quick, improved, laborsaving, preprepared food. The symbolic aspects of our eating culture should not be disregarded, and the industry should focus on offering healthy food adapted to the needs of modern life: fresh, clean, cut, preprocessed vegetables in manageable portions. If healthy food products do not adapt to our times and manners of commensality, we are asking too much of cooking mothers. Moreover, we need to reconstruct a positive image of healthy food, for a brightly colored box filled with junk food enjoys more prestige among a child's peers than does an apple. Therefore, the box is an easier-to-share object of desire. Food does not serve just to quench hunger but to indicate the eater's social standing, so discredited foods do not make good choices. The material aspects of nutrition generate inclusion principles, as we have seen in the Argentine example.

Lifestyle should not be reduced to an individual problem when it originates from the social (economic and symbolic) structure and is shared by millions of people. By reducing the lifestyle to individual conducts and neglecting the characteristics of the social milieu, we turn the tables on the victims and blame them for their own suffering while freeing the society from guilt. Despite empirical evidence, there are still those who insist on detaching individual behavior from its social base, as if each individual were a Robinson confined to his own desert island and isolated from the surrounding dynamics. In fact, social processes like economics and demography will determine a particular constellation of risk factors (an abundance of cheap energy, architectural obstacles to movement) that will lead to the obesity epidemic and its comorbidities. Such critical social processes, all of them consequences of a particular history and culture, make one particular individual prone to this or that risk factor. An individual's choices are neither free nor infinite; they are strongly conditioned by the society's structure of rights, which, in turn, determines the individual's economic status, education, and quality of life. Within these constraints, we can choose *some* parameters about how to live and how to eat. In the market society, each level of income generates a lifestyle within boundaries.

Equals choose among the possible options pertaining to that style. Bourdieu *(72)* explained how the different lifestyles develop, survive, conceal, justify, and reproduce themselves and how limited individual decisions tend to be, as they always choose, as if it were an original decision, something that agrees with the groups' style. Raised in "that" lifestyle, their perception of reality can conceive of only one handful of possible choices for each particular situation.

At present, public health policies are posited as if an individual's decision to go against the stream could be rewarded with good health, without taking into account that the said individual has, since early childhood, lived in a society that stimulates excessive food consumption while barring physical movement. It does not seem likely that people will choose a type of individual behavior that disagrees with that of their peer group, or that he will voluntarily become excluded from his present social life for the sake of future health.

The task awaiting us is not easy. American researcher Marion Nestlé *(45)* points out the difficulty of imagining that the large food companies and their satellites will continue to profit if consumption dwindles. The economists working at the American Department of Agriculture have declared that if people ate more healthily, agriculture and processed food industries would undergo "serious adjustments." Perhaps that is why the answer to the Surgeon General of the United States' 2001 Call for Action is delayed.

As long as the obesity epidemic is regarded as the patient's problem, freeing from responsibility the society that hands him the tools for obesity on a platter, *there will be no political action to transform the social forces that determine obesity*. While addressing the social causes, it should be remembered that we humans eat both nutrients and meanings, so the organization of values in the market society, the logic of profit that legitimizes nonsustainable production, unequal distribution, and induced consumption should all be regarded as serious hindrances to the development of healthy actions to the social aggregate.

This logic gives rise to hunger in poor rural areas and obesity in poor urban areas. By legitimizing the prevailing logic of profit-making, we are consenting to overproduction at any cost, even if it means tricking those who cannot choose, as is the case with children and poor people. Within this logic, health criteria are not worthwhile; thus they should be introduced from the State, regulating the interests of the market for the sake of the common good. It is also necessary to bring some rationality in the agrofood chain with the aim of "caring" for both the environment and the humans who inhabit it with a view to achieve sustainable production, equitable distribution, and commensal consumption.

REFERENCES

1. NHANES – National Health and Nutrition Examination Surveys. Available at http://www.cdc.gov/nchs/nhanes.htm

2. WHO. Ministerial Conference on Counteracting Obesity. European Charter on Counter-acting Obesity. EUR/06/5062700/8. Istanbul, Copenhagen, WHO. Regional Office for Europe, November 16, 2006

3. Caballero B. A nutrition paradox-underweight and obesity in developing countries. N Engl J Med 2005; 352(15): 1514

4. ENNYS – Encuesta Nacional de Nutrición y Factores de Riesgo. Ministerio de Salud, Buenos Aires, 2004

5. INTA – Instituto de Nutrición y Tecnología de los Alimentos. Universidad de Chile, Santiago, 2004

6. Monteiro A, Mondini I. The Nutrition transition in Brazil. Eur J Clin Nutr 1995; 49: 105–113

7. Monteiro C, Moura E, Popkin B. Socioeconomic status and obesity in adult populations of developing countries: a review. Bull World Health Organ 2004; 82: 12

8. Popkin B. The nutrition transition and obesity in the developing world. J. Nutr 2001; 131: 871S–873S

9. Menendez MA, Monteiro CA, Popkin BM. Overweight now exceeds underweight among women in most developing countries. Am J Clin Nutr 2005; 81: 714–721

10. Aguirre P. Gordos de Escasez: las consecuencias de la cocina de la pobreza. In: Maronese L y Alvarez M (eds.) La Cocina como Patrimonio Intangible. 1° Jornada de Patrimonio Gastronómico. Secretaría de Cultura, Gobierno de la Ciudad de Buenos Aires. 2001, pp. 169–189

11. Eaton SB, Konner M. Paleolithic nutrition, a consideration of its nature and current implications. N Engl J Med 1985; 312: 283–290

12. Lev-Ran A. Thrifty genotype: how applicable is it to obesity and type 2 diabetes? Diabetes Rev 1999; 7: 1–22

13. Ross E. Una revisión de las Tendencias dietéticas desde los cazadores-recolectores hasta las sociedades capitalistas modernas. In: Contreras J (ed.) Alimentación y Cultura. Universitat de Barcelona, Necesidades, gustos y costumbres, 1995, pp. 259–307

14. Neel JV. Looking ahead: some genetic issues of the future. Perspect Biol Med 1997; 40: 328–347

15. Aguirre P. Alimentación Humana. Aspectos Culturales. In: Braguinsky J (ed.) Obesidad Saberes y Conflictos, 1st edn. ACINDES-AWWE, Buenos Aires, 2007, pp. 207–237

16. Hayes M, Pietrobelli A, Heymsfield S. Low physical activity levels of modern homo sapiens among free ranging mammals-International. J Obes 2005; 29: 151–156

17. Uliajaszek SJ. Physical activity lifestyle and health of urban populations. In: Schell LM, Ulijaszek SM (eds.) Urbanism, Health, and Human Biology in Industrialized Countries. Cambridge University Press, Cambridge, 1999, pp. 250–279

18. Roberts SB, Dietz W, et al. Multiple laboratory comparison of the doubly labeled water technique. Obes Res 1995; 3(Suppl 1): 3–13

19. Braguinsky J. Gasto energético. In: Braguinsky J. (ed.) Obesidad, Saberes y Conflictos. Un tratado de Obesidad. ACINDES-AWWE, Buenos Aires, 2007, pp. 237–255

20. Heymsfield S. Preface. Am J Clin Nutr 2004; 79(5): 897S–898S

21. Bleich S, Cutler DM, Murray CJ, Adams A. Why is the developed world obese? NBER Working Paper No. W12954, March 2007

22. Braguinsky J. Una Visión Epidemiológica de la Obesidad. In: Braguinsky J (ed.) Obesidad Saberes y Conflictos. Un Tratado de obesidad. ACINDES-AWWE, Buenos Aires, 2007, pp. 45–62

23. Report of a joint WHO/FAO Expert Consultation. Diet, Nutrition, and the Prevention of Chronic Disease. WHO Technical Report Series 196, Geneve, 2003

24. Swinburn BA, Egger G, Raza F. Dissecting obesogenic environments. The development and application of a framework for identifying and prioritizing environmental interventions for obesity. Prev Med 1999; 29: 563–570

25. Office of the United Nations High Commissioner on Human Rights on the Right to Food. Special Reporter of the Commission on Human Rights on the Right to Food. October 2006. Available at http://www.ohchr.org/English/issues/food/htm

26. Smil V. Feeding the World. A Challenge for the Twenty-First Century. Massachussets Institute of Technology Press, Cambridge, MA, 2000

27. Benoit D. Quelques faits marquants de la dynamique récente des échanges de produits alimentaires en Economie Rurale, 234/5, Paris, 1996, pp. 11–35

28. Gallo A. The Food Marketing System in 1996. Agriculture Information Bulletin No. 743. Department of Agriculture - Economic Research Service, Washington, DC, September 5, 1998, pp. 19–21

29. Fritscher M. Los límites de la Agricultura Industrial.¿Hacia un nuevo paradigma? Polis. Departamento de Sociología, UNAM, México, 2001, p. 127

30. USDA Conference "On the Farm Hill and the Implications for World Trade". Washington, DC, May 22, 2002

31. Aguirre P. Seguridad Alimentaria. En: Plan de Acción para la Alimentación y Nutrición en Argentina. FAO-Ministerio de Salud, Buenos Aires, 1996, pp. 65–79

32. OECD. Agricultural Policies. At a Glance. OECD, Paris, 2004

33. FAO. World Agriculture Towards 2015/2030. Summary Report. FAO, Rome, 2002

34. Schäfer Elinder L. Obesity, hunger, and agriculture: the damaging role of subsidies. BMJ 2005; 331: 1333–1336

35. OXFAM. Milking the CAP. How European Dairy Regime is Devastating Livelihoods in the Developing World. Oxfam, Oxford, 2002

36. Trueba I (ed.) El Fin del Hambre en 2025. Un Desafío para Nuestra Generación. FAO, Grupo Mundi-Prensa, 2006

37. Swedish National Food Administration. In: Schäfer Elinder L. op cit: p. 1334

38. Ricardo D. Principios de Economía Política y tributación. Fondo de Cultura Económica, Buenos Aires, 1998

39. Piermartini R. The Role of Export Taxes in the Field of Primary Commodities. OMC, Ginebra, Suiza, 2004

40. Mintz S. Dulzura y Poder. El lugar del Azúcar en la Historia Moderna. Siglo XXI Editores, México, 1996

41. Aguirre P. La Cocina, Comida y Comensales en el Río de la Plata. En Población y Bienestar. Una historia Social del siglo XX. Torrado S. Compiladora. Tomo 2. EDHASA, Buenos Aires, 2007, pp. 469–505

42. Giddens A. Modernity and Self-Identity. Self and Society in the Late Modern Age. Polity Press and Blackwell, London, 1991

43. Henderson D. Between the farm gate and the dinner plate: motivations for industrial change in the processed food sector. In: The Future of Food. OECD, Paris, 1998, pp. 126–148

44. Harris M. Good to Eat. Simon and Shuster, New York, 1985

45. Fischler C. El (H)omnívoro: el gusto, la cocina, el cuerpo. Anagrama, Barcelona, 1995

46. Young L, Nestle M. Expanding portion sizes in the U.S. marketplace: implications for nutrition counseling. J Am Diet Assoc 2003; 103(2): 231–234

47. Chopra M, Galbraith S, Darnton-Hill I. A global response to a global problem: the epidemic of overnutrition. Bull World Health Organ 2002; 80(12): 952–958

48. Koplan JP, Liverman CT, Kraak VI (eds.) Preventing Childhood Obesity. Health in the Balance. National Academies Press, Washington, DC, 2005

49. Nestle M. Food marketing and childhood obesity. A matter of policy. N Engl J Med 2006; 354(24): 2527–2529

50. Story M, French S. Food advertising and marketing direct as childrens and adolescents in the US. Int J Behav Nutr Phys Act 2004; 1(1): 3

51. MCGinnis JM, Gootman JA, Kraak VI (eds.) Food Marketing to Children and Youth: Threat or Opportunity? National Academies Press, Washington, DC, 2006

52. Getting a handle on obesity. The Lancet 2002; 359(9322): 1955

53. China: A Study of Smoking Habits. Horizon Consultancy Group, Beijing, 2006

54. Ziegler J. The Right to Food. Commission of Human Right Resolution 2006/25. Special Consultant about Food Rights, UN, 2007

55. Breier BH, Vickers MH, Ikenasio BA, Chan KY, Wong PS. Fetal programming of appetite and obesity. Mol Cell Endocrinol 2001; 185(1–2): 73–79

56. Sachs JD, Mc Arthur JW. The millennium project. A plan for meeting the millennium development goals. Lancet 2005; 365: 347–353

57. Darmon N, Ferguson AL, Briend A. A cost constraint alone has adverse effects on food selection and nutrient density: an analysis of human diets by linear programming. J Nutr 2002; 132: 3764–3771

58. French SA. Pricing effects on food choice. J Nutr 2003; 133: 841S–843S

59. Drewnowsky A, Darmon N. The economic of obesity: dietary energy density and energy cost. Am J Clin Nutr 2005; 82: 265S–273S

60. Strurm R. Childhood obesity. What we can learn from existing data on societal trends. Part 2. Prev Chronic Dis 2005; 2: A20

61. Calvo E, Aguirre P. Crisis de la seguridad alimentaria en la Argentina y estado nutricional en una población vulnerable. Arch Argent Pediatr SAP Buenos Aires 2005; 103(1): 77–91

62. Aguirre P. Estrategias de Consumo Qué comen los argentinos que comen. CIEPP-Miño y Dávila Eds, Buenos Aires, 2005

63. Aguirre P. Ricos-Flacos. Gordos-Pobres. La Alimentación en Crisis. Ed Capital Intelectual, Colección Claves para Todos, Buenos Aires, 2004. p. 90

64. Doeler E. The Welfare of Food. Blackwell, London, 2003

65. Drewnowski A. Obesity and the food environment. Dietary energy density and diet cost. Am J Prevent Med 2004; 27: 154–162

66. Drewnowsky A, Popkin B. The nutrition transition: new trends in the global diet. Nutr Rev 1997; 55(2): 31–44

67. Keith SW, Redden DT, Katzmarzyk PT, Boggiano MM, Hanlon EC, Benca RM, Ruden D, Pietrobelli A, Barger JL, Fontaine KR, Wang C, Aronne LJ, Wright SM, Baskin M, Dhurandhar NV, Lijoi MC, Grilo CM, DeLuca M, Westfall AO, Allison DB. Putative contributors to the secular increase in obesity: exploring the roads less traveled. Int J Obes 2006; 30: 1565–1594

68. Christakis NA, Fowler J. The spread of obesity in a large social network over 32 years. N Engl J Med 2007; 357: 370–379

69. DeLong B. Estimating World GDP. One Million BC. Present. University of Berkeley, California. Available at http://www.econ.berkeley.edu/TCEH/estimatingworldGDP.htm

70. Pickett KE, Nelly S, Brunner E, Lobstein T, Wilkinson RG. Wider income gaps, wide waistbands? An ecological study of obesity and income inequality. J Epidemiol Community Health 2005; 59: 670–674

71. McCarthy M. The economics of obesity. Lancet 2004; 364: 2169–2170, http://www.thelancet.com

72. Bourdieu P. La Distinción. Criterios y Bases Sociales del Gusto. Taurus, Madrid, 1985

7

Eating Disorders and Depression in Women with Diabetes

Patricia A. Colton and Gary Rodin

Abstract

The close relationship between the physical and mental health of individuals with diabetes has been clearly demonstrated. This is most evident in eating disorders and depression, two common mental health problems in women with diabetes. The presence of either or both of these problems can interfere significantly with the ability to achieve optimal metabolic control and can lead to an increased risk of diabetes-related medical complications. There is a substantial female preponderance in the occurrence of eating disorders, due to gender-related factors. Depression is also more common in women, an association that has been linked to socioeconomic factors and adverse life events experienced more frequently by women. Effective treatments are available for both of these comorbid conditions, although evidence suggests that they are often overlooked in medical settings. Treatment of these mental health problems in individuals with diabetes has the potential to improve outcomes with regard to diabetes and other health states, as well as overall well-being.

This chapter provides an introduction to eating disorders and depression in association with diabetes, the potential mechanisms that account for this association and the detection and management of these comorbid conditions.

Key words: Mental health and diabetes; Eating disorders; Depression; Psychosocial adjustment to diabetes.

From: *Diabetes in Women: Pathophysiology and Therapy*
Edited by: A. Tsatsoulis et al. (eds.), DOI 10.1007/978-1-60327-250-6_7
© Humana Press, a part of Springer Science+Business Media, LLC 2009

EATING DISORDERS AND DEPRESSION: AN INTRODUCTION

Eating disorders are a group of psychosomatic conditions characterized by disturbed eating behavior and a constellation of psychological traits and symptoms. "Disturbed eating behavior" refers to dieting and fasting, binge eating episodes and compensatory behavior for weight control. The latter includes excessive exercise for weight loss, and purging behavior, such as self-induced vomiting and the abuse of laxatives, diuretics and diet pills. Individuals with diabetes have an additional purging behavior available to them, namely, the dangerous practice of deliberate insulin dosage manipulation or omission to promote weight loss. This behavior has more recently been named "diabulimia." By decreasing, delaying or eliminating prescribed insulin doses, an individual can induce hyperglycemia and rapidly lose calories in the urine, termed glycosuria. Less dramatic neglect of insulin therapy, such as irregular blood sugar monitoring and inadequate adjustment of insulin dosage to compensate for fluctuations in food intake, is very common and may occur with varying degrees of intentionality.

Although dietary dysregulation is the most obvious manifestation of eating disorders, these conditions are also associated with underlying disturbances in the body image, self-concept and emotional life of individuals affected. Individuals with these disturbances may manifest high levels of concern and distress about body weight and shape, distortions of body image (for example, believing that they are overweight when at a normal or low weight), overvaluation of weight and shape in the determination of self-concept, fears of gaining weight or becoming fat, and disturbed attitudes toward food, calories and eating (1). Mood, substance use and personality disorders are all substantially more common in those with full-syndrome and subthreshold eating disorders than in the general population (2–5). Indeed, significant depressive symptoms have been identified in 40–70% of individuals with eating disorders (6–10).

The comorbid association of eating disorders and depression could arise for a variety of reasons. Negative emotional states, including intense feelings of depression, anger or anxiety, may precipitate the full range of disturbed eating behavior (11, 12), in addition to other maladaptive behavior. It has also been suggested that binge eating, vomiting, extreme food restriction and other weight-control behavior may be used to help modulate or to distract oneself from depressed mood, or to give the illusion of control or mastery by focusing on a specific aspect of self-regulation (11, 12). Severe eating disorders are also associated with frequent medical complications and a significant mortality rate. In a meta-analysis of outcome studies of anorexia nervosa, crude mortality rate was found to be 5% at 4–10-year follow-up, and 9% at follow-up after 10 years (13).

Disturbed body image, eating attitudes, eating behavior and the associated emotional distress and functional impairment occur along a continuum of severity. More severe symptoms at one end of this continuum may meet DSM-IV-TR (Diagnostic and Statistical Manual of Mental Disorders, fourth edition, text revision) (1) diagnostic criteria for a "full-syndrome" eating disorder. These disorders are categorized into three primary groupings, namely anorexia nervosa, bulimia nervosa and eating disorder not otherwise specified (ED-NOS). The diagnosis of anorexia nervosa requires significant weight loss, amenorrhea and severely disturbed body image. Bulimia nervosa involves binge eating episodes and compensatory behavior, both of which must occur, on average, twice weekly, as well as body image disturbance. ED-NOS encompasses a heterogeneous group of disorders, including binge eating disorder and other disorders that are of clinical significance, but which do not meet exact criteria for anorexia nervosa or bulimia nervosa. There are also milder, subthreshold variants of all of the above that do not meet full DSM-IV criteria, but which may still represent a significant health risk and deserve clinical attention in individuals with diabetes.

Eating disorders may be the most gender-specific psychological problem, with a frequency in adult females in the general population estimated to be 10–12 times greater than that of males (14, 15).

The etiology of these conditions appears to be complex and multifactorial, likely involving the influence of genetic, individual, family, peer group and sociocultural factors (16, 17). In that regard, body dissatisfaction and disturbed eating behavior are more common in social or cultural contexts in which a thin, fit female ideal is highly valued, and in which obesity is considered unacceptable or unattractive in women (18, 19). Bulimia nervosa and its subthreshold variants are more common in Western countries, although their prevalence has been increasing in non-Western countries; anorexia nervosa, by contrast, does not appear to be culture bound (20). Many girls and women, with and without diabetes, now experience contradictory environmental pressures regarding dietary intake. There are pervasive influences for women in many cultures to enhance their self-worth by striving for an unrealistic body weight and shape through dieting, while they are simultaneously exposed to large quantities of high calorie, palatable foods that promote overeating and weight gain

Prospective longitudinal studies in the general population have consistently identified a number of individual risk factors for the development of eating disorders. These include the following: dietary restraint and dieting; weight gain and being overweight; early puberty compared to peers; low self-esteem; disturbed family functioning; disturbed parental eating attitudes; peer and cultural influences, and a range of personality traits (21–25). Considerable evidence, reviewed later in the chapter, has also accumulated to suggest that living with DM1 is a risk factor for disturbed eating behavior and eating disorders.

The increased risk of eating disorders in girls and young women with DM1 appears to be due to multiple, interacting factors related to diabetes and its management. These postulated factors include: the increased body mass and consequent body dissatisfaction that may result from effective insulin therapy (26, 27); the perceived dietary restraint related to diabetes dietary management (28); the availability of deliberate insulin omission as a ready means of controlling weight (29), and the effects of diabetes on self-concept, body image (30) and family interactions (31). Developmental issues, related to the balance between autonomy and confidence in one's ability to care for oneself and the development of meaningful relationships and emotional closeness, are often central psychological concerns of individuals with eating disorders (32). Associated conflicts about mastery, control and decision-making may emerge in the family dynamics of individuals with diabetes and eating disorders (31).

The most consistent longitudinal predictor of the emergence of eating disorders is dieting and disturbed eating behavior, (33, 34) which tend to persist and worsen over time (35–38). For example, teenage girls who diet "severely" are at 18-fold risk, compared with nondieters, to develop an eating disorder in the subsequent 3 years, and moderate dieters are at 5-fold risk (34). Similarly, the presence of a range of eating problems in childhood and adolescence strongly predicts the development of eating disorders in adulthood (39). Longitudinal findings indicate that dieting may be considered either a risk factor for the onset of a clinically significant eating disorder or an early stage in its development. Although the majority of dieters never go on to develop an eating disorder, dieting is an almost universal first step in those who do eventually develop a full-syndrome eating disorder. Diabetes management may be an iatrogenic factor that encourages prolonged attention to food intake and dietary restraint, which can eventually trigger dietary dysregulation with overeating and binge eating episodes. A vulnerable individual may then intensify efforts to control food intake and weight, thereby becoming trapped in a cycle of dieting, further binge eating, weight-control and purging behavior.

Although recent innovations in diabetes management have enabled many individuals to adopt a more flexible eating plan, carbohydrate counting still commonly underlies diabetes meal planning. Individuals with diabetes, particularly those with DM2 and/or metabolic syndrome, often receive medical recommendations to reduce body weight and to limit cholesterol and carbohydrate intake. Diabetes meal plans are now more flexible than many weight-loss diets, but they still increase the focus on food and calories, and may be experienced as restrictive. Although an optimal diabetes meal plan is well balanced and has adequate calories, the restriction of certain foods resembles that of many weight-loss diets. This encouragement to follow an imposed eating plan, rather than to eat in response to internal cues for hunger and satiety, may constitute a pathway of risk for the development of disturbed eating behavior.

Appropriate diabetes management may contribute to an increased risk of eating disorders, in part, because intensive insulin therapy is associated with weight gain *(27)*. In that regard, it has been shown that adolescent girls and adult women with DM1, on average, have significantly higher BMI values than their nondiabetic peers *(26, 27, 40, 41)*. This increased weight may heighten body dissatisfaction in young women and increase the risk of dieting and binge eating. This risk appears to be relatively specific to females, since girls are more likely than boys to believe that they are overweight or to be dissatisfied with their weight *(42, 43)*.

Diabetes may lower the threshold for the development of disturbed eating behavior through the dietary restraint imposed by diabetes management. However, food or bodily preoccupation alone may not be a sufficient risk factor for the development of eating disorders. Eating disorders have not been shown to occur at increased rates in conditions such as cystic fibrosis, in which there is pressure to increase food intake *(44)*, nor in adolescents with scoliosis *(45)*, who have an altered body appearance. There is a gender-related gradient of risk for disturbed eating attitudes in individuals with and without DM1, with the highest disturbances in females with DM1, the lowest in males without DM1, and intermediate disturbances in nondiabetic females and males with DM1 *(46–48)*. Gender may also interact with other risk factors for eating disturbances. For example, although adolescent boys with DM1 have higher BMI values and an elevated drive for thinness than their nondiabetic peers, they do not appear to be at increased risk to suffer from an eating disorder *(49)*. The gender-specific risk of eating disorders appears to be due to individual, family and sociocultural factors that amplify the body dissatisfaction and distress related to an elevated BMI in girls and women with diabetes.

DIABETES AND EATING DISORDERS: EPIDEMIOLOGY AND CLINICAL FEATURES

There has been controversy in the literature about the association of eating disorders and DM1 *(50)*. However, the evidence from methodologically rigorous studies and from a meta-analytic review *(51)* supports the view that there is an increased risk for both subthreshold and full-syndrome eating disorders in girls and women with DM1. In studies using a diagnostic interview, the prevalence of full-syndrome eating disorders in girls and women with DM1 ranged from 0 to 11%, and the prevalence of subthreshold eating disorders from 7 to 35% *(52–60)*. An increased risk of disturbed eating behavior in girls with DM1 can be detected even in the preteen years, with disturbed eating behavior reported by girls as young as 9 and 10 years of age *(52)*.

There is no clear association between DM2 and disturbed eating behavior, although this relationship has been less extensively investigated in DM2 than in DM1. Binge eating disorder appears to be the most common eating disorder in those with DM2 *(61)*. It has been suggested that the diagnosis and management of DM2 does not generally worsen or precipitate an eating disorder *(62)*, but eating disorders are more likely to be found in those with DM2 because of its association with being overweight.

Metabolic control in DM1 often worsens during the adolescent period, particularly in girls *(63, 64)*. Although hormonal factors may be partially responsible for this deterioration *(65)*, our research group and others have postulated that disturbed eating behavior, often including deliberate insulin omission, is a common behavioral cause of this worsening of metabolic control. Deliberate insulin dosage manipulation or omission, which induces high blood sugar levels and the spilling of glucose in the urine, is the most common method of purging in girls with DM1, and becomes progressively more common through the teen years. This behavior is reported by only 2% of preteen girls *(52)*, but its prevalence increases to rates as high as 15% by the midteen years *(29, 55, 60, 66, 67)*, and to 30–39% in the late teenage and early adult years *(66, 68)*. The reason most frequently cited by young women with DMI for deliberate insulin omission is weight control, although other motivating factors include fear of hypoglycemia, denial of having diabetes, embarrassment about blood sugar testing or insulin administration in front of others, desire to have a "holiday" from diabetes management, fear of needles and secondary gain *(68, 69)*. One or all of these other motivating factors can operate, in combination with a desire to control weight, to reinforce or rationalize the insulin omission behavior.

There are currently four published longitudinal studies of disturbed eating behavior in individuals with DM1 *(66, 67, 70, 71)*, but none in individuals with DM2. Bryden and colleagues' study *(70)* had a small sample size (*n* = 33) and insufficient power to detect a significant association between disturbed eating behavior and diabetes-related medical outcomes. Colton and colleagues' 5-year follow-up study showed that disturbed eating behavior is common and persistent in pre-teen and teenage girls with DM1 *(67)*. Of girls with disturbed eating behavior early in the study, 92% continued to report disturbed eating behavior at subsequent follow-up. By age 14–18, half of the participants reported current disturbed eating behavior, and 13% of the sample met criteria for a full-syndrome or subthreshold eating disorder. Our group also conducted a 4-year follow-up of 91 young women with DM1 *(66)*, in which disturbed eating behavior at baseline was associated with a tripled rate of diabetic retinopathy 4 years later. Peveler and colleagues *(71)* also found high rates of medical complications and significant mortality in young women with DM1 and antecedent eating disorders. Others have reported similar findings in smaller, cross-sectional samples of young women with DM1 *(72–75)*.

Disturbed eating behavior is of great clinical concern because it increases the risk of diabetic ketoacidosis, hospitalization and diabetes-related medical complications, particularly retinopathy and neuropathy *(66, 69, 73, 74)*. Both subthreshold and full-syndrome eating disorders have been shown to be associated with poor metabolic control *(54, 55, 66, 76)* and blood lipid abnormalities *(72, 77)*. Each of these effects can independently increase the risk of long-term diabetes-related complications, affecting multiple body systems. Eating disorders are also associated with elevated mortality in those with DMI *(51, 71, 78)*. In Nielsen's registry-based study *(78)*, after approximately 10 years of follow-up, mortality rates were 2.2 (per 1,000 person-years) for individuals with DM1, 7.3 for individuals with anorexia nervosa, and 34.6 for individuals with both DM1 and anorexia nervosa.

DEPRESSION AND DIABETES

The term "depression" refers both to a mood state and, when severe, persistent, and associated with a number of other symptoms, to a clinical syndrome or disorder. Depressive disorders include major depressive disorder, bipolar disorder and dysthymic disorder, a more chronic, less severe form of depression. The term "minor depression" or subthreshold depression refers to depressive symptoms of at least 2 weeks duration that fall short of full diagnostic criteria for a major depressive episode or dysthymic disorder. Symptoms that meet diagnostic criteria for a major depressive episode include some or all of the following characteristics present for at least 2 weeks: a sustained period of low, sad mood, a loss of interest and enjoyment, low energy, sleep disruption, changes in appetite and weight, poor concentration, low self-esteem, feelings of hopelessness and guilt, and, in some cases, thoughts about death and suicide. The lifetime prevalence of major depressive disorder in the general population is more than 15% *(79)*, and is higher in women than in men. Between 2 and 4% of adults in the general population are experiencing a current major depressive episode at any given time *(80)*. Rates of depression are higher in individuals with most major medical conditions, including both DM1 and

DM2. In these conditions, depression is linked to factors such as physical distress and disability, disease severity, prior history of depression and low social support *(81)*. Like eating disorders, depressive symptoms occur along a continuum of severity, and the threshold for clinical concern and intervention should be lower when associated with diabetes than in nonmedical populations.

It has been shown in a variety of studies that depressive disorders are at least twice as common in those with DM1 or DM2, including in children, teens and adults with diabetes, as in the general population *(82–86)*. These findings were supported by a recent meta-analysis of 39 studies including more than 20,000 subjects, which indicated that the risk of depression in diabetes is twice that of the general population *(87)*, and that 29% of adults with either DM1 or DM2 meet lifetime criteria for major depressive disorder. Some studies suggest that depression in individuals with diabetes is characterized by longer episodes, higher recurrence rates and lower recovery rates *(88, 89)*. The association of depression with DM2 appears to be reciprocal, since depression has been identified as a risk factor for the onset of DM2 *(90)*. Further, depression has been associated not only with impaired metabolic control but also with increased mortality in patients with DM2 *(91–93)*.

Women with diabetes are more likely to suffer both from depression and from its consequences. A large meta-analysis *(87)* demonstrated that the female preponderance of depression in association with diabetes mirrors the increased prevalence of depression in women in the general population *(94, 95)*. Other evidence also suggests that, among those with diabetes, women and those with less education and social support are more likely to be depressed *(96, 97)*. Although biological factors have been proposed to account for the increased risk of depression in women, evidence from the general population suggests that the gender effect may be largely attributed to sociocultural factors, psychological attributes and adverse life events that disproportionately affect women *(94)*.

Both biological and psychological mechanisms have been postulated to account for the relationship between depression and impaired metabolic control in diabetes. The impact of depression on blood sugar levels may be due to its adverse effect on treatment adherence, including managing diabetes self-care tasks and attending medical appointments *(98)*. The relationship between depression and poor compliance with diabetes treatment may be reciprocal. Depression can lead to lower self-efficacy and to self-neglecting and self-defeating behaviors, such as poor adherence to blood glucose monitoring, meal plan and exercise recommendations, while variations in blood sugar level can contribute to depressive symptoms *(99)*. It has also been postulated, but not confirmed, that the metabolic abnormalities associated with diabetes lead to changes in brain structure and function, which then render individuals more susceptible to developing a depressive disorder *(100)*.

The presence of depressive symptoms in patients with diabetes should be of clinical concern for a number of reasons, including their effect on quality of life, health status and healthcare utilization. Major depressive disorder has been estimated to be the fourth leading global cause of disability *(101)*, and is associated with greater decrements in global health scores than asthma, angina or diabetes itself. The combination of diabetes and depression is associated with particularly severe impairment in global health scores and quality of life *(102)*. A recent study of people with diabetes indicated that depression is associated with a 50–75% increase in health services costs, only 15% of which is related to mental health services costs *(103)*. Similar findings were reported by Kalsekar et al. who found that patients with diabetes and depression had nearly 65% higher overall health costs than those without depression *(104)*. A review of cross-sectional, longitudinal and treatment studies of patients with a variety of chronic medical conditions *(105)* indicated that depression significantly increases functional impairment in these populations, and that its treatment reduces both disability and health service costs. Depressive symptoms have also been associated with impaired metabolic control in patients with DM1 *(82, 106, 107)*, and both minor and major depression are associated with increased mortality in patients with DM2 *(92)*.

It has been argued that the threshold for the diagnosis of major depression in current psychiatric diagnostic criteria, such as in the DSM-IV, is too low, and that diagnosing cases of mild to moderate major depressive disorder might be pathologizing normal sadness. In that vein, it has been reported that the majority of individuals with diabetes who have elevated scores on self-report measures of depression do not meet full diagnostic criteria for major depressive disorder (97). However, while this categorical distinction has relevance for psychiatric nosology, evidence suggests that continuous measures of depression best predict difficulties with adherence to diet, exercise and glucose self-monitoring regimens. Further, even low levels of depressive symptoms are associated with nonadherence to important aspects of diabetes self-care (107).

Depression may also be of concern in individuals with diabetes because of its association with health risk behaviors and medical morbidity. The health risk behaviors with which depression is associated include cigarette smoking, overeating, physical inactivity and obesity. The adverse effects of which are amplified in those with comorbid diabetes. Whatever the mechanism that accounts for the comorbidity of depression and diabetes, depression has also been associated with an increased risk of diabetes-related medical complications, including sexual dysfunction, retinopathy, nephropathy, heart disease, and stroke (82, 108). Because of the reciprocal relationship between depression and metabolic control, attention to both mood disturbances and to diabetes management may be necessary in order to prevent or delay the progression of diabetes complications.

The emerging Western epidemics of diabetes and obesity are linked (109) and demonstrate some gender effects. The prevalence of obesity is estimated to have increased by 60% in the United States in the past decade (110), and it has been estimated that nearly one in three adults and one in six children and adolescents are now overweight (111). Some research suggests that women have higher obesity rates across all age groups, although these rates are also affected by racial, ethnic and socio-economic factors (112). It has been suggested that a consistent relationship between obesity and depression has not been demonstrated because of the influence of gender (113). In that regard, in a large study, Istvan and colleagues (114) found a relationship between obesity and depression in women but not in men. Similarly, obesity was associated with a 37% increase in the prevalence of major depressive disorder in women but with a reduction in the prevalence of major depressive disorder in men (115). Other evidence suggests that the association of depression with obesity in women may be mediated through the impact of the latter on self-esteem and body dissatisfaction (113).

The increased health risks associated with depression when comorbid with either eating disorders and/or diabetes is likely due to both biological and behavioral mechanisms. Both depressive symptoms (99, 116) and eating disorders (55, 66) can independently have adverse effects on metabolic control, likely via both behavioral and neuroendocrine pathways. Impaired memory, motivation and problem-solving in either condition, intentional insulin omission in those with eating disorders, and effects of depression on the hypothalamic-adrenal axis and the degree of insulin resistance (86) can all affect metabolic control. Both depression (91) and eating disorders (51, 71) independently increase medical morbidity and mortality rates in individuals with diabetes. In women with either DM1 or DM2, depression is associated with an earlier time to onset of coronary artery disease, independent of other identified risk factors (117). In addition, both depression (118) and disturbed eating behavior (66) are associated with an increased risk of progressive retinopathy.

An enduring significant stressful childhood experience is an established risk factor for depression (119). The ongoing challenges of living with both diabetes may contribute to such stress through its effects on family functioning, social relationships and morale (85). This may account for the finding that teenage girls and women with both diabetes and an eating disorder are more depressed than diabetic controls without an eating disorder (59, 120), and have poorer metabolic control (59). This is of particular concern as early onset depression is more likely to be chronic and severe (121).

The presence of a medical condition, such as diabetes, can adversely affect the body image and self-concept of some women and contribute to a lowering of mood. Those with the onset of diabetes during or prior to childbearing years may worry about their partner's reaction to the condition, its influence on their ability to bear children or the genetic transmission of the disease. Having a chronic medical condition can also contribute to a lack of a sense of control or predictability in relation to the body, to feelings of bodily defectiveness, or to enduring feelings of grief and unfairness related to the diagnosis and burden of the disease. These factors, together with the multiple and complex daily tasks of diabetes management, the difficulty optimizing blood sugar levels the family strain related to managing diabetes, and the risk of diabetes-related medical complications, all may contribute to feelings of frustration, helplessness and depression.

EATING DISORDERS AND DEPRESSION: SCREENING AND TREATMENT

In view of the high rates of both depression and eating disorders and their medical consequences in girls and women with diabetes, regular screening for these problems should be incorporated into their primary medical care, beginning in the preteen years. Questions about persistent mood alterations, loss of interest in activities, lowering of motivation or energy level, or sleep problems, can reveal the presence of a mood disturbance. Enquiry about satisfaction with weight and shape, dieting, binge eating and weight-control behavior can uncover difficulties with body image and eating behavior. There are well-validated self-report screening measures for both depression and eating disorders that can be useful in the medical clinic setting. Scales commonly used to screen for depressive symptoms in this context include the Center for Epidemiologic Studies Depression Scale *(122)*, the Beck Depression Inventory-II *(123)* and the PHQ-9 *(124)*. Appropriate screening measures for eating disorders include the Eating Attitudes Test *(125)* and the modified Diagnostic Survey for Eating Disorders (DSED) *(126)*, both of which have been used in individuals with diabetes. Diagnoses should be confirmed by clinical interview in those individuals whose scores on a self-report measure indicate the possibility of a clinically significant disturbance.

In women with diabetes, several warning signs may suggest the presence of either depression or an eating disorder. These include the following: overall deterioration in psychosocial functioning (including school attendance and performance, work functioning and interpersonal relationships); worsening in metabolic control; increasing neglect of diabetes management, including blood sugar monitoring, insulin titration and adherence to other medications; erratic clinic attendance; significant weight gain or weight loss; increased concern about meal planning and food composition; and somatic complaints, including low energy, fatigue, disrupted sleep and increased worries about physical health. In some cases, family members will raise concerns about depression or disturbed eating before the individual with diabetes does so. If worsening metabolic control is due to intentional insulin omission, the individual may appear surprisingly unconcerned, and may initially deny that she has engaged in this behavior. Such denial may allow the individual to avoid reactions of disappointment, criticism, fear, or anger from their family or their diabetes team. It may also help them to avoid the threat of weight gain often associated with improving metabolic control. Indeed, it is often challenging for family and care-givers to tolerate the knowledge that the individual with diabetes continues to engage in disturbed eating behavior, particularly insulin omission, with such dangerous health consequences. Although individuals with either depression or an eating disorder may be reluctant to seek treatment, defensiveness about or refusal of treatment has been more commonly described in association with eating disorders. Adopting a nonjudgmental stance and using motivation enhancement techniques to facilitate exploration of the benefits and dangers of an eating disorder and recovery is often more helpful than warnings or "scare tactics" to engage these individuals in treatment for their eating disorder. If an eating disorder is known or suspected to be present, early referral to a mental health professional with experience working with individuals with eating disorders is warranted.

Both antidepressant medication and some modalities of psychotherapy have proven useful in decreasing or eradicating binge eating and purging symptoms, in studies conducted in nondiabetic populations. There have been several positive randomized controlled trials of cognitive-behavioral therapy for bulimia nervosa and binge eating disorder (127). Cognitive-behavioral therapy is a time-limited psychotherapy, usually 16–20 1-hour sessions, which is intended to help the individual to better understand the links between distorted thought patterns, negative emotions, and maladaptive behavioral patterns. Through this intervention, patients learn and practice ways of challenging negative thoughts and altering their environment and behavior in order to stop engaging in eating disorder behavior. There is a strong focus in this intervention on normalizing eating patterns. This includes eating in a planned way and at regular intervals during the day, as well as incorporating a broad variety of foods into the meal plan, which serves to diminish food cravings and binge eating of "forbidden foods." In our clinical experience, having an explicit treatment contract (e.g., number of planned sessions, consultation with their endocrinologist, and use of urgent care services if necessary), with negotiated and concrete treatment goals (e.g., related to specific aspects of diabetes management, such as checking blood glucose regularly and taking insulin appropriately) is important. Interpersonal therapy is another time-limited (e.g., 16–20 1-hour sessions) psychotherapy in which the patient and her therapist choose a specific interpersonal area of current difficulty on which to focus throughout the therapy. The problem area is grouped into one of the four major themes (a) unresolved grief, (b) interpersonal role disputes, (c) role transitions, or (d) deficits in social relationships (128). The goal of therapy is to work toward resolving current difficulties in that interpersonal area by developing and practising skills in effective communication and conflict resolution, and by strengthening meaningful social relationships. Interestingly, in randomized controlled trials of interpersonal therapy, improvements in eating behavior occur even without overt focus on eating or body image (129). Those with more severe disturbances may require more intensive treatment, including either day hospitalization or inpatient hospitalization, to achieve full remission of bulimic symptoms. We have found that intensive treatment of more severe eating disorders associated with diabetes is most likely to achieve sustained optimization of blood sugar levels. There is a paucity of evidence for effective treatment of anorexia nervosa, although some of the most promising results have been obtained with family therapy for adolescents, with benefit sustained at 5-year follow-up (130). Treatment of anorexia nervosa generally focuses on medical stabilization, nutritional rehabilitation and weight gain into a healthy range, along with a variety of individual and family psychotherapeutic approaches (131), including motivation enhancement and cognitive-behavioral therapy.

Evidence-based treatment guidelines for the management of both depression and eating disorders have been published, including those from the American Psychiatric Association (131) and the Canadian Psychiatric Association (132). However, there is limited evidence regarding the effectiveness and efficacy of the various treatment modalities to support the application of these guidelines in special populations, such as women with diabetes. There are few treatment studies in this population; although a small, uncontrolled study of cognitive-behavioral therapy for an eating disorder in women with DM1 (133) suggested that treatment may be more difficult in women with DM1 and an eating disorder than in those without DM1. A small study of "integrated inpatient treatment" of individuals with DM1 and an eating disorder showed promising reductions in eating disorder symptoms (134) maintained at 3-year follow-up. However, validation of these results would require a study with a larger sample and with inclusion of a control group. Our group conducted the first randomized controlled treatment study for disturbed eating attitudes and behavior in individuals with diabetes (135). We found that a brief psychoeducational intervention offered to girls 12–19 years of age with DM1 was associated with reductions in dieting, body dissatisfaction, and preoccupation with thinness and eating, and that these improvements were maintained at 12-month follow-up. However, the intervention did not result in significant improvements in metabolic control or insulin omission for weight control.

There is some evidence for the effectiveness of the treatment of depression in association with diabetes. Antidepressant medication, cognitive-behavioral therapy and problem-solving therapy have been shown to improve depression outcomes in individuals with diabetes *(136–139)*, as they have in general population studies *(132)*. Those with depression and more severe medical complications may benefit most from collaborative care, which may better allow the multiple needs of these patients to be addressed *(140)*. Collaborative care, including a stepped care approach delivered by specialized nurses, has also been shown to be associated with a reduction of healthcare costs in the context of an organized healthcare system *(141)*. Lustman and colleagues *(137)* demonstrated in patients with DM2 that an intervention that included cognitive-behavioral therapy and diabetes education produced more than a 3-fold higher remission rate from depression, compared to a control condition. This treatment was associated with a significant improvement in metabolic control 6 months after the end of treatment. There is also some evidence that fluoxetine may help to improve metabolic control in patients with diabetes *(138)*.

There are no published guidelines regarding choice of antidepressant therapy for individuals with DM1 or DM2. However, differences in metabolic side effects, including changes in weight, insulin sensitivity, and lipid profile, can guide medication choice to some extent. The selective serotonin reuptake inhibitors (SSRIs), the serotonin and norepinephrine reuptake inhibitors (SNRIs; e.g., venlafaxine and duloxetine), mirtazapine, moclobemide, monoamine oxidase inhibitors, tricyclic agents and bupropion are all indicated for the treatment of depression *(132)*. The SSRIs and SNRIs are also first-line agents for the treatment of anxiety disorders, and so these agents should likely be used in cases that involve both depression and an anxiety disorder *(132)*.

Of the antidepressants currently in widespread clinical use, venlafaxine and duloxetine appear to be, on average, weight-neutral, while bupropion is often associated with no weight gain or a small amount of weight loss. SSRIs are weight-neutral or promote only small amounts of weight gain, with the exception of paroxetine, which appears to promote more weight gain than the other agents in this class. Mirtazapine, monoamine oxidase inhibitors and tricyclic agents are the most likely to promote weight gain, and so are not ideal first-line agents in individuals with diabetes *(142, 143)*. Differential effects of various antidepressants on lipid profile have been little studied, but available findings to date suggest that those medications most strongly associated with weight gain (tricyclic agents, mirtazapine as well as paroxetine) are also associated with a less favorable lipid profile *(144)*.

Individuals with diabetes should be counseled to be vigilant in monitoring their blood sugar levels when antidepressants are initiated or their dosage changed, as some of these medications affect glucose homeostasis *(145)*. A synthesis of the available literature *(146)* indicated that SSRIs tend to increase insulin sensitivity and reduce hyperglycemia, so that individuals with DM1 overall require less insulin. Some tricyclic agents can decrease insulin sensitivity and thereby raise blood sugar levels and insulin requirements. SNRIs and bupropion do not usually affect glucose metabolism, while monoamine oxidase inhibitors are sometimes associated with hypoglycemia *(146)*.

Antipsychotic agents are occasionally used in individuals with depression, either to augment a primary antidepressant's effectiveness or in the treatment of depression with psychotic features. Atypical antipsychotics (i.e., risperidone, olanzapine, clozapine, quetiapine, aripiprazole and ziprasidone) are now used more frequently than older antipsychotic medication. It has become clear that these medications can have significant negative effects on weight, lipid metabolism, and glucose homeostasis, contributing to the constellation of cardiac risk factors that constitutes metabolic syndrome *(147)*. Of these medications, aripiprazole and ziprasidone appear to be least likely to promote weight gain, and, to date, have not been found to be associated with an increased risk of worsening glucose homeostasis, although there have been occasional case reports of sudden onset diabetic ketoacidosis or worsening of the lipid profile *(147)*. Both risperidone and quetiapine have an intermediate propensity to promote weight gain, with some potential to precipitate new-onset diabetes or to worsen lipid profiles. Olanzapine and clozapine are associated with the highest weight gain, on average in the range of 4–10 kg *(148)*, and appear to confer the highest risk of worsening lipid profiles and precipitating diabetes in nondiabetic individuals. There are clear clinical guidelines for clinicians to adequately monitor these metabolic risk factors in individuals taking these medications. This involves assessing weight, waist circumference, blood pressure, fasting glucose and fasting lipid profile at baseline and at regular intervals during treatment *(147)*. Given these findings, when an antipsychotic medication is warranted in an individual with DM1, first-line choices should include the medications less likely to contribute to a metabolic syndrome namely, quetiapine, risperidone, aripiprazole or ziprasidone, and the individual's cardiac risk factors should be closely monitored.

Antidepressant medication, cognitive-behavioral or interpersonal therapy, or a combination of these modalities, all appear to be appropriate treatment approaches in women with diabetes and depression. However, there is an urgent need to evaluate and tailor interventions to prevent and treat depression and eating disorders in girls and women with diabetes because of the adverse effects of these conditions on metabolic control and on diabetes-related health outcomes. Further, close collaboration between diabetes and mental healthcare providers is crucial in helping individuals with diabetes and depression and/ or an eating disorder to integrate both the psychological and behavioral changes needed to improve overall well-being as well as diabetes management.

CONCLUSION

Eating disorders and depression are both common mental health problems in women with diabetes. Both affect women disproportionately, though the gender bias is much greater in the case of eating disorders. These conditions significantly affect the physical and emotional health of women with diabetes, and both are associated with impaired metabolic control and a higher risk of medical complications, including higher mortality rates. Disturbances of mood or eating that are in the subthreshold range may escape detection or treatment, although they may significantly affect the quality of life, physical health and survival of those affected. Brief self-report screening measures are available for the detection of both depression and eating disorders, and clinicians should also maintain an index of suspicion for both conditions, particularly when there is unexplained poor metabolic control. Brief interventions may be effective for both eating disorders and depression, and a low threshold for referral to mental health professionals is warranted. Psychotherapeutic interventions are the primary modality for the less severe disorders, and antidepressant medications may also be helpful for depression with or without comorbid eating disorders. Attention to such disturbances may be life saving in a condition such as diabetes in which outcomes are so dependent on behavioral compliance. Indeed, there are few medical conditions in which the early detection and treatment of behavioral and psychological disturbances can make such an important difference to health outcomes.

REFERENCES

1. American Psychiatric Association. Diagnostic and Statistical Manual of Mental Disorders, 4th edn, Text Revision. Washington, DC: American Psychiatric Association; 2000
2. Garfinkel PE, Lin E, Goering P, et al. Bulimia nervosa in a Canadian community sample: prevalence and comparison of subgroups. Am J Psychiatry 1995;152:1052–8
3. Gartner AF, Marcus RN, Halmi K, Loranger AW. DSM-III-R personality disorders in patients with eating disorders. Am J Psychiatry 1989;146:1585–91

4. Keel PK, Mitchell JE, Miller KB, Davis TL, Crow SJ. Predictive validity of bulimia nervosa as a diagnostic category. Am J Psychiatry 2000;157:136–8

5. Wilson JR. Bulimia nervosa: occurrence with psychoactive substance use disorders. Addict Behav 1992;17:603–7

6. Fornari V, Kaplan M, Sandberg D, Matthews M, Skolnick N, Katz J. Depressive and anxiety disorders in anorexia nervosa and bulimia nervosa. Int J Eat Disord 1992;12:21–9

7. Kennedy SH, Kaplan AS, Garfinkel PE, Rockert W, Toner B. Depression in anorexia nervosa and bulimia nervosa: discriminating depressive symptoms and episodes. J Psychosom Res 1994;38:773–82

8. Kruger S, McVey G, Kennedy SH. The changing profile of anorexia nervosa at the Toronto Programme for Eating Disorders. J Psychosom Res 1998;45:533–47

9. Sullivan PF, Bulik CM, Carter FA, Gendall KA, Joyce PR. The significance of a prior history of anorexia in bulimia nervosa. Int J Eat Disord 1996;20:253–61

10. Wiederman M, Pryor T. Body dissatisfaction, bulimia, and depression among women: the mediating role of drive for thinness. Int J Eat Disord 2000;27:90–5

11. Connors ME, Johnson CL. Epidemiology of bulimia and bulimic behaviors. Addict Behav 1987;12:165–79

12. Kaye WH, Gwirtsman HE, George DT, Weiss SR, Jimerson DC. Relationship of mood alterations to bingeing behaviour in bulimia. Br J Psychiatry 1986;149:479–85

13. Steinhausen HC. The outcome of anorexia nervosa in the 20th century. Am J Psychiatry 2002;159:1284–93

14. Dorian BJ, Garfinkel PE. The contributions of epidemiologic studies to the etiology and treatment of the eating disorders. Psychiatr Ann 1999;29:187–92

15. Woodside DB, Kennedy S. Gender differences in eating disorders. In: Seeman M, (ed.). Gender and Psychopathology. Washington, DC: American Psychiatric Press; 1995, pp. 253–68

16. Gowers SG, Shore A. Development of weight and shape concerns in the aetiology of eating disorders. Br J Psychiatry 2001;179:236–42

17. Striegel-Moore R. Etiology of binge eating: a developmental perspective. In: Fairburn CG, Wilson GT, (eds.). Binge Eating: Nature, Treatment and Assessment. New York, NY: Guilford Press; 1993, pp. 144–72

18. Crisp AH. Anorexia Nervosa: Let Me Be. Hillsdale, USA: Lawrence Erlbaum Associates; 1995

19. Pumariega AJ. Acculturation and eating attitudes in adolescent girls: a comparative and correlational study. J Am Acad Child Psychiatry 1986;25:276–9

20. Keel PK, Klump KL. Are eating disorders culture-bound syndromes? Implications for conceptualizing their etiology. Psychol Bull 2003;129:747–69

21. Graber JA, Brooks-Gunn J, Paikoff RL, Warren MP. Prediction of eating problems: an 8-year study of adolescent girls. Dev Psychol 1994;30:823–34

22. Huon GF, Walton CJ. Initiation of dieting among adolescent females. Int J Eat Disord 2000;28:226–30

23. Leon GR, Fulkerson JA, Perry CL, Cudeck R. Personality and behavioral vulnerabilities associated with risk status for eating disorders in adolescent girls. J Abnorm Psychol 1993;102:438–44

24. Pike KM, Rodin J. Mothers, daughters, and disordered eating. J Abnorm Psychol 1991;100:198–204

25. Swarr AE, Richards MH. Longitudinal effects of adolescent girls' pubertal development, perceptions of pubertal timing, and parental relations on eating problems. Dev Psychol 1996;32:636–46

26. Diabetes Control and Complications Trial (DCCT) Research Group. Weight gain associated with intensive therapy in the Diabetes Control and Complications Trial. Diabetes Care 1988;11:567–73

27. Diabetes Control and Complications Trial (DCCT) Research Group. Influence of intensive diabetes treatment on body weight and composition of adults with type I diabetes in the Diabetes Control and Complications Trial. Diabetes Care 2001;24:1711–21

28. Rodin GM, Daneman D. Eating disorders and IDDM. A problematic association. Diabetes Care 1992;15:1402–12

29. Rodin G, Craven J, Littlefield C, Murray M, Daneman D. Eating disorders and intentional insulin undertreatment in adolescent females with diabetes. Psychosomatics 1991;32:171–6

30. Colton PA, Rodin GM, Olmsted MP, Daneman D. Eating disturbances in young women with type 1 diabetes mellitus: mechanisms and consequences. Psychiatr Ann 1999;29:213–8

31. Maharaj S, Rodin G, Connolly J, Olmsted M, Daneman D. Eating problems and the observed quality of mother-daughter interactions among girls with type 1 diabetes. J Consult Clin Psychol 2001;69:950–8

32. de Groot J, Rodin G. Coming alive: the psychotherapeutic treatment of women with eating disorders. Can J Psychiatry 1998;43:359–66

33. Killen JD, Taylor CB, Hayward C, et al. Pursuit of thinness and onset of eating disorder symptoms in a community sample of adolescent girls: a three-year prospective analysis. Int J Eat Disord 1994;16:227–38

34. Patton GC, Selzer R, Coffey C, Carlin JB, Wolfe R. Onset of adolescent eating disorders: population based cohort study over 3 years. Br Med J 1999;318:765–8

35. Attie I, Brooks-Gunn J. Development of eating problems in adolescent girls: a longitudinal study. Dev Psychol 1989;25:70–9

36. Gardner RM, Stark K, Friedman BN, Jackson NA. Predictors of eating disorder scores in children ages 6 through 14: a longitudinal study. J Psychosom Res 2000;49:199–205

37. King MB. The natural history of eating pathology in attenders to primary medical care. Int J Eat Disord 1991;10:379–87

38. Patton GC, Johnson-Sabine E, Wood K, Mann AH, Wakeling A. Abnormal eating attitudes in London schoolgirls – a prospective epidemiological study: outcome at twelve month follow-up. Psychol Med 1990;20:383–94

39. Kotler LA, Cohen P, Davies M, Pine DS, Walsh BT. Longitudinal relationships between childhood, adolescent, and adult eating disorders. J Am Acad Child Adolesc Psychiatry 2001;40:1434–40

40. Domargard A, Sarnblad S, Kroon M, Karlsson I, Skeppner G, Aman J. Increased prevalence of overweight in adolescent girls with type 1 diabetes mellitus. Acta Paediatr Scand 1999;88:1223–8

41. Holl RW, Grabert M, Sorgo W, Heinze E, Debatin KM. Contributions of age, gender and insulin administration to weight gain in subjects with IDDM. Diabetologia 1998;41:542–7

42. Field AE, Camargo CA, Taylor CB, et al. Overweight, weight concerns, and bulimic behaviors among girls and boys. J Am Acad Child Adolesc Psychiatry 1999;38:754–60

43. Richards MH, Casper RC, Larson R. Weight and eating concerns among pre- and young adolescent boys and girls. J Adolesc Health Care 1990;11:203–9

44. Shearer JE, Bryon M. The nature and prevalence of eating disturbances and eating disorders in adolescents with cystic fibrosis. J R Soc Med 2004;97(Suppl. 4):36–42

45. Smith FM, Latchford GJ, Dickson RA. Do chronic medical conditions increase the risk of eating disorders? A cross-sectional investigation of eating pathology in adolescent females with scoliosis and diabetes. J Adolesc Health 2008;42:58–63

46. Rosmark B, Berne C, Holmgren S, Lago C, Renholm G, Sohlberg S. Eating disorders in patients with insulin-dependent diabetes mellitus. J Clin Psychiatry 1986;47:547–50

47. Steel JM, Young RJ, Lloyd GG, Macintyre CCA. Abnormal eating attitudes in young insulin-dependent diabetics. Br J Psychiatry 1989;155:515–21

48. Wing RR, Nowalk MP, Marcus MD, Koeske R, Finegold D. Subclinical eating disorders and glycemic control in adolescents with type I diabetes. Diabetes Care 1986;9:162–7

49. Svensson M, Engstrom I, Aman J. Higher drive for thinness in adolescent males with insulin-dependent diabetes mellitus compared with healthy controls. Acta Paediatr 2003;92:114–7

50. Daneman D, Rodin G, Jones J, et al. Eating disorders in adolescent girls and young adult women with type 1 diabetes. Diabetes Spectrum 2002;15:83–106

51. Nielsen S. Eating disorders in females with type 1 diabetes: an update of a meta-analysis. Eur Eat Disord Rev 2002;10:241–54

52. Colton P, Olmsted M, Daneman D, Rydall A, Rodin G. Disturbed eating behavior and eating disorders in pre-teen and early teenage girls with type 1 diabetes: a case-controlled study. Diabetes Care 2004;27:1654–9

53. Engstrom I, Kroon M, Arvidsson CG, Segnestam K, Snellman K, Aman J. Eating disorders in adolescent girls with insulin-dependent diabetes mellitus: a population-based case-control study. Acta Paediatr 1999;88:175–80

54. Fairburn CG, Peveler RC, Davies B, Mann JI, Mayou RA. Eating disorders in young adults with insulin dependent diabetes mellitus: a controlled study. Br Med J 1991;303:17–20

55. Jones JM, Lawson ML, Daneman D, Olmsted MP, Rodin G. Eating disorders in adolescent females with and without type 1 diabetes: cross sectional study. Br Med J 2000;320:1563–6

56. Mannucci E, Ricca V, Mezzani B, et al. Eating attitude and behavior in IDDM patients. Diabetes Care 1995;18:1503–4

57. Striegel-Moore RH, Nicholson TJ, Tamborlane WV. Prevalence of eating disorder symptoms in preadolescent and adolescent girls with IDDM. Diabetes Care 1992;15:1361–8

58. Vila G, Nollet-Clemencon C, Vera L, Crosnier H, Robert J-J, Mouren-Simeoni M-C. Étude des troubles des conduites alimentaires dans une population d'adolescentes souffrant de diabète insulino-dépendant. Revue Canadienne de Psychiatrie 1993;38:606–10

59. Vila G, Robert JJ, Nollet-Clemencon C, et al. Eating and emotional disorders in adolescent obese girls with insulin-dependent diabetes mellitus. Eur Child Adolesc Psychiatry 1995;4:270–9

60. Peveler RC, Fairburn CG, Boller I, Dunger DB. Eating disorders in adolescents with IDDM: a controlled study. Diabetes Care 1992;15:1356–60

61. Herpertz S, Albus C, Lichtblau K, Kohle K, Mann K, Senf W. Relationship of weight and eating disorders in type 2 diabetes patients: a multicenter study. Int J Eat Disord 2000;28:68–77

62. Mannucci E, Tesi F, Ricca V, et al. Eating behavior in obese patients with and without type 2 diabetes mellitus. Int J Obes Relat Metab Disord 2002;26:848–53

63. Bryden KS, Peveler RC, Stein A, Neil A, Mayou RA, Dunger DB. Clinical and psychological course of diabetes from adolescence to young adulthood: a longitudinal cohort study. Diabetes Care 2001;24:1536–40

64. Mortensen HB, Hougaard P. Comparison of metabolic control in a cross-sectional study of 2,873 children and adolescents with IDDM from 18 countries. The Hvidore Study Group on Childhood Diabetes. Diabetes Care 1997;20:714–20

65. Amiel SA, Sherwin RS, Simonson DC, Lauritano AA, Tamborlane WV. Impaired insulin action in puberty: a contributing factor to poor glycemic control in adolescents with diabetes. N Engl J Med 1986;315:215–9

66. Rydall AC, Rodin GM, Olmsted MP, Devenyi RG, Daneman D. Disordered eating behavior and microvascular complications in young women with insulin-dependent diabetes mellitus. N Engl J Med 1997;336:1849–54

67. Colton PA, Olmsted MP, Daneman D, Rydall AC, Rodin GM. 5-Year prevalence and persistence of disturbed eating behavior and eating disorders in girls with type 1 diabetes. Diabetes Care 2007;30:2861–2

68. Biggs MM, Basco MR, Patterson G, Raskin P. Insulin withholding for weight control in women with diabetes. Diabetes Care 1994;17:1186–9

69. Polonsky WH, Anderson BJ, Lohrer PA, Aponte JE, Jacobson AM, Cole CF. Insulin omission in women with IDDM. Diabetes Care 1994;17:1178–85

70. Bryden KS, Neil A, Mayou R, Peveler R, Fairburn C, Dunger D. Eating habits, body weight and insulin misuse: a longitudinal study of teenagers and young adults with type 1 diabetes. Diabetes Care 1999;22:1956–60

71. Peveler RC, Bryden KS, Neil HA, et al. The relationship of disordered eating habits and attitudes to clinical outcomes in young adult females with type 1 diabetes. Diabetes Care 2005;28:84–8

72. Affenito SG, Backstrand JR, Welch GW, Lammi-Keefe CJ, Rodriguez NR, Adams CH. Subclinical and clinical eating disorders in IDDM negatively affect metabolic control. Diabetes Care 1997;20:182–4

73. Colas C, Mathieu P, Tchobroutsky G. Eating disorders and retinal lesions in type 1 (insulin-dependent) diabetic women. Diabetologia 1991;34:288

74. Steel JM, Young RJ, Lloyd GG, Clarke BF. Clinically apparent eating disorders in young diabetic women: associations with painful neuropathy and other complications. Br Med J (Clin Res Ed) 1987;294:859–62

75. Ward A, Troop N, Cachia M, Watkins P, Treasure J. Doubly disabled: diabetes in combination with an eating disorder. Postgrad Med J 1995;71:546–50

76. Friedman S, Vila G, Timsit J, Boitard C, Mouren-Simeoni MC. Eating disorders and insulin-dependent diabetes mellitus (IDDM): relationships with glycaemic control and somatic complications. Acta Psychiatr Scand 1998;97:206–12

77. Affenito SG, Lammi-Keefe CJ, Vogel S, Backstrand JR, Welch GW, Adams CH. Women with insulin-dependent diabetes mellitus (IDDM) complicated by eating disorders are at risk for exacerbated alterations in lipid metabolism. Eur J Clin Nutr 1997;51:462–6

78. Nielsen S, Emborg C, Molbak AG. Mortality in concurrent type 1 diabetes and anorexia nervosa. Diabetes Care 2002;25(2):309–12

79. Kessler RC, Berglund P, Demler O, et al. The epidemiology of major depressive disorder: results from the National Comorbidity Survey Replication (NCS-R). J Am Med Assoc 2003;289:3095–105

80. Burvill PW. Recent progress in the epidemiology of major depression. Epidemiol Rev 1995;17(1):21–31

81. Rodin G, Nolan RP, Katz MR. Depression (in the Medically Ill). In: Levenson J, (ed.). Textbook of Psychosomatic Medicine. Washington, DC: American Psychiatric Press; 2004. pp. 113–217

82. de Groot M, Anderson R, Freedland KE, Clouse RE, Lustman PJ. Association of depression and diabetes complications: a meta-analysis. Psychosom Med 2001;63:619–30

83. Eaton WW. Epidemiologic evidence on the comorbidity of depression and diabetes. J Psychosom Res 2002;53:903–6

84. Egede LE, Zheng D, Simpson K. Comorbid depression is associated with increased health care use and expenditures in individuals with diabetes. Diabetes Care 2002;25:464–70

85. Grey M, Whittemore R, Tamborlane W. Depression in type 1 diabetes in children: natural history and correlates. J Psychosom Res 2002;53:907–11

86. Lustman PJ, Clouse RE. Depression in diabetic patients: the relationship between mood and glycemic control. J Diabetes Complications 2005;19:113–22

87. Anderson RJ, Freedland KE, Clouse RE, Lustman PJ. The prevalence of comorbid depression in adults with diabetes: a meta-analysis. Diabetes Care 2001;24:1069–78

88. Kovacs M, Goldston D, Obrosky DS, Bonar LK. Psychiatric disorders in youths with IDDM: rates and risk factors. Diabetes Care 1997;20:36–44

89. Peyrot M, Rubin RR. Persistence of depressive symptoms in diabetic adults. Diabetes Care 1999;22:448–52

90. Eaton WW, Armenian H, Gallo J, Pratt L, Ford DE. Depression and risk for onset of type II diabetes. A prospective population-based study. Diabetes Care 1996;19:1097–102

91. Zhang X, Norris SL, Gregg EW, Cheng YJ, Beckles G, Kahn HS. Depressive symptoms and mortality among persons with and without diabetes. Am J Epidemiol 2005;161:652–60

92. Katon WJ, Rutter C, Simon G, et al. The association of comorbid depression with mortality in patients with type 2 diabetes. Diabetes Care 2005;28:2668–72

93. Egede LE, Nietert PJ, Zheng D. Depression and all-cause and coronary heart disease mortality among adults with and without diabetes. Diabetes Care 2005;28:1339–45

94. Piccinelli M, Wilkinson G. Gender differences in depression: critical review. Br J Psychiatry 2000;177:486–92

95. Nau DP, Aikens JE, Pacholski AM. Effects of gender and depression on oral medication adherence in persons with type 2 diabetes mellitus. Gend Med 2007;4:205–13

96. Peyrot M, Rubin RR. Levels and risks of depression and anxiety symptomatology among diabetic adults. Diabetes Care 1997;20:585–90

97. Fisher L, Skaff MM, Mullan JT, et al. Clinical depression versus distress among patients with type 2 diabetes: not just a question of semantics. Diabetes Care 2007;30:542–8

98. Wing RR, Phelan S, Tate D. The role of adherence in mediating the relationship between depression and health outcomes. J Psychosom Res 2002;53:877–81

99. Van Tilburg MA, McCaskill CC, Lane JD, et al. Depressed mood is a factor in glycemic control in type 1 diabetes. Psychosom Med 2001;63:551–5

100. Jacobson AM, Samson JA, Weinger K, Ryan CM. Diabetes, the brain, and behavior: is there a biological mechanism underlying the association between diabetes and depression? Int Rev Neurobiol 2002;51:455–79

101. Murray CJ, Lopez AD. Alternative projections of mortality and disability by cause 1990–2020: Global Burden of Disease Study. Lancet 1997;349:1498–504

102. Moussavi S, Chatterji S, Verdes E, Tandon A, Patel V, Ustun B. Depression, chronic diseases, and decrements in health: results from the World Health Surveys. Lancet 2007;370:851–8

103. Simon GE, Katon WJ, Lin EHB, et al. Diabetes complications and depression as predictors of health services costs. Gen Hosp Psychiatry 2005;27:344–51

104. Kalsekar ID, Madhavan ASM, Amonkar MM, Scott V, Douglas SM, Makela E. The effect of depression on health care utilization and costs in patients with type 2 diabetes. Manag Care Interface 2006;19:39–46

105. Simon GE. Social and economic burden of mood disorders. Biol Psychiatry 2003;54:208–15

106. Lustman PJ, Anderson RJ, Freedland KE, de Groot M, Carney RM, Clouse RE. Depression and poor glycemic control: a meta-analytic review of the literature. Diabetes Care 2000;23:934–42

107. Gonzalez JS, Safren SA, Cagliero E, et al. Depression, self-care, and medication adherence in type 2 diabetes. Diabetes Care 2007;30:2222–7

108. Kinder LS, Kamarck TW, Baum A, Orchard TJ. Depressive symptomatology and coronary heart disease in Type I diabetes mellitus: a study of possible mechanisms. Health Psychol 2002;21:542–52

109. Mokdad AH, Bowman BA, Ford ES, Vinicor F, Marks JS, Koplan JP. The continuing epidemics of obesity and diabetes in the United States. J Am Med Assoc 2001;286:1195–200

110. US Department of Health and Human Services. Healthy People 2010: Understanding and Improving Health, 2nd edn. Washington, DC: U.S. Government Printing Office; 2000

111. Baskin ML, Ard J, Franklin F, Allison DB. Prevalence of obesity in the United States. Obes Rev 2005;6:5–7

112. Hedley AA, Ogden CL, Johnson CL, Carroll MD, Curtin LR, Flegal KM. Prevalence of overweight and obesity among US children, adolescents and adults, 1999–2002. J Am Med Assoc 2004;291:2847–50

113. Lim W, Thomas KS, Bardwell WA, Dimsdale JE. Which measures of obesity are related to depressive symptoms and in whom? Psychosomatics 2008;49:23–8

114. Istvan J, Zavela K, Weidner G. Body weight and psychological distress in NHANES, I. Int J Obes Relat Metab Disord 1992;16:999–1003

115. Carpenter KM, Hasin DS, Allison DB, Faith MS. Relationships between obesity and DSM-IV major depressive disorder, suicide ideation, and suicide attempts: results from a general population study. Am J Public Health 2000;90:251–7

116. de Groot M, Jacobson AM, Samson JA, Welch G. Glycemic control and major depression in patients with type 1 and type 2 diabetes mellitus. J Psychosom Res 1999;46:425–35

117. Lustman PJ, Clouse RE. Treatment of depression in diabetes: impact on mood and medical outcome. J Psychosom Res 2002;53:917–24

118. Kovacs M, Mukerji P, Drash A, Iyengar S. Biomedical and psychiatric risk factors for retinopathy among children with IDDM. Diabetes Care 1995;18:1592–9

119. Moskvina V, Farmer A, Swainson V, et al. Interrelationship of childhood trauma, neuroticism, and depressive pheno-type. Depress Anxiety 2007;24:163–8

120. Takii M, Komaki G, Uchigata Y, Maeda M, Omori Y, Kubo C. Differences between bulimia nervosa and binge-eating disorder in females with type 1 diabetes: the important role of insulin omission. J Psychosom Res 1999;47:221–31

121. Oldehinkel AJ, Wittchen H-U, Schuster P. Prevalence, 20-month incidence and outcome of unipolar depressive disorders in a community sample of adolescents. Psychol Med 1999;29:655–68

122. Radloff LS. The CES-D: a self-report depression scale for research in the general population. Appl Psychol Meas 1977;1(3):385–401

123. Beck AT, Steer RA, Brown GK. Manual for the Beck Depression Inventory-II. San Antonio, TX: Psychological Corporation; 1996

124. Kroenke K, Spitzer RL, Williams JB. The PHQ-9: validity of a brief depression severity measure. J Gen Intern Med 2001;16(9):606–13

125. Garner DM, Olmsted MP, Bohr Y, Garfinkel PE. The eating attitudes test: psychometric features and clinical correlates. Psychol Med 1982;12:871–8

126. Johnson C. Diagnostic Survey for Eating Disorders (DSED). In: Johnson C, Connors ME, (eds.). The Etiology and Treatment of Bulimia Nervosa. New York: Basic Books; 1987

127. Laessle RG, Zoettle C, Pirke KM. Meta-analysis of treatment studies for bulimia. Int J Eat Disord 1987;6:647–54

128. Weissman MM, Markowitz JC, Klerman GL. Comprehensive Guide to Interpersonal Psychotherapy. New York: Basic Books; 2000

129. Agras WS, Walsh T, Fairburn CG, Wilson GT, Kraemer HC. A multicenter comparison of cognitive-behavioral therapy and interpersonal psychotherapy for bulimia nervosa. Arch Gen Psychiatry 2000;57:459–66

130. Eisler I, Simic M, Russell GFM, Dare C. A randomised controlled treatment trial of two forms of family therapy in adolescent anorexia nervosa: a five-year follow-up. J Child Psychol Psychiatry 2007;48:552–60

131. Work Group on Eating Disorders. Practice guideline for the treatment of patients with eating disorders, 3rd edition. Am J Psychiatry 2006;163:5–54

132. Canadian Psychiatric Association. Clinical guidelines for the treatment of depressive disorders. Can J Psychiatry 2001;46:5S–90S

133. Peveler RC, Fairburn CG. The treatment of bulimia nervosa in patients with diabetes mellitus. Int J Eat Disord 1992;11:45–53

134. Takii M, Uchigata Y, Komaki G, et al. An integrated inpatient therapy for type 1 diabetic females with bulimia nervosa: a 3-year follow-up study. J Psychosom Res 2003;55:349–56

135. Olmsted MP, Rodin G, Rydall AC, Lawson ML, Daneman D. The effects of psychoeducation on disturbed eating attitudes and behavior in young women with type 1 diabetes mellitus. Int J Eat Disord 2002;32:230–9

136. Lustman PJ, Griffith LS, Freedland KE, Clouse RE. The course of major depression in diabetes. Gen Hosp Psychiatry 1997;19:138–43

137. Lustman PJ, Griffith LS, Freedland KE, Kissel SS, Clouse RE. Cognitive behavior therapy for depression in type 2 diabetes mellitus: a randomized, controlled trial. Ann Intern Med 1998;129:613–21

138. Lustman PJ, Freedland KE, Griffith LS, Clouse RE. Fluoxetine for depression in diabetes: a randomized double-blind placebo-controlled trial. Diabetes Care 2000;23:618–23

139. Williams JW, Katon W, Lin EHB, et al. The effectiveness of depression care management on diabetes-related outcomes in older patients. Ann Intern Med 2004;140:1015–24

140. Kinder LS, Katon WJ, Ludman E, et al. Improving depression care in patients with diabetes and multiple complications. J Gen Intern Med 2006;21:1036–41

141. Simon GE, Katon WJ, Lin EHB, et al. Cost-effectiveness of systematic depression treatment among people with diabetes mellitus. Arch Gen Psychiatry 2007;64:65–72

142. Vanina Y, Podolskaya A, Sedky K, et al. Body weight changes associated with psychopharmacology. Psychiatr Serv 2002;53(7):842–7

143. Papakostas GI. Tolerability of modern antidepressants. J Clin Psychiatry 2008;69(Suppl E1):8–13

144. McIntyre RS, Soczynska JK, Konarski JZ, Kennedy SH. The effect of antidepressants on lipid homeostasis: a cardiac safety concern? Expert Opin Drug Saf 2006;5(4):523–37

145. Zimmermann U, Kraus T, Himmerich H, Schuld A, Pollmacher T. Epidemiology, implications and mechanisms underlying drug-induced weight gain in psychiatric patients. J Psychiatr Res 2003;37(3):193–220

146. McIntyre RS, Soczynska JK, Konarski JZ, Kennedy SH. The effect of antidepressants on glucose homeostasis and insulin sensitivity: synthesis and mechanisms. Expert Opin Drug Saf 2006;5(1):157–68

147. American Diabetes Association; American Psychiatric Association; American Association of Clinical Endocrinologists; North American Association for the Study of Obesity. Consensus development conference on antipsychotic drugs and obesity and diabetes. J Clin Psychiatry 2004;65(2):267–72

148. Newcomer JW, Haupt DW. The metabolic effects of antipsychotic medications. Can J Psychiatry 2006;51(8):480–91

8

Sexual Health in Women with Diabetes

Andrea Salonia, Roberto Lanzi, Emanuele Bosi,
Patrizio Rigatti, and Francesco Montorsi

CONTENTS

ABSTRACT

Women's sexual dysfunction (SD) is defined as a disorder of sexual desire, arousal, orgasm, and/or sexual pain, which results in significant personal distress and may have a negative effect on a woman's health and quality of life. Although previously published data suggest that sexual complaints are highly prevalent among women with diabetes mellitus (DM), the scientific community has scarcely investigated the potential correlation between diabetes mellitus and women's SD. In case-control studies, SD was reported at a significantly greater rate in women with DM type 1 (DM1) than among controls – arousal difficulties being most common. Interestingly, sexual complaints were not isolated in occurrence, because women with DM often reported at least two sexual problems. Sexual disorders are also highly prevalent in women with DM type 2 (DM2), with low sexual desire being most commonly reported. Few treatment options and no specific compounds have been investigated to address the various types of SD in women with diabetes.

Therefore, additional medical research, education and training are needed to improve the identification and management of SD in diabetic women. In this context, it is of paramount importance that both researchers and clinicians address the issue of sexuality and sexual health among diabetic women in well-designed longitudinal studies that have sufficient statistical power and are free of bias.

Key words: Diabetes mellitus; Female sexual dysfunction; Sexual health; Sexual desire; Sexual arousal; Dyspareunia; Menstrual cycle.

From: *Diabetes in Women: Pathophysiology and Therapy*
Edited by: A. Tsatsoulis et al. (eds.), DOI 10.1007/978-1-60327-250-6_8
© Humana Press, a part of Springer Science+Business Media, LLC 2009

INTRODUCTION

Women's SD is defined as a disorder of sexual desire, arousal, orgasm, and/or sexual pain, which results in significant personal distress and may have a negative effect on a woman's health and quality of life. Women's SD is a prevalent, multifaceted problem that continues to be under-recognized and under-treated *(1)*. Healthcare professionals are aware of the high prevalence of SD among women but infrequently initiate a discussion of sexual function (SF) with their female patients or conduct a comprehensive evaluation for SD *(1)*.

Many recent studies have investigated the prevalence of female SD. Among women with SD, 64% (range: 16–75%) experienced desire difficulty, 35% (16–48%) experienced orgasm difficulty, 31% (12–64%) experienced arousal impairment, and 26% (7–58%) complained of sexual pain. Only a few epidemiological studies assessed the proportion of women with SD who were actually distressed by it, showing a prevalence ranging between 21% and 67% *(2)*.

Sexual symptoms may signal serious underlying disease, and this confirms the importance of sexual enquiry as an integral component of medical assessment *(3)*. Many common medical disorders have negative effects on women's SF, including diabetes mellitus. Increased scientific knowledge of the central and peripheral physiology of sexual response should help to identify the pathophysiology of SD from disease and to ameliorate or prevent some dysfunction. Unfortunately, rigorous data on the epidemiology of these disorders, their pathophysiology, and potential effective and safe treatments for SD among diabetic women are scant and inadequately documented. Therefore, in this chapter, which is based on everyday clinical practice according to the most updated peer-reviewed publications, we focus on the potential correlation between women's SF and DM1 or DM2 as comorbid conditions.

FEMALE SEXUAL DYSFUNCTION: DEFINITIONS, CLINICAL CLASSIFICATION, AND EPIDEMIOLOGY

Sexual dysfunction in women has been defined as a multifactorial condition with anatomical, physiological, medical, psychological and social components. Sexual complaints are common among women within the general population *(4–7)*.

The classic definitions of women's sexual disorders were based mainly on genitally focused events in a linear sequence model (desire, arousal and orgasm). More recently, SD has been considered a disturbance in SF involving one or multiple phases of the sexual response cycle or pain associated with sexual activity *(7–9)*. A sexual disorder is SD that meets the Diagnostic and Statistical Manual of Mental Disorders, 4th Edition criteria for sexual disorders; however, a problem becomes a SD only if it causes distress, as opposed to a normal physiological response to difficult circumstances *(7–9)*.

Therefore, a sexual symptom that does not result in distress may not require treatment. However, it is important to screen for sexual symptoms as they may signal serious underlying disease.

Based on the previous classification criteria and recent reconsideration of the American Foundation of Urologic Disease, an International Definitions Committee of 13 experts from seven countries proposed new definitions that were presented in July 2003 at the Second International Consultation on Sexual Medicine in Paris *(7–9)*. Sexual dysfunctions were thus subdivided into (1) sexual desire/interest disorder, (2) subjective sexual arousal disorder, (3) genital sexual arousal disorder, (4) combined sexual arousal disorder (with a marked or absent subjective sexual arousal [feelings of excitement and pleasure] combined with either reduced or impaired genital sexual arousal [vulvar swelling, lubrication]), (5) persistent sexual arousal disorder syndrome, (6) orgasmic disorder, (7) vaginismus, and (8) dyspareunia *(7–11)*. The rationale for this classification system is that it considers a woman's SF as a consequence of the current psychosocial and interpersonal context, which is determined to some degree by her sexual history medical history and medication history *(7, 8)*.

Objective prevalence of these categories in the general population is poorly known *(9)*. According to the National Health and Social Life Survey, approximately 43% of American women suffer from sexual disorders of some type *(4)*, and SD is associated with various psychodemographic characteristics such as age, education, and poor physical and emotional health. The Global Study of Sexual Attitudes and Behaviors (GSSAB) is the first large, multinational survey to systematically study attitudes, beliefs and behaviours associated with sexual relationships among middle-aged and older adults *(5)*. The survey involved 13,882 women and 13,618 men aged 40–80 years in 29 countries that represented many world regions. The GSSAB showed that for women lack of interest in sex and difficulty in reaching orgasm were the most common sexual problems across the world, ranging between 26% and 48% and 18% and 41%, respectively. Hypoactive sexual desire disorder (HSDD) certainly represents the most widely reported female SD worldwide.

Investigators have also debated the prevalence and predictors of female SD across Europe *(6, 12–15)*. For instance, in a cohort of Austrian women aged 43 ± 15 years, 22% complained of sexual desire disorders, 35% of arousal disorders, and 39% of orgasmic disorders *(6)*, and these complaints increased with age *(6, 16)*. Graziottin *(13)* recently published prevalence data collected on 2,467 women (age: 20–70 years) from France, Germany, Italy and the United Kingdom, via the Women's International Survey on Health and Sexuality. The survey, which included women with surgical and natural menopausal status and those with premenopausal status, showed that sexual activity decreased with age, coupled with an increase in SD, particularly loss of sexual desire, which was directly correlated with increasing age. However, the distress associated with loss of sexual desire was inversely correlated with age. Cultural and context-dependent factors in the different European countries affected the prevalence of women's SD, mainly in women aged 20–49 years with normal ovarian function. However, when women underwent surgical menopause, the culture-related differences were blunted *(13)*.

Large cohort studies have clearly identified that diabetes is strongly associated with SD in men, with the incidence of SD in diabetic men approaching 50% *(17–19)*. SD in men has been linked to vascular alterations, endocrine abnormalities, psychological problems and neurologic deficits. However, the SF of women with diabetes has only recently received attention. The scientific literature lacks accurate prevalence rates of SD in women with diabetes mellitus and vice versa from random, population-based samples; most reported data have been derived from selected clinic populations. Moreover, older data were gathered in studies with methodological flaws, small numbers of subjects, absence of controls, failure to differentiate DM1 and DM2, incomplete assessment of diabetic complications, or failure to distinguish either premenopausal from postmenopausal women or hormone-replaced from oestrogen-depleted subjects *(20–24)*. Moreover, most of the published series do not use the more updated classifications *(7, 8)*, making the data interpretation difficult.

In more recent studies, the most commonly reported SD in women with diabetes is decreased sexual arousal often associated with inadequate vaginal lubrication *(23–26)*. Diabetic women, however, may also suffer from hypoactive libido and dyspareunia *(23–26)*.

Sexual Disorders Among Women with Type 1 Diabetes Mellitus

Prevalence and predictors of SD among DM1 women were elegantly reported by Enzlin et al. *(19, 26)*. This case-control epidemiological survey performed at the University Hospitals of the Catholic University of Leuven, Belgium included 120 consecutive women with DM1 with a stable heterosexual relationship lasting at least 1 year, who were surveyed during a 2-year period *(26)*.

The final analysed subset was 97 women with DM1 (response rate: 80.8%; mean duration of diabetes: 14.3 ± 10.1 years; mean HbA_{1c} value: $8.0 \pm 1.4\%$) who were compared with 145 age-matched women who had a stable heterosexual relationship and who visited the outpatient gynecology clinic for routine screening. Among the DM1 group, 52% had no diabetic complications, 28% had at least one complication, and 20% had multiple complications. According to the results of a modified version of the Udvalg for Kliniske Undersoegelser questionnaire, a validated 48-item instrument with a specific four-item domain covering SF *(27)*, SD was reported at a significantly greater rate in women with DM1 than among controls (27% vs. 15%; $\chi^2 = 4.5$, df = 1, $p = 0.04$). Sexual complaints were not isolated in occurrence, because 11% of the women with diabetes and 7% of the controls reported at least two sexual problems ($\chi^2 = 0.16$, df = 2, $p = 0.92$). By segregating sexual problems, women with DM1 reported a higher prevalence of sexual arousal disorder than controls (14% vs. 6%, respectively; $\chi^2 = 3.8$, df = 1, $p = 0.05$), whereas no significant differences were found for desire (17% vs. 9%; $p = 0.09$), dyspareunia (12% vs. 6%; $p = 0.15$), or orgasmic disorders (14% vs. 10%, $p = 0.52$) *(26)*. A weakness of the analyses of prevalence rates was poor statistical power due to the small numbers studied.

However, Enzlin et al.'s results were in accordance with other reports on sexual disorders among women with DM1 *(28–32)*. For instance, in two different studies on women with DM1, Jensen found that 28–29% mentioned SD as compared with 25% of the controls *(28, 29)*. Similar rates were found subdividing the groups for each sexual disorder *(28–34)*.

Although Enzlin et al.'s study was the largest ever to compare diabetic women with 'healthy' nondiabetic controls and provided good information in terms of prevalence of the actual disorders, the analysis did not consider a cohort of solely pre- vs. postmenopausal women, did not segregate results according to the specific phase of the menstrual cycle, and did not use a gender-specific psychometric instrument to objectively assess SF.

Interestingly, Enzlin et al. *(19)* subsequently reported that among 222 patients with DM1 (95 men, 97 women) who consecutively visited the same facilities in Belgium during a comparable 2-year period, a similar rate of sexual disorders was reported by both genders (27% vs. 22% for women and men, respectively; $\chi^2 = 0.61$, $p = 0.49$). Moreover, no significant differences were found in the distribution of the type of SD between sexes.

Using the Brief Sexual Function Inventory questionnaire *(35)* and the Derogatis Interview for Sexual Functioning *(36)*, Basson et al. *(37)* reported 40%, 38%, and 31% rate of reduced lubrication, orgasm difficulties, and sexual pain, respectively, among a small cohort of both pre- and postmenopausal DM1 women, aged 20–76 years. Doruk et al. *(38)* also investigated the effect of diabetes mellitus upon female SF, aiming to detect possible risk factors that might predict SD in a cohort of 127 pre- and postmenopausal married women: 21 DM1, 50 DM2 and 56 healthy women. Among the women with DM1 the overall prevalence of SD was 71% compared with 37% among controls. Sexual desire disorders were reported in 85% of the women with DM1, following by low arousal (76%), reduced lubrication (57%), orgasm difficulties (66%), pain (61%), and dissatisfaction (52%). The prevalence and severity of sexual disorders was objectively defined with the Female Sexual Function Index (FSFI), a multidimensional instrument for the self-reported assessment of women's SF that includes 19 items compiled in six domains (desire, arousal, lubrication, orgasm, satisfaction, and pain) *(39)*. The FSFI scores for sexual desire, arousal, and lubrication were significantly lower in the DM1 group than in the controls ($p < 0.05$), whereas scores for orgasm, satisfaction, dyspareunia, and total SF domains were only slightly lower in the DM1 group than in the healthy subjects. Interestingly, SD prevalence was significantly higher among the DM1 subjects than in DM2 subjects and controls *(38)*.

Sexual Disorders Among Women with Type 2 Diabetes Mellitus

The study by Doruk et al. *(38)* showed a SD prevalence of 42% within the DM2 women. Low sexual desire was reported in 82% of the DM2 women, whereas 68% complained of low arousal, 38% of reduced lubrication, 38% of orgasm difficulties, 46% of coital pain, and 50% of sexual dissatisfaction. Troubles in sexual arousal, lubrication, and orgasmic function were significantly more prevalent among DM2 subjects than among the healthy controls *(23, 38)*.

Erol et al. *(40)* assessed the SF profile in 72 premenopausal DM2 women (mean age: 38.8 years; range: 25–47) with no other systemic disease as compared with 60 age-matched healthy women. The FSFI was used to assess the prevalence of sexual disorders throughout the analysis. Overall, DM2 patients had a significantly lower FSFI total score than controls (29.3 ± 6.4 vs. 37.7 ± 3.5; $p < 0.05$). Low sexual desire was the most frequently reported SD, being observed in 77% of the DM2 patients. Reduced lubrication (defined as vaginal dryness) was observed in 37.5%, whereas orgasm difficulties, vaginal discomfort (pain), and sexual dissatisfaction were reported by 49%, 42%, and 42% of the DM2 women, respectively. Similarly, Basson et al. *(37)* reported reduced lubrication in 47% of the DM2 women in their cohort, as well as a 31% rate for orgasm difficulties and a 42% rate of coital pain as compared with a 34%, 33%, and 26% prevalence among healthy controls *(23, 37)*.

More recently, Olarinoye et al. *(41)* assessed the SF of 51 DM2 women attending the Diabetes Clinic, University of Ilorin Teaching Hospital, Nigeria. Patients' FSFI scores were compared with those of 39 nondiabetic controls. The FSFI total score for the DM2 women was significantly lower than that for controls (20.5 ± 8.3 vs. 31.2 ± 8.8; $p = 0.001$). Similarly, FSFI domain scores for arousal, pain, orgasm, and overall satisfaction were also lower for the diabetics (all $p < 0.05$). Interestingly, there was no significant difference for the sexual desire domain between the two groups. Overall, DM2 women attempted sex less frequently than healthy subjects ($p < 0.05$). Once more, a negative correlation between age and all the FSFI domain scores was found ($p < 0.05$). Although the authors acknowledged the study's limitations (namely, small sample size and lack of data about both insulin resistance and HbA_{1c}), this study is important because this geographical area has not been previously considered among multinational studies assessing women's SF, either within general or special populations.

PREDICTORS OF SEXUAL DYSFUNCTION AMONG WOMEN WITH DIABETES

Age

Sexual dysfunction is widely recognized as increasing with age in the general population *(4–6, 42, 43)*. In this context, Lindau et al. *(42)* reported the prevalence of sexual activity, behaviours, and problems in a national sample of 3,005 US adults (1,550 women and 1,455 men) aged 57–85 years, recruited between July 2005 and March 2006. Although the prevalence of sexual activity declined with age, many older adults remained sexually active. Within the analysed population, women were less likely than men to have an intimate relationship and to be sexually active at all ages. Among respondents who were sexually active, about half of both sexes reported at least one bothersome sexual problem, with low sexual desire (43%), difficulty with vaginal lubrication (39%), and inability to climax (34%) the most prevalent problems among women. Women with diabetes were less likely to be sexually active (OR: 0.61, 95% CI: 0.46–0.81) than those without.

Data regarding a potential pathophysiologic correlation between age and impaired SF among women with diabetes are controversial, with most not showing any significant detrimental association *(9, 19, 21, 23, 25, 37, 38, 40, 41)*. For instance, in their case-control survey on DM1, Enzlin et al. observed that women with SD were not significantly different for age, BMI, duration of diabetes, or

HbA_{1c} compared with those without SD *(19, 26)*. In the same study, the subanalysis of women with diabetes either with or without complications did not reveal significant differences for age ($p = 0.28$ and 0.36, respectively). Similar findings were also reported by Doruk et al. *(38)* in their subanalysis of their subset of women with DM1.

In contrast, Erol et al. noted that the incidence of all reported SDs was significantly higher in DM2 women than in age-comparable controls *(40)*. Likewise, data from Nigeria supported this finding: age was a significant determinant ($p = 0.003$) of the FSFI among DM2 women *(41)*. Indeed, women who were younger than 40 years reported a mean FSFI total score of 30.67 ± 8.4, while those above that age had a mean score of 18.36 ± 7.4 ($p = 0.001$).

Overall, the scientific literature lacks a well-designed, multinational, prospective survey aimed at assessing the impact of the ageing process on SF in women with diabetes.

Duration of Diabetes, Diabetes-Related Complications, and Diabetes Control

The effect of diabetes on women's SF is complex. Overall, the literature suggests that there is poor correlation between sexual difficulties and either duration of diabetes or diabetes complications *(23)*. In this context, Enzlin et al.'s survey observed that women who reported SD were not significantly different in duration of diabetes ($p = 0.36$) and HbA_{1c} values ($p = 0.47$). The subanalysis of women with or without diabetes complications also did not reveal significant differences for HbA_{1c} values between those with and without SD ($p = 0.052$ and 0.29, respectively) *(19)*.

Duration of diabetes is usually associated with a greater rate of diabetic complications. Neuropathy, vascular impairment and psychological complaints have been shown to be implicated in the pathogenesis of decreased libido, low arousability, decreased vaginal lubrication, orgasmic dysfunction, and dyspareunia, but discrepancies exist among reports *(25, 44, 45)*. In Enzlin et al.'s case-control survey *(19, 26)*, the rate of women with diabetic complications (33%) – such as peripheral neuropathy, autonomic neuropathy, nephropathy, and retinopathy – who reported sexual problems was not significantly higher than the rate of their counterparts without complications (22%; $\chi^2 = 1.3$, df = 1, $p = 0.34$). An overall comparison of the percentages of women reporting a specific SD showed that only decreased lubrication was more prevalent among women with diabetes complications ($\chi^2 = 6.5$, df = 2, $p = 0.04$). A specific subanalysis revealed that the latter finding was due to the significant difference between the percentage of women with diabetes with complications and healthy controls *(19, 26)*. In contrast, there was an association between the number of complications and the occurrence of SD: subjects with more complications were more likely to report greater SD ($p = 0.002$), for both the men and women enrolled in their survey *(19, 26)*.

Likewise, Olarinoye et al. *(41)* observed a nearly significant association between the FSFI total score and the duration of diabetes ($p = 0.05$). In contrast, duration of diabetes was negatively correlated with lubrication ($p = 0.03$) as well as orgasmic function ($p = 0.04$). Glycaemic control and diabetic complications were not significantly correlated with any of the FSFI domain scores *(41)*.

Few objective data are available on the pathophysiology of diabetic complications that underlie SD in women. Consequently, the effects of diabetes on genital tissue structure, innervation and function remain poorly characterized. Rutherford and Collier *(21)* conducted a comprehensive literature review as it pertained to the etiology of SD among diabetic women. An alteration in blood supply secondary to diabetes mellitus, also coupled with reduced vasocongestion due to lower nitric oxide, was hypothesized as a key factor in determining genital arousal difficulties in diabetic women *(21)*. In a case-control study, Wincze et al. *(23, 46)* measured vaginal vasocongestion in response to erotic stimuli in women with diabetes, using vaginal photoplethysmography to measure the capillary engorgement at the vaginal wall, while subjects individually viewed counterbalanced erotic and nonerotic videotapes. Women with diabetes demonstrated significantly less physiological genital arousal to erotic stimuli than controls, whereas their subjective responses were comparable. Although they did not consider the more recently published clinical classification for female SD *(7, 8)*, their objective, physiological findings supported the idea of a causal diabetes-related genital sexual arousal disorder. The psychometric profile revealed no difference in terms of subjectively experienced sexual difficulties in diabetic women as compared with the control group *(46)*.

Peripheral and autonomic neuropathies have been frequently associated with and are considered an important cause of erectile dysfunction in diabetic men. With the specific aim to assess whether peripheral neuropathy may be causally associated with the development of sexual disorders among diabetic women, Erol et al. *(44)* experimentally evaluated the genital and extragenital somatic sensory system using biothesiometry. In this case-control survey of 30 premenopausal diabetic women and 20 healthy sexually active women, women with diabetes showed a mean FSFI total score significantly lower than that of controls (23.6 vs. 38.3; $p < 0.0005$). Moreover, for each genital and extragenital site, the mean biothesiometric values were significantly higher in diabetics, with the sensation at the vaginal introitus, the labium minora, and the clitoris the most deteriorated in diabetic women. A correlation was not found in women with diabetes, because the difference between women with or without SD was not significant in terms of biothesiometric values.

Several interesting basic studies assessing the impact of diabetes on SF have been conducted in animal models. To better understand the reduction in vaginal lubrication that is frequently reported by diabetic women in real-life clinical practice, Park et al. *(47)* studied the vascular impairment at the vaginal level in a streptozotocin-induced diabetic rat model. Their hypothesis was that reduced vaginal lubrication in diabetic women may result from structural changes of the vagina. They investigated the vaginal structures using histochemistry and the expression of transforming growth factor β1 (TGF-β1) using immunohistochemistry. In the diabetic animals, vaginal tissue revealed reduced epithelial layers and decreased vaginal submucosal vasculatures as compared with the control animals. The collagen connective tissue in the submucosal area of the diabetic animals' tissue showed a dense, irregular and distorted arrangement. The TGF-β1 immunoreactivity in the diabetic animals was prominent in the collagen connective tissue, fibroblasts and smooth muscle fibres, whereas no immunoreactivity was detected in the vaginal structures of the controls. Therefore, in the rat model, Park et al. concluded that diabetes mellitus may induce vaginal tissue fibrosis by TGF-β1 expression, with a consequently reduced sexually driven local vasocongestion.

A recent study by Kim et al. *(48)* supported these findings. Indeed, they observed that in streptozotocin-treated female rats, the vaginal blood flow response to pelvic nerve stimulation was significantly reduced as compared with healthy controls. Moreover, the histological examination of vaginal tissue from diabetic animals showed reduced epithelial thickness and atrophy of the muscular layer. Diabetic animals also had reduced vaginal levels of endothelial nitric oxide synthase and arginase I, but elevated levels of cyclic guanosine monophosphate-dependent protein kinase (three key enzymes that regulate smooth muscle relaxation). These alterations were accompanied by a reduction in both estrogen receptor alpha and androgen receptor expression in nuclear extracts of vaginal tissue from diabetic animals. The authors reported that similar changes were also found previously in ovariectomized animals; therefore, they hypothesized that diabetes may lead to multiple disruptions in sex steroid hormone synthesis, metabolism and action. These pathological events may cause dramatic changes in tissue structure and key enzymes that regulate cell growth and smooth muscle contractility, ultimately affecting the genital response during sexual arousal. In a different study of streptozotocin-induced diabetic rats *(49)*, diabetes was confirmed to be associated with vaginal fibrosis, as evidenced by increased collagen, TGF-β1, plasminogen activator inhibitor, apoptosis, and by decreased α-smooth muscle actin. The increment of reactive oxygen species and the reduction of superoxide dismutase indicated oxidative stress in diabetic tissue, accompanied by inducible nitric oxide synthase induction and increased reaction between nitric oxide and reactive oxygen species.

Park et al. *(50)* also investigated the effect of diabetes on clitoral hemodynamics and structures in the alloxan-induced diabetic female rabbit. After having verified the development of diabetes, clitoral cavernous blood flow was measured with a laser Doppler flowmeter. Mean baseline flaccid and peak clitoral cavernous blood flow was significantly decreased in the diabetic group than in the control group ($p < 0.05$). Moreover, histology revealed diffuse clitoral fibrosis in the diabetic group, with a significant reduction of the clitoral cavernous smooth muscle ($p < 0.05$). The authors concluded that diabetes mellitus may produce significant adverse effects on the hemodynamic mechanism of clitoral engorgement and lead to diffuse clitoral cavernous fibrosis in the animal model, and this finding may be related with decreased sexual arousal in diabetic women.

Unfortunately, there are few human studies that have explored the sexually related functional vascular anatomy in women. Park et al. *(51, 52)* also demonstrated that the angiotensin (ANG) system is a potent modulator for the maintenance of smooth muscle tone of the rabbit clitoral cavernosum, as the clitoral cavernosum contracted dose-dependently by the addition of ANG I, ANG II, ANG III and ANG IV. More recently, they reported that the contractile responses to all four ANG peptides are significantly enhanced in the diabetic clitoral cavernosum *(53)*. Enhancement of contractility in diabetic clitoral cavernosum may be related to the increased affinity to ANG II receptors for ANG peptides, which was the epiphenomenon of impaired clitoral vasocongestion in the analysed diabetic animals.

Giraldi et al. *(54)* characterized the effect of experimental streptozotocin-induced diabetes on neurotransmission in rat vagina. Diabetes was demonstrated to interfere with adrenergic-, cholinergic- and nonadrenergic, noncholinergic (NANC) neurotransmitter mechanisms in the smooth muscle of the rat vagina, leading to impairment in vaginal SF. Such an elegant demonstration is not available for diabetic women, where the actual potential impact of peripheral neuropathy is still not adequately studied and understood.

Menopausal Status and the Androgen Milieu

The correlation between menopausal status and sexual health among diabetic women has been poorly investigated. Data seem to suggest, however, that the postmenopausal condition does not cause a significantly negative impact on women's sexuality particularly because of the diabetes mellitus itself *(9, 23, 37, 38, 40)*.

Similarly, the potential associations among the circulating androgen milieu [total and free testosterone, dehydroepiandrosterone (DHEA), DHEA sulphate (DHEAS), and Δ_4-androstenedione ($\Delta4A$)] and SF in diabetic women have been scarcely analysed, especially when studies adequately segregating both the type of diabetes and the pre- vs. postmenopausal population are considered. In contrast, several studies have analysed the concept that endogenous sex hormones may have a role in sex-dependent aetiologies of DM2, such that hyperandrogenism may increase risk in women while decreasing risk in men *(55–63)*. In their comprehensive review, Ding et al. *(56)* reported that cross-sectional studies indicated that testosterone level was significantly lower in DM2 men but higher in DM2 women than in controls ($p < 0.001$, for sex difference). Similarly, prospective studies showed that men with higher testosterone levels had a 42% lower risk of DM2 (RR: 0.58; 95% CI: 0.39–0.87), while there was suggestion that testosterone increased risk in women ($p = 0.06$, for sex difference). These authors concluded that endogenous sex hormones may differentially modulate glycaemic status and risk of DM2 in men and women *(56)*. Likewise, data from the cross-sectional Multi-Ethnic Study of Atherosclerosis on 1973 postmenopausal women not taking hormone replacement therapy showed that endogenous bioavailable testosterone, estradiol, and DHEA were positively associated, whereas sex hormone-binding globulin was negatively associated with insulin resistance *(57)*. Moreover, Korytkowski et al. *(58)* showed that DM2 postmenopausal women have both clinical and biochemical evidence of androgen excess that may contribute to more adverse cardiovascular risk profiles. Similarly, Phillips et al. *(62)* analysed the correlation between androgens and coronary heart disease among DM2 postmenopausal Hispanic women. These patients had both hyperandrogenemia and hyperestrogenemia, with total or free testosterone positively correlated with a greater risk for coronary heart disease. Thus, Phillips et al. concluded that hyperandrogenemia may be a link between diabetes and coronary heart disease in women *(62)*. Indeed, hypoandrogenism, coronary heart disease, and diabetes are all significant independent predictors of sexual disorders in men. Thus, the actual pathophysiology of the relationship between diabetes mellitus, menopause and women's SF certainly needs to be adequately investigated.

The role of endogenous androgens in women's SF among the general population is still controversial *(23, 64–66)*. Androgens play a key role in determining sexual desire and satisfaction, as well as in conditioning mood, energy and psychological well-being *(64, 67)*. Androgens are necessary for the development of female reproductive function and hormonal homeostasis, and they are the immediate precursors of estrogens. In pre- and postmenopausal women, a low serum-free testosterone level has been proposed as a diagnostic marker of the female androgen insufficiency syndrome, which is characterized by reduced libido, diminished well-being and depressed mood *(64, 66–68)*. There is increasing awareness of the impact of low androgen levels on the emotional, social, psychological and sexual well-being of women. Several studies have shown that testosterone substitution therapy in women may improve sexual desire, orgasm and satisfaction after either physiological *(65, 66, 69, 70)* or surgical menopause *(65, 66, 70–75)*.

However, the diagnosis of female androgen insufficiency syndrome is not unequivocal, because there is currently no reliable and inexpensive assay to measure circulating levels of free testosterone in the range observed in women *(23, 76)*, nor is there agreement on the serum-free testosterone threshold that defines the hypoandrogenism associated with impaired SF *(23, 77, 78)*. In addition, we must note that the levels of circulating androgens associated with symptomatic hypoandrogenism have not been unequivocally defined even for men *(23, 76, 79–81)*.

Moreover, recent data show that endogenous androgens are not independent predictors of well-being in postmenopausal women. Only DHEAS is associated with greater vitality in premenopausal women *(78)*. In addition, a recent community-based, cross-sectional study including more than 1,400 women failed to show a relationship between low serum levels of either free or total testosterone or Δ4A and low psychometric scores for SF. Interestingly, the same study demonstrated that among premenopausal women low DHEAS levels were associated with lower scores for sexual desire, sexual arousal, and sexual responsiveness *(82)*. The Endocrine Society recently recommended against diagnosing androgen deficiency in women because a widely accepted definition of female androgen insufficiency syndrome and normative total or free testosterone levels in women throughout their lifespan are still not available *(23, 65)*.

Labrie et al. *(83, 84)* demonstrated that steroid hormones can be produced within cells in peripheral target tissues, where they can exert effects without release into systemic circulation, thus making unreliable the measurement of serum testosterone as a marker of total androgenic activity. This implies that serum levels of androgenic hormone might not accurately reflect the actual androgenic activity in tissue *(84)*. This may have implications for women with androgen deficiency involving osteoporosis, obesity, DM2, SD or a loss of muscular strength. Therefore, the role of androgens in both glucose homeostasis and SF in postmenopausal women requires further study.

Menstrual Cycle and the Endocrine Profile Among Reproductive-Aged Women with Type 1 Diabetes

In women with diabetes, SF may vary according to the phase of the menstrual cycle. Our recent study investigated SF in reproductive-aged DM1 women, compared these results with those of age-matched normally cycling healthy fertile women with an objectively assessed normal SF, compared the endocrine profile of both groups, and analysed the correlation between endocrine milieu and SF according to the phase of the menstrual cycle *(85)*. The findings suggested that DM1 may affect several aspects of women's SF. In addition, the results emphasized that both psychosexual and endocrine parameters must be assessed according to the different phases of the menstrual cycle. Indeed, when comparing the FSFI scores recorded independently of the phases of the menstrual cycle, a significant impairment of the overall SF as well as lower values on the desire, arousal, lubrication, orgasm and pain domains were found in the DM1 group compared to the control group. In contrast, a menstrual phase-related analysis revealed lack of any significant difference between the two groups for each domain of the FSFI during the midfollicular phase, but decreased arousal and lubrication, decreased capability of reaching orgasm, decreased satisfaction, and increased sexual pain in DM1 patients during the midluteal phase *(85)*. Sexual desire did not seem to be affected by diabetes according to the phase of the menstrual cycle, which is in accordance with Kolodny *(86)* but is contrary to other studies *(25, 87)*.

The impairment of arousal, lubrication and orgasm observed in patients with diabetes is not exclusively related to psychosexual issues. A reduction in lubrication has been reported in 10–34% of the cases. Orgasmic difficulties are also frequently described, with a prevalence of 11–14% in women with diabetes *(25, 26, 28, 33, 34)*. Interestingly, in our study *(85)*, the major differences were found when comparing either the overall values of the sexual pain domain (independent of the specific phase of the menstrual cycle) or the midluteal-phase values. In the literature, pain or discomfort during coitus was reported by 10–12% of diabetic women *(25, 26, 28, 33, 34)*.

Widom et al. *(88)* reported that the menstrual cycle may influence glucose metabolism in women with DM1. A subgroup of patients exhibits worsening premenstrual hyperglycaemia and a decline in insulin sensitivity during the luteal phase, and the deterioration in glucose uptake in this subgroup has been associated with a greater increment in estradiol levels from the follicular to the luteal phase. In our study, glycaemic control did not directly affect the different domains of FSFI. In fact, we did not find any significant correlations between HbA_{1c} levels and the FSFI domains. This finding is in accord with previous reports *(19)* and confirmed that poor glycaemic control probably has a minor impact on SF in women. In contrast, a positive correlation was found between HbA_{1c} values and both midfollicular-phase total testosterone and midluteal progesterone levels. This finding was contrary to those of Widom et al. *(88)*, who reported changes in reproductive hormones not related to differing glucose uptake throughout the menstrual cycle.

Interesting results emerged from analysis of the endocrine profile of the DM1 women *(85)*. Patients and controls showed similar circulating levels of follicle-stimulating hormone, luteinizing hormone and prolactin. As far as gonadotropins are concerned, our data were in line with previous observations of Bestetti et al. in diabetic rats *(89)*. Other researchers, however, have shown that impairment of gonadotropin release in diabetic rats may be appreciated only after stimulation with gonadotropin-releasing hormone *(90)*. This test was not performed in our study. However, according to previous reports *(91–95)*, oestrogen levels during both the midfollicular and the midluteal phase were reduced in comparison with those of controls and the same occurred for progesterone during the luteal phase. A decrease in estradiol had a negative impact on mood profile scores, as defined by means of the Beck's Inventory for Depression (BDI) scores *(96, 97)*, and we found a significant negative correlation between estradiol and sexual pain.

Both overall and midluteal total testosterone levels were higher in diabetes patients than in controls. However, the relevance of this result remained doubtful, because both the sex hormone-binding globulin and free testosterone levels were comparable in the two groups during all phases. The increased total testosterone levels might be related to a positive modulatory effect of exogenous insulin on the expression of the luteinizing hormone receptor in the granulosa cell of the ovaries (98), which differentiate into androgen-producing interstitial cells. High levels of circulating testosterone bring about follicular atresia and, lead to a loss of estrogen-secreting cells and the development of polycystic ovaries and hirsutism (99). Patients also showed an overall reduction in adrenocortical androgen production, as previously stated by Couch (100).

Of note was the finding of low triiodothyronine/thyroxine (T3/T4) levels during both the midfollicular and the midluteal phase in DM1 patients (85). In addition, we found that the worse the glycaemic control, the more compromised the thyroid function. During the midfollicular phase, free triiodothyronine (fT3) was positively associated to sexual desire, lubrication, and sexual satisfaction. A higher rate of mood deflection was also related to lower values of fT3. We also found a significant association between fT3 and the FSFI full scale as well as the arousal, lubrication, orgasm, and sexual satisfaction domains during the midluteal phase. The fT3 plasma levels were also positively correlated with arousal, lubrication, orgasm, and satisfaction in controls.

Our findings suggested that DM1 reproductive-aged women are at an increased risk for SD, with an endocrine milieu characterized by reduced estrogenic tone, adrenocortical androgen production, and low T3/T4. The role of the endocrine milieu in the pathogenesis of SD related to diabetes remains to be clarified. Moreover, our findings highlighted that investigations of the sexuality of premenopausal women with diabetes mellitus require examination of all the parameters in relation to the different phases of the menstrual cycle (85).

Psychological Factors

Therapy of diabetes-associated SD in women must include consideration of the psychometric profile, including mood deflection and major depression, interpersonal issues and the psychological aspects of living with diabetes, since all these factors are correlates of woman's sexual health (19, 23, 25, 26, 37, 38, 85, 101, 102). The two major studies by Enzlin et al. (19, 26) showed that women with DM1 either with or without SD reported more depressive symptoms than men with and without SD, respectively. Moreover, women with SD suffered from a greater amount of depressive complaints than those without SD. Enzlin et al. (25) reported a significantly higher incidence of depressive symptoms in women with DM1 who had sexual problems than in women without SD. Based on the clinically defined cut-off score for depression of the BDI (≥ 16), four times more women with SD had scores suggestive of clinical depression than those without SD (37.7% vs. 8.3%, respectively; $p < 0.001$) (19). A significant association was found between depression and SD, decreased libido and arousal impairment, whereas data from Enzlin et al.'s cohort do not reveal any correlation with orgasmic functioning. In our study, we did not find any significant difference between subjects and controls in terms of either mood deflection or clinically significant depression, regardless of the specific phases of the menstrual cycle (85). Thus, our findings suggested that alterations in SF could not be totally ascribed to a depressive state. However, depression is a well-known determinant of decreased desire and impaired arousability in women (28, 29, 103), and we found a significant negative correlation between the BDI scores and the desire and arousal scores during both analysed phases of the menstrual cycle. A similar correlation was found between BDI and the lubrication, orgasm and sexual satisfaction domains as well, but only during the midfollicular phase. These latter results confirmed that it is mandatory to distinguish sexual behaviours and sexual complaints according to the different phases of the menstrual cycle in order to reduce an important bias (104).

In Enzlin et al.'s analyses *(19, 25, 26)*, the overall quality of marital relationship was significantly lower for women with diabetes than for controls. In addition, diabetic women with SD reported a significantly lower overall quality of marital relationship than women without SD ($p < 0.001$), but this difference was not found among men *(19)*. Similarly, women with DM1 with SD were found to have a more negative appraisal of their diabetes ($p = 0.01$), have more problems with emotional adjustment to diabetes ($p = 0.01$), be less satisfied with the treatment ($p = 0.01$), and experience more impact of treatment on daily life ($p = 0.04$). Because psychological adjustment to diabetes and SD are related, the authors concluded that disease acceptance is a crucial factor in predicting the SF outcome within a couple. They also observed that there is a relationship between SD and psychological adjustment to diabetes: the addition of any diabetic complication altered the perception of the psychological impact of SD in women with diabetes *(19, 25, 26)*. In accordance with Enzlin et al. *(19)* but in contrast to Tyrer et al. *(34)*, our findings suggested that SD may also be psychogenic in diabetic women and occur independently of the disease-related complications *(85)*. However, we did not find any correlation between number or types of complications or between the duration of the disease and number or types of sexual disorders *(85)*.

Moreover, according to the Female Sexual Distress Scale, a 12-item instrument to measure sexually related personal distress in women *(105)*, we found that sexual distress was similar between patients and control subjects during the follicular phase, while patients complained of significantly greater sexually related distress during the luteal phase of the menstrual cycle *(85)*. In women with DM1 sexual distress was significantly correlated to a reduction in libido scores ($r = -0.44$, $p = 0.034$) and to lower lubrication scores ($r = -0.45$, $p = 0.032$) during the midfollicular phase *(85)*. Likewise, sexual distress was significantly correlated to a decreased sexual desire during the luteal phase ($r = -0.42$, $p = 0.041$) *(85)*.

TREATMENT OF SEXUAL DISORDERS IN WOMEN WITH DIABETES

Few treatment options have been investigated to address SD in diabetic women. Moreover, no compounds have been specifically developed for the therapy of SD in diabetic women.

Genital Sexual Arousal Disorders Among Women with Diabetes

Data from epidemiological studies support the finding that sexual arousal disorder is the most commonly reported sexual problem among diabetic women *(9, 19, 23, 25, 26)*. In physiological terms, genital sexual excitement is characterized by pelvic vasocongestion and swelling of the external genitalia, including clitoral and vaginal engorgement *(106–109)*. Clitoral engorgement is a highly complex phenomenon, mainly characterized by hemodynamic modifications consequent to local smooth muscle relaxation. At least in an animal model, diabetes mellitus produces significant adverse effects on the hemodynamic mechanism of clitoral engorgement and leads to diffuse clitoral cavernous fibrosis *(50)*. Indeed, diabetes is associated with atherosclerosis and microangiopathy, leading to an impairment of the clitoral hemodynamics. This might imply that decreased sexual arousal in diabetic women may result from hemodynamic-driven structural changes in the clitoris. Although controversial, vaginal photoplethysmography and color Doppler ultrasonography represent the most widely used assessment modalities to measure physiological sexual arousal and sexually generated genital responses in women. These measures should not be used in isolation, rather women's SF should be evaluated using vaginal vasocongestion measures in conjunction with subjective indices *(110–114)*.

Although published guidelines on diagnosing SD in diabetic women are still not available, we personally recommend a comprehensive assessment of the external genitalia; it would particularly be important to look for vasocongestion and swelling of the genitalia, including clitoral and vaginal engorgement immediately after mechanically promoted genital sexual excitement *(106–109)*.

The development of phosphodiesterase-type-5 (PDE5) inhibitors, such as sildenafil, tadalafil and vardenafil, has revolutionized the treatment of SD in men. Preclinical studies with clitoral tissue baths suggested a rationale for using these agents to treat women's SD *(115, 116)*. However, clinical investigations regarding vasocongestive therapies for women's sexual complaints have yielded inconsistent results *(116)*.

Caruso et al. presented the largest peer-reviewed series regarding the use of sildenafil in both diabetic *(117, 118)* and nondiabetic *(119, 120)* women complaining of genital sexual arousal disorder. They assessed whether sildenafil was effective in modifying clitoral blood flow in a group of 30 premenopausal women with DM1 as compared with 39 healthy premenopausal women. A direct comparison showed that the DM1 patients had significantly lower scores for the arousal, orgasm and frequency of sexual activity domains of the Personal Experience Questionnaire. Moreover, diabetic women suffered from dyspareunia more frequently than the healthy controls. Likewise, the baseline clitoral blood flow of the DM1 women was significantly lower than that of the control group. Each DM1 woman received a single oral dose of 100-mg sildenafil and underwent a translabial colour Doppler of the clitoral arteries 1 and 4 h after sildenafil absorption *(117)*. At 1 h after the administration of sildenafil, several hemodynamic parameters at the clitoral arteries were significantly changed and were greater than the baseline and the 4-h postsildenafil evaluation. Although we are skeptical that the latter results might actually have clinical significance in a real-life setting, Caruso et al. concluded that sildenafil seemed to improve the clitoral blood flow of premenopausal DM1 women, even without any erotic stimulus *(117)*. They also attributed the local changes as a potential consequence of the direct vasodilator effect of sildenafil on the women's genital tissues. The rationale for using sildenafil to treat women's sexual arousal disorder was that this compound, like tadalafil and vardenafil, is an orally active, potent, selective inhibitor of cyclic guanosine monophosphate-specific PDE5. PDEs catalyse the hydrolysis of the secondary messengers, cyclic adenosine monophosphate and cyclic guanosine monophosphate, which are involved in signal pathways of cavernous smooth muscle in men. In this context, several reports described the presence of nitric oxide synthase and PDE5 in both animal models and the human clitoral and vaginal tissues *(121–125)*.

Subsequently, Caruso et al. *(118)* confirmed their original finding in a double-blind, placebo-controlled, cross-over, independent study aimed at verifying the effectiveness of sildenafil in a larger cohort of DM1 premenopausal women with sexual arousal disorder. Each woman received either 100 mg of sildenafil or placebo to be taken no more than once a day at 1 h prior to sexual intercourse for eight consecutive weeks. After a 1-week washout period, the participants received the other compound (that is, placebo or sildenafil). As expected, women did not obtain improvement in libido. However, sildenafil was able to significantly improve the subjective experience of arousal, orgasmic function and sexual enjoyment. Likewise, the active drug significantly improved both the experience of arousal and orgasm over the placebo. Sildenafil also promoted a reduction in dyspareunia with respect to both the baseline condition and the placebo period. These subjective improvements were coupled with the objective finding of significantly improved clitoral hemodynamics after sildenafil intake. Therefore, the authors concluded that sildenafil was apparently able to improve both the subjective and the genital component of the sexual arousal domain of premenopausal DM1 women *(118)*. No further study has been published either corroborating these results or showing a significant effect of any PDE5 inhibitor in either pre- and postmenopausal diabetic women.

Hormonal Replacement Therapy, Women's Sexual Health, and Diabetes

Upon natural menopause, sex hormones, physical and mental well-being and feelings for the partner are extremely relevant for women's sexuality. Even a significant lack of androgens, as more frequently occurs in surgical menopause, has a negative impact on women's desire and sexual responsiveness (126).

Although menopause has been identified as a significant risk factor for SD among the general population (127–131), the same issue has been scarcely investigated among women with diabetes (19–26, 37, 38, 40, 41, 57, 58, 62). All the reports described earlier seem to support the idea that menopause per se should not be considered as an independent predictor of SD in diabetic women. Moreover, no studies have investigated the potential use of specific compounds for the treatment of SD among postmenopausal diabetic women, not even hormone replacement therapy.

Local estrogen supplementation need not be withheld in postmenopausal women with diabetes. Indeed, vulvovaginal atrophy may be a significant consequence of local estrogen deficiency, potentially leading to dyspareunia and to dryness, pruritus, loss of sexual sensitivity and recurrent vaginal and urinary tract infections. Data have shown that oestrogen replacement therapy significantly improves symptomatic vulvovaginal atrophy, strictly linked to dyspareunia and vulval atrophy (23). According to our finding that a lower estrogenic basal tone characterized even premenopausal women with DM1 (85), we believe that further investigations are urgently needed to assess the potential role of hormone replacement therapy for this special population.

Studies of estrogen deficiency in women within the general population have highlighted a prevalence rate of 32–41% for dyspareunia (23). Data on specific populations, such as in women with diabetes mellitus, are scant. However, findings seem to support the idea that diabetes may predispose women to dyspareunia from low estrogen. Dyspareunia due to vaginal dryness appears to be most responsive to estrogen replacement therapy via restoration of vaginal cells, pH and blood flow (132, 133). Progestins can oppose these changes and lead to a recurrence of dryness and dyspareunia depending on their biochemical properties (134, 135). However, even though estrogen therapy and estrogen/progestin therapy may be effective treatments for vaginal atrophy and increasing vaginal lubrication, they have not been shown to consistently increase sexual desire or activity, and many women with SD remain unresponsive (133, 136). There is a significant subgroup of women whose sexual difficulties respond initially to estrogen therapy but who subsequently revert to their initial problems, especially when the specific problem was loss of libido (133, 137).

Collectively, these data highlight the evidence that estrogen and estrogen/progestin therapies are not universally efficacious in treating women's SD (126, 138). However, it is necessary to investigate the differences, mainly on the plasma sex steroid and sex hormone-binding globulin levels, among various schemes of conventional hormone therapies in terms of type of molecule, route of administration, mechanism of action and metabolism. Moreover, it is necessary to develop such prospective studies for special populations, such as women with diabetes.

In this context, it is of paramount importance to highlight that hormone replacement therapy is controversial in general, since a number of recent studies have demonstrated an increase in the risk of cardiovascular events among postmenopausal women (139–143). This controversy is even more pertinent to the women with diabetes since they are at higher risk for cardiovascular events than the general population. Therefore, the risks and benefits of hormone replacement therapy on all aspects of a woman's health need to be always considered carefully.

Testosterone Substitution Therapy

As previously discussed, the role of endogenous androgens in women's sexual health is still controversial (64, 65). Although, several studies have shown that testosterone replacement may improve sexual desire, orgasm and satisfaction among postmenopausal women *(65, 66, 69–74, 144)*, the Endocrine Society has recommended against both diagnosing androgen deficiency in women and against general use of testosterone by women, because of the paucity of data for long-term safety and effectiveness *(65)*.

A comprehensive Cochrane review of randomised trials that compared testosterone plus estrogen vs. estrogen alone both in pre- and in postmenopausal women showed that such a combination improved SF scores for postmenopausal women within the general population *(69)*. No data are available on the efficacy of testosterone treatment without estrogen. Likewise, there are no specific studies regarding the potential use of either testosterone substitution or tibolone, a synthetic steroid with estrogenic, androgenic and progestogenic activity that is able to improve SF in postmenopausal women *(23, 144, 145)* for the treatment of SD among diabetic women.

CONCLUSIONS

Since 1974 the World Health Organization has recognized that human sexuality is an important element of an individual's health and well-being: 'Sexual health is a state of physical, emotional, mental and social well-being in relation to sexuality; it is not merely the absence of disease, dysfunction or infirmity. Sexual health requires a positive and respectful approach to sexuality and sexual relationships, as well as the possibility of having pleasurable and safe sexual experiences, free of coercion, discrimination and violence. For sexual health to be attained and maintained, the sexual rights of all persons must be respected, protected and fulfilled' *(146)*. Sexual rights embrace human rights that are already recognized in national laws, international human rights documents and other consensus statements.

Having stated this cornerstone point and despite published data suggesting that sexual complaints are highly prevalent among both women with DM1 and DM2, the scientific community has still barely begun to investigate the relationship between diabetes mellitus and women's SF impairment. In this context, a number of studies highlight both biological/functional and psychological aspects related with the pathophysiology of sexual complaints among diabetic women. In contrast, only a few reports comprehensively debate potential treatment modalities.

Therefore, it is of paramount importance that both researchers and clinicians address the issue of sexuality and sexual health among diabetic women in well-designed longitudinal studies that have sufficient statistical power and are free of biases. Moreover, additional medical education and training are needed to improve the identification and management of SD in diabetic women.

Acknowledgements   The authors thank BoldFace Editors for reviewing the language of the manuscript

REFERENCES

1. Bachmann G. Female sexuality and sexual dysfunction: are we stuck on the learning curve? J Sex Med 2006;3:639–645
2. Hayes RD, Bennett CM, Fairley CK, Dennerstein L. What can prevalence studies tell us about female sexual difficulty and dysfunction? J Sex Med 2006;3:589–595
3. Basson R, Schultz WW. Sexual sequelae of general medical disorders. Lancet 2007;369:409–424
4. Laumann EO, Paik A, Rosen RC. Sexual dysfunction in the United States: prevalence and predictors. JAMA 1999;281:537–544
5. Laumann EO, Nicolosi A, Glasser DB, Paik A, Gingell C, Moreira E, Wang T for the GSSAB Investigators' Group. Sexual problems among women and men aged 40–80 y: prevalence and correlates identified in the Global Study of Sexual Attitudes and Behaviors. Int J Impot Res 2005;17:39–57

6. Ponholzer A, Roehlich M, Racz U, Temml C, Madersbacher S. Female sexual dysfunction in a healthy Austrian cohort: prevalence and risk factors. Eur Urol 2005;47:366–374

7. Basson R, Leiblum S, Brotto L, Derogatis L, Fourcroy J, Fugl-Meyer K, Graziottin A, Heiman JR, Laan E, Meston C, Schover L, van Lankveld J, Schultz WW. Definitions of women's sexual dysfunction reconsidered: advocating expansion and revision. J Psychosom Obstet Gynaecol 2003;24:221–229

8. Basson R, Leiblum S, Brotto L, Derogatis L, Fourcroy J, Fugl-Meyer K, Graziottin A, Heiman JR, Laan E, Meston C, Schover L, van Lankveld J, Schultz WW. Revised definitions of women's sexual dysfunction. J Sex Med 2004;1:40–48

9. Clayton AH. Epidemiology and neurobiology of female sexual dysfunction. J Sex Med 2007;4(Suppl 4):260–268

10. Basson R. Clinical practice: sexual desire and arousal disorders in women. N Engl J Med 2006;354:1497–1506

11. Basson R, Brotto LA, Laan E, Redmond G, Utian WH. Assessment and management of women's sexual dysfunctions: problematic desire and arousal. J Sex Med 2005;2:291–300

12. Cayan S, Akbay E, Bozlu M, Canpolat B, Acar D, Ulusoy E. The prevalence of female sexual dysfunction and potential risk factors that may impair sexual function in Turkish women. Urol Int 2004;72:52–57

13. Graziottin A. Prevalence and evaluation of sexual health problems: HSDD in Europe. J Sex Med 2007;4(Suppl 3):211–219

14. Eplov L, Giraldi A, Davidsen M, Garde K, Kamper-Jørgensen F. Sexual desire in a nationally representative Danish population. J Sex Med 2007;4:47–56

15. Dennerstein L, Koochaki P, Barton I, Graziottin A. Hypoactive sexual desire disorder in menopausal women: a survey of Western European women. J Sex Med 2006;3:212–222

16. Hayes R, Dennerstein L. The impact of ageing on sexual function and sexual dysfunction in women: a review of population-based studies. J Sex Med 2005;2:317–330

17. Fedele D, Coscelli C, Santeusanio F, Bortolotti A, Chatenoud L, Colli E, Landoni M, Parazzini F. Gruppo Italiano Studio Deficit Erettile nei Diabetici. Erectile dysfunction in diabetic subjects in Italy. Diabetes Care 1998;21:1973–1977

18. Penson DF, Latini DM, Lubeck DP, Wallace KL, Henning JM, Lue TF, Comprehensive Evaluation of Erectile Dysfunction (ExCEED) database. Do impotent men with diabetes have more severe erectile dysfunction and worse quality of life than the general population of impotent patients? Results from the Exploratory Comprehensive Evaluation of Erectile Dysfunction (ExCEED) database. Diabetes Care 2003;26:1093–1099

19. Enzlin P, Mathieu C, Van den Bruel A, Vanderschueren D, Demyttenaere K. Prevalence and predictors of sexual dysfunction in patients with type 1 diabetes. Diabetes Care 2003;26:409–414

20. Sarkadi A, Rosenqvist U. Intimacy and women with type 2 diabetes: an exploratory study using focus group interviews. Diabetes Educ 2003;29:641–652

21. Rutherford D, Collier A. Sexual dysfunction in women with diabetes mellitus. Gynecol Endocrinol 2005;21:189–192

22. Grandjean C, Moran B. The impact of diabetes mellitus on female sexual well-being. Nurs Clin N Am 2007;42:581–592

23. Bhasin S, Enzlin P, Coviello A, Basson R. Sexual dysfunction in men and women with endocrine disorders. Lancet 2007;369:597–611

24. Thomas A, Lo Piccolo J. Sexual functioning in persons with diabetes: issues in research, treatment and education. Clin Psychol Rev 1994;14:61–86

25. Enzlin P, Mathieu C, Vanderschueren D, Demyttenaere K. Diabetes mellitus and female sexuality: a review of 25 years' research. Diabet Med 1998;15:809–815

26. Enzlin P, Mathieu C, Van den Bruel A, Bosteels J, Vanderschueren D, Demyttenaere K. Sexual dysfunction in women with type 1 diabetes. Diabetes Care 2002;25:672–677

27. Lingjaerde O, Ahlfors UG, Bech P, Dencker SJ, Elgen K. The UKU side effect rating scale: a new comprehensive rating scale for psychotropic drugs and a cross-sectional study of side effects in neuroleptic-treated patients. Acta Psychiatr Scand Suppl 1987;334:1–100

28. Jensen S. Diabetic sexual dysfunction: a comparative study of 160 insulin treated diabetic men and women and an age-matched control group. Arch Sex Behav 1981;10:493–504

29. Jensen S. Sexual relationships in couples with a diabetic partner. J Sex Marital Ther 1985;11:259–270

30. Diemont WL, Vruggink PA, Meuleman EJH, Doesburg WH, Lemmens WAJG, Berden JHM. Sexual dysfunction after renal replacement therapy. Am J Kidney Dis 2000;35:845–851

31. Levine SB, Yost MA. Frequencies of sexual dysfunction in a general gynaecological clinic: an epidemiological approach. Arch Sex Behav 1976;5:229–238

32. Bachman GA, Leiblum SR, Grill J. Brief sexual inquiry in gynaecologic practice. Obstet Gynecol 1989;73:425–427

33. Schreiner-Engel P, Schiavi R, Vietorisz D, Smith H. The differential impact of diabetes type on female sexuality. J Psychosom Res 1987;31:23–33

34. Tyrer G, Steel J, Ewing D, Bancroft J, Warner P, Clarke B. Sexual responsiveness in diabetic women. Diabetologia 1983;24:166–171

35. Taylor JF, Rosen RC, Leiblum SR. Self-report assessment of female sexual function: psychometric evaluation of the Brief Index of Sexual Functioning for Women. Arch Sex Behav 1994;23:627–643

36. Derogatis LR. The Derogatis Interview for Sexual Functioning (DISF/DISF-SR): an introductory report. J Sex Marital Ther 1997;23:291–304

37. Basson RJ, Rucker BM, Laird PG, Conry R. Sexuality of women with diabetes. J Sex Reprod Med 2001;1:11–20

38. Doruk H, Akbay E, Cayan S, Akbay E, Bozlu M, Acar D. Effect of diabetes mellitus on female sexual function and risk factors. Arch Androl 2005;51:1–6

39. Rosen RC, Brown C, Heiman J, Leiblum S, Meston CM, Shabsigh R, Ferguson D, D'Agostino R Jr. The Female Sexual Function Index (FSFI): a multidimensional self-report instrument for the assessment of female sexual function. J Sex Marital Ther 2000;26:191–208

40. Erol B, Tefekli A, Ozbey I, Salman F, Dincag N, Kadioglu A, Tellaloglu S. Sexual dysfunction in type II diabetic females: a comparative study. J Sex Marital Ther 2002;28(Suppl 1):55–62

41. Olarinoye J, Olarinoye A. Determinants of sexual function among women with type 2 diabetes in a Nigerian population. J Sex Med 2007;5(4):878–876

42. Lindau ST, Schumm LP, Laumann EO, Levinson W, O'Muircheartaigh CA, Waite LJ. A study of sexuality and health among older adults in the United States. N Engl J Med 2007;357:762–774

43. Arshag D, Mooradian MD, Greiff V. Sexuality in older women. Arch Intern Med 1990;150:1033–1038

44. Erol B, Tefekli A, Sanli O, Ziylan O, Armagan A, Kendirci M, Eryasar D, Kadioglu A. Does sexual dysfunction correlate with deterioration of somatic sensory system in diabetic women? Int J Impot Res 2003;15:198–202

45. Duby JJ, Campbell RK, Setter SM, White JR, Rasmussen KA. Diabetic neuropathy: an intensive review. Am J Health Syst Pharm 2004;61:160–173

46. Wincze JP, Albert A, Bansal S. Sexual arousal in diabetic females: physiological and self-report measures. 1. Arch Sex Behav 1993;22:587–601

47. Park K, Ryu SB, Park YI, Ahn K, Lee SN, Nam JH. Diabetes mellitus induces vaginal tissue fibrosis by TGF-beta 1 expression in the rat model. J Sex Marital Ther 2001;27:577–587

48. Kim NN, Stankovic M, Cushman TT, Goldstein I, Munarriz R, Traish AM. Streptozotocin-induced diabetes in the rat is associated with changes in vaginal hemodynamics, morphology and biochemical markers. BMC Physiol 2006;6:4

49. Ferrini MG, Nolazco G, Vernet D, Gonzalez-Cadavid NF, Berman J. Increased vaginal oxidative stress, apoptosis, and inducible nitric oxide synthase in a diabetic rat model: implications for vaginal fibrosis. Fertil Steril 2006;86(Suppl 4):1152–1163

50. Park K, Ahn K, Chang JS, Lee SE, Ryu SB, Park YI. Diabetes induced alteration of clitoral hemodynamics and structure in the rabbit. J Urol 2002;168:1269–1272

51. Park JK, Kim SZ, Kim SH, Kim YG, Cho KW. Renin angiotensin system of rabbit clitoral cavernosum: interaction with nitric oxide. J Urol 2000;164:556–561

52. Park JK, Kim SZ, Kim JU, Kim YG, Kim SM, Cho KW. Comparison of effects of angiotensin peptides in the regulation of clitoral cavernosum smooth muscle tone. Int J Impot Res 2002;14:72–80

53. Park JK, Lee SO, Cui WS, Kim SZ, Koh GY, Cho KW. Activity of angiotensin peptides in clitoral cavernosum of alloxan induced diabetic rabbit. Eur Urol 2005;48:1042–1050

54. Giraldi A, Persson K, Werkström V, Alm P, Wagner G, Andersson KE. Effects of diabetes on neurotransmission in rat vaginal smooth muscle. Int J Impot Res 2001;13:58–66

55. Haffner SM. Sex hormones, obesity, fat distribution, type 2 diabetes and insulin resistance: epidemiological and clinical correlation. Int J Obes Relat Metab Disord 2000;24(Suppl 2):S56–S58

56. Ding EL, Song Y, Malik VS, Liu S. Sex differences of endogenous sex hormones and risk of type 2 diabetes: a systematic review and meta-analysis. JAMA 2006;295:1288–1299

57. Golden SH, Dobs AS, Vaidya D, Szklo M, Gapstur S, Kopp P, Liu K, Ouyang P. Endogenous sex hormones and glucose tolerance status in postmenopausal women. J Clin Endocrinol Metab 2007;92:1289–1295

58. Korytkowski MT, Krug EI, Daly MA, Deriso L, Wilson JW, Winters SJ. Does androgen excess contribute to the cardiovascular risk profile in postmenopausal women with type 2 diabetes? Metabolism 2005;54:1626–1631

59. Joffe HV, Ridker PM, Manson JE, Cook NR, Buring JE, Rexrode KM. Sex hormone-binding globulin and serum testosterone are inversely associated with C-reactive protein levels in postmenopausal women at high risk for cardiovascular disease. Ann Epidemiol 2006;16:105–112

60. Golden SH, Ding J, Szklo M, Schmidt MI, Duncan BB, Dobs A. Glucose and insulin components of the metabolic syndrome are associated with hyperandrogenism in postmenopausal women: the atherosclerosis risk in communities study. Am J Epidemiol 2004;160:540–548

61. Rexrode KM, Manson JE, Lee IM, Ridker PM, Sluss PM, Cook NR, Buring JE. Sex hormone levels and risk of cardio-vascular events in postmenopausal women. Circulation 2003;108:1688–1693

62. Phillips GB, Tuck CH, Jing TY, Boden-Albala B, Lin IF, Dahodwala N, Sacco RL. Association of hyperandrogenemia and hyperestrogenemia with type 2 diabetes in Hispanic postmenopausal women. Diabetes Care 2000;23:74–79

63. Hak AE, Westendorp IC, Pols HA, Hofman A, Witteman JC. High-dose testosterone is associated with atherosclerosis in postmenopausal women. Maturitas 2007;56:153–160

64. Bachmann G, Bancroft J, Braunstein G, Burger H, Davis S, Dennerstein L, Goldstein I, Guay A, Leiblum S, Lobo R, Notevolitz M, Rosen RC, Sarrel P, Sherwin B, Simon J, Simpson E, Shifren J, Spark R, Traish A. Female androgen insuf-ficiency: the Princeton consensus statement on definition, classification, and assessment. Fertil Steril 2002;77:660–665

65. Wierman ME, Basson R, Davis SR, Khosla S, Miller KK, Rosner W, Santoro N. Androgen therapy in women: an Endocrine Society Clinical Practice Guideline. J Clin Endocrinol Metab 2006;91:3697–3710

66. Kingsberg S. Testosterone treatment for hypoactive sexual desire disorder in postmenopausal women. J Sex Med 2007;4(Suppl 3):227–234

67. Miller KK, Rosner W, Lee H, Hier J, Sesmilo G, Schoenfeld D, Neubauer G, Klibanski A. Measurement of free testo-sterone in normal women and women with androgen deficiency: comparison of methods. J Clin Endocrinol Metab 2004;89:525–533

68. Cameron DR, Braunstein GD. Androgen replacement therapy in women. Fertil Steril 2004;82:273–289

69. Shifren JL, Davis SR, Moreau M, Waldbaum A, Bouchard C, DeRogatis L, Derzko C, Bearnson P, Kakos N, O'Neill S, Levine S, Wekselman K, Buch A, Rodenberg C, Kroll R. Testosterone patch for the treatment of hypoactive sexual desire disorder in naturally menopausal women: results from the INTIMATE NM1 Study. Menopause 2006;13:770–779

70. Shifren JL, Braunstein GD, Simon JA, Casson PR, Buster JE, Redmond GP, Burki RE, Ginsburg ES, Rosen RC, Leiblum SR, Caramelli KE, Mazer NA. Transdermal testosterone treatment in women with impaired sexual function after oophorectomy. N Engl J Med 2000;343:682–688

71. Simon J, Braunstein G, Nachtigall L, Utian W, Katz M, Miller S, Waldbaum A, Bouchard C, Derzko C, Buch A, Rodenberg C, Lucas J, Davis S. Testosterone patch increases sexual activity and desire in surgically menopausal women with hypoactive sexual desire disorder. J Clin Endocrinol Metab 2005;90:5226–5233

72. Miller KK, Biller BM, Beauregard C, Lipman JG, Jones J, Schoenfeld D, Sherman JC, Swearingen B, Loeffler J, Klibanski A. Effects of testosterone replacement in androgen-deficient women with hypopituitarism: a randomized, double-blind, placebo-controlled study. J Clin Endocrinol Metab 2006;91:1683–1690

73. Braunstein GD, Sundwall DA, Katz M, Shifren JL, Buster JE, Simon JA, Bachman G, Aguirre OA, Lucas JD, Rodenberg C, Buch A, Watts NB. Safety and efficacy of a testosterone patch for the treatment of hypoactive sexual desire disorder in surgically menopausal women: a randomized, placebo-controlled trial. Arch Intern Med 2005;165:1582–1589

74. North American Menopause Society. The role of testosterone therapy in postmenopausal women: position statement of The North American Menopause Society. Menopause 2005;12:496–511

75. Kingsberg S, Shifren J, Wekselman K, Rodenberg C, Koochaki P, Derogatis L. Evaluation of the clinical relevance of benefits associated with transdermal testosterone treatment in postmenopausal women with hypoactive sexual desire disorder. J Sex Med 2007;4:1001–1008

76. Lazarou S, Reyes-Vallejo L, Morgentaler A. Wide variability in laboratory reference values for serum testosterone. J Sex Med 2006;3:1085–1089

77. Rivera-Woll LM, Papalia M, Davis SR, Burger HG. Androgen insufficiency in women: diagnostic and therapeutic implications. Hum Reprod Update 2004;10:421–432

78. Bell RJ, Donath S, Davison SL, Davis SR. Endogenous androgen levels and well-being: differences between premeno-pausal and postmenopausal women. Menopause 2006;13:65–71

79. Bhasin S, Cunningham GR, Hayes FJ, Matsumoto AM, Snyder PJ, Swerdloff RS, Montori VM. Testosterone therapy in adult men with androgen deficiency syndromes: an endocrine society clinical practice guideline. J Clin Endocrinol Metab 2006;91:1995–2010

80. Maggi M, Schulman C, Quinton R, Langham S, Uhl-Hochgraeber K. The burden of testosterone deficiency syndrome in adult men: economic and quality-of-life impact. J Sex Med 2007;4:1056–1069

81. Santoro N, Torrens J, Crawford S, Allsworth JE, Finkelstein JS, Gold EB, Korenman S, Lasley WL, Luborsky JL, McConnell D, Sowers MF, Weiss G. Correlates of circulating androgens in mid-life women: the study of women's health across the nation. J Clin Endocrinol Metab 2005;90:4836–4845

82. Davis SR, Davison SL, Donath S, Bell RJ. Circulating androgen levels and self-reported sexual function in women. JAMA 2005;294:91–96

83. Labrie F, Luu-The V, Labrie C, Bélanger A, Simard J, Lin SX, Pelletier G. Endocrine and intracrine sources of androgens in women: inhibition of breast cancer and other roles of androgens and their precursor dehydroepiandrosterone. Endocr Rev 2003;24:152–182

84. Labrie F, Bélanger A, Bélanger P, Bérubé R, Martel C, Cusan L, Gomez J, Candas B, Castiel I, Chaussade V, Deloche C, Leclaire J. Androgen glucuronides, instead of testosterone, as the new markers of androgenic activity in women. J Steroid Biochem Mol Biol 2006;99:182–188

85. Salonia A, Lanzi R, Scavini M, Pontillo M, Gatti E, Petrella G, Licata G, Nappi RE, Bosi E, Briganti A, Rigatti P, Montorsi F. Sexual function and endocrine profile in fertile women with type 1 diabetes. Diabetes Care 2006;29:312–316

86. Kolodny RC. Sexual dysfunction in diabetic females. Diabetes 1971;20:557–559

87. Zrustova M, Rostlapid J, Kabshelova A. Sexual disorders in diabetic women. Ches Gunekol 1978;43:277–280

88. Widom B, Diamond MP, Simonson DC. Alterations in glucose metabolism during menstrual cycle in women with IDDM. Diabetes Care 1992;15:213–220

89. Bestetti G, Locatelli V, Tirone F, Rossi GL, Muller EE. One month of streptozotocin-diabetes induces different neuroendocrine and morphological alterations in the hypothalamo-pituitary axis of male and female rats. Endocrinology 1985;117:208–216

90. Djursing H, Haan C, Nylholm HC, Carstensen L, Andersen A. Gonadotropin responses to gonadotropin-releasing hormone and prolactin responses to thyrotropin-releasing hormone and metoclopramide in women with amenorrhea and insulin-treated diabetes mellitus. J Clin Endocrinol Metab 1983;46:1016–1021

91. Valimaki M, Liewendahl K, Nikkanen P, Peldkonen R. Hormonal changes in severely uncontrolled type 1 (insulin-dependent) diabetes mellitus. Scand J Clin Lab Invest 1991;51:385–393

92. Kjaer K, Hagen C, Sando SH, Eshoj O. Epidemiology of menarche and menstrual disturbances in an unselected group of women with insulin-dependent diabetes mellitus compared with controls. J Clin Endocrinol Metab 1992;75:524–529

93. Rosenfield RL. Evidence that idiopathic functional adrenal hyperandrogenism is caused by dysregulation of adrenal steroidogenesis and that hyperinsulinemia may be involved. J Clin Endocrinol Metab 1996;81:878–880

94. Cara JF, Rosenfield RL. Insulin-like growth factor-I and insulin potentiate luteinizing hormone-induced androgen synthesis by rat ovarian theca-interstitial cells. Endocrinology 1988;123:733–739

95. O'Hare JA, Eichold BH, II, Vignati L. Hypogonadotropic secondary amenorrhea in diabetes: effects of central opiate blockade and improved metabolic control. Am J Med 1987;83:1080–1084

96. Schwab J, Bialow M, Clemmons R, Martin P, Holzer G. The Beck Depression Inventory with medical inpatients. Acta Psychiatr Scand 1967;43:255–266

97. Beck A, Beamersderfer A. Assessment of depression: the depression inventory. Mod Probl Pharmacopsychiatry 1974;7:151–169

98. Erickson GF, Magoffin DA, Dyer CA, Hofeditz C. The ovarian androgen producing cells: a review of structure/function relationships. Endocr Rev 1985;6:371–399

99. Escobar-Morreale HF, Roldan B, Barrio R, Alonso M, Sancho J, de la Calle H, Garcia-Robles R. High prevalence of the polycystic ovary syndrome and hirsutism in women with type 1 diabetes mellitus. J Clin Endocrinol Metab 2000;85:4182–4187

100. Couch RM. Dissociation of cortisol and adrenal androgen secretion in poorly controlled insulin-dependent diabetes mellitus. Acta Endocrinol 1992;127:115–117

101. de Groot M, Anderson R, Freedland KE, Clouse RE, Lustman PJ. Association of depression and diabetes complications: a meta-analysis. Psychosom Med 2001;63:619–630

102. Newman A, Bertelson A. Sexual dysfunction in diabetic women J Behav Med 1986;9:261–270

103. Leedom L, Feldman M, Warner P, Zeidler A. Symptoms of sexual dysfunction and depression in diabetic women. J Diabetes Complicat 1991;5:38–41

104. Apaydin KC, Akar Y, Akar ME, Zorlu GC, Ozer HO. Menstrual cycle dependent changes in blue-on-yellow visual field analysis of young diabetic women with severe non-proliferative diabetic retinopathy. Clin Experiment Ophthalmol 2004;32:265–269

105. Derogatis LR, Rosen R, Leiblum S, Burnett A, Heiman J. The Female Sexual Distress Scale (FSDS): initial validation of a standardized scale for assessment of sexually related personal distress in women. J Sex Marital Ther 2002;28:317–330

106. Gragasin FS, Michelakis ED, Hogan A, Moudgil R, Hashimoto K, Wu X, Bonnet S, Haromy A, Archer SL. The neurovascular mechanism of clitoral erection: nitric oxide and cGMP-stimulated activation of BKCa channels. FASEB J 2004;18:1382–1391

107. Garcia S, Talakoub L, Maitland S, Dennis A, Goldstein I, Munarriz R. Genital duplex Doppler ultrasonography before and after sexual stimulation in women with sexual dysfunction: gray scale, volumetric, and hemodynamic findings. Fertil Steril 2005;83:995–999

108. Yang CC, Cao YY, Guan QY, Heiman JR, Kuffel SW, Peterson BT, Maravilla KR. Influence of PDE5 inhibitor on MRI measurement of clitoral volume response in women with FSAD: a feasibility study of a potential technique for evaluating drug response. Int J Impot Res 2008;20:105–110

109. Levin RJ, Wylie K. Vaginal vasomotion: its appearance, measurement, and usefulness in assessing the mechanisms of vasodilatation. J Sex Med 2008;5:377–386

110. Laan E, Everaerd W. Physiological measures of vaginal vasocongestion. Int J Impot Res 1998;10(Suppl 2):S107–S110

111. Prause N, Cerny J, Janssen E. The labial photoplethysmograph: a new instrument for assessing genital hemodynamic changes in women. J Sex Med 2005;2:58–65

112. McCall KM, Meston CM. The effects of false positive and false negative physiological feedback on sexual arousal: a comparison of women with or without sexual arousal disorder. Arch Sex Behav 2007;36:518–530

113. Khalifé S, Binik YM, Cohen DR, Amsel R. Evaluation of clitoral blood flow by color Doppler ultrasonography. J Sex Marital Ther 2000;26:187–189

114. Paulus WE, Strehler E, Zhang M, Jelinkova L, El-Danasouri I, Sterzik K. Benefit of vaginal sildenafil citrate in assisted reproduction therapy. Fertil Steril 2002;77:846–847

115. Park K, Moreland RB, Goldstein I, Atala A, Traish A. Sildenafil inhibits phosphodiesterase type 5 in human clitoral corpus cavernosum smooth muscle. Biochem Biophys Res Commun 1998;249:612–617

116. Perelman MA. Clinical application of CNS-acting agents in FSD. J Sex Med 2007;4(Suppl 4):280–290

117. Caruso S, Rugolo S, Mirabella D, Intelisano G, Di Mari L, Cianci A. Changes in clitoral blood flow in premenopausal women affected by type 1 diabetes after single 100-mg administration of sildenafil. Urology 2006;68: 161–165

118. Caruso S, Rugolo S, Agnello C, Intelisano G, Di Mari L, Cianci A. Sildenafil improves sexual functioning in premenopausal women with type 1 diabetes who are affected by sexual arousal disorder: a double-blind, crossover, placebo-controlled pilot study. Fertil Steril 2006;85:1496–1501

119. Caruso S, Intelisano G, Lupo L, Agnello C. Premenopausal women affected by sexual arousal disorder treated with sildenafil: a double-blind, cross-over, placebo-controlled study. BJOG 2001;108:623–628

120. Caruso S, Intelisano G, Farina M, Di Mari L, Agnello C. The function of sildenafil on female sexual pathways: a double-blind, cross-over, placebo-controlled study. Eur J Obstet Gynecol Reprod Biol 2003;110:201–206

121. Burnett AL, Calvin DC, Silver RI, Peppas DS, Docimo SG. Immunohistochemical description of nitric oxide synthase isoforms in human clitoris. J Urol 1997;158:75–78

122. D'Amati G, di Gioia CR, Bologna M, Giordano D, Giorgi M, Dolci S, Jannini EA. Type 5 phosphodiesterase expression in the human vagina. Urology 2002;60:191–195

123. Munarriz R, Kim SW, Kim NN, Traish A, Goldstein I. A review of the physiology and pharmacology of peripheral (vaginal and clitoral) female genital arousal in the animal model. J Urol 2003;170:S40–S44

124. Gragasin FS, Michelakis ED, Hogan A, Moudgil R, Hashimoto K, Wu X, Bonnet S, Haromy A, Archer SL. The neurovascular mechanism of clitoral erection: nitric oxide and cGMP-stimulated activation of BKCa channels. FASEB J 2004;18:1382–1391

125. Mayer M, Stief CG, Truss MC, Uckert S. Phosphodiesterase inhibitors in female sexual dysfunction. World J Urol 2005;23:393–397

126. Nappi RE. New attitudes to sexuality in the menopause: clinical evaluation and diagnosis. Climacteric 2007;10(Suppl 2):105–108

127. Alexander JL, Kotz K, Dennerstein L, Kutner SJ, Wallen K, Notelovitz M. The effects of postmenopausal hormone therapies on female sexual functioning: a review of double-blind, randomized controlled trials. Menopause 2004;11:749–765

128. Dennerstein L, Lehert P, Burger H. The relative effects of hormones and relationship factors on sexual function of women through the natural menopausal transition. Fertil Steril 2005;84:174–180

129. Dennerstein L, Hayes RD. Confronting the challenges: epidemiological study of female sexual dysfunction and menopause. J Sex Med 2005;2(Suppl 3):118–132

130. Alexander JL, Dennerstein L, Woods NF, Kotz K, Halbreich U, Burt V, Richardson G. Neurobehavioral impact of menopause on mood. Expert Rev Neurother 2007;7(11 Suppl):S81–S91

131. Dennerstein L, Lehert P, Guthrie JR, Burger HG. Modeling women's health during the menopausal transition: a longitudinal analysis. Menopause 2007;14:53–62

132. Sarrel PM. Sexuality and menopause. Obstet Gynecol 1990;75:26S–35S

133. Nappi R, Salonia A, Traish AM, van Lunsen RH, Vardi Y, Kodiglu A, Goldstein I. Clinical biologic pathophysiologies of women's sexual dysfunction. J Sex Med 2005;2:4–25

134. Sherwin BB. The impact of different doses of estrogen and progestin on mood and sexual behavior in postmenopausal women. J Clin Endocrinol Metab 1991;72:336–343

135. Bachmann GA. The hyperandrogenic woman: pathophysiologic overview. Fertil Steril 2002;77:S72–S76

136. Sarrel PM. Androgen deficiency: menopause and estrogen-related factors. Fertil Steril 2002;77:S63–S67

137. Sarrel PM. Effects of hormone replacement therapy on sexual psychophysiology and behaviour in postmenopause. J Womens Health Gend Based Med 2000;9:S25–S32

138. Cayan F, Dilek U, Pata O, Dilek S. Comparison of the effects of hormone therapy regimens, oral and vaginal estradiol, estradiol + drospirenone and tibolone, on sexual function in healthy postmenopausal women. J Sex Med 2008;5:132–138

139. Rossouw JE, Anderson GL, Prentice RL, LaCroix AZ, Kooperberg C, Stefanick ML, Jackson RD, Beresford SA, Howard BV, Johnson KC, Kotchen JM, Ockene J; Writing Group for the Women's Health Initiative Investigators. Risks and benefits of estrogen plus progestin in healthy postmenopausal women: principal results From the Women's Health Initiative randomized controlled trial. JAMA 2002;288:321–333

140. Anderson GL, Limacher M, Assaf AR, Bassford T, Beresford SA, Black H, Bonds D, Brunner R, Brzyski R, Caan B, Chlebowski R, Curb D, Gass M, Hays J, Heiss G, Hendrix S, Howard BV, Hsia J, Hubbell A, Jackson R, Johnson KC, Judd H, Kotchen JM, Kuller L, LaCroix AZ, Lane D, Langer RD, Lasser N, Lewis CE, Manson J, Margolis K, Ockene J, O'sullivan MJ, Phillips L, Prentice RL, Ritenbaugh C, Robbins J, Rossouw JE, Sarto G, Stefanick ML, Van Horn L, Wactawski-Wende J, Wallace R, Wassertheil-Smoller S; Women's Health Initiative Steering Committee. Effects of conjugated equine estrogen in postmenopausal women with hysterectomy: the Women's Health Initiative randomized controlled trial. JAMA 2004;291:1701–1712

141. Vickers MR, MacLennan AH, Lawton B, Ford D, Martin J, Meredith SK, DeStavola BL, Rose S, Dowell A, Wilkes HC, Darbyshire JH, Meade TW; WISDOM group. Main morbidities recorded in the women's international study of long duration oestrogen after menopause (WISDOM): a randomised controlled trial of hormone replacement therapy in postmenopausal women. BMJ 2007;335:239

142. Heiss G, Wallace R, Anderson GL, Aragaki A, Beresford SA, Brzyski R, Chlebowski RT, Gass M, LaCroix A, Manson JE, Prentice RL, Rossouw J, Stefanick ML; WHI Investigators. Health risks and benefits 3 years after stopping randomized treatment with estrogen and progestin. JAMA 2008;299:1036–1045

143. Kublickiene K, Fu XD, Svedas E, Landgren BM, Genazzani AR, Simoncini T. Effects in postmenopausal women of estradiol and medroxyprogesterone alone and combined on resistance artery function and endothelial morphology and movement. J Clin Endocrinol Metab 2008;93:1874–1883

144. Braunstein GD. Management of female sexual dysfunction in postmenopausal women by testosterone administration: safety issues and controversies. J Sex Med 2007;4:859–866

145. Kenemans P, Speroff L, International Tibolone Consensus Group. Tibolone: clinical recommendations and practical guidelines. A report of the International Tibolone Consensus Group. Maturitas 2005;51:21–28

146. World Health Organization. Education and treatment in human sexuality: the training of health professionals. Available at: http://www.who.int/reproductive-health/gender/sexualhealth.html Accessed 27 January 2008

9 Contraception for Women with Diabetes

Siri L. Kjos

ABSTRACT

Today, diabetic women have an increasing variety of safer and effective contraceptive methods. While more contraceptive trials in diabetic women are needed, data from existing studies and extrapolation from clinical trials in healthy women support the use of most contraceptive methods. This chapter will review contraception in women with type 1 (DM1) and type 2 (DM2) diabetes mellitus, with or without sequelae. It will also review contraception in prediabetic women, e.g., with previous gestational diabetes mellitus to augment the limited studies in women with DM2. The goal will be to provide a simple question-based approach to individualized counseling, considering diabetic sequelae and comorbidities, metabolic effects, and lifestyle demands.

Key words: Diabetes mellitus; Contraception; Oral contraceptives; Intrauterine device; Hormonal contraception; Contraception and breastfeeding; Progestin-only contraception; Estrogen.

INTRODUCTION

Offering women with diabetes a safe contraceptive method that they will reliably use is key to successfully preventing and planning pregnancy. Effective contraception enables women to work with their health care team to optimize their health prior to pregnancy, to switch to nonteratogenic medications, and to achieve euglycemia prior to pregnancy and during early embryogenesis, thereby reducing risks of congenital anomalies and abortions. Yet preconception health care occurs in only 15–30% of pregnancies in women with DM1 and even less in DM2 *(1)*. The real risks to the fetus and mother

From: *Diabetes in Women: Pathophysiology and Therapy*
Edited by: A. Tsatsoulis et al. (eds.), DOI 10.1007/978-1-60327-250-6_9
© Humana Press, a part of Springer Science+Business Media, LLC 2009

from poorly controlled glucose and vascular disease far exceed the risks from using any effective contraceptive method. Today, diabetic women have an increasing variety of safer and effective contraceptive methods. While more contraceptive trials in diabetic women are needed, data from existing studies and extrapolation from clinical trials in healthy women support the use of most contraceptive methods. This chapter will review contraception in women with DM1 and DM2, with or without sequelae. It will also review contraception in prediabetic women, e.g., with previous gestational diabetes mellitus to augment the limited studies in women with DM2. The goal will be to provide a simple question-based approach to individualized counseling, considering diabetic sequelae and comorbidities, metabolic effects, and lifestyle demands.

COUNSELING AND SELECTING A METHOD

A woman's reproductive desires and contraceptive preferences change throughout her reproductive life, irrespective of whether she has diabetes. Thus, the discussion of pregnancy plans and contraceptive preferences needs to be ongoing. A woman with diabetes should be encouraged that with preparation, good medical and prenatal care, most likely she will be able to have a successful pregnancy and reduce her risk to have an anomalous or premature baby. Importantly, she must know the positive steps she can make to prepare for pregnancy or to keep healthy until she desires pregnancy. While it is important for her provider to explain to her the increased risk of congenital anomalies, miscarriage, and morbidity, it is more productive to harness her motivation by helping her set reachable health and glycemic goals to reduce these risks. The more she takes charge of her general and diabetic health, the safer any pregnancy, planned or unplanned, will be for her and her baby (see Chap. 15).

Successful contraception depends on a woman's and/or her partner's willingness to consistently and properly use their chosen method. It must suit her/their individual lifestyle and sexual practices that are subject to change. Many women will have successfully used a method for years that has a higher failure rate, such as condoms or diaphragms. Some find that methods that need daily administration, such as the pill, do not work for them. Others may prefer a simple, no thought method, such as the intrauterine device (IUD) or implant. Thus, it is important to coordinate her contraceptive history with her daily habits.

Another important component of counseling that needs to be addressed is possible contraceptive failure and suspected early pregnancy. Despite contraceptive prescription, roughly half of pregnancies remain unplanned or unintended. Therefore, it is crucial to discuss what she should do if she believes she may be pregnant. Should she stop any of her medications? Diabetic women often take many medications, not only for diabetes, but for hypertension, hyperlipidemia, and renal disease. Each medication needs to be reviewed for its safety during early pregnancy. Commonly, women stop oral antidiabetic medication prior to obtaining medical care with the belief that these drugs may harm their baby. They need to be counseled that elevated glucose levels, resulting from stopping such medications before initiating insulin therapy, are likely to increase their risk of congenital malformations (see Chap. 15). While data are inadequate to conclude that any oral-diabetic medications are safe during embryogenesis, both sulfonylureas (2) and metformin (3) do not appear to increase the risk of malformations.

Another important safeguard to prescribe all contracepting women is emergency contraception, often referred to as the "morning after pill," to use within 72 h after recognized method failure, e.g., unprotected coitus, broken condom, several missed oral contraceptive pills, etc. The shorter the time interval from method failure to administration of emergency contraception, the more effective the pregnancy protection, that is, 0.5% pregnancy rate within first 12 h to 4.1% pregnancy rate within last 12 h of the 72-h window (4). In diabetic women, the progestin-only regimen, levo-norgestrel (1.5 mg total dose), is recommended and has no contraindications to use. It is recommended that all contracepting women should be offered (and prescribed) an emergency contraceptive regimen in advance.

BARRIER METHODS

Barrier methods block fertilization by preventing access of the sperm into the womb. Except for the diaphragm and cervical cap, they are obtainable without prescription, e.g., male and female condoms, contraceptive sponges, cervical shields, spermicidal jellies, and suppositories. Barrier methods are metabolically neutral and have no medical contraindications to their use. Their typical use failure rate is relatively high (16–21%) as success is dependent on proper application with each coitus and may expose her to an unacceptable pregnancy risk. Barrier method failure rates can be reduced by prescribing emergency contraception.

Condom use, in addition to pregnancy prevention, also decreases the transmission risk of HIV and sexually transmitted diseases. Sexual history is an important component of gynecologic care and needs to be reviewed. Women in nonmonogamous relationships should be encouraged to use condoms irrespective of contraceptive benefits to reduce this risk.

HORMONAL CONTRACEPTION

Hormonal contraception contains either a progestin compound alone or in conjunction with estrogen. They can be administered orally, intramuscularly, transdermally, and transvaginally. Some IUDs also contain progestin. Estrogen does not affect glucose tolerance (5), but progestins do increase insulin resistance and decrease glucose tolerance in a dose and potency fashion (6–8). Estrogen slightly increases blood pressure (9) by increasing angiotensin production while progestins have no effect. Estrogens produce an increase in clotting factors while progestins have no effect (10–14). Estrogens favorably affect lipid profiles, decreasing LDL-cholesterol and increasing HDL-cholesterol, while progestins produce an opposite effect (15–19). Estrogen increases triglycerides, while progestins have no effect. When estrogens and progestins are combined as in combination oral contraceptives (COC), the lower doses and less androgenic progestins generally produce milder and a more estrogen-dominant effect on carbohydrate and lipid metabolism with no effect on glucose tolerance and favorable changes in serum lipids. Table 1 gives an overview of general metabolic effects on glucose tolerance, serum

Table 1
Metabolic Effects of Hormonal Contraceptive Components

	Oral estrogen	Oral progestin	Progestin intramuscular injections and implants
Glucose tolerance	Neutral	↑ Insulin resistance, ↑ glucose tolerance	↑ Insulin resistance, ↑ glucose tolerance
Serum lipids	↑ HDL-Chol ↓ LDL-Chol ↑ Triglyceride	↓ HDL-Chol ↑ LDL-Chol	↓ Triglyceride Minimal effect on HDL-C and Chol
Blood pressure	Slight ↑	Neutral	Neutral
Coagulation factors	↑ Globulins: dose-dependent ↑	Neutral	Neutral

↑ increase; ↓ decrease; *HDL* High-density lipoprotein; *LDL* low-density lipoprotein lipids, blood pressure, and coagulation factors. In women with diabetes, these metabolic effects become important considerations when comorbidities exist, particularly hypertension or hyperlipidemia. Serum lipids and blood pressure need to be assessed to select the best formulation with the least possible metabolic effect. As a rule the lowest possible dose and potency formulations should be selected.

COC, containing both estrogen and progestin, have been extensively studied for over 40 years. Today's formulations contain lower doses of both ethinyl estradiol (20–35 µg) and various formulations of progestins. They have an excellent safety profile and can be prescribed in healthy women without physical examination, except for a blood pressure measurement. Newer combination methods deliver estrogen plus progestin via injection, transdermally or intravaginally. These methods will be considered similar to COC in risks and benefits, but they lack long-term safety data and have limited metabolic data. These methods offer an advantage of longer duration of coverage, weeks to monthly dosing. Short-term and limited studies in healthy women show a neutral effect on blood pressure, coagulation factors, and lipid metabolism with combination injectable contraception (CIC) *(20, 21)*. Minimal information is available regarding metabolic effects of the transdermal patch *(22)* or vaginal ring. Data are also limited regarding the newer progestin-only implant containing etonogestrel, and therefore it will be considered together with well-studied levonorgestrel (LVN) implant and injectable depo-medroxyprogesterone acetate (DMPA).

Studies examining contraceptive use in diabetic or prediabetic women are similarly limited and generally retrospective *(23)*, necessitating extrapolation from the vast number of clinical trials and epidemiological studies in healthy women as well as the World Health Organization classification of categories of contraceptive risk *(24)*. Thus, most of the data presented will be a combination of level C evidence, expert opinion, and practitioner experience (Table 2).

The following series of questions will help the provider decide which methods of contraception are best suited to the patient with diabetes.

Question: Can She Use Hormonal Contraception?

Women of reproductive age produce estrogen and progesterone. Most women with diabetes can safely use hormonal contraception. The few exceptions that exist are generally unrelated to diabetes and include liver disease (active hepatitis, cirrhosis, or cholestasis associated with prior hormone contraception use), malignant or benign liver tumors (focal nodular hyperplasia or adenomas), or estrogen- or progesterone-sensitive malignancies (breast cancer).

Question: Can She Use Estrogen-Containing Contraception?

It is the progestin component of hormonal contraceptives that prevents pregnancy. Estrogen is added to decrease intermenstrual bleeding. To prescribe an estrogen-containing contraceptive, the diabetic woman's cardiovascular risks need to be evaluated due to the estrogen-induced changes in her metabolic profile. Estrogen produces a dose-dependent increase in globulin production, increasing coagulation factors and angiotensin II levels, thereby increasing thromboembolic risk and a slight increase in mean arterial blood pressure *(9, 25)*. With low estrogen dose COC (≤35 mg), the absolute increase in arterial thromboembolism associated with COC in women is very low (1:12,000) *(26)*. Data from large case-control studies examining COC use and stroke suggest that the excess thromboembolic risk is related to the presence of cardiovascular risk factors. In two large case-control studies from the USA *(27)* and Europe *(28)*, the adjusted risk for ischemic or hemorrhagic stroke was not increased with current or former use of low-estrogen COCs. However, the risk was increased when cardiovascular risk factors, e.g., hypertension, diabetes, smoking, migraine, or prior thrombotic disease,

Table 2
Guide to Contraceptive Methods and Women with Diabetes

	Type 1 diabetes	Type 2 diabetes	Diabetes with vascular disease	Postpartum and breastfeeding
I. Combination hormonal (Estrogen/Progestin) Oral (pill) Transdermal (patch) Transvaginal (ring) Intramuscular (injectable)	**Acceptable with risk:** - Evaluate cardiovascular risk factors - Select lowest dose estrogen (↓ thrombotic risk, minimize BP effect) - Select lowest dose/potency progestin (↓ insulin resistance, minimize adverse lipid changes) - Short-term use supported in studies	**Acceptable with risk:** - Evaluate cardiovascular risk factors - Select lowest dose estrogen (↓ thrombotic risk, minimize BP effect) - Select lowest dose/potency progestin (↓ insulin resistance, minimize adverse lipid changes)	**Avoid in microvascular disease:** - No evidence that low-dose COC accelerates retinopathy **Contraindicated in macrovascular disease** ↑ risk stroke, myocardial infarction in hypertensive disease	**May initiate 6 weeks after delivery in breastfeeding and nonbreastfeeding women** Product license does not support COC use in breastfeeding women
II. Progestin-only Hormonal Oral (pill) Injectable Subcutaneous implants	**Acceptable with risk:** - no effect on BP and coagulation factors - Short-term PO-OC use supported in studies	**Acceptable with risk:** - no effect on BP and coagulation factors - No data available in diabetic women	**Acceptable with risk:** - no effect on BP and coagulation factors - No data available in diabetic women - Evaluate cardiovascular risk	**May initiate 21 days after delivery** - May be started postpartum in high-risk women - PO-OC and DMPA may accelerate development of diabetes in breastfeeding women with prior GDM

Table 2
(continued)

	Type 1 diabetes	Type 2 diabetes	Diabetes with vascular disease	Postpartum and breastfeeding
III. Intrauterine Device/system Copper-medicated Levonorgestrel IUS	**No restriction:** - General guidelines apply - LVN-IUS and copper-medicated IUD have no effect on glucose metabolism (level 1 evidence) - Copper-medicated IUD: no ↑ risk in pelvic inflammatory disease	**No restriction:** - General guidelines apply - LVN-IUS and copper-medicated IUD have no effect on glucose metabolism (level 1 evidence) - Copper-medicated IUD: no ↑ risk in pelvic inflammatory disease	**No restriction** General guidelines apply	**No restriction** - Copper-medicated IUD insertion <48 h or [34] weeks postdelivery - LVN IUS insertion [34] weeks postdelivery
Barrier Condoms (male /female) Diaphragm Spermicide	**No restriction** - Condoms effectively prevent HIV and sexually transmitted disease	**No restriction** - Condoms effectively prevent HIV and sexually transmitted disease	**No restriction** - Condoms effectively prevent HIV and sexually transmitted disease	**No restriction** - Condoms effectively prevent HIV and sexually transmitted disease

↑ increase; ↓ decrease; *BP* blood pressure; *LVN IUS* levonorgestrel intrauterine system; *COC* combination oral contraceptive; *PO-OC* progestin-only oral contraceptive; *DMPA* depo medroxyprogesterion acetate; *IUD* Intrauterine devise were present. The presence of hypertension appears to be a particularly strong risk factor, being associated with hemorrhagic stroke in hypertensive women using COCs (29) and with myocardial infarction (30, 31). In the Collaborative Study for Stroke in Young Women, the risk for hemorrhagic stroke was also shown to be increased with increasing blood pressure (32) and with higher doses of estrogen (≥50 mg) (33, 34). Another international case-control study also found an increased risk of ischemic stroke related to the use of oral contraceptives, primarily in hypertensive women, smokers, and women whose blood pressure was not measured prior to oral contraceptive prescription (34). Currently, no studies have examined COC use in women with DM2 who are likely to have other cardiovascular risk factors and/or the metabolic syndrome. Estrogen has a mixed effect on serum lipids. While producing desirable effects on HDL- and LDL-cholesterol levels, estrogen can also increase serum triglyceride levels, which often are elevated in women with DM2 particularly those with poor glycemic control and thyroid disease. Prescribing the lowest possible estrogen dose (20 mg) COC or progestin-only oral contraceptive (PO-OC) should be considered.

In summary, women with diabetes and vascular sequelae, hypertension, and/or cardiovascular disease should not be prescribed estrogen-containing contraceptives due to the possible exacerbation of thromboembolic risk and hypertension. Diabetic women who smoke or have migraines should also avoid COC. An estrogen-containing method is considered a second-choice method as it could further increase her thromboembolic risk and/or blood pressure. Progestin-only methods are preferable. Should she have another strong reason or desire for estrogen-containing methods, such as severe acne, hirsuitism, she should undergo regular monitoring of glucose, lipids, blood pressure, and urinary microalbumin.

As women with diabetes approach the latter decade of reproductive life, e.g., >35 years of age, the risk of diabetic macrovascular and microvascular disease increases as well as dyslipidemia, obesity, and other cardiovascular risks (35). Currently, no studies exist that examine estrogen-containing hormonal methods in older women with diabetes. Progestin-only methods, IUDs, and barrier methods offer safer alternatives that are not associated with increased thromboembolic risk.

Combination hormonal contraception can be prescribed in women without micro- or macrovascular disease. The lowest possible dose/potency of both estrogen and progestin should be selected. Short-term (<1 year) prospective studies in women with DM1 have evaluated lower doses of older progestins, norethindrone (NET, ≤0.75-mg mean daily dose) or triphasic LVN preparation, and newer progestins (gestodene, desogestrel). These studies demonstrated no or minimal effect on glycemic parameters, serum lipids (36–38), and cardiovascular risk factors (39, 40). Currently there are several COC that contain very low-dose estrogen (≤20 mg) and less androgenic progestins, which would be expected to perform better than formulations examined in the older studies.

COC formulations are not generally recommended when microvascular disease is present. Clear evidence for or against the use of COC in women with diabetic microvascular disease is lacking. Some retrospective cross-sectional studies (41) and case-control trials (42) have not found any increase in risk of, or progression of diabetic sequelae (retinopathy, renal disease, or hypertension) with past or current use of COCs. A recent cross-sectional study suggested that OC use may increased renal plasma flow and increase the risk of microalbuminuria; however, the study did not assess glucose control, diabetic treatment, and type of diabetes (43). Thus COC formulations should be prescribed with care and close monitoring in women with microvascular disease. The use of PO-OC avoids possible estrogen effects on the renin–angiotensin system and elevations in blood pressure.

In women with prior GDM who share many risk factors for DM2, short-term prospective studies have not demonstrated any adverse effect of low dose/potency COCs on glucose or lipid metabolism (44–46). A long-term, controlled study found that continued use of two COCs, one with monophasic norethindrone (40 mg) and the other with triphasic LVN (50–125 µg), did not influence the development of diabetes, with virtually identical 3-year cumulative incidence rates for those using oral contraceptives (25.4%) compared with nonhormonal methods (26.5%) *(47)*. Thus COCs do not appear to increase the diabetes rates in women at high risk to develop type 2 diabetes.

Currently, it is unclear whether the monthly combination injectable contraceptive (CIC; Lunelle™; estradiol cypionate 5 mg/medroxyprogesterone 25 mg), or the weekly transdermal patches (OrthoEvra®, norelgestromin 6 mg/ethinyl estradiol 0.75 mg), or the 3-week intravaginal ring (NuvaRing®, etonogestrel 125 µg/ethinyl estradiol 15 µg) offers any metabolic advantages over COC. The benefit of these methods is the less frequent application due to the longer duration of protection. No studies exist evaluating these methods in women with diabetes or prediabetes. The route of combination contraceptives should be based on patient preference and expected reliability in administration of the method (daily, weekly, or monthly).

Question: What Progestin Dose and Formulation Should be Selected in Prescribing COC?

COCs contain a wide variety of progestin formulations and doses. Most progestins are testosterone derivatives and have varying degrees of androgenic effects, e.g., decreasing sex-binding globulin, increasing insulin resistance, and adverse changes in serum lipids *(3)*. Newer formulations of oral progestins (desogestrel, gestodene) or older lower dose/potency norethindrone formulations minimize androgenic side effects and, therefore, generally are preferable. Their net effect is estrogen-dominant and may improve metabolic states in women in whom increased insulin resistance, unfavorable lipid profiles, and hirsuitism should be minimized, such as those with prior gestational diabetes and polycystic ovarian syndrome.

Question: Should She Use Progestin-Only Contraception?

Women desiring hormonal contraception but who are unable to use estrogen are candidates for progestin-only hormonal methods. Progestin-only formulations do not increase blood pressure *(9, 48)* or coagulation factors *(10, 13–14)*, and thus these are the first-choice methods for women with diabetes and vascular disease, hypertension, and cardiovascular or thromboembolic risk factors.

There are two formulations of PO-OC that are taken continuously with no pill-free intervals, one containing norethindrone (0.35 mg daily) and the other LVN (0.75 mg daily), currently not marketed in the USA. Longer acting options include an injection every 3 months (DMPA) or every month (NET or EN), an implant (etonogestrel) every 3 years, or an intrauterine system containing levonorgestrel (LNG-IUS) every 5 years. The LVN implant (Norplant®) currently off the US market has an excellent safety record.

Few studies compare metabolic effects of the various routes of administration in either healthy or diabetic women. DMPA may have a less desirable effect on serum lipids and insulin resistance *(7, 11)* compared with Norplant®*(10, 12)*. It has also been associated with significant weight gain and reversible bone demineralization. Although an observational study comparing DMPA with COC use in women with prior GDM for up to 9 years after delivery found higher annual diabetes incidence rates in DMPA users (19% vs. 12%), this appears to be explained by the fact that women with initial higher risk were selected for DMPA administration *(49)*. After adjusting for baseline imbalances of BMI, breastfeeding, family history of diabetes, and HDL-cholesterol and triglyceride levels and for weight gain, the differences in development of diabetes were no longer significant. Subsets of women appear to be at higher risk for diabetes. Women with elevated triglycerides levels (>150 mg/dl) and women breastfeeding had a 2.3 and 2.3-fold increase in adjusted risk, respectively, for developing diabetes. Therefore, DMPA would not be the first choice for women with diabetes or prediabetes who are likely to have other cardiovascular risk factors, coexisting polycystic ovarian syndrome, metabolic syndrome, or obesity. In contrast, oral progestins have been widely studied in healthy women and studied short term in women with DM1. They have a documented safety profile and can be rapidly discontinued if side effects occur. However, in select patients where daily compliance may be problematic, such as a sexually active teenager with DM1, a highly efficacious long-acting method such as DMPA may be preferable. When prescribing these methods in either women with diabetes or with prediabetes, periodic glucose and lipid monitoring similar to that recommended for oral contraceptives is recommended.

QUESTION: CAN SHE USE INTRAUTERINE CONTRACEPTION?

The intrauterine contraceptives have little or no systemic or metabolic effects. It is an ideal, long-term method for diabetic women, especially those with vascular disease, hypertension, retinopathy, or hyperlipidemia. Most women with diabetes are excellent candidates for IUDs, and the prescription of IUDs follows the same guideline as for healthy women, that is, those at low risk for sexually transmitted infections, parous, and without recent pelvic inflammatory disease. General gynecological principles should be adhered to for proper patient selection, insertion, and monitoring in women with diabetes. None of the studies involving women with diabetes used prophylactic antibiotics with insertion or removal, and it seems unlikely that prophylaxis would add any benefit.

Question: Which Intrauterine Contraceptive Should She Use: The Copper-Containing Intrauterine Device or the Levonorgestrel-Containing Intrauterine System?

The copper-medicated IUD (Cu-IUD) is a first-choice method. It is metabolically neutral and highly efficacious with 10-year duration of use. In a large meta-analysis of several prospective WHO trials, the overall incidence of pelvic inflammatory disease associated with Cu-IUD use was 1.6 per 1,000 women-years of IUD use (50). Daily iron supplementation or preferably a multivitamin with folate is recommended to counteract any increase in menstrual blood loss. Three prospective studies examined Cu-IUDs in women with DM1 (51, 52) and DM2 (53), and older studies examined non-medicated devices (54–56) in women with diabetes. None found any evidence for an increased rate of pelvic infection or decreased efficacy with IUD use. However, because of the low incidence of pelvic inflammatory disease, it is unlikely that a large enough study in diabetic women will ever be conducted to demonstrate the absence of increased risk of pelvic infection (53).

A second medicated intrauterine contraceptive contains levonorgestrel (LVN-IUS), making it a mixed hormonal plus intrauterine "system." LVN is released directly into the uterine cavity and reaches plasma levels that are 5% of the levels seen with a 105-mg dose of oral LNG. Thus, systemic metabolic effects are minimal but there is beneficial local progestin effect on the endometrium with decreased menstrual blood loss (57). A 1-year randomized trial in women with diabetes compared the LVN-IUS with the Cu-IUD and found no significant differences in fasting glucose levels, glyco-sylated hemoglobin, or daily insulin requirements at 6 weeks, 6 or 12 months postinsertion (58). The hemoglobin levels were slightly but significantly increased from baseline while the Cu-IUD resulted in a slight but significant decrease. Thus, the LVN-IUS is also a first-choice method for women with diabetes, especially those with anemia from renal disease or heavy menses.

BREASTFEEDING AND POSTPARTUM CONTRACEPTION: STEPWISE QUESTIONS

Question: Does She Need Contraception During the Postpartum Period if She Is Breastfeeding?

After delivery, the estrogen and progesterone levels drastically drop, removing the inhibitory effect on prolactin action, permitting breast milk production. Breast engorgement and full milk secretion starts 3–4 days after delivery. Newborn suckling further stimulates the release of prolactin, sustaining milk production and interrupting the cyclic release of pulsatile GnRH from the hypothalamus. This in turn interrupts the pulsatile release of LH, blocking FSH-mediated stimulation of the ovary and ovulation. The earliest return of ovulation after delivery in nonbreastfeeding women has been documented to be 25 days *(59)*. Thus, 4 weeks after delivery fertility can return necessitating the need for contraception after 21 days.

In contrast, exclusive breastfeeding reliably delays ovulation for up to 6 months, providing a 98% contraceptive efficacy *(60–63)*. While a woman is exclusively breastfeeding, ovulation is delayed and all methods used have a low failure rate when used correctly. Exclusive breastfeeding when used as birth control is called lactation amenorrhea method (LAM). To use LAM properly, women need to start exclusive breastfeeding immediately postpartum, breastfeed at least every 4 h during daytime and 6 h during nighttime, and avoid milk supplementation. Another method should be used if menses resumes or 6 months have passed since delivery or if supplemental feeding is used. The cumulative pregnancy rate at 6 months with LAM is up to 1.2% (95% CI, 0–2.4%) *(62)*. During the newborn period, the contraceptive needs of the mother should be assessed. Intercourse may be less frequent with the demands of motherhood. Women may be reluctant to take unnecessary medication while breastfeeding. Encouraging the use of LAM plus condoms during this period will effectively provide pregnancy protection and will encourage exclusive breastfeeding, which has many benefits for the newborn.

Question: Can Hormonal Contraception Be Used During Breastfeeding?

The level of steroid hormones transferred to breast milk is less than 1% of the maternal dose and is comparable to hormone levels observed during ovulatory cycles. A review examining the limited available studies comparing the effect of COC and PO-OC on breast milk found that PO-OC use during the first 6 weeks postpartum had no effect on breast milk volume but the evidence was inconclusive for COC use *(64)*. Importantly, neither PO-OC, COC, nor progestin implants affect infant growth and weight. Lacking evidence-based data, the recommendations for when to initiate hormonal contraception in breastfeeding women come from expert committees *(65–67)*. In breastfeeding women, PO-OCs can be started on day 21 postpartum without additional protection, noting that using PO-OC before 6 weeks is outside of the product license. The ACOG states that COCs should not be started before 6 weeks postpartum, after lactation is well established and the infant's nutritional status is well monitored. In contrast, the WHO advocates delaying COC use until after 6 months postpartum. Prior to 6 months, the use of COCs should be restricted to those cases when no acceptable alternatives are available *(66, 67)*. The use of COC while breastfeeding is outside product license. Besides the possible effect on quantity of breast milk, estrogen-containing methods are contraindicated during the first 6 weeks to avoid further increased risk of postpartum thromboembolic events.

Progestin-only injectable methods, e.g., DMPA, also are not recommended until 6 weeks postdelivery *(66)* but may be given as early as 21 days postpartum if the risk of immediate pregnancy is high

(67). Emergency contraception, given within 72 h of unprotected coitus, is not indicated before 21 days postpartum, after which time the standard use guidelines can be followed.

Question: When Should Intrauterine Contraception Be Used After Delivery?

Cu-IUD and other nonmedicated IUDs can either be inserted within 48 h after delivery or delayed until 4 weeks postpartum *(67)*. The LVN-IUS may be inserted 4 weeks after delivery. Diaphragms and cervical caps should not be fitted or used until 6 weeks postpartum to allow for uterine involution and proper fitting. IUDs are also effective when inserted as emergency contraception within 5 days after unprotected intercourse with a pregnancy rate ≤0.2% *(68)*.

Question: Which Methods Can Be Used in Postpartum Women with Diabetes?

Encouraging breastfeeding in women with diabetes should be a priority for her physician. Studies in women with diabetes found that only half had received information about breastfeeding during pregnancy *(69)*. In addition to decreasing childhood allergies by decreasing exposure to cow's milk antigens and improving bonding, breastfeeding importantly appears to reduce childhood obesity in offspring of women with prior gestational diabetes *(70)* and obesity *(71)*, and it reduces the risk of type 2 diabetes in mothers with prior gestational diabetes *(72)*. Thus, promoting LAM with condom use offers excellent pregnancy protection, promotes exclusive breastfeeding, and removes the woman's worry of ingesting additional medication.

When hormonal methods or IUD methods are desired by women with diabetes, they should be initiated according to the standard guidelines for postpartum prescription. In nonbreastfeeding women with diabetes, stepwise evaluation with aforementioned questions can be utilized.

Special exceptions related to breastfeeding should be noted in women with prior gestational diabetes. The use of PO-OC while breastfeeding was associated with an increased adjusted risk of development of type 2 diabetes (HR 2.87; 95% CI, 1.57–5.87) compared with COC use in nonbreastfeeding women with prior GDM *(50)*. This risk increased with duration of use: use greater than 8 months was associated with almost a fivefold increase in risk. Similarly the use of DMPA while breastfeeding was associated with over a twofold increase in risk compared with either COC use or DMPA use in nonbreastfeeding women *(49)*. Thus, breastfeeding women with recent GDM should consider either nonhormonal contraception, such as LAM with condoms or IUDs, or wait to start COCs 6 weeks after delivery and continue nursing on COC.

REFERENCES

1. Clausen TD, Mathiesen E, Ekbom P, Hellmuth E, Mandrup-Poulsen T, Damm P. Poor pregnancy outcome in women with type 2 diabetes. Diabetes Care 28:323–328, 2005
2. Towner D, Kjos SL, Leung B, Montoro MM, Xiang A, Mestman JH, Buchanan TA. Congenital malformations in pregnancies complicated by NIDDM. Diabetes Care 18:1446–1451, 1995
3. Gilbert C, Valois M, Koren G. Pregnancy outcome after first trimester exposure to metformin: a meta-analysis. Fertil Steril 86:658–663, 2006
4. Piaggio G, Grimes DA, Van Look PFA. Task Force on Postovulatory Methods of Fertility Regulation Timing of emergency contraception with levonorgestrel or the Yuzpe regimen. Lancet 353:721, 1999
5. Spellacy WN, Buhi WC, Birk SA. The effect of estrogens on carbohydrate metabolism: glucose, insulin and growth hormone studies on one hundred seventy-one women ingesting premarin, mestranol and ethinyl estradiol for six months. Am J Obstet Gynecol 114:388–392, 1971
6. Perlman JA, Russell-Briefel R, Ezzati T, Lieberknecht. Oral glucose tolerance and the potency of contraceptive progestins. J Chronic Dis 338:857–864, 1985

7. Fahmy K, Abdel-Razik, Shaaraway M, et al. Effect of long-acting progestagen-only injectable contraceptives on carbohydrate metabolism and its hormonal profile. Contraception 44:419–429, 1991

8. Konje JC, Otolorin EO, Ladipo AO. The effect of continuous subdermal levonorgestrel (Norplant) on carbohydrate metabolism. Am J Obstet Gynecol 166(1 Pt 1):15–19, 1992

9. Wilson ES, Cruickshank J, McMaster M, et al. A prospective controlled study of the effect on blood pressure of contraceptive preparations containing different types of dosages and progestogen. Br J Obstet Gynaecol 91:1254–1260, 1984

10. Singh K, Viegas OA, Koh SC, Ratnam SS. The effect of long-term use of Norplant implants on haemostatic function. Contraception 45:141–153, 1992

11. Fajumi JO. Alterations in blood lipids and side effects induced by depo-provera in Nigerian women. Contraception 27:161–175, 1983

12. Shaaban MM, Elwan SI, Abdalla SA, Darwish HA. Effect of subdermal levonorgestrel contraceptive implants, Norplant, on serum lipids. Contraception 30:413–419, 1984

13. Meade TW. Oral contraceptives, clotting factors and thrombosis. Am J Obstet Gynecol 142:758–761, 1982

14. Shaaban M, Elwan SI, El-Kabsh MY, Farghaly SA, Thabet N. Effect of levonorgestrel contraceptive implants, Norplant, on blood coagulation. Contraception 30:421–430, 1984

15. Godsland IF, Crook D, Simpson R, et al. The effects of different formulations of oral contraceptive agents on lipid and carbohydrate metabolism. N Engl J Med 323:1375–1381, 1990

16. Liew DFM, Ng CSA, Yong YM, et al. Long term effects of depo-provera on carbohydrate and lipid metabolism. Contraception 31:51, 1985

17. Speroff L, DeCherney A. Evaluation of a new generation of oral contraceptives. The Advisory Board of the New Progestins. Obstet Gynecol 81:1034–1047, 1993

18. Fahraeus L, Sydsjo A, Wallentin L. Lipoprotein changes during treatment of pelvic endometriosis with medroxyprogesterone acetate. Fertil Steril 45:501–506, 1986

19. Deslypere JP, Thiery N, Vermeulen A. Effect of long-term hormonal contraception in plasma lipids. Contraception 31:633–642, 1985

20. Haiba NA, et al. Clinical evaluation of two monthly injectable contraceptives and their effects on some metabolic parameters. Contraception 39:619–632, 1989

21. Kesserü EV, et al. A multicentered, two-year, phase III clinical trial of norethisterone enanthate 50 mg plus estradiol valerate 5 mg as a monthly injectable contraceptive. Contraception 44:589–598, 1991

22. Smallwood GH, et al. Efficacy and safety of a transdermal contraceptive system. Obstet Gynecol 98:799–805, 2001

23. Visser J, Snel M, Van Vliet HAAM. Hormonal versus non-hormonal contraceptives in women with diabetes mellitus type 1 and 2 (review). The Cochrane Collaboration, http://www.thecochranelibrary.com., Issue 1, 2008

24. The World Health Organization Medical Eligibility Criteria for Contraceptive Use, 3rd edition 2004, http://www.who.int/reproductive-health

25. Dong W, Colhoun HM, Poulter NR. Blood pressure in women using oral contraceptives: results from the Health Survey for England 1994. J Hypertens 15:1063, 1997

26. Heimemann LA, Lewis MA, Thorogood M, et al. Case-control study of oral contraceptives and risk of thromboembolic stroke: results from International Study on Oral Contraceptives and Health of Young Women. BMJ 315:1502, 1997

27. Petitti DB, Sidney S, Bernstein A, et al. Stroke in users of low-dose oral contraceptives. N Engl J Med 335:8, 1996

28. Lidegaard O. Oral contraceptives, pregnancy and the risk of cerebral thromboembolism: the influence of diabetes, hypertension, migraine and previous thrombotic disease. Br J Obstet Gynaecol 102:153, 1995

29. Gillum LA, Mamidipudi SK, Johnston SC. Ischemic stroke risk with oral contraceptives: a meta-analysis. JAMA 284:72–78, 2000

30. Khader YS, et al. Oral contraceptives use and the risk of myocardial infarction: a meta-analysis. Contraception 68:11–17, 2003

31. Tanis BC, et al. Oral contraceptives and the risk of myocardial infarction. N Engl J Med 345:1787–1193, 2001

32. Collaborative Group for the Study of Stroke in Young Women. Oral contraceptives and stroke in young women: associated risk factors. JAMA 231:718, 1975

33. Lidegaard O. Oral contraceptives and risk of cerebral thromboembolic attack: Results of a case-control study. BMJ 306:956, 1993

34. WHO Collaborative Study of Cardiovascular Disease and Steroid Hormone Contraception. Ischaemic stroke and combined oral contraceptives: results of an international, multicentre, case-control study. Lancet 348:498, 1996

35. Selber C, Babrouche E, Fagan J, Myint E, Wetterneck T, Wittemyer M. Prescribing oral contraceptives for women older than 35 years of age. Ann Intern Med 138:54–64, 2003

36. Skouby SO, Jensen BM, Kuhl C, et al. Hormonal contraception in diabetic women: acceptability and influence on diabetes control of a nonaldkylated estrogen/progestogen compound. Contraception 32:23–31, 1985

37. Skouby SO, Molsted-Pedersen, Kuhl C, et al. Oral contraceptives in diabetic women: metabolic effects of four compounds with different estrogen/progestogen profiles. Fertil Steril 46:858–864, 1986

38. Radberg T, Gustafson A, Skryten A, et al. Oral contraception in diabetic women. Diabetes control, serum and high density lipoprotein lipids during low-dose progestogen, combined oestrogen/progestogen and non-hormonal contraception. Acta Endocrinol 98:246–251, 1981

39. Peterson KR, Skouby SO, Sidelmann J, Molsted-Pedersen L, Jespersen J. Effects of contraceptive steroids on cardiovascular risk factors in women with insulin-dependent diabetes mellitus. Am J Obstet Gynecol 171: 400–405, 1994

40. Peterson KR, Skouby SO, Vedel P, Haaber AB. Hormonal contraception in women with IDDM. Diabetes Care 18: 800–806, 1995

41. Klein BEK, Moss SE, Klein R. Oral contraceptives in women with diabetes. Diabetes Care 13:895–898, 1990

42. Garg SK, Chase HP, Marshal G, Hoops S, Holmes DL, Jackson WE. Oral contraceptives and renal and retinal complications in young women with insulin-dependent diabetes mellitus. JAMA 271:1099–1102, 1994

43. Ahmed SB, Hovind P, Prving H-H, Rossing P, Price DA, Laffel LM, Lansang MC, Fisher NDL, Hollenberg NK. Oral contraceaptives, angiotensin-dependent renal vasoconstriction, and risk of diabeteic nephropathy. Diabetes Care 28:1988–1994, 2005

44. Skouby SO, Anderson O, Saurbrey N, et al. Oral contraception and insulin sensitivity: in vivo assessment in normal women and women with previous gestational diabetes. J Clin Endocrinol Metab 64:519–523, 1987

45. Skouby SO, Kuhl C, Molsted-Pedersen, et al. Triphasic oral contraception: metabolic effects in normal women and those with previous gestational diabetes. Am J Obstet Gynecol 153:495–500, 1985

46. Kjos SL, Shoupe D, Douyan S, et al. Effect of low-dose oral contraceptives on carbohydrate and lipid metabolism in women with recent gestational diabetes: results of a controlled, randomized, prospective study. Am J Obstet Gynecol 163:1822–1827, 1990

47. Kjos SL, Peters RK, Xiang A, Thomas D, Schaefer U, Buchanan TA. Contraception and the risk of type 2 diabetes mellitus in Latina women with prior gestational diabetes mellitus. JAMA 280:533–538, 1998

48. Chasan-Taber L, Willett WC, Manson JE, Spiegelman D, Hunter DJ, Curham G, et al. Prospective study of oral contraceptives and hypertension among women in the United States. Circulation 94:483–489, 1996

49. Xiang AH, Kawakubo M, Kjos SL, Buchanan TA. Long-acting injectable progestin contraception and risk of type 2 diabetes in Latino women with prior gestational diabetes mellitus. Diabetes Care 29(3):613–617, 2006

50. Farley TMM, Rosenberg MJ, Rowe PJ, Chen J-H, Meirek O. Intrauterine devices and pelvic inflammatory disease: an international perspective. Lancet 339:785–788, 1992

51. Skouby SO, Molsted-Pedersen L, Kosonen A. Consequences of intrauterine contraception in diabetic women. Fert Steril 42:568–572, 1984

52. Kimmerle R, Weiss R, Berger M, Kurz K-H. Effectiveness, safety and acceptablilty of a copper intrauterine device (CU Safe 300) in type I diabetic women. Diabetes Care 16:1227–1230, 1993

53. Kjos SL, Ballagh SA, La Cour M, Xiang A, Mishell DR Jr. The copper T380A intrauterine device in women with type II diabetes mellitus. Obstet Gynecol 84:1006–1009, 1994

54. Gosen C, Steel J, Ross A, Springerbett A. Intrauterine contraception in diabetic women. Lancet 1:530–535, 1982

55. Lawless M, Vessey MP. Intrauterine device use by diabetic women. Br J Fam Plann 7:110–111, 1982

56. Wiese J. Intrauterine contraception in diabetic women. Fert Steril 28:422–425, 1977

57. Stewart A, et al. The effectiveness of the levonorgestrel-releasing intrauterine systems in menorrhagia: a systemic review. BJOG 108:74–86, 2001

58. Rogovskay S, Rivera R, Grimes DA, Chen P-L, Bosny P-L, Prilepskaya V, Kulakov V. Effect of levonorgestrel intrauterine system on women with type 1 diabetes: a randomized trial. Obstet Gynecol 105:811–815, 2005

59. Campbell OM, Gray RH. Characteristics and determinants of postpartum ovarian function in women in the United States. Am J Obstet Gynecol 169:55–60 1993

60. Perez A, Labbok MH, Queenan JT. Clinical study of the lactational amenorrhoea method for family planning. Lancet 339:968–970, 1992

61. Kennedy KI, Rivera R, McNeilly AS. Consensus statement on the use of breastfeeding as a family planning method. Contraception 39:477–496, 1989

62. Labbok M, Perez A, Valdes V, et al. The lactational amenorrhea method (LAM): a postpartum introductory family planning method with policy and program implications. Adv Contracept 10:93–109, 1994

63. Quality Care in Family Planning. Medical Eligibility Criteria for Contraceptive Use. Geneva: World Health Organization Reproductive Health and Research, 2000

64. Truit ST, Fraser AB, Grimes DA, Gallo MF, Schulz KF. Combined hormonal versus nonhormonal versus progestin-only contraception in lactation. Cochrane Database Syst Rev (2):CDC003988, 2003
65. World Health Organization (WHO). Selected Practice Recommendations for Contraceptive Use. Geneva, Switzerland: WHO, 2002
66. Faculty of Family Planning and Reproductive Health Care Clinical Effectiveness Unit. Family Planning and Reproductive Health Care Guidance (July 2004). Contraceptive choices for breastfeeding women. J Fam Plann Reprod Health Care 30:181–189, 2004
67. ACOG Educational Bulletin No 258. Breastfeeding: Maternal and Infant Aspects. Washington DC: American College of Obstetricians and Gynecologists 2004 Compendium of Selected Publications, 2004
68. Zhou L, Xiao B. Emergency contraception with Multiload Cu-375 SL IUD: a multicenter clinical trial. Contraception 64:107–112, 2001
69. Stage E, Nøgård, Damm P, Mathiesen E. Long-term breast-feeding in women with type 1 diabetes. Diabetes Care 29:7714, 2006
70. Schaefer-Graf UM, Hartmann R, Pawliczik J, Passow D, About-Dakn M, Vetter K, Kordonouri O. Association of breast-feeding and early childhood overweight in children from mothers with gestational diabetes mellutis. Diabetes Care 29:1105–1107, 2006
71. Public Affairs Committee of Teratology Society. Teratology Public Affairs Committee Position Paper: maternal obesity and pregnancy. Birth Defects Res A Clin Mol Teratol 76:73–77, 2006
72. Stuebe AM, Rich-Edwards JW, Willett WC, Manson JE, Michels KB. Duration of lactation and incidence of type 2 diabetes. JAMA 294:2601–2610, 2005

10

The Effect of PCOS on Fertility and Pregnancy

Kelsey E.S. Salley and John E. Nestler

Contents

Abstract

Polycystic ovary syndrome (PCOS) affects 5–10% of women of reproductive age. One of the hallmarks of the syndrome is chronic oligo- or anovulation, making it one of the most common causes of infertility. While infertile PCOS patients have traditionally undergone conventional fertility treatments, insulin-sensitizing agents are also being explored because of the hyperinsulinemic insulin resistance intrinsic to the syndrome. Once women with PCOS become pregnant they are at increased risk for complications including early pregnancy loss, gestational diabetes and pregnancy-induced hypertension. Because pregnancy is a state of heightened insulin resistance and compensatory hyperinsulinemia, insulin-sensitizing agents, particularly metformin, are being investigated for prevention of these complications.

Key words: Polycystic ovary syndrome; Fertility; Pregnancy; Infertility; Early pregnancy loss; Gestational diabetes; Pregnancy-induced hypertension.

INTRODUCTION

Polycystic ovary syndrome (PCOS) affects 5–10% of women of reproductive age (*1, 2*). It is characterized by hyperandrogenism, often presenting as hirsutism, alopecia or acne, and chronic oligo- or anovulation, which typically presents as oligomenorrhea or amenorrhea and infertility (*3*). In addition, hyperinsulinemic insulin resistance is intrinsic to the syndrome, increasing the risk of type 2 diabetes mellitus (*4*), metabolic syndrome and cardiovascular risk (*5*).

From: *Diabetes in Women: Pathophysiology and Therapy*
Edited by: A. Tsatsoulis et al. (eds.), DOI 10.1007/978-1-60327-250-6_10
© Humana Press, a part of Springer Science+Business Media, LLC 2009

Given its prevalence, it is not surprising that 75% of women with infertility due to anovulation are diagnosed with PCOS *(6)*. Women with PCOS have traditionally undergone conventional fertility treatments, such as ovulation induction using clomiphene citrate or gonadotropins and in-vitro fertilization (IVF). Newer treatment options have focused on insulin-sensitizing medications, including metformin.

Once they become pregnant, women with PCOS appear to be more susceptible to pregnancy complications. Increased rates of early first trimester pregnancy loss (EPL), gestational diabetes mellitus (GDM) and pregnancy-induced hypertension (PIH) have been reported in this population, and insulin resistance has been implicated in the genesis of these pregnancy-related complications. Because of the hyperinsulinemic insulin resistance of patients with PCOS, particularly those who are obese, insulin-sensitizing drugs, especially metformin, have been explored as treatments to reduce the risk of miscarriage and the risk of GDM.

PATHOGENESIS OF INFERTILITY

Serum luteinizing hormone (LH) levels are elevated in many patients with PCOS, especially in those who are lean *(7)*. Abnormal regulation of LH was previously implicated as the cause of chronic anovulation in patients with PCOS. Studies have shown that increased LH levels during the follicular phase in patients with PCOS have deleterious effects on conception rates *(8)* and may contribute to higher miscarriage rates *(9)* although the mechanism remains controversial. However, up to 50% of women with clinical and biochemical manifestations of PCOS have normal LH levels, rendering its measurement of limited diagnostic value *(3)*.

Hyperinsulinemia is present in about 80% of obese women with PCOS and 30–40% of normal weight women with PCOS *(10)*. Disturbances of insulin secretion or action are more prominent in women with PCOS complicated by amenorrhea or anovulation than in equally hyperandrogenemic women with regular cycles *(11, 12)*. Hyperinsulinemic insulin resistance plays a key role in the pathogenesis of infertility in PCOS by inhibiting follicle maturation and increasing ovarian androgen production with stimulation of P450c17α *(13)*. Paradoxically, although patients with PCOS have peripheral insulin resistance, ovarian tissue appears to remain sensitive or even hypersensitive to insulin *(14–16)*. Additionally, increased insulin levels inhibit the hepatic production of sex hormone binding globulin (SHBG), contributing to hyperandrogenism by increasing the fraction of testosterone that is free or unbound *(17)*.

PCOS is characterized on pelvic ultrasound by the presence of more than 12 small follicles (2–9 mm) in the ovary due to the arrest of growth of follicles at earlier stages. Granulosa cells from individual follicles obtained from anovulatory polycystic ovaries were found to be prematurely responsive to LH, typically at a diameter of 4 mm as opposed to normal follicles that are responsive to LH only once the diameter reaches 9.5 mm or greater *(14)*. The hyperinsulinemic state may render follicles in PCOS ovaries responsive to LH at an earlier stage, contributing to premature arrest of development and anovulation.

INFERTILITY TREATMENT IN PCOS

Inducing ovulation in patients with PCOS can be accomplished through several approaches: reducing insulin concentrations, follicle stimulating hormone (FSH) stimulation or reducing LH concentrations *(6)*. Reducing insulin concentrations can be accomplished by either weight loss or insulin-sensitizing agents, like metformin. Clomiphene citrate or gonadotrophin therapies have traditionally been used to stimulate FSH; more recently, aromatase inhibitors have been investigated for this purpose. Laparoscopic ovarian drilling (LOD), gonadotrophin releasing hormone (GnRH) agonists and GnRH antagonists work through reducing LH concentrations and are second- or third-line agents for the treatment of infertility.

Weight Loss

Excess body fat accentuates insulin resistance in patients with PCOS, and obese women with PCOS are more likely than lean women to manifest menstrual irregularities (12). Furthermore, increased body mass index (BMI) is associated with impaired response to standard doses of clomiphene citrate (18, 19). Obesity, independent from hyperinsulinemia, is related to lower oocyte retrieval in IVF and increased total FSH requirements for ovarian stimulation (20, 21).

Weight loss has been found to enhance fertility through improving ovarian function, reducing androgen concentrations, and increasing SHBG. Crosignani et al. studied 33 anovulatory overweight patients with PCOS who were recommended to follow a 1,200 kcal/day diet and increase their physical exercise for a study period of 12 months (22). Twenty-five patients (76%) lost at least 5% of their body weight and 11 patients (33%) had a 10% decrease. Eighteen patients (72% of compliant subjects) resumed regular menstrual cycles, including 15 patients who developed ovulatory cycles during the 12-month study period, and 10 patients (33%) became pregnant within 12 months.

Improved diet and exercise alone, without significant weight loss, may improve ovulation rates. Huber-Buchholz et al. studied the relationship between insulin sensitivity and ovulation in 18 anovulatory obese PCOS women with infertility before and after a 6-month intervention of gradual dietary changes and a moderate exercise regimen (23, 24). Anovulatory subjects who regained ovulation during the study showed an 11% reduction in central fat, a 39% reduction in LH levels and improved insulin sensitivity. This was achieved with moderate lifestyle modification that did not result in significant weight loss.

Whether diet or exercise has a more important role in weight loss in infertile obese PCOS patients is currently being investigated. A recent pilot study by Palombo et al. showed improved fertility in 40 obese PCOS patients with anovulatory infertility who underwent either a structured exercise training program or a hypocaloric high-protein diet (25). After 24 weeks of intervention, improved menstrual cyclicity was seen in both groups. However, the ovulation rate was significantly higher ($p < 0.05$) in the exercise training group than in the diet group, despite significantly more weight loss in the ovulatory diet group vs. the ovulatory exercise training group (−10.5 vs. −5.6 kg). The authors postulate that the improved ovulation in the exercise group was due to improved waist circumference, which reflects visceral adipose tissue as well as cellular muscle metabolism enhancement, thus improving insulin sensitivity (25). While not statistically significant, there was also a trend toward higher pregnancy rates in the exercise vs. diet group with cumulative pregnancy rates of 35% and 10%, respectively ($p = 0.058$).

While lifestyle modification can be challenging to achieve and maintain for many patients, it can be effective in restoring fertility in overweight women with PCOS. In obese women, a loss of 5–10% of their body weight can improve or restore reproductive function (22, 26). Diet and exercise are relatively inexpensive compared to other fertility treatments and do not carry an increased risk of multiple gestations. Improvements in mood and self-esteem that may be achieved by weight loss may also improve fertility (27). Because obese women have lower pregnancy rates and higher risks of pregnancy complications, losing weight can help improve outcomes even if fertility treatments are needed

(28). Weight loss is not known to be of benefit for fertility in lean patients with PCOS, and because there are detrimental effects on fertility in patients who are underweight, weight loss should not be recommended in this population *(29).* Drug therapy is usually warranted in these patients.

Clomiphene Citrate

Clomiphene citrate, an indirect stimulator of FSH secretion, has been the traditional approach to ovulation induction in infertile patients with PCOS. It is typically given at a dose of 50 mg per day for 5 days starting from day 2 to day 5 of spontaneous or induced menses. The dose of clomiphene can be increased in increments of 50 mg per day each cycle if ovulation is not achieved up to a maximum dose of 250 mg, although doses in excess of 150 mg are not typically prescribed *(6).* Ovulation occurs in 60–85% of patients given clomiphene, 30–40% of whom become pregnant *(9, 30, 31).* Approximately 75% of those who conceive on clomiphene become pregnant during the first three cycles of treatment *(32–34).* There is an increased risk of ovarian and uterine cancer in patients continuing prolonged ovulation induction with clomiphene *(35–37).* Therefore, treatment is usually attempted for 3–6 cycles but no more than 12 cycles *(9).*

While clomiphene increases the number of follicles attaining ovulation, it also has antiestrogenic effects on the endometrium and cervical mucous, which may inhibit sperm penetration and implantation of the embryo *(38);* these effects may account for the discrepancy between the ovulation and conception rates *(39).* In addition, some studies have found a diminished effect of clomiphene on ovulation rates over time *(32, 40).* However, the hyperinsulinemic state of PCOS may reduce endometrial expression of the binding proteins, glycodelin and insulin-like growth factor (IGF) binding-protein-1, which may also impair conception and/or increase early miscarriage rates *(41).* Clomiphene has also been associated with the development of ovarian cysts, risk of ovarian hyperstimulation syndrome (OHSS), and an increase in the multiple gestation rate (4–10%) *(9).* The risks of OHSS and multiple gestations underscore the need for careful monitoring, usually with ultrasound, of patients undergoing their first treatment cycle with clomiphene *(9).*

Several studies have shown that increased BMI is predictive of poor response to ovulation induction and that overweight patients require higher doses of clomiphene to ovulate *(9, 42, 43).* In addition to obesity, Imani et al. found that anovulatory patients with amenorrhea, increased ovarian volume, and increased androgen levels are less likely to respond to ovulation induction with clomiphene *(31, 44).* Finally, age is also known to be a predictor of response to clomiphene, with younger patients having higher success rates with treatment *(32, 44–46).* LH concentrations have not been predictive of ovarian response to treatment *(9, 31).*

Approximately 20–25% of anovulatory women with PCOS will not ovulate despite treatment with increasing doses of clomiphene citrate *(6, 31).* A few studies suggest that the addition of dexamethasone to suppress adrenal androgen production and decrease LH levels may improve follicular development and conception rates *(47–50).* Daly et al. reported that this may be most helpful in women with raised dehydroepiandrosterone sulfate (DHEAS) levels but subsequent studies have shown benefit in PCOS women with normal DHEAS levels *(50).* Contrary to the statement of a recent consensus workshop that dexamethasone added to clomiphene had no beneficial effect *(51),* the cited study *(47)* did, in fact, show benefit as have subsequent studies *(48–50).* In a small, prospective, placebo-controlled study, Elnashar et al. found improved ovulation (75% vs. 15%, $p < 0.001$) and pregnancy rates (40% vs. 5%, $p < 0.05$) in clomiphene-resistant women with PCOS who were given dexamethasone on days 3–12 in addition to clomiphene compared with placebo plus clomiphene *(48).* While dexamethasone may be beneficial for the short term, the long-term use of corticosteroids can cause weight gain, so, this adjunctive treatment may be less desirable in the PCOS population and further studies are needed to further examine the efficacy (6).

Metformin

Because of the increasing evidence of the role of insulin resistance in the pathogenesis of PCOS, medications that improve insulin sensitivity and lower circulating insulin have been investigated for treatment of anovulatory infertility. Metformin, an oral biguanide used to treat type 2 diabetes mellitus, has proven effective in decreasing ovarian androgen secretion in women with PCOS (52–57). Metformin may also decrease adrenal steroidogenesis, which may also be elevated due to hyperinsulinemia (58). Studies have shown that it is effective in improving ovulation rates in patients naïve to fertility treatments as well as those with clomiphene resistance (59–61). Several studies have found that metformin's effects to improve ovulation may require several months (up to 3–6) of treatment in many patients, likely because metformin is a metabolic drug that acts indirectly to improve insulin sensitivity, which subsequently improves reproductive function (40, 62). The starting dose is typically 500 mg daily, which can be titrated up to 1,000 mg twice daily as tolerated. The main limiting side effects of metformin are nausea and diarrhea, which occur in 10–25% of patients (63). In most cases, these effects are transient and improve with a reduction in dose.

Metformin, Clomiphene Citrate or Both for Ovulation Induction in PCOS

Given the demonstrated efficacy of metformin as monotherapy in increasing ovulation, the question arises whether it might constitute first-line therapy in the treatment of the anovulatory infertility of PCOS. The literature on this issue is conflicting and controversial. Palombo et al. performed a prospective, randomized, double-blind trial of metformin compared with clomiphene 150 mg in 100 nonobese PCOS patients (40). While there was no difference in ovulation rates, the pregnancy rate was significantly higher in the metformin group (15.5%) than in the clomiphene group (7.2%) ($p = 0.009$) (40). The cumulative pregnancy rate was 68.9% for the metformin group as compared with 34% for the clomiphene group ($p < 0.001$). Moll et al. performed a randomized, double-blind trial that examined the effects of metformin compared with placebo given with clomiphene in 228 women with PCOS and found no significant differences in ovulation or pregnancy rates between the two groups (64).

In the largest study to date, Legro et al. performed a randomized, controlled trial of metformin, clomiphene or both for treatment of infertility in PCOS. The study included 626 women, including obese patients and those with prior fertility treatments, and the primary outcome was live birth rate (19). Live birth rate was significantly lower in the metformin group than in the clomiphene group and the combination therapy group ($p < 0.001$). While ovulation rates were significantly higher in the combination group than in either single drug group, there was no significant improvement in the live birth rate in the combination therapy group over clomiphene alone. Most recently, Palomba et al. performed a multicenter, nonrandomized, prospective, controlled study examining metformin alone compared with clomiphene alone in 80 patients with PCOS and found no significant differences in ovulation or cumulative pregnancy rates between the two groups (65). It is difficult to compare the various studies due to their considerable heterogeneity, including differences in patient inclusion criteria and treatment protocols. As mentioned previously, metformin's beneficial effects on ovulation rates take considerable time to occur and most studies either start metformin concurrently with clomiphene or allow just 1 month for metformin to take effect.

Several meta-analyses have also investigated this issue and have found metformin to be beneficial for ovulation rates when added to clomiphene. Lord et al. found an odds ratio (OR) of 4.41 for ovulation rates in patients who were treated with metformin in addition to clomiphene (66). There was a similar improvement in pregnancy rate as well although the studies had significant heterogeneity. Kashyap et al. performed a meta-analysis of four randomized controlled trials, which revealed an improvement in ovulation and pregnancy rates [relative risk (RR) = 3.04 and 3.65, respectively] in patients receiving clomiphene plus metformin as compared with clomiphene alone (67). Additionally, a recent meta-analysis by Creanga et al. found that metformin plus clomiphene increased the odds of ovulation and pregnancy (OR 4.39 and 2.67, respectively with number-needed-to-treat of 3.7 and 4.6, respectively) when compared with clomiphene alone (68).

Eisenhardt et al. found that metformin may be most beneficial in women with significant insulin resistance (69). Guidelines of a recent consensus conference state that metformin should be used to treat infertility in PCOS only in the presence of impaired glucose tolerance (51). However, a subsequent challenge to that recommendation suggests that the use of metformin be more widespread and tailored to the time lines and preferences of the patient (70). While clomiphene results in ovulation more rapidly than metformin, it also carries the possible adverse effects of multiple gestations and OHSS. The patient's age and tolerance for multiple gestations are important factors to consider when choosing between metformin and clomiphene. Finally, further studies are needed to determine if there are certain subgroups of women who may benefit more from insulin-sensitizing treatment than from clomiphene.

Metformin has also been compared with second-line treatments in patients who are clomiphene resistant. Two studies have found metformin to be as effective or more effective than LOD in clomiphene-resistant women, with metformin administration 20-fold less expensive than LOD and not carrying the risk of general anesthesia and possible adhesions (71, 72).

Thiazolidenediones

Thiazolidenediones (TZDs) have also been examined for their possible role in the treatment of infertility in PCOS. The main mechanism of action is through activation of the nuclear peroxisome proliferator-activated receptor gamma (PPAR-γ), which decreases peripheral insulin resistance (73, 74). Troglitazone was the first drug of this class that was shown to improve ovulation rates, hyperandrogenemia and insulin resistance compared with placebo (75). It has been shown in vitro to impede LH and insulin stimulation of ovarian androgen production as thecal cells also possess PPAR-γ receptors (76). Troglitazone has since been withdrawn from the market due to concerns of hepatotoxicity.

Two of the newer TZDs, rosiglitazone and pioglitazone, have also demonstrated improved reproductive function in women with PCOS. A prospective study by Belli et al. examining the effects of rosiglitazone showed improved menstrual regularity and decreased insulin resistance (77). A randomized, controlled, double-blind trial by Baillargeon et al. showed increased ovulatory frequency and reduced hyperandrogenemia following treatment with rosiglitazone in nonobese patients with normal insulin sensitivity (78). A recent randomized controlled trial found adding rosiglitazone to clomiphene to be more effective in ovulation induction than adding metformin in clomiphene-resistant PCOS (79).

In a randomized, double-blind, controlled trial, Brettenthaler et al. showed significantly improved insulin sensitivity, hyperandrogenism and ovulation rates during treatment with pioglitazone (80). When pioglitazone was added in a small sample of patients nonresponsive to metformin, patients were found to have improved menstrual regularity and decreased insulin resistance (81). TZDs are a category C medication, which has limited their clinical use in the treatment of infertility. Larger randomized controlled trials are needed to determine the utility and safety of TZDs in the treatment of anovulatory infertility in PCOS.

Gonadotropin Therapy

A second-line option for infertility treatment is direct gonadotropin therapy with either FSH or human menopausal gonadotropin (hMG). Because of the increased number of FSH-responsive follicles in polycystic ovaries, patients with PCOS are more at risk for OHSS and multiple gestations (82–84). A low-dose, step-up protocol has been developed, which yields an increased pregnancy rate while reducing the incidence of OHSS and multiple gestations (83, 85, 86). Treatment consists of employing a low starting dose, typically 50 or 75 international units (IU) per day, and using small incremental dose increases when necessary to initiate and continue follicular development, up to maximum of 225 IU (6, 85). Ultrasounds are performed every 3–4 days to monitor follicle development, and ovulation is triggered by intramuscular human chorionic gonadotropin (hCG) injection (85). Treatment is typically discontinued if more than three follicles develop to reduce the risk of OHSS and multiple gestations (85). In patients who develop excessive follicles, smaller starting doses and/or smaller incremental increases are used for subsequent cycles (85). No significant differences in ovulation and pregnancy rates have been found between treatment with FSH and (hMG) in patients with PCOS, although FSH may be associated with a lower risk of OHSS (87, 88). Patients with a higher BMI are likely to require higher doses of gonadotropins and are less likely to conceive than lean patients (85). Alternatively, a step-down protocol has been designed, although it is less frequently used due to the need for more intensive monitoring during the first few days of treatment (85, 89).

Aromatase Inhibitors

Aromatase inhibitors, such as letrozole and anastrozole, have been used for ovulation induction in anovulatory infertility or as adjunctive treatment to gonadotropins for induction of multiple follicles for assisted reproduction (90). Their mechanism of action is through preventing conversion of androgen to estrogen. Aromatase inhibitors have a relatively short half-life (approximately 45 h) and therefore cause less adverse effects on estrogen target tissues and no downregulation of estrogen receptors as is seen with clomiphene citrate (90, 91). Begum et al. compared the efficacy of letrozole 7.5 mg to clomiphene 150 mg in patients with PCOS who did not respond to 100 mg of clomiphene (91). Patients treated with letrozole had significantly higher ovulation and pregnancy rates. Bayar et al. compared the use of letrozole 2.5 mg with clomiphene 100 mg in a prospective randomized study of 74 infertile PCOS women and found the two treatments to be comparable in ovulation and pregnancy rates (92).

While a recent study by Badawy et al. showed an increased number of follicles in clomiphene-resistant PCOS patients treated with anastrozole than with letrozole, pregnancy rates and miscarriage rates were similar between the two groups (93). Some authors have argued that letrozole is unlikely to have teratogenic effects due to its rapid elimination before fetal organogenesis (90). Limited data have found the incidence of anomalies to be slightly lower than in all births (90) but more studies are needed to further assess the safety of aromatase inhibitors in pregnancy. Miscarriage and ectopic pregnancy rates for aromatase inhibitors have been comparable to clomiphene citrate, with a lower rate of multiple gestations (90). However, a recent study found no advantage in pregnancy rate in the use of letrozole over clomiphene citrate as a first-line treatment for ovulation induction in women with PCOS (94). Infertility treatments with aromatase inhibitors remain a second-line agent for patients who are resistant to first-line treatments.

Laparoscopic Ovarian Drilling

Surgical ovarian wedge resection was the first surgical treatment for anovulatory PCOS but fell out of favor due to the risk of postsurgical adhesion formation *(95–97)*. Alternatively, LOD involves cautery of the ovarian surface using electrocoagulation or laser, which can be done on an outpatient basis, results in fewer postoperative adhesions, and requires no ongoing monitoring *(98–100)*. It has been used as an alternate therapy in patients who do not conceive with clomiphene or gonadotropin therapy or in women who hyperrespond to gonadotropins and are therefore at increased risk of developing OHSS *(101)*.

The mechanism involved in improvement in ovulation is unclear although it appears to be related to decreased LH concentrations, which are lowered significantly within days of the procedure *(6)*. In patients with hyperandrogenemia, serum testosterone rates are also lowered following LOD *(100, 101)*. Spontaneous ovulation rates following electrocautery LOD are 71–92% and pregnancy rates are 52–84% (spontaneous and stimulated) *(102)*. While retrospective studies have shown no significant difference in ovulation rates following LOD with electrocoagulation and laser (83% vs. 77.5%), cumulative pregnancy rates at 12 months were higher following electrocautery (65% vs. 54.5%) *(102)*. Laser therapy may produce more postprocedure adhesions than electrocautery *(100)*. Spontaneous ovulation is presumed to continue for years following LOD, as it did in patients who underwent ovarian wedge resection *(96)*.

To induce ovulation, LOD appears to most benefit lean PCOS women with high LH concentrations *(103)*. Following LOD, previously clomiphene-resistant patients are more responsive to treatment with clomiphene citrate *(104, 105)* and patients may have more successful pregnancy rates with gonadotropin treatment.

A recent Cochrane review revealed no significant difference in live birth or clinical pregnancy rate between LOD and gonadotropins while multiple gestation rates were lower with ovarian drilling (1% vs. 16%) *(98)*. Miscarriage rates appear to be similar between the two groups. While one LOD procedure is less expensive than gonadotropin therapy, it carries the risks of general anesthesia and postoperative adhesions, although less than with traditional ovarian wedge resection. Furthermore, it is unclear if there are long-term effects of LOD on ovarian function *(98)*.

A recent prospective randomized clinical trial by Youssef and Atallah found unilateral ovarian drilling to be as effective as bilateral LOD at lowering LH concentrations in patients with PCOS as well as similar ovulation and pregnancy rates, which could result in less time required for the procedure and fewer complications *(106)*.

Gonadotropin Releasing Hormone

Both GnRH agonists and antagonists are being investigated for their roles in ovulation induction in patients with PCOS. While GnRH agonists in conjunction with gonadotropins may increase pregnancy rates, reduce the risk of miscarriage, and may be of use in patients with high LH levels who have either failed gonadotropin therapy alone or who have had recurrent miscarriages, the concern for multiple follicle development has hampered their use in these patients *(6, 107, 108)*. Only small studies have been completed using GnRH antagonist treatment in conjunction with gonadotropins in patients with PCOS, and randomized controlled trials are needed to further define their role *(109)*. Finally, pulsatile GnRH treatment has also been explored but due to the small size and short duration of studies, it needs further investigation *(110)*.

In Vitro Fertilization

IVF represents a last resort for PCOS patients with infertility. A meta-analysis examining IVF outcomes in patients with PCOS compared with normal controls found an increased cycle cancellation rate and lower fertilization rates among patients with PCOS *(111)*. However, they were also found to have more oocytes per retrieval and comparable pregnancy and live birth rates when compared with the control group.

In vitro maturation of oocytes in which immature oocytes are retrieved without stimulation is being investigated for its utility in PCOS patients who have failed other treatments or couples who have additional causes of infertility. Studies so far have shown similar pregnancy, live birth and miscarriage rates to IVF, and the technique reduces the risk of OHSS compared with traditional IVF cycles *(112–114)*.

PREGNANCY

Normal pregnancy is a state of heightened insulin resistance and hyperinsulinemia, with progesterone, cortisol and estradiol contributing to the insulin resistance and human placental lactogen to augmented insulin production and hyperinsulinemia *(39)*. Markers of insulin resistance are elevated during normal pregnancy including triglycerides, small dense LDL particles, free fatty acids, plasminogen activator inhibitor-1 (PAI-1), tissue plasminogen activator antigen, vascular cell adhesion molecules, leptin, and tumor necrosis factor (TNFα) *(115)*. Some of these markers may be factors in the development of GDM or PIH, whereas others may be indicators of the underlying disease process *(115)*.

Early Pregnancy Loss

Early pregnancy loss (EPL) is defined as miscarriage of a clinically recognized pregnancy during the first trimester *(39)*. While EPL occurs in 10–15% of normal women *(116)*, rates in women with PCOS are as high as 30–50% *(117)*. Because of the prevalence of infertility in patients with PCOS, many women require fertility treatments which in themselves increase the prevalence of miscarriage *(118)*. However, several studies in women undergoing fertility treatment with IVF have demonstrated that women with PCOS have a higher miscarriage rate than controls *(107, 108, 119, 120)*. Although there has been considerable research interest in this area, the exact mechanisms underlying the increased risk of EPL in women with PCOS are not clearly elucidated.

LH AND EPL

Initially, EPL in PCOS was thought to be due to elevated LH levels *(8, 107, 117, 121, 122)*. A prospective study of women by Regan et al. revealed that regularly menstruating women with higher LH values were less likely to conceive (67% vs. 88%) and were more likely to miscarry (65% vs. 12%) than women with normal LH values *(121)*. Watson et al. demonstrated raised urinary LH levels or a premature LH surge in 81% of women with recurrent fetal loss *(122)*. Subsequent studies in women with PCOS have found an increased risk of EPL among women with elevated LH levels. Homburg et al. examined LH levels in women with PCOS undergoing fertility treatments and found a significantly elevated serum LH level in patients with early loss of pregnancy compared with those whose pregnancies progressed *(8)*. In a later study, Homburg et al. demonstrated a decreased miscarriage rate in PCOS patients who underwent long-term pituitary suppression with a GnRH agonist *(107)*. Balen et al. similarly found a decreased miscarriage rate among women with polycystic ovaries undergoing IVF who were treated with a GnRH agonist compared with clomiphene *(108)*.

However, a subsequent study by Clifford et al. found that LH suppression with a LH releasing hormone analogue before conception did not improve live birth rate in women with polycystic ovaries, elevated LH levels and a history of recurrent miscarriage *(123)*. Most recently, Rai et al. followed a cohort of 2,199 women with a history of recurrent miscarriage who conceived spontaneously and found no increased miscarriage rate among patients with an elevated serum LH *(124)*. It should be noted, however, that the two latter studies included only patients with a normal BMI, so the differing results from earlier studies may be confounded by the effects of obesity on pregnancy outcome.

ANDROGENS AND EPL

Because of the contradictory results of studies examining LH hypersecretion in the pathogenesis of EPL, alternative hypotheses have been explored. Because hyperandrogenemia is common in PCOS, it has been considered as a possible cause of EPL. Aksoy et al. found elevated ratios of maternal free testosterone (expressed in pg/mL) to total testosterone (expressed in ng/mL) greater than 1.05 during 6–12 weeks of gestation to be predictive of subsequent miscarriage *(125)*. In a prospective study of 50 women with a history of at least three consecutive miscarriages, Tulpalla et al. found higher levels of total and free testosterone as well as dehydroepiandrosterone sulfate (DHEA-S) among women who miscarried their next pregnancy *(126)*. Interestingly, the presence of polycystic ovaries did not predict miscarriage. Okon et al. found higher testosterone concentrations among patients (with and without PCOS) with recurrent miscarriages than in normal fertile controls *(127)*. There were no differences in plasma LH levels between the two groups. The authors postulated that high androgen levels antagonize estrogen, which may adversely affect endomctrial development and implantation *(127)*.

PLASMINOGEN ACTIVATOR INHIBITOR ACTIVITY AND EPL

High PAI-1 activity has also been postulated as a cause of EPL in women with PCOS. PAI-1 activity has been found to be associated with recurrent pregnancy loss in women with unexplained recurrent miscarriages *(128)* and has also been found to be significantly higher in women with PCOS, regardless of BMI *(129)*. Glueck et al. studied 41 women with PCOS and at least one pregnancy and found PAI-1 activity to be an independent risk factor for miscarriage, possibly due to hypofibrinolysis, which results in placental insufficiency through increased thrombosis as the placenta is forming *(130)*. Palombo et al. found that metformin significantly reduced PAI-1 activity levels resulting in improved pregnancy outcomes in overweight women with PCOS *(131)*. Conversely, LOD had no significant effect on PAI-1 levels. Additionally, a prospective study on a larger cohort of women with PCOS showed that PAI-1 activity was positively associated with first trimester miscarriage in women with PCOS and that BMI was a positive independent determinant of PAI-1 activity *(132)*. There was also a reduction in EPL in patients who had reduced PAI-1 levels during treatment with metformin. Patients who received metformin but did not have reductions in PAI-1 continued to have increased miscarriage rates. The authors postulated that metformin reduces PAI-1 activity, reduces placental insufficiency, and therefore reduces the risk of EPL *(132)*.

OBESITY, HYPERINSULINEMIA, AND EPL

Obesity itself appears to increase the risk of EPL *(119, 133, 134)*, and women with PCOS are more likely to be obese than the general population. Moderate obesity has been shown to increase the risk of miscarriage in PCOS women undergoing treatments with low-dose gonadotropin *(28)*. A subsequent study found obesity to be an independent risk factor for EPL in women undergoing IVF or intracytoplasmic sperm injection (ICSI) although patients who were obese had fewer oocytes retrieved as well, which may have affected the risk *(135)*. A meta-analysis by Metwally et al. found that obesity increased the general risk of miscarriage (OR 1.67) and increased the risk of miscarriage after oocyte donation and ovulation induction, although they did not find a significantly increased risk of miscarriage in patients undergoing IVF-ICSI *(134)*.

Hyperinsulinemia is a prominent feature of PCOS *(136)*, and it may play a role in the increased EPL in women with PCOS. Tian et al. recently showed insulin resistance to be an independent risk factor for miscarriage in patients undergoing assisted reproduction technology treatment *(137)*. In addition to causing hyperandrogenemia and increased PAI-1 activity, insulin resistance may affect the expression of endometrial proteins, including glycodelin and insulin growth factor binding protein 1 (IGFBP-1), which may be involved in embryonic implantation. Levels of these proteins were found to be significantly lower during the first trimester of pregnancy in PCOS patients who had a miscarriage *(41)*. Furthermore, insulin resistance is associated with decreased uterine vascularity, which could further affect implantation and increase the risk for EPL among patients with PCOS *(41)*. Metformin is known to decrease insulin resistance, and evidence suggests that it increases glycodelin and IGFBP-1 levels and improves uterine vascularity, all of which may improve implantation success *(138)*.

PREVENTION OF EPL WITH METFORMIN

Several studies have examined the effect of metformin on reducing EPL. Jakubowicz et al. performed a retrospective study of women with PCOS who had become pregnant and found an EPL rate of 8.8% in patients who had taken metformin throughout pregnancy and 41.9% in the control group, which consisted of PCOS women who never received metformin ($p < 0.001$) *(117)*. In a subgroup analysis of women with a prior history of miscarriage, EPL remained significantly decreased in the metformin group. Insulin sensitivity improved and testosterone levels decreased in patients taking metformin during pregnancy as compared with controls.

Glueck et al. performed a prospective cohort pilot study of women with PCOS and found the first trimester miscarriage rate to be 39% in historical controls who had not received metformin compared with 11% in patients who received metformin throughout pregnancy *(139)*. Patients treated with metformin for a median of 6 months were noted to have a reduction in fasting serum insulin levels, which positively correlated with reduced PAI-1 activity. In a follow-up prospective study, Glueck et al. again found a reduced rate of EPL (17%) among 72 PCOS women given metformin preconceptually and continued during pregnancy *(140)*. The study's control group consisted of historical controls of 40 women with PCOS who had conceived off metformin previously, who had a very high EPL rate of 62%. Among these women, EPL rates dropped from 62 to 26% when the women were treated with metformin. Pregnancy outcomes did not differ in women who stopped metformin at the end of the first trimester compared with those who continued it throughout pregnancy. Study entry fasting serum insulin, but not PAI-1 activity, was a significant independent variable by logistic regression for first trimester loss [OR 1.32 for each 5 μIU/mL increment in insulin, confidence intervals (CI) 1.09–1.60, $p = 0.005$].

Finally, impaired glucose tolerance that is more common in women with PCOS may be an important risk factor for EPL. A small prospective clinical trial by Zolghadri et al. found that women who had a history of recurrent spontaneous abortion were more likely to have an abnormal glucose tolerance test (17.6% vs. 5.4%, $p = 0.017$). Subsequently, 29 patients with recurrent EPL with and without PCOS who had impaired glucose tolerance were randomized to receive metformin or placebo and monitored during pregnancy. Patients without PCOS who were treated with metformin had a reduced first trimester abortion rate from 55 to 15% (OR 2.4, 95% CI 0.35–4.4) *(141)*. Although the EPL rate decreased in PCOS patients given metformin, it was not statistically significant (25% vs. 66%, $p = 0.42$). Larger studies are needed to determine if impaired glucose tolerance alone is an independent risk factor for EPL.

Controversy remains regarding when to discontinue metformin once a woman conceives. In a nonrandomized prospective cohort study, Khattab et al. examined the use of metformin in 200 women with PCOS. EPL among women who continued metformin throughout pregnancy at a dose of 1,000–2,000 mg daily was decreased compared with those who discontinued it at the time of conception or during pregnancy, including after the first trimester (11.6% vs. 36.3%, $p < 0.0001$) (142). Further studies are needed to determine if metformin should be continued for the first trimester or throughout pregnancy.

METFORMIN AND PREGNANCY RISKS

The majority of evidence so far has found metformin to be safe when taken during pregnancy. In a report that initially raised concerns about metformin's safety, Hellmuth et al. performed a small cohort study to examine the maternal and neonatal complications in pregnant diabetic women treated with metformin or a sulfonylurea compared with those treated with insulin (143). While there was no difference in neonatal mortality, the authors found an increased risk of preeclampsia and perinatal mortality among women taking metformin. However, patients in the metformin group had a significantly higher BMI and worse diabetic control, both of which increase the risk of preeclampsia. Further studies have not substantiated this increased risk.

Metformin is classified as a pregnancy category B drug, indicating that no teratogenic effects were seen in animal studies. A number of studies have supported this claim (117, 139–141, 144–146). Glueck et al. performed a prospective analysis of growth and development in infants born to women who took metformin throughout pregnancy (147). The study found no teratogenic effects of metformin and no effect on growth or motor-social development in the first 18 months of life. While female infants exposed to metformin were shorter (48.9 ± 5.4 vs. 50.6 ± 2.7 cm, $p = 0.006$) and weighed less (3.09 ± 0.85 vs. 3.29 ± 0.52 kg, $p = 0.04$) at birth, the biological significance of these differences is unknown. There were no significant differences in height or weight at 6, 12, and 18 months. In the Jakubowicz et al. study, one infant was found to have achondroplasia, a hereditary condition thought to be unrelated to metformin (117). A small study by Kovo et al. found a marginally significant decreased birth weight percentile among infants born to women who had taken metformin during the first trimester, although the study consisted of only 33 patients in the treatment group and was retrospectively performed (148). A recent meta-analysis by Gilbert et al. found no increased risk of major fetal malformations in women who were treated with metformin during the first trimester (149). Overall, metformin does not appear to increase the risk of congenital malformations, and most studies support its safety in the first trimester. There is limited data on use in the third trimester, although a recently published randomized controlled trial of metformin use in women with GDM was reassuring (150). Metformin may be effective in reducing EPL in women with PCOS but large, randomized controlled trials are needed to definitively assess its efficacy.

Gestational Diabetes

GDM is defined as diabetes or impaired glucose tolerance that develops during pregnancy (39). It affects 4–7% of pregnant women (151, 152) and carries considerable perinatal risk including macrosomia, hypoglycemia, stillbirth, jaundice and respiratory distress syndrome (153). A randomized controlled trial has shown that rates of serious perinatal complications were reduced, birth weight was lower, and macrosomia was less frequent in patients who were treated intensively for impaired glucose tolerance in pregnancy than in those who received conventional treatment (154). In addition to perinatal risks, women with GDM are at increased risk for birth trauma, cesarean section, pregnancy-induced hypertensive disorders and developing type 2 diabetes mellitus later in life (39, 155).

In normal women, pregnancy is known to increase insulin resistance, which is compensated by hyperinsulinemia; effects are maximal in the third trimester *(115, 156)*. Women with PCOS have greater insulin resistance than normal women and their pancreatic beta cells may be unable to fully compensate for the additional insulin resistance of pregnancy, making them more prone to the development of GDM *(157)*. They are also more likely to be obese and due to the increased rate of infertility in women with PCOS, they frequently conceive at an older age. Both obesity and advanced age increase the risk for GDM *(152)*. Studies have sought to determine if the increased risk for GDM in women with PCOS is due to insulin resistance or other factors that are associated with the syndrome.

POLYCYSTIC OVARIES AND GDM

Several studies have found an increased prevalence of polycystic ovaries in women with a history of GDM. Holte et al. compared 34 women with GDM 3–5 years prior to 36 controls with uncomplicated pregnancies *(158)*. Women with a history of GDM were more likely to have polycystic ovaries by ultrasound (41% vs. 3%, $p < 0.0001$), hirsutism, irregular menses and a higher BMI. In a subgroup analysis of the women with previous GDM, those with polycystic ovaries had higher androstenedione and testosterone concentrations, higher LH/FSH ratios, and higher levels of triglycerides and total cholesterol, all independent of age and BMI, despite similar glucose tolerance and prevalence of diabetes. The polycystic ovary group also had lower insulin sensitivity ($p < 0.05$), independent of BMI, than the group with normal ovaries. Similarly, Anttila et al. found polycystic ovaries to be more common among women with a history of GDM than among age- and BMI-matched controls *(159)*. However, because polycystic ovaries can also be found in normal women, using ultrasound evidence of polycystic ovaries is not a definitive surrogate for PCOS and examining rates of polycystic ovaries can overestimate the true prevalence of PCOS in GDM *(39)*.

BMI AND GDM

Several studies have found BMI to be predictive of GDM. In a multiethnic group of women, Kousta et al. found that women with a history of GDM had a higher prevalence of polycystic ovaries, higher fasting glucose, higher BMI, increased waist/hip ratio and lower insulin sensitivity than control women *(160)*. In addition, women with a history of GDM and polycystic ovaries were more likely to have irregular menstrual cycles. Koivunen et al. found that women with a history of GDM were more likely to have polycystic ovaries as well as lower early phase insulin response to glucose and impaired insulin sensitivity *(161)*. However, they were also more likely to be obese and when corrected for waist/hip ratio (but not BMI), the difference in insulin sensitivity was abolished.

PCOS AND GDM

Additional studies have sought to further define the association between PCOS and GDM. Urman et al. examined pregnancy outcomes in patients with known PCOS compared with that in healthy controls *(162)*. Women with PCOS had higher rates of GDM than controls ($p < 0.05$); the difference remained even when lean PCOS patients were compared with lean controls. In a retrospective cohort study, Radon et al. found an increased risk of glucose intolerance among patients with PCOS than among normal controls (OR 22.2, CI 3.8–170) *(163)*. However, there was no comparison performed to determine if obesity or PCOS were independent predictors of GDM.

In a larger retrospective analysis, Mikola et al. found that 20% of PCOS patients developed GDM compared with 8.9% of controls ($p < 0.001$) *(164)*. After logistic regression analysis, PCOS remained an independent predictor (adjusted OR 1.9, CI 1.0–3.5) but BMI > 25 appeared to be the greatest predictor for GDM (adjusted OR 5.1, CI 3.2–8.3). Similarly, in a retrospective comparison of PCOS patients and controls, Turhan et al. found PCOS to be the main predictor of impaired glucose tolerance ($p = 0.01$); however, logistic regression analysis revealed that a prepregnancy BMI > 25 was the main predictor of GDM ($p = 0.002$) *(165)*.

A large population-based study by Lo et al. showed a more than twofold increased odds of GDM (adjusted OR 2.44, CI 2.10–2.83) among women with a documented diagnosis of PCOS, independent of age, race, ethnicity and multiple gestations *(152)*. In addition, they found an intermediate increased risk of GDM (OR 1.40, CI 1.27–1.54) among women with PCOS symptoms by chart review. Unfortunately, the study did not control for obesity rendering it unclear if these results would remain independent of BMI.

Not all studies have found PCOS to be associated with GDM. In a retrospective case-control study comparing age- and weight-matched women, Haakova et al. found no increased incidence in GDM in patients with PCOS when compared with controls *(166)*. While the studies vary in diagnostic criteria and selection of a control group, both the majority of studies and the larger studies support an association between PCOS and GDM. Further support comes from a meta-analysis done by Boomsma et al. comprising 720 women with PCOS who were found to have a significantly higher risk of developing GDM (OR 2.94, CI 1.7–5.08) *(167)*. In addition, a family history of diabetes increases the risk for GDM, and studies have shown that 30–40% of women with PCOS and glucose intolerance have a first degree relative with diabetes *(168)*. Obesity further exacerbates the propensity for developing GDM, again emphasizing the importance of weight loss prior to conception.

PREVENTION OF GDM WITH METFORMIN

Metformin has been investigated for its ability to reduce the incidence of GDM in women with PCOS. Glueck et al. studied development of GDM in nondiabetic women with PCOS who conceived while taking metformin and had live births compared with historical controls who conceived without metformin *(144)*. Development of GDM was 3% in the metformin group vs. 23% in the control group. Of the women in the metformin group with prior pregnancies, 67% had previously developed GDM, suggesting that metformin may also be effective for secondary prevention. The cohorts did not differ in height, weight or insulin resistance. When all live births were combined, the odds ratio for GDM with metformin vs. GDM without metformin was 0.093 (CI 0.011–0.795). No adverse effects were noted on fetal outcomes. An additional study by Glueck et al. found no increase in preeclampsia during pregnancy in women given metformin during pregnancy *(169)*.

Glueck's group further examined the effects of metformin combined with a high-protein diet in preventing GDM and found a similar reduction in rates of GDM in patients taking metformin for both primary and secondary prevention *(170)*. Metformin did not result in any congenital malformations or fetal hypoglycemia. The authors hypothesized that metformin reduces development of GDM by reducing pregnancy-associated insulin resistance and that prevention of GDM with metformin may reduce the subsequent development of type 2 diabetes later in life, although this remains speculative *(170)*. Metformin plus a high-protein, low-carbohydrate diet may also help prevent excessive weight gain during pregnancy, which can also reduce the risk of GDM *(170)*. Nutrition during pregnancy is reviewed in detail in Chap. 14 of this text.

While these results are promising, randomized controlled trials are needed to fully assess the efficacy of metformin in the prevention of GDM. There is limited information regarding the use of other insulin sensitizers in pregnancy. TZDs are pregnancy class C and should be not be taken during pregnancy.

Pregnancy-Induced Hypertension

During normal pregnancy, blood pressure usually falls in the late first to early second trimester and rises again to prepregnancy levels in the third trimester *(115)*. PIH complicates 5–10% of pregnancies in the USA, including 3–5% of pregnancies in previously normotensive women *(115)*. Gestational hypertension is defined as elevated blood pressure on two occasions that develops after the twentieth week of pregnancy, without systemic symptoms, in previously normotensive women *(171)*. Preeclampsia is the development of gestational hypertension plus proteinuria of greater than 300 mg protein in 24 h. Complications of preeclampsia include hepatic dysfunction, hemolysis, disseminated intravascular coagulation and seizures *(115)*.

HYPERINSULINEMIA AND PIH

While many factors influence a woman's likelihood of developing PIH, there has been considerable interest in metabolic factors that may contribute. Studies have shown that women with PIH demonstrate exaggerated hyperinsulinemia compared with those with normal pregnancy. In a prospective cohort study, Hamasaki et al. found that the incidence of gestational hypertension was higher among patients with hyperinsulinemia than among controls (24.1% vs. 7.3%, $p < 0.005$) *(172)*. The risk remained after controlling for BMI, age and parity (RR 1.19, CI 1.03–1.38). Laivuori et al. found that women with a history of preeclamptic pregnancy 17 years prior had higher insulin levels, regardless of BMI *(173)*. In a case control study by Solomon et al., women who developed PIH had higher fasting insulin levels even after adjustment for BMI and age (RR 1.12, $p = 0.03$) *(174)*.

Hyperinsulinemia may increase renal reabsorption of sodium and stimulate the sympathetic nervous system, both of which can increase the risk of developing hypertension *(115)*. Furthermore, insulin resistance and/or its associated factors have been shown to be associated with PIH even years after pregnancy *(175–180)*. Insulin resistance or associated hyperglycemia may impair endothelial function, which may decrease prostacyclin production *(39)*. The hyperinsulinemic insulin resistance intrinsic to PCOS may therefore increase the risk of PIH.

Further support for this hypothesis comes from several studies that have found an association between GDM and PIH *(181–184)*. Some of the studies had small sample sizes and did not account for confounders such as race and BMI. However, in a large, population-based study, Bryson et al. found a significantly increased risk of gestational hypertension (OR 1.4, CI 1.2–1.6) and preeclampsia among women with GDM that persisted even after adjusting for BMI *(185)*. The association was stronger among women who received less prenatal care and among African-American women.

PCOS AND PIH

Given the risk for PIH in those with insulin resistance, it is not surprising that studies have found an association between women with PCOS and PIH. Diamant et al. found that preeclampsia was 11 times more common in anovulatory patients with PCOS undergoing ovulation induction than in normal controls *(186)*. PCOS women were also more likely to have preeclampsia than anovulatory women without PCOS. The study did not control for BMI. Gjonnaess followed 62 pregnancies of PCOS women who conceived after LOD and found the prevalence of preeclampsia to be 12.9%, which is higher than the risk in the general population *(187)*. While the most overweight women had the highest risk and normal weight women did not differ from the general population, even women who were mildly overweight had an increased risk of preeclampsia, implicating increased weight as a risk factor *(187)*. However, Urman et al. also found an increased risk of PIH even when lean PCOS patients were compared with lean controls *(162)*.

To further investigate the role of obesity in PIH in women with PCOS, de Vries et al. performed a retrospective case-control study examining the incidence of PIH in patients with and without PCOS who were treated for infertility *(188)*. While the overall incidence of PIH was similar in both groups, PCOS patients had a higher incidence of preeclampsia (14% vs. 2.5%, $p = 0.02$) regardless of BMI, ovulation induction, age and parity. A retrospective cohort study by Radon et al. found that women with PCOS had an increased risk of preeclampsia during pregnancy (OR 15.0, CI 1.9–121.5) compared to age- and weight-matched controls *(163)*. In a prospective cohort study, Bjercke et al. found an increased incidence of gestational hypertension among PCOS women compared to controls who had undergone assisted reproduction (11.5% vs. 0.3%, $p < 0.01$) *(189)*. Additionally, preeclampsia was increased among insulin-resistant PCOS patients compared to noninsulin-resistant PCOS patients and controls, supporting the association between hyperinsulinemia and PIH.

While some authors have postulated that PCOS patients are more likely to have PIH due to ovulation induction, several studies have found PCOS to be associated with PIH even when controlling for infertility treatment. A retrospective case-control study of patients who had undergone ovulation induction by Kashyap et al. showed a higher incidence of PIH among PCOS patients than among controls (31.8% vs. 3.7%, $p = 0.016$) *(190)*. Additionally, de Vries et al. stratified women according to treatment regimens for ovulation induction and found no relationship between the method used and preeclampsia *(188)*.

Blood pressure readings during pregnancy in PCOS women provide further support for the association between PCOS and PIH. While a retrospective case control study found no differences in blood pressure during the first and second trimester between PCOS and control women, a significant increase in blood pressure occurred during the third trimester and labor in PCOS women *(191)*. Similarly, in a prospective case-control study, Hu et al. demonstrated that women with PCOS had higher blood pressure throughout pregnancy than controls who were matched for age, BMI, parity and ethnicity *(192)*. In addition, 27% (6/22) of the women with PCOS developed PIH compared with none in the control group ($p = 0.011$). The authors postulated that women with PCOS have decreased arterial elasticity, which worsens as gestation progresses, causing vascular maladaptation and elevated blood pressure *(192)*.

Not all studies have found an association between PCOS and PIH. Turhan et al. found the prevalence of preeclampsia to be higher in PCOS women than in controls, although it did not reach statistical significance *(165)*. In a retrospective case-control study, Haakova et al. reported no significant difference in the prevalence of PIH between PCOS patients and controls matched by age and weight *(166)*. Overall, the studies support an association that was confirmed in the meta-analysis by Boomsma et al., which demonstrated a significantly higher chance of developing PIH (OR 3.67, CI 1.98–6.81) for women with PCOS *(167)*. The increased risk remained in a subgroup analysis of two higher validity studies (OR 3.71, CI 1.72–17.49). Furthermore, women with PCOS demonstrated a higher risk of preeclampsia. The authors suggested that the association of PCOS with PIH suggested an increase in placental insufficiency, which could confer considerable risk to the fetus. While the initial analysis found a higher risk of premature deliveries, perinatal mortality and admission to the neonatal intensive care unit, a subgroup analysis of higher validity studies did not support this association.

ANDROGENS AND PIH

Hyperandrogenemia has also been examined as a possible contributor to the increased risk of PIH in PCOS patients. Laivuori et al. found mild hyperandrogenism among women with a history of preeclampsia 17 years after delivery, suggesting that the patients may have had PCOS *(193)*. Hu et al. noted a possible role for the hyperandrogenemia of PCOS in the pathogenesis of PIH in that androgens induce production of vasoconstrictors such as endothelin and angiotensinogen *(192)*. They found elevated total testosterone levels in PCOS patients than in controls, but no differences in DHEAS. Furthermore, studies in animal models have shown that androgens decrease the production of prostacyclin *(194)*, which could also be a factor in the development of PIH.

PREVENTION OF PIH IN PCOS

Gestational hypertension and preeclampsia have important short- and long-term implications. Women with gestational hypertension have higher rates of induction of labor and cesarean delivery than the general population (171). Even more consequentially, severe preeclampsia is associated with increased perinatal and maternal mortality and morbidity, particularly if the condition develops before 32-weeks gestation (171). Furthermore, studies have shown that women with a history of PIH have an increased risk of developing chronic hypertension and cardiovascular disease than women who remain normotensive during pregnancy (195–198). This may be due to endothelial dysfunction and insulin resistance along with effects of hyperandrogenism (195). For these reasons it is important to minimize the risk of PIH in patients with PCOS. Preconception counseling should include lifestyle interventions to promote weight loss in obese patients. Whether insulin-sensitizing agents, such as metformin, could be used for prevention of PIH in patients with PCOS remains to be determined.

CONCLUSION

Infertility in patients with PCOS appears to be multifactorial. First-line treatments include weight loss, clomiphene and metformin, and management should be based on individualized patient goals and preferences. Patients should be informed of the additional risks of pregnancy, including EPL, GDM and PIH, and receive appropriate preconception and prenatal screening and care. Patients should be counseled regarding lifestyle modification and weight loss prior to conception in an effort to improve chances of conceiving and reduce their risk of adverse pregnancy outcomes.

Further research is needed to investigate the risk of maternal and perinatal complications in PCOS pregnancies. Most studies to date have been done retrospectively, including only small numbers of patients and have yielded conflicting results. Because of the confounding factors associated with PCOS, including obesity, age and a higher multiple gestation rate, future studies should match for BMI and other factors or analyze whether they are independent predictors of outcome in PCOS patients. Studies to determine treatment strategies have been limited due to methodological challenges. Further randomized controlled trials are needed to assess the efficacy and safety of metformin and other treatment possibilities during pregnancy for reducing the risk of EPL, GDM and PIH in patients with PCOS.

REFERENCES

1. Suncion M, Calvo RM, San Millan JL, Sancho J, Avila S, Escobar-Morreale HF, A prospective study of the prevalence of the polycystic ovary syndrome in unselected Caucasian women from Spain. J Clin Endocrinol Metab 2000; 85(7):2434–2438
2. Knochenhauer ES, Key TJ, Kahsar-Miller M, Waggoner W, Boots LR, Azziz R. Prevalence of the polycystic ovary syndrome in unselected black and white women of the southeastern United States: a prospective study. J Clin Endocrinol Metab 1998; 83(9):3078–3082
3. Franks S. Polycystic ovary syndrome. N Engl J Med 1995; 333(13):853–861
4. Legro RS, Kunselman AR, Dodson WC, Dunaif A. Prevalence and predictors of risk for type 2 diabetes mellitus and impaired glucose tolerance in polycystic ovary syndrome: a prospective, controlled study in 254 affected women. J Clin Endocrinol Metab 1999; 84(1):165–169
5. Orio F, Jr, Palomba S, Spinelli L, Cascella T, Tauchmanova L, Zullo F et al. The cardiovascular risk of young women with polycystic ovary syndrome: an observational, analytical, prospective, case-control study. J Clin Endocrinol Metab 2004; 89(8):3696–3701
6. Homburg R. The management of infertility associated with polycystic ovary syndrome. Reprod Biol Endocrinol 2003; 1:109
7. Balen AH, Conway GS, Kaltsas G, Techatrasak K, Manning PJ, West C et al. Polycystic ovary syndrome: the spectrum of the disorder in 1741 patients. Hum Reprod 1995; 10(8):2107–2111

8. Homburg R, Armar NA, Eshel A, Adams J, Jacobs HS. Influence of serum luteinising hormone concentrations on ovulation, conception, and early pregnancy loss in polycystic ovary syndrome. BMJ 1988; 297(6655):1024–1026

9. Kousta E, White DM, Franks S. Modern use of clomiphene citrate in induction of ovulation. Hum Reprod Update 1997; 3(4):359–365

10. Dunaif A, Segal KR, Futterweit W, Dobrjansky A. Profound peripheral insulin resistance, independent of obesity, in polycystic ovary syndrome. Diabetes 1989; 38(9):1165–1174

11. Dunaif A, Graf M, Mandeli J, Laumas V, Dobrjansky A. Characterization of groups of hyperandrogenic women with acanthosis nigricans, impaired glucose tolerance, and/or hyperinsulinemia. J Clin Endocrinol Metab 1987; 65(3):499–507

12. Robinson S, Kiddy D, Gelding SV, Willis D, Niththyananthan R, Bush A et al. The relationship of insulin insensitivity to menstrual pattern in women with hyperandrogenism and polycystic ovaries. Clin Endocrinol (Oxf) 1993; 39(3):351–355

13. Nestler JE, Jakubowicz DJ. Lean women with polycystic ovary syndrome respond to insulin reduction with decreases in ovarian P450c17 alpha activity and serum androgens. J Clin Endocrinol Metab 1997; 82(12):4075–4079

14. Franks S, Gilling-Smith C, Watson H, Willis D. Insulin action in the normal and polycystic ovary. Endocrinol Metab Clin North Am 1999; 28(2):361–378

15. Baillargeon JP, Carpentier A. Role of insulin in the hyperandrogenemia of lean women with polycystic ovary syndrome and normal insulin sensitivity. Fertil Steril 2007; 88(4):886–893

16. Baillargeon JP, Nestler JE. Commentary: polycystic ovary syndrome: a syndrome of ovarian hypersensitivity to insulin? J Clin Endocrinol Metab 2006; 91(1):22–24

17. Nestler JE, Powers LP, Matt DW, Steingold KA, Plymate SR, Rittmaster RS et al. A direct effect of hyperinsulinemia on serum sex hormone-binding globulin levels in obese women with the polycystic ovary syndrome. J Clin Endocrinol Metab 1991; 72(1):83–89

18. Crosignani PG, Ragni G, Parazzini F, Wyssling H, Lombroso G, Perotti L. Anthropometric indicators and response to gonadotrophin for ovulation induction. Hum Reprod 1994; 9(3):420–423

19. Legro RS, Barnhart HX, Schlaff WD, Carr BR, Diamond MP, Carson SA et al. Clomiphene, metformin, or both for infertility in the polycystic ovary syndrome. N Engl J Med 2007; 356(6):551–566

20. Fedorcsak P, Dale PO, Storeng R, Tanbo T, Abyholm T. The impact of obesity and insulin resistance on the outcome of IVF or ICSI in women with polycystic ovarian syndrome. Hum Reprod 2001; 16(6):1086–1091

21. Fedorcsak P, Dale PO, Storeng R, Ertzeid G, Bjercke S, Oldereid N et al. Impact of overweight and underweight on assisted reproduction treatment. Hum Reprod 2004; 19(11):2523–2528

22. Crosignani PG, Colombo M, Vegetti W, Somigliana E, Gessati A, Ragni G. Overweight and obese anovulatory patients with polycystic ovaries: parallel improvements in anthropometric indices, ovarian physiology and fertility rate induced by diet. Hum Reprod 2003; 18(9):1928–1932

23. Clark AM, Ledger W, Galletly C, Tomlinson L, Blaney F, Wang X et al. Weight loss results in significant improvement in pregnancy and ovulation rates in anovulatory obese women. Hum Reprod 1995; 10(10):2705–2712

24. Huber-Buchholz MM, Carey DG, Norman RJ. Restoration of reproductive potential by lifestyle modification in obese polycystic ovary syndrome: role of insulin sensitivity and luteinizing hormone. J Clin Endocrinol Metab 1999; 84(4):1470–1474

25. Palomba S, Giallauria F, Falbo A, Russo T, Oppedisano R, Tolino A et al. Structured exercise training programme versus hypocaloric hyperproteic diet in obese polycystic ovary syndrome patients with anovulatory infertility: a 24-week pilot study. Hum Reprod 2008; 23(3):642–650

26. Kiddy DS, Hamilton-Fairley D, Bush A, Short F, Anyaoku V, Reed MJ et al. Improvement in endocrine and ovarian function during dietary treatment of obese women with polycystic ovary syndrome. Clin Endocrinol (Oxf) 1992; 36(1):105–111

27. Clark AM, Thornley B, Tomlinson L, Galletley C, Norman RJ. Weight loss in obese infertile women results in improvement in reproductive outcome for all forms of fertility treatment. Hum Reprod 1998; 13(6):1502–1505

28. Hamilton-Fairley D, Kiddy D, Watson H, Paterson C, Franks S. Association of moderate obesity with a poor pregnancy outcome in women with polycystic ovary syndrome treated with low dose gonadotrophin. Br J Obstet Gynaecol 1992; 99(2):128–131

29. Davies MJ. Evidence for effects of weight on reproduction in women. Reprod Biomed Online 2006; 12(5):552–561

30. Hughes E, Collins J, Vandekerckhove P. Clomiphene citrate for ovulation induction in women with oligo-amenorrhoea. Cochrane Database Syst Rev 2000;(2):CD000056

31. Imani B, Eijkemans MJ, te Velde ER, Habbema JD, Fauser BC. Predictors of patients remaining anovulatory during clomiphene citrate induction of ovulation in normogonadotropic oligoamenorrheic infertility. J Clin Endocrinol Metab 1998; 83(7):2361–2365

32. Imani B, Eijkemans MJ, te Velde ER, Habbema JD, Fauser BC. Predictors of chances to conceive in ovulatory patients during clomiphene citrate induction of ovulation in normogonadotropic oligoamenorrheic infertility. J Clin Endocrinol Metab 1999; 84(5):1617–1622

33. Garcia J, Jones GS, Wentz AC. The use of clomiphene citrate. Fertil Steril 1977; 28(7):707–717

34. Gysler M, March CM, Mishell DR, Jr, Bailey EJ. A decade's experience with an individualized clomiphene treatment regimen including its effect on the postcoital test. Fertil Steril 1982; 37(2):161–167

35. Althuis MD, Moghissi KS, Westhoff CL, Scoccia B, Lamb EJ, Lubin JH et al. Uterine cancer after use of clomiphene citrate to induce ovulation. Am J Epidemiol 2005; 161(7):607–615

36. Brinton LA, Lamb EJ, Moghissi KS, Scoccia B, Althuis MD, Mabie JE et al. Ovarian cancer risk after the use of ovulation-stimulating drugs. Obstet Gynecol 2004; 103(6):1194–1203

37. Rossing MA, Daling JR, Weiss NS, Moore DE, Self SG. Ovarian tumors in a cohort of infertile women. N Engl J Med 1994; 331(12):771–776

38. Gonen Y, Casper RF. Sonographic determination of a possible adverse effect of clomiphene citrate on endometrial growth. Hum Reprod 1990; 5(6):670–674

39. Patel SM, Nestler JE. Fertility in polycystic ovary syndrome. Endocrinol Metab Clin North Am 2006; 35(1):137–155, vii

40. Palomba S, Orio F, Jr, Falbo A, Manguso F, Russo T, Cascella T et al. Prospective parallel randomized, double-blind, double-dummy controlled clinical trial comparing clomiphene citrate and metformin as the first-line treatment for ovulation induction in nonobese anovulatory women with polycystic ovary syndrome. J Clin Endocrinol Metab 2005; 90(7):4068–4074

41. Jakubowicz DJ, Essah PA, Seppala M, Jakubowicz S, Baillargeon JP, Koistinen R et al. Reduced serum glycodelin and insulin-like growth factor-binding protein-1 in women with polycystic ovary syndrome during first trimester of pregnancy. J Clin Endocrinol Metab 2004; 89(2):833–839

42. Lobo RA, Gysler M, March CM, Goebelsmann U, Mishell DR, Jr. Clinical and laboratory predictors of clomiphene response. Fertil Steril 1982; 37(2):168–174

43. Polson DW, Kiddy DS, Mason HD, Franks S. Induction of ovulation with clomiphene citrate in women with polycystic ovary syndrome: the difference between responders and nonresponders. Fertil Steril 1989; 51(1):30–34

44. Imani B, Eijkemans MJ, te Velde ER, Habbema JD, Fauser BC. A nomogram to predict the probability of live birth after clomiphene citrate induction of ovulation in normogonadotropic oligoamenorrheic infertility. Fertil Steril 2002; 77(1):91–97

45. Eimers JM, te Velde ER, Gerritse R, Vogelzang ET, Looman CW, Habbema JD. The prediction of the chance to conceive in subfertile couples. Fertil Steril 1994; 61(1):44–52

46. Scott RT, Opsahl MS, Leonardi MR, Neall GS, Illions EH, Navot D. Life table analysis of pregnancy rates in a general infertility population relative to ovarian reserve and patient age. Hum Reprod 1995; 10(7):1706–1710

47. Daly DC, Walters CA, Soto-Albors CE, Tohan N, Riddick DH. A randomized study of dexamethasone in ovulation induction with clomiphene citrate. Fertil Steril 1984; 41(6):844–848

48. Elnashar A, Abdelmageed E, Fayed M, Sharaf M. Clomiphene citrate and dexamethazone in treatment of clomiphene citrate-resistant polycystic ovary syndrome: a prospective placebo-controlled study. Hum Reprod 2006; 21(7):1805–1808

49. Trott EA, Plouffe L, Jr, Hansen K, Hines R, Brann DW, Mahesh VB. Ovulation induction in clomiphene-resistant anovulatory women with normal dehydroepiandrosterone sulfate levels: beneficial effects of the addition of dexamethasone during the follicular phase. Fertil Steril 1996; 66(3):484–486

50. Parsanezhad ME, Alborzi S, Motazedian S, Omrani G. Use of dexamethasone and clomiphene citrate in the treatment of clomiphene citrate-resistant patients with polycystic ovary syndrome and normal dehydroepiandrosterone sulfate levels: a prospective, double-blind, placebo-controlled trial. Fertil Steril 2002; 78(5):1001–1004

51. The Thessaloniki ESHRE/ASRM Sponsored PCOS Consens. Consensus on infertility treatment related to polycystic ovary syndrome. Hum Reprod 2008; 23(3):462–477

52. Arslanian SA, Lewy V, Danadian K, Saad R. Metformin therapy in obese adolescents with polycystic ovary syndrome and impaired glucose tolerance: amelioration of exaggerated adrenal response to adrenocorticotropin with reduction of insulinemia/insulin resistance. J Clin Endocrinol Metab 2002; 87(4):1555–1559

53. Nestler JE, Jakubowicz DJ. Decreases in ovarian cytochrome P450c17 alpha activity and serum free testosterone after reduction of insulin secretion in polycystic ovary syndrome. N Engl J Med 1996; 335(9):617–623

54. Salley KE, Wickham EP, Cheang KI, Essah PA, Karjane NW, Nestler JE. POSITION STATEMENT: Glucose intolerance in polycystic ovary syndrome – a position statement of the Androgen Excess Society. J Clin Endocrinol Metab 2007; 92(12):4546–4556

55. Sharma ST, Nestler JE. Prevention of diabetes and cardiovascular disease in women with PCOS: treatment with insulin sensitizers. Best Pract Res Clin Endocrinol Metab 2006; 20(2):245–260

56. Sharma ST, Wickham EP, III, Nestler JE. Changes in glucose tolerance with metformin treatment in polycystic ovary syndrome: a retrospective analysis. Endocr Pract 2007; 13(4):373–379

57. Unluhizarci K, Kelestimur F, Bayram F, Sahin Y, Tutus A. The effects of metformin on insulin resistance and ovarian steroidogenesis in women with polycystic ovary syndrome. Clin Endocrinol (Oxf) 1999; 51(2):231–236

58. la Marca A, Morgante G, Paglia T, Ciotta L, Cianci A, De Leo V. Effects of metformin on adrenal steroidogenesis in women with polycystic ovary syndrome. Fertil Steril 1999; 72(6):985–989

59. Fleming R, Hopkinson ZE, Wallace AM, Greer IA, Sattar N. Ovarian function and metabolic factors in women with oligomenorrhea treated with metformin in a randomized double blind placebo-controlled trial. J Clin Endocrinol Metab 2002; 87(2):569–574

60. Pirwany IR, Yates RW, Cameron IT, Fleming R. Effects of the insulin sensitizing drug metformin on ovarian function, follicular growth and ovulation rate in obese women with oligomenorrhoea. Hum Reprod 1999; 14(12):2963–2968

61. Siebert TI, Kruger TF, Steyn DW, Nosarka S. Is the addition of metformin efficacious in the treatment of clomiphene citrate-resistant patients with polycystic ovary syndrome? A structured literature review. Fertil Steril 2006; 86(5):1432–1437

62. Neveu N, Granger L, St Michel P, Lavoie HB. Comparison of clomiphene citrate, metformin, or the combination of both for first-line ovulation induction and achievement of pregnancy in 154 women with polycystic ovary syndrome. Fertil Steril 2007; 87(1):113–120

63. Nestler JE. Metformin for the treatment of the polycystic ovary syndrome. N Engl J Med 2008; 358(1):47–54

64. Moll E, Bossuyt PM, Korevaar JC, Lambalk CB, van d, V. Effect of clomifene citrate plus metformin and clomifene citrate plus placebo on induction of ovulation in women with newly diagnosed polycystic ovary syndrome: randomised double blind clinical trial. BMJ 2006; 332(7556):1485

65. Palomba S, Orio F, Jr, Falbo A, Russo T, Tolino A, Zullo F. Clomiphene citrate versus metformin as first-line approach for the treatment of anovulation in infertile patients with polycystic ovary syndrome. J Clin Endocrinol Metab 2007; 92(9):3498–3503

66. Lord JM, Flight IH, Norman RJ. Metformin in polycystic ovary syndrome: systematic review and meta-analysis. BMJ 2003, 327(7421):951–953

67. Kashyap S, Wells GA, Rosenwaks Z. Insulin-sensitizing agents as primary therapy for patients with polycystic ovarian syndrome. Hum Reprod 2004; 19(11):2474–2483

68. Creanga AA, Bradley HM, McCormick C, Witkop CT. Use of metformin in polycystic ovary syndrome: a meta-analysis. Obstet Gynecol 2008; 111(4):959–968

69. Eisenhardt S, Schwarzmann N, Henschel V, Germeyer A, von Wolff M, Hamann A et al. Early effects of metformin in women with polycystic ovary syndrome: a prospective randomized, double-blind, placebo-controlled trial. J Clin Endocrinol Metab 2006; 91(3):946–952

70. Palomba S, Pasquali R, Orio JF, Nestler JE. Clomiphene citrate, metformin or both as first-step approach in treating anovulatory infertility in patients with polycystic ovary syndrome (PCOS): a systematic review of head-to-head randomized controlled studies and meta-analysis. Clin Endocrinol (Oxf) 2008

71. Malkawi HY, Qublan HS, Hamaideh AH. Medical vs. surgical treatment for clomiphene citrate-resistant women with polycystic ovary syndrome. J Obstet Gynaecol 2003; 23(3):289–293

72. Palomba S, Orio F, Jr, Nardo LG, Falbo A, Russo T, Corea D et al. Metformin administration versus laparoscopic ovarian diathermy in clomiphene citrate-resistant women with polycystic ovary syndrome: a prospective parallel randomized double-blind placebo-controlled trial. J Clin Endocrinol Metab 2004; 89(10):4801–4809

73. Checa MA, Requena A, Salvador C, Tur R, Callejo J, Espinos JJ et al. Insulin-sensitizing agents: use in pregnancy and as therapy in polycystic ovary syndrome. Hum Reprod Update 2005; 11(4):375–390

74. Froment P, Touraine P. Thiazolidinediones and fertility in polycystic ovary syndrome (PCOS). PPAR Res 2006; 2006:73986

75. Azziz R, Ehrmann D, Legro RS, Whitcomb RW, Hanley R, Fereshetian AG et al. Troglitazone improves ovulation and hirsutism in the polycystic ovary syndrome: a multicenter, double blind, placebo-controlled trial. J Clin Endocrinol Metab 2001; 86(4):1626–1632

76. Veldhuis JD, Zhang G, Garmey JC. Troglitazone, an insulin-sensitizing thiazolidinedione, represses combined stimulation by LH and insulin of de novo androgen biosynthesis by thecal cells in vitro. J Clin Endocrinol Metab 2002; 87(3):1129–1133

77. Belli SH, Graffigna MN, Oneto A, Otero P, Schurman L, Levalle OA. Effect of rosiglitazone on insulin resistance, growth factors, and reproductive disturbances in women with polycystic ovary syndrome. Fertil Steril 2004; 81(3):624–629

78. Baillargeon JP, Jakubowicz DJ, Iuorno MJ, Jakubowicz S, Nestler JE. Effects of metformin and rosiglitazone, alone and in combination, in nonobese women with polycystic ovary syndrome and normal indices of insulin sensitivity. Fertil Steril 2004; 82(4):893–902

79. Rouzi AA, Ardawi MS. A randomized controlled trial of the efficacy of rosiglitazone and clomiphene citrate versus metformin and clomiphene citrate in women with clomiphene citrate-resistant polycystic ovary syndrome. Fertil Steril 2006; 85(2):428–435

80. Brettenthaler N, De Geyter C, Huber PR, Keller U. Effect of the insulin sensitizer pioglitazone on insulin resistance, hyperandrogenism, and ovulatory dysfunction in women with polycystic ovary syndrome. J Clin Endocrinol Metab 2004; 89(8):3835–3840

81. Glueck CJ, Moreira A, Goldenberg N, Sieve L, Wang P. Pioglitazone and metformin in obese women with polycystic ovary syndrome not optimally responsive to metformin. Hum Reprod 2003; 18(8):1618–1625

82. Hamilton-Fairley D, Franks S. Common problems in induction of ovulation. Baillieres Clin Obstet Gynaecol 1990; 4(3):609–625

83. Homburg R, Levy T, Ben Rafael Z. A comparative prospective study of conventional regimen with chronic low-dose administration of follicle-stimulating hormone for anovulation associated with polycystic ovary syndrome. Fertil Steril 1995; 63(4):729–733

84. Van Der MM, Hompes PG, De Boer JA, Schats R, Schoemaker J. Cohort size rather than follicle-stimulating hormone threshold level determines ovarian sensitivity in polycystic ovary syndrome. J Clin Endocrinol Metab 1998; 83(2):423–426

85. Gorry A, White DM, Franks S. Infertility in polycystic ovary syndrome: focus on low-dose gonadotropin treatment. Endocrine 2006; 30(1):27–33

86. Hedon B, Hugues JN, Emperaire JC, Chabaud JJ, Barbereau D, Boujenah A et al. A comparative prospective study of a chronic low dose versus a conventional ovulation stimulation regimen using recombinant human follicle stimulating hormone in anovulatory infertile women. Hum Reprod 1998; 13(10):2688–2692

87. Hughes E, Collins J, Vandekerckhove P. Ovulation induction with urinary follicle stimulating hormone versus human menopausal gonadotropin for clomiphene-resistant polycystic ovary syndrome. Cochrane Database Syst Rev 2000;(2):CD000087

88. Sagle MA, Hamilton-Fairley D, Kiddy DS, Franks S. A comparative, randomized study of low-dose human menopausal gonadotropin and follicle-stimulating hormone in women with polycystic ovarian syndrome. Fertil Steril 1991; 55(1):56–60

89. van Santbrink EJ, Donderwinkel PF, van Dessel TJ, Fauser BC. Gonadotrophin induction of ovulation using a step-down dose regimen: single-centre clinical experience in 82 patients. Hum Reprod 1995; 10(5):1048–1053

90. Casper RF. Aromatase inhibitors in ovarian stimulation. J Steroid Biochem Mol Biol 2007; 106(1–5):71–75

91. Begum MR, Ferdous J, Begum A, Quadir E. Comparison of efficacy of aromatase inhibitor and clomiphene citrate in induction of ovulation in polycystic ovarian syndrome. Fertil Steril 2008;

92. Bayar U, Basaran M, Kiran S, Coskun A, Gezer S. Use of an aromatase inhibitor in patients with polycystic ovary syndrome: a prospective randomized trial. Fertil Steril 2006; 86(5):1447–1451

93. Badawy A, Mosbah A, Shady M. Anastrozole or letrozole for ovulation induction in clomiphene-resistant women with polycystic ovarian syndrome: a prospective randomized trial. Fertil Steril 2008; 89(5):1209–1212

94. Badawy A, Abdel Aal I, Abulatta M. Clomiphene citrate or letrozole for ovulation induction in women with polycystic ovarian syndrome: a prospective randomized trial. Fertil Steril 2007; epub

95. Kistner RW. Peri-tubal and peri-ovarian adhesions subsequent to wedge resection of the ovaries. Fertil Steril 1969; 20(1):35–41

96. Lunde O, Djoseland O, Grottum P. Polycystic ovarian syndrome: a follow-up study on fertility and menstrual pattern in 149 patients 15–25 years after ovarian wedge resection. Hum Reprod 2001; 16(7):1479–1485

97. STEIN IF, COHEN MR, ELSON R. Results of bilateral ovarian wedge resection in 47 cases of sterility; 20 year end results; 75 cases of bilateral polycystic ovaries. Am J Obstet Gynecol 1949; 58(2):267–274

98. Farquhar C, Lilford RJ, Marjoribanks J, Vandekerckhove P. Laparoscopic 'drilling' by diathermy or laser for ovulation induction in anovulatory polycystic ovary syndrome. Cochrane Database Syst Rev 2007;(3):CD001122

99. Gurgan T, Kisnisci H, Yarali H, Develioglu O, Zeyneloglu H, Aksu T. Evaluation of adhesion formation after laparoscopic treatment of polycystic ovarian disease. Fertil Steril 1991; 56(6):1176–1178

100. Felemban A, Tan SL, Tulandi T. Laparoscopic treatment of polycystic ovaries with insulated needle cautery: a reappraisal. Fertil Steril 2000; 73(2):266–269

101. Shibahara H, Hirano Y, Kikuchi K, Suzuki T, Takamizawa S, Suzuki M. Postoperative endocrine alterations and clinical outcome of infertile women with polycystic ovary syndrome after transvaginal hydrolaparoscopic ovarian drilling. Fertil Steril 2006; 85(1):244–246

102. Saleh AM, Khalil HS. Review of nonsurgical and surgical treatment and the role of insulin-sensitizing agents in the management of infertile women with polycystic ovary syndrome. Acta Obstet Gynecol Scand 2004; 83(7):614–621

103. Gjonnaess H. Ovarian electrocautery in the treatment of women with polycystic ovary syndrome (PCOS). Factors affecting the results. Acta Obstet Gynecol Scand 1994; 73(5):407–412

104. Kato M, Kikuchi I, Shimaniki H, Kobori H, Aida T, Kitade M et al. Efficacy of laparoscopic ovarian drilling for polycystic ovary syndrome resistant to clomiphene citrate. J Obstet Gynaecol Res 2007; 33(2):174–180

105. Palomba S, Orio F, Jr, Falbo A, Russo T, Caterina G, Manguso F et al. Metformin administration and laparoscopic ovarian drilling improve ovarian response to clomiphene citrate (CC) in oligo-anovulatory CC-resistant women with polycystic ovary syndrome. Clin Endocrinol (Oxf) 2005; 63(6):631–635

106. Youssef H, Atallah MM. Unilateral ovarian drilling in polycystic ovarian syndrome: a prospective randomized study. Reprod Biomed Online 2007; 15(4):457–462

107. Homburg R, Levy T, Berkovitz D, Farchi J, Feldberg D, Ashkenazi J et al. Gonadotropin-releasing hormone agonist reduces the miscarriage rate for pregnancies achieved in women with polycystic ovarian syndrome. Fertil Steril 1993; 59(3):527–531

108. Balen AH, Tan SL, MacDougall J, Jacobs HS. Miscarriage rates following in-vitro fertilization are increased in women with polycystic ovaries and reduced by pituitary desensitization with buserelin. Hum Reprod 1993; 8(6):959–964

109. Griesinger G, Diedrich K, Tarlatzis BC, Kolibianakis EM. GnRH-antagonists in ovarian stimulation for IVF in patients with poor response to gonadotrophins, polycystic ovary syndrome, and risk of ovarian hyperstimulation: a meta-analysis. Reprod Biomed Online 2006; 13(5):628–638

110. Bayram N, van Wely M, van dee Veen F. Pulsatile gonadotrophin releasing hormone for ovulation induction in subfertility associated with polycystic ovary syndrome. Cochrane Database Syst Rev 2004;(1):CD000412

111. Heijnen EM, Eijkemans MJ, Hughes EG, Laven JS, Macklon NS, Fauser BC. A meta-analysis of outcomes of conventional IVF in women with polycystic ovary syndrome. Hum Reprod Update 2006; 12(1):13–21

112. Cha KY, Chung HM, Lee DR, Kwon H, Chung MK, Park LS et al. Obstetric outcome of patients with polycystic ovary syndrome treated by in vitro maturation and in vitro fertilization-embryo transfer. Fertil Steril 2005; 83(5):1461–1465

113. Child TJ, Phillips SJ, Abdul-Jalil AK, Gulekli B, Tan SL. A comparison of in vitro maturation and in vitro fertilization for women with polycystic ovaries. Obstet Gynecol 2002; 100(4):665–670

114. Le Du A, Kadoch IJ, Bourcigaux N, Doumerc S, Bourrier MC, Chevalier N et al. In vitro oocyte maturation for the treatment of infertility associated with polycystic ovarian syndrome: the French experience. Hum Reprod 2005; 20(2):420–424

115. Seely EW, Solomon CG. Insulin resistance and its potential role in pregnancy-induced hypertension. J Clin Endocrinol Metab 2003; 88(6):2393–2398

116. Gray RH, Wu LY. Subfertility and risk of spontaneous abortion. Am J Public Health 2000; 90(9):1452–1454

117. Jakubowicz DJ, Iuorno MJ, Jakubowicz S, Roberts KA, Nestler JE. Effects of metformin on early pregnancy loss in the polycystic ovary syndrome. J Clin Endocrinol Metab 2002; 87(2):524–529

118. Homburg R. Pregnancy complications in PCOS. Best Pract Res Clin Endocrinol Metab 2006; 20(2):281–292

119. Wang JX, Davies MJ, Norman RJ. Obesity increases the risk of spontaneous abortion during infertility treatment. Obes Res 2002; 10(6):551–554

120. Winter E, Wang J, Davies MJ, Norman R. Early pregnancy loss following assisted reproductive technology treatment. Hum Reprod 2002; 17(12):3220–3223

121. Regan L, Owen EJ, Jacobs HS. Hypersecretion of luteinising hormone, infertility, and miscarriage. Lancet 1990; 336(8724):1141–1144

122. Watson H, Kiddy DS, Hamilton-Fairley D, Scanlon MJ, Barnard C, Collins WP et al. Hypersecretion of luteinizing hormone and ovarian steroids in women with recurrent early miscarriage. Hum Reprod 1993; 8(6):829–833

123. Clifford K, Rai R, Watson H, Franks S, Regan L. Does suppressing luteinising hormone secretion reduce the miscarriage rate? Results of a randomised controlled trial. BMJ 1996; 312(7045):1508–1511

124. Rai R, Backos M, Rushworth F, Regan L. Polycystic ovaries and recurrent miscarriage – a reappraisal. Hum Reprod 2000; 15(3):612–615

125. Aksoy S, Celikkanat H, Senoz S, Gokmen O. The prognostic value of serum estradiol, progesterone, testosterone and free testosterone levels in detecting early abortions. Eur J Obstet Gynecol Reprod Biol 1996; 67(1):5–8

126. Tulppala M, Stenman UH, Cacciatore B, Ylikorkala O. Polycystic ovaries and levels of gonadotrophins and androgens in recurrent miscarriage: prospective study in 50 women. Br J Obstet Gynaecol 1993; 100(4):348–352

127. Okon MA, Laird SM, Tuckerman EM, Li TC. Serum androgen levels in women who have recurrent miscarriages and their correlation with markers of endometrial function. Fertil Steril 1998; 69(4):682–690

128. Gris JC, Ripart-Neveu S, Maugard C, Tailland ML, Brun S, Courtieu C et al. Respective evaluation of the prevalence of haemostasis abnormalities in unexplained primary early recurrent miscarriages. The Nimes Obstetricians and Haematologists (NOHA) Study. Thromb Haemost 1997; 77(6):1096–1103

129. Orio F, Jr, Palomba S, Cascella T, Tauchmanova L, Nardo LG, Di Biase S et al. Is plasminogen activator inhibitor-1 a cardiovascular risk factor in young women with polycystic ovary syndrome? Reprod Biomed Online 2004; 9(5):505–510

130. Glueck CJ, Wang P, Fontaine RN, Sieve-Smith L, Tracy T, Moore SK. Plasminogen activator inhibitor activity: an independent risk factor for the high miscarriage rate during pregnancy in women with polycystic ovary syndrome. Metabolism 1999; 48(12):1589–1595

131. Palomba S, Orio F, Jr, Falbo A, Russo T, Tolino A, Zullo F. Plasminogen activator inhibitor 1 and miscarriage after metformin treatment and laparoscopic ovarian drilling in patients with polycystic ovary syndrome. Fertil Steril 2005; 84(3):761–765

132. Glueck CJ, Sieve L, Zhu B, Wang P. Plasminogen activator inhibitor activity, 4G5G polymorphism of the plasminogen activator inhibitor 1 gene, and first-trimester miscarriage in women with polycystic ovary syndrome. Metabolism 2006; 55(3):345–352

133. Maheshwari A, Stofberg L, Bhattacharya S. Effect of overweight and obesity on assisted reproductive technology – a systematic review. Hum Reprod Update 2007; 13(5):433–444

134. Metwally M, Ong KJ, Ledger WL, Li TC. Does high body mass index increase the risk of miscarriage after spontaneous and assisted conception? A meta-analysis of the evidence. Fertil Steril 2007; 90(3):714–726

135. Fedorcsak P, Storeng R, Dale PO, Tanbo T, Abyholm T. Obesity is a risk factor for early pregnancy loss after IVF or ICSI. Acta Obstet Gynecol Scand 2000; 79(1):43–48

136. Ehrmann DA, Liljenquist DR, Kasza K, Azziz R, Legro RS, Ghazzi MN. Prevalence and predictors of the metabolic syndrome in women with polycystic ovary syndrome. J Clin Endocrinol Metab 2006; 91(1):48–53

137. Tian L, Shen H, Lu Q, Norman RJ, Wang J. Insulin resistance increases the risk of spontaneous abortion after assisted reproduction technology treatment. J Clin Endocrinol Metab 2007; 92(4):1430–1433

138. Jakubowicz DJ, Seppala M, Jakubowicz S, Rodriguez-Armas O, Rivas-Santiago A, Koistinen H et al. Insulin reduction with metformin increases luteal phase serum glycodelin and insulin-like growth factor-binding protein 1 concentrations and enhances uterine vascularity and blood flow in the polycystic ovary syndrome. J Clin Endocrinol Metab 2001; 86(3):1126–1133

139. Glueck CJ, Phillips H, Cameron D, Sieve-Smith L, Wang P. Continuing metformin throughout pregnancy in women with polycystic ovary syndrome appears to safely reduce first-trimester spontaneous abortion: a pilot study. Fertil Steril 2001; 75(1):46–52

140. Glueck CJ, Wang P, Goldenberg N, Sieve-Smith L. Pregnancy outcomes among women with polycystic ovary syndrome treated with metformin. Hum Reprod 2002; 17(11):2858–2864

141. Zolghadri J, Tavana Z, Kazerooni T, Soveid M, Taghieh M. Relationship between abnormal glucose tolerance test and history of previous recurrent miscarriages, and beneficial effect of metformin in these patients: a prospective clinical study. Fertil Steril 2008; 90(3):727–730

142. Khattab S, Mohsen IA, Foutouh IA, Ramadan A, Moaz M, Al Inany H. Metformin reduces abortion in pregnant women with polycystic ovary syndrome. Gynecol Endocrinol 2006; 22(12):680–684

143. Hellmuth E, Damm P, Molsted-Pedersen L. Oral hypoglycaemic agents in 118 diabetic pregnancies. Diabet Med 2000; 17(7):507–511

144. Glueck CJ, Wang P, Kobayashi S, Phillips H, Sieve-Smith L. Metformin therapy throughout pregnancy reduces the development of gestational diabetes in women with polycystic ovary syndrome. Fertil Steril 2002; 77(3):520–525

145. Turner MJ, Walsh J, Byrne KM, Murphy C, Langan H, Farah N. Outcome of clinical pregnancies after ovulation induction using metformin. J Obstet Gynaecol 2006; 26(3):233–235

146. Thatcher SS, Jackson EM. Pregnancy outcome in infertile patients with polycystic ovary syndrome who were treated with metformin. Fertil Steril 2006; 85(4):1002–1009

147. Glueck CJ, Goldenberg N, Pranikoff J, Loftspring M, Sieve L, Wang P. Height, weight, and motor-social development during the first 18 months of life in 126 infants born to 109 mothers with polycystic ovary syndrome who conceived on and continued metformin through pregnancy. Hum Reprod 2004; 19(6):1323–1330

148. Kovo M, Weissman A, Gur D, Levran D, Rotmensch S, Glezerman M. Neonatal outcome in polycystic ovarian syndrome patients treated with metformin during pregnancy. J Matern Fetal Neonatal Med 2006; 19(7):415–419

149. Gilbert C, Valois M, Koren G. Pregnancy outcome after first-trimester exposure to metformin: a meta-analysis. Fertil Steril 2006; 86(3):658–663

150. Rowan JA, Hague WM, Gao W, Battin MR, Moore MP. Metformin versus insulin for the treatment of gestational diabetes. N Engl J Med 2008; 358(19):2003–2015

151. Ferrara A, Hedderson MM, Quesenberry CP, Selby JV. Prevalence of gestational diabetes mellitus detected by the National Diabetes Data Group or the Carpenter and Coustan plasma glucose thresholds. Diabetes Care 2002; 25(9):1625–1630

152. Lo JC, Feigenbaum SL, Escobar GJ, Yang J, Crites YM, Ferrara A. Increased prevalence of gestational diabetes mellitus among women with diagnosed polycystic ovary syndrome: a population-based study. Diabetes Care 2006; 29(8):1915–1917

153. Pettitt DJ, Knowler WC, Baird HR, Bennett PH. Gestational diabetes: infant and maternal complications of pregnancy in relation to third-trimester glucose tolerance in the Pima Indians. Diabetes Care 1980; 3(3):458–464

154. Crowther CA, Hiller JE, Moss JR, McPhee AJ, Jeffries WS, Robinson JS. Effect of treatment of gestational diabetes mellitus on pregnancy outcomes. N Engl J Med 2005; 352(24):2477–2486

155. Henry OA, Beischer NA. Long-term implications of gestational diabetes for the mother. Baillieres Clin Obstet Gynaecol 1991; 5(2):461–483

156. Buchanan TA, Metzger BE, Freinkel N, Bergman RN. Insulin sensitivity and B-cell responsiveness to glucose during late pregnancy in lean and moderately obese women with normal glucose tolerance or mild gestational diabetes. Am J Obstet Gynecol 1990; 162(4):1008–1014

157. Paradisi G, Fulghesu AM, Ferrazzani S, Moretti S, Proto C, Soranna L et al. Endocrino-metabolic features in women with polycystic ovary syndrome during pregnancy. Hum Reprod 1998; 13(3):542–546

158. Holte J, Gennarelli G, Wide L, Lithell H, Berne C. High prevalence of polycystic ovaries and associated clinical, endocrine, and metabolic features in women with previous gestational diabetes mellitus. J Clin Endocrinol Metab 1998; 83(4):1143–1150

159. Anttila L, Karjala K, Penttila RA, Ruutiainen K, Ekblad U. Polycystic ovaries in women with gestational diabetes. Obstet Gynecol 1998; 92(1):13–16

160. Kousta E, Cela E, Lawrence N, Penny A, Millauer B, White D et al. The prevalence of polycystic ovaries in women with a history of gestational diabetes. Clin Endocrinol (Oxf) 2000; 53(4):501–507

161. Koivunen RM, Juutinen J, Vauhkonen I, Morin-Papunen LC, Ruokonen A, Tapanainen JS. Metabolic and steroidogenic alterations related to increased frequency of polycystic ovaries in women with a history of gestational diabetes. J Clin Endocrinol Metab 2001; 86(6):2591–2599

162. Urman B, Sarac E, Dogan L, Gurgan T. Pregnancy in infertile PCOD patients: complications and outcome. J Reprod Med 1997; 42(8):501–505

163. Radon PA, McMahon MJ, Meyer WR. Impaired glucose tolerance in pregnant women with polycystic ovary syndrome. Obstet Gynecol 1999; 94(2):194–197

164. Mikola M, Hiilesmaa V, Halttunen M, Suhonen L, Tiitinen A. Obstetric outcome in women with polycystic ovarian syndrome. Hum Reprod 2001; 16(2):226–229

165. Turhan NO, Seckin NC, Aybar F, Inegol I. Assessment of glucose tolerance and pregnancy outcome of polycystic ovary patients. Int J Gynaecol Obstet 2003; 81(2):163–168

166. Haakova L, Cibula D, Rezabek K, Hill M, Fanta M, Zivny J. Pregnancy outcome in women with PCOS and in controls matched by age and weight. Hum Reprod 2003; 18(7):1438–1441

167. Boomsma CM, Eijkemans MJ, Hughes EG, Visser GH, Fauser BC, Macklon NS. A meta-analysis of pregnancy outcomes in women with polycystic ovary syndrome. Hum Reprod Update 2006; 12(6):673–683

168. Ehrmann DA, Kasza K, Azziz R, Legro RS, Ghazzi MN. Effects of race and family history of type 2 diabetes on metabolic status of women with polycystic ovary syndrome. J Clin Endocrinol Metab 2005; 90(1):66–71

169. Glueck CJ, Bornovali S, Pranikoff J, Goldenberg N, Dharashivkar S, Wang P. Metformin, pre-eclampsia, and pregnancy outcomes in women with polycystic ovary syndrome. Diabet Med 2004; 21(8):829–836

170. Glueck CJ, Pranikoff J, Aregawi D, Wang P. Prevention of gestational diabetes by metformin plus diet in patients with polycystic ovary syndrome. Fertil Steril 2008; 89(3):625–634

171. Sibai BM. Diagnosis and management of gestational hypertension and preeclampsia. Obstet Gynecol 2003; 102(1):181–192

172. Hamasaki T, Yasuhi I, Hirai M, Masuzaki H, Ishimaru T. Hyperinsulinemia increases the risk of gestational hypertension. Int J Gynaecol Obstet 1996; 55(2):141–145

173. Laivuori H, Tikkanen MJ, Ylikorkala O. Hyperinsulinemia 17 years after preeclamptic first pregnancy. J Clin Endocrinol Metab 1996; 81(8):2908–2911

174. Solomon CG, Carroll JS, Okamura K, Graves SW, Seely EW. Higher cholesterol and insulin levels in pregnancy are associated with increased risk for pregnancy-induced hypertension. Am J Hypertens 1999; 12(3):276–282

175. Caruso A, Ferrazzani S, De Carolis S, Lucchese A, Lanzone A, De Santis L et al. Gestational hypertension but not pre-eclampsia is associated with insulin resistance syndrome characteristics. Hum Reprod 1999; 14(1):219–223

176. Fuh MM, Yin CS, Pei D, Sheu WH, Jeng CY, Chen YI et al. Resistance to insulin-mediated glucose uptake and hyperinsulinemia in women who had preeclampsia during pregnancy. Am J Hypertens 1995; 8(7):768–771

177. Nisell H, Erikssen C, Persson B, Carlstrom K. Is carbohydrate metabolism altered among women who have undergone a preeclamptic pregnancy? Gynecol Obstet Invest 1999; 48(4):241–246

178. He S, Silveira A, Hamsten A, Blomback M, Bremme K. Haemostatic, endothelial and lipoprotein parameters and blood pressure levels in women with a history of preeclampsia. Thromb Haemost 1999; 81(4):538–542

179. Kaaja R, Laivuori H, Laakso M, Tikkanen MJ, Ylikorkala O. Evidence of a state of increased insulin resistance in preeclampsia. Metabolism 1999; 48(7):892–896

180. Bartha JL, Romero-Carmona R, Torrejon-Cardoso R, Comino-Delgado R. Insulin, insulin-like growth factor-1, and insulin resistance in women with pregnancy-induced hypertension. Am J Obstet Gynecol 2002; 187(3):735–740

181. Conde-Agudelo A, Belizan JM. Risk factors for pre-eclampsia in a large cohort of Latin American and Caribbean women. BJOG 2000; 107(1):75–83

182. Jensen DM, Sorensen B, Feilberg-Jorgensen N, Westergaard JG, Beck-Nielsen H. Maternal and perinatal outcomes in 143 Danish women with gestational diabetes mellitus and 143 controls with a similar risk profile. Diabet Med 2000; 17(4):281–286

183. Joffe GM, Esterlitz JR, Levine RJ, Clemens JD, Ewell MG, Sibai BM et al. The relationship between abnormal glucose tolerance and hypertensive disorders of pregnancy in healthy nulliparous women. Calcium for Preeclampsia Prevention (CPEP) Study Group. Am J Obstet Gynecol 1998; 179(4):1032–1037

184. Suhonen L, Teramo K. Hypertension and pre-eclampsia in women with gestational glucose intolerance. Acta Obstet Gynecol Scand 1993; 72(4):269–272

185. Bryson CL, Ioannou GN, Rulyak SJ, Critchlow C. Association between gestational diabetes and pregnancy-induced hypertension. Am J Epidemiol 2003; 158(12):1148–1153

186. Diamant YZ, Rimon E, Evron S. High incidence of preeclamptic toxemia in patients with polycystic ovarian disease. Eur J Obstet Gynecol Reprod Biol 1982; 14(3):199–204

187. Gjonnaess H. The course and outcome of pregnancy after ovarian electrocautery in women with polycystic ovarian syndrome: the influence of body-weight. Br J Obstet Gynaecol 1989; 96(6):714–719

188. de Vries MJ, Dekker GA, Schoemaker J. Higher risk of preeclampsia in the polycystic ovary syndrome: a case control study. Eur J Obstet Gynecol Reprod Biol 1998; 76(1):91–95

189. Bjercke S, Dale PO, Tanbo T, Storeng R, Ertzeid G, Abyholm T. Impact of insulin resistance on pregnancy complications and outcome in women with polycystic ovary syndrome. Gynecol Obstet Invest 2002; 54(2):94–98

190. Kashyap S, Claman P. Polycystic ovary disease and the risk of pregnancy-induced hypertension. J Reprod Med 2000; 45(12):991–994

191. Fridstrom M, Nisell H, Sjoblom P, Hillensjo T. Are women with polycystic ovary syndrome at an increased risk of pregnancy-induced hypertension and/or preeclampsia? Hypertens Pregnancy 1999; 18(1):73–80

192. Hu S, Leonard A, Seifalian A, Hardiman P. Vascular dysfunction during pregnancy in women with polycystic ovary syndrome. Hum Reprod 2007; 22(6):1532–1539

193. Laivuori H, Kaaja R, Rutanen EM, Viinikka L, Ylikorkala O. Evidence of high circulating testosterone in women with prior preeclampsia. J Clin Endocrinol Metab 1998; 83(2):344–347

194. Wakasugi M, Noguchi T, Kazama YI, Kanemaru Y, Onaya T. The effects of sex hormones on the synthesis of prostacyclin (PGI2) by vascular tissues. Prostaglandins 1989; 37(4):401–410

195. Paradisi G, Biaggi A, Savone R, Ianniello F, Tomei C, Caforio L et al. Cardiovascular risk factors in healthy women with previous gestational hypertension. J Clin Endocrinol Metab 2006; 91(4):1233–1238

196. Sibai BM, el Nazer A, Gonzalez-Ruiz A. Severe preeclampsia-eclampsia in young primigravid women: subsequent pregnancy outcome and remote prognosis. Am J Obstet Gynecol 1986; 155(5):1011–1016

197. Smith GC, Pell JP, Walsh D. Pregnancy complications and maternal risk of ischaemic heart disease: a retrospective cohort study of 129,290 births. Lancet 2001; 357(9273):2002–2006

198. Irgens HU, Reisaeter L, Irgens M, Lie RT. Long term mortality of mothers and fathers after pre-eclampsia: population based cohort study. BMJ 2001; 323(7323):1213–1217

11

The Effect of Pregnancy on Energy Metabolism, Body Composition, and Endothelial Function

Dilys J. Freeman and Naveed Sattar

CONTENTS

ABSTRACT

Maternal adaptations in energy metabolism are required to respond to the additional energy demands of pregnancy, and these adaptations are influenced by the degree of maternal obesity. Glucose intolerance does not influence the adaptation of maternal energy metabolism to pregnancy. Pregnancy is associated with increased maternal insulin resistance, which is further increased in obese and glucose-intolerant mothers. Endothelial function is improved in pregnancy but to a lesser extent in obese and glucose-intolerant mothers. While these changes in maternal metabolism and physiology in response to pregnancy have been described, the timing and the resulting impact on the quality of circulating maternal metabolites are poorly understood. An appreciation of the detail of these processes is important in order to inform our understanding of how obesity and glucose intolerance may contribute to adverse pregnancy outcome and to allow the development of sensible, evidence-based prevention strategies.

Key words: Metabolism; Obesity; Glucose intolerance; Insulin resistance; Endothelium.

From: *Diabetes in Women: Pathophysiology and Therapy*
Edited by: A. Tsatsoulis et al. (eds.), DOI 10.1007/978-1-60327-250-6_11
© Humana Press, a part of Springer Science+Business Media, LLC 2009

INTRODUCTION

In pregnancy, there are important adaptations to maternal metabolism in order to support the growing fetus. Energy is required to support the increase in metabolically active tissue including placenta, mammary gland, uterus, increased maternal blood volume, and the fetus. Compared with other mammalian species the daily energy needs of a human pregnancy are very small because the cost is spread over a long gestation [reviewed in (1)]. This means that metabolic or behavioral adjustments to energy usage can contribute to energy economy during pregnancy. However, because of the length of gestation, total energy costs are high in comparison to other mammals. Many of the changes in maternal metabolism reflect the requirement for the mother to provide sufficient energy and essential nutrients to her growing fetus. There is increased fat deposition in pregnancy to provide a source of energy for maintaining the fetus (2), and these maternal fat depots can buffer short- or medium-term changes in energy supply. Maintenance of a supply of glucose, which is transferred across the placenta by facilitated diffusion (3), and of essential and nonessential fatty acids, which are transferred across the placenta via specific binding proteins (4), is achieved by maternal insulin resistance and gestational hyperlipidemia. Increased vasodilatation occurs to accommodate the changed circulatory requirements. In situations where the maternal metabolic response to pregnancy is exaggerated or abnormal, such as in obesity or glucose intolerance, the metabolic dysregulation could, in some women, impact negatively on vascular function, and optimal nutrient supply to the fetus may be compromised.

ENERGY METABOLISM IN PREGNANCY

The Energy Cost of Pregnancy

The energy costs of supporting a pregnancy have been estimated (5) as 20 MJ deposited as new tissue, 150 MJ deposited as fat, and 150 MJ to maintain the new tissue. However, the average increase in energy intake during pregnancy of 0.3 MJ/day (1) is apparently insufficient to support this energy cost. Attempts to directly measure the energy costs of pregnancy have indicated that there is a huge interindividual variability (6). A large retrospective analysis of 360 pregnancies from ten studies incorporating a wide range of geographical and nutritional settings (6) showed that maintenance energy costs (cumulative change in basal metabolic rate) ranged from −45 to 210 MJ, energy deposition as fat ranged from −23 to 267 MJ, and total energy costs (the sum of maintenance costs, energy deposited as fat, and energy content of the conceptus) ranged from −20 to 523 MJ. Energy expenditure during pregnancy is contributed to by basal metabolic rate (BMR), thermogenesis, and maternal physical activity. Changes in energy expenditure, particularly BMR, which represents 70–80% of total daily energy expenditure in sedentary women (7), might partly explain the mismatch between the total energy cost of pregnancy and increase in energy intake (8).

Basal Metabolic Rate in Pregnancy

The large differences in calculated energy costs of pregnancy between studies can be attributed to a high level of intrapopulation variability (9) and also to the level of affluence of the country from which the population was selected (6). Women from affluent, developed countries showed a rapid early increase in BMR in response to pregnancy (1). In contrast, women from less affluent countries either show a delayed increase in BMR, or in some there is an initial rapid fall in BMR during the first weeks of pregnancy (10). Total energy costs of pregnancy also varied according to the affluence of the population with the least nourished population showing a net reduction in BMR, fat loss rather than accumulation, and a resulting negative total energy cost (6). Birth weight was lowest in the least affluent population but was highest when expressed as a proportion of the maternal weight gain during pregnancy resulting in a fairly constant birth weight/maternal weight ratio across populations.

If mothers from the least affluent population had dietary energy supplements they had a reduced initial fall in BMR and increased fat deposition (10). These studies demonstrate that poorly nourished women become less active in order to achieve a saving in energy expenditure during pregnancy. Many groups studying well-nourished populations show around a 30% increase in basal energy expenditure expressed as both basal oxygen consumption (VO_2) and kcal/day from prepregnancy to late gestation (11), and this increase in BMR is suggested to be the biggest contributor to the total energy cost of pregnancy (12). Reducing energy expenditure due to physical activity in later pregnancy (13) has been observed and may help compensate for the energy gap in well-nourished populations. Early studies indicated that there is reduced diet-induced thermogenesis in the second (14) and the third trimester of pregnancy (15), although the physiological relevance of the size of the effect has been questioned (16). This physiological adaptation could also reduce the gap between the total energy cost of pregnancy and the energy intake. However, it is clear that increased energy intake during pregnancy is required (17).

The Impact of Maternal Obesity on the Energy Cost of Pregnancy

The total energy cost of pregnancy is positively associated with prepregnancy fat mass, % body fat, and pregnancy weight gain (6), but maintenance costs are only associated with prepregnancy fatness. This might be explained by the fact that prepregnancy fatness is a marker of overall nutritional status or that prepregnancy fatness may indicate a positive energy balance before conception, and this energy balance might be maintained throughout pregnancy. Either mechanism would explain the wide variability in metabolic response to pregnancy and serve to match energy requirements to energy availability, hence optimizing fetal growth. Leptin has been suggested to be the signal that may link prepregnancy fatness with the maternal metabolic response to pregnancy (5).

Butte et al. (13) compared energy metabolism in women with a low, normal, and high body mass index (BMI). The increase in BMR during pregnancy was highest in a high BMI (≥ 26 kg/m^2) group at 16.3 (5.4) kcal/week compared with a normal BMI (19.8–26.0 kg/m^2) group at 9.5 (4.6) kcal/week and a low BMI (≤ 19.8 kg/m^2) group at 8.8 (4.5) kcal/week (13). Increments in BMR and 24-h energy expenditure were correlated with change in weight and fat-free mass but also with prepregnancy BMI or percentage fat (13). The change in BMR at 24 weeks gestation was significantly correlated with maternal obesity prior to pregnancy. Women who were lean prepregnancy were more likely to attenuate the increase in BMR in order to spare energy, whereas obese women had larger increases in BMR in response to energy excess (8).

The Energy Cost of Pregnancy in Gestational Diabetes Mellitus

In common with others, Okereke et al. (11) observed an increase in BMR from the prepregnant state to late pregnancy in obese women with normal glucose tolerance (NGT) and obese women with gestational diabetes mellitus (GDM). There were no significant differences in basal energy expenditure between NGT and GDM obese women (11). Obese GDM women had total energy expenditure similar to that of obese NGT women (11). Similar observations were made for lean GDM and NGT women (18). GDM women had oxygen consumption, CO_2 production, total energy expenditure, and BMR similar to that of controls after correction for higher body mass (19). It is, therefore, suggested that the adaptations of energy metabolism to pregnancy are not influenced by glucose intolerance. This is possibly due to the placental production of hormones overriding any localized influence of maternal metabolic abnormalities (11).

BODY COMPOSITION

Gestational weight gain ranges from 10 to 30% of prepregnancy weight *(5)*. Amongst women with good pregnancy outcome the total weight gain and pattern of weight gain during pregnancy were highly variable *(20)*. Some have observed that changes in body fat are not correlated with changes in body weight during pregnancy *(21)*. Others, however, have observed that the correlation between BMI and percent body fat is maintained throughout pregnancy, although there is a wide range in the 95% confidence interval for predicting percent body fat from mean BMI *(22)*.

Assessment of Body Composition in Pregnancy

Body composition measurements are difficult during pregnancy because of the disproportionate amount of water accumulating in the fat-free mass component during pregnancy *(23)*. A large longitudinal study of 170 women during pregnancy using bioimpedance analysis indicated that total body water and extracellular water were significantly increased during the second and third trimesters of pregnancy *(24)*. These researchers also found a small increase in intracellular water, which peaked in the third trimester. These changes are due to the enlargement of the vascular bed that occurs in pregnancy and the subsequent increase in blood volume *(24)*. Standard methods of assessing body composition such as bioelectrical impedance and hydrostatic weighing may be influenced by these pregnancy-related changes in hydration *(25)*. Thus, it is not possible to use models or equations for estimation of fat mass that have been derived in the nonpregnant population and then apply them to studies of body composition in pregnancy *(26)*. Specific equations validated in pregnancy should be applied. A number of methods and models for determining maternal body composition are available [reviewed in *(27)*], but it is clear that the means of accurately assessing maternal body composition are cumbersome and often impractical [skinfold thickness, dual-energy X-ray absorptiometry (DEXA), computed tomography (CT), magnetic resonance imaging (MRI), or ultrasound].

Weight Gain in Pregnancy

Very similar mean increases in body weight of around 12 kg have been observed by a number of groups *(9, 23, 28)*. Prentice and Goldberg *(5)* observed that women from poorer countries have a lower percentage weight gain and have a wide variation in absolute weight gain (0–23 kg in women of moderate nutritional status). Women who gain weight prior to 20 weeks gestation were more likely to retain this weight postpartum than women who gained weight after 20 weeks when fetal growth rate is higher *(29)*.

Changes in Body Composition Associated with Pregnancy

Bioimpedance analysis in a large cohort of women indicated an increase in fat mass during pregnancy, but the investigators did not quantify it due to the inaccuracy of bioimpedance analysis in estimating fat mass *(24)*. Those studies where fat mass accumulation has been quantified using a variety of methods show a wide variation in the accumulation of fat during pregnancy of between 0 and >5 kg *(5, 9–11, 23, 30–32)*. Studies following women from preconception until 15 weeks gestation observed that body fat had accumulated by the seventh week of gestation *(33)*. Some studies indicate that the increase in maternal fat mass is complete by the end of the second trimester *(23, 34)* with a decline thereafter. Skinfold thickness, but not fat cell diameter correlated with these changes *(34)*. Other studies indicate that most of the fat mass is deposited between 13 and 35 weeks of gestation *(11)*. It has been suggested that during the third trimester, the fetus may require such a large proportion of energy that women do not deposit any additional fat *(23)*. Fat gain during pregnancy may be required to provide sufficient energy for subsequent lactation, and women who have less than optimal energy intake during pregnancy cannot maintain bodyweight during lactation *(35)*.

Baseline energy intake and change in energy intake during pregnancy were not correlated with the gestational fat gain during pregnancy. Prepregnancy weight, fat mass, and fat-free mass also did not predict the amount of fat deposited. There was some evidence that women with higher resting metabolic rates prepregnancy gained more fat *(5, 23)*.

Location of Fat Deposition in Pregnancy

The location of fat deposition, visceral or subcutaneous, is important because of regional variation in adipocyte metabolism. However, this has not yet been fully explored in pregnancy. It has been observed that in pregnancy fat accumulates predominantly in the central compartment *(36)*. A study using ultrasound to differentiate abdominal visceral fat (the preperitoneal fat layer) and subcutaneous fat showed that intra-abdominal visceral fat accumulation increases during pregnancy resulting in a change in regional fat distribution *(37)*. However, a magnetic resonance imaging (MRI) study *(32)* found the majority of additional adipose volume (76%) to be placed subcutaneously predominantly in the trunk (68%) and thighs (16%). Obviously further work is required to resolve these discrepancies. The location of fat deposition is important, as there is some evidence that centrally deposited fat is associated with glucose intolerance/gestational diabetes mellitus *(38)* and gestational hypertension/preeclampsia *(39, 40)*. Furthermore, Bartha et al. *(41)* observed that first trimester (11–14 weeks of gestation) visceral fat thickness correlated better than BMI with metabolic risk factors such as blood pressure, insulin sensitivity, and plasma lipids.

Although pregnancy influences the site of fat deposition, it does not affect the functionality of the regional adipose tissue *(42)*. In early pregnancy, basal lipolysis tends to be higher in femoral rather than abdominal fat, similar to the nonpregnant situation *(43)*. Consistently for pregnant and nonpregnant women, there is higher lipoprotein lipase activity and lower norepinephrine-stimulated lipolysis in femoral fat than in abdominal fat, and there are similar rates of fatty acid esterification and acylglyceride synthesis between pregnant and nonpregnant women *(42, 43)*.

Fat Deposition in Obese Pregnancy

Lean women gained more percent body fat than obese women *(36)* but gained similar amounts of fat mass. Butte et al. *(13)* found that fat deposition differed between BMI groups with 5.3 kg fat deposited in women with low BMI ($\leq$19.8 kg/m^2), 4.6 kg in women with normal BMI (19.8–26.0 kg/m^2), and 8.4 kg in women with high BMI ($\geq$26 kg/m^2). A greater gain in percentage fat, absolute fat mass, and absolute lean body mass was also seen during pregnancy in adolescents than in mature women *(44)*. Using skinfold thickness measurements it was observed that lean women gained most of their adipose tissue peripherally, whereas obese women did not *(36)*.

Gestational Diabetes Mellitus and Fat Deposition

Lean women with abnormal glucose tolerance before pregnancy had a smaller increase in fat mass (1.3 kg, $P = 0.04$) than lean women with NGT *(18)*. Change in fat mass was inversely associated with change in insulin sensitivity *(18)*. There is an increase in fat mass from the prepregnant state to late pregnancy in both obese NGT and GDM women, but there was no difference between NGT and GDM women in the amount of fat accumulated *(11)*. A wide range of fat mass and fat-free mass gain was observed *(11)*.

The distribution of accumulated fat throughout pregnancy was similar for glucose tolerance and GDM women using skinfold thickness *(36)*.

INSULIN RESISTANCE IN PREGNANCY

An early gestation (weeks 6–10) decrease in maternal fasting glucose of 2 mg/dL has been observed with little further decrease by the third trimester *(45)*. Since the decline occurs before fetal utilization can contribute, this suggests that maternal metabolic and hormonal factors may alter plasma glucose concentration independently of fetal glucose utilization. Late pregnancy is associated with more than 50% decrease in peripheral insulin sensitivity assessed by euglycemic hyperinsulinemic clamp tests *(46)*. There was also a significant 3–3.5-fold increase in insulin release in response to an intravenous glucose tolerance test *(46)*. Furthermore, in this same group of women it was shown that there was a 30% increase in basal endogenous glucose production independent of fat-free mass despite a 65% increase in fasting insulin concentrations by late gestation *(47)*. The endogenous glucose production was still sensitive to suppression by insulin infusion. These findings have been confirmed in a much larger study (*n* = 298) in late pregnancy using oral glucose tolerance tests *(48)*. Glucose tolerance was significantly impaired, and insulin resistance increased at 32 weeks, gestation compared to 17 weeks, gestation. Data from euglycemic hyperinsulinemic clamp tests carried out prior to pregnancy and at around 13 and 35 weeks of gestation *(49)* demonstrated a 65% increase in both basal insulin and C-peptide with advancing gestation, and the metabolic clearance of insulin increased significantly. These changes in insulin kinetics may partly explain the hyperinsulinemia of pregnancy and may be a physiological response to the insulin resistance of pregnancy. Changes in insulin sensitivity related to later pregnancy are primarily at the peripheral level and secondarily at the hepatic level *(50)*. It has been suggested that the elevated levels of nonesterified free fatty acids in later pregnancy contribute to the peripheral insulin resistance *(51, 52)*.

Pancreatic islet cells make adaptations to pregnancy [reviewed in *(53)*] under the control of placental lactogens and prolactin *(54, 55)*. These adaptations include lowering the threshold for glucose-stimulated insulin secretion as well as enhanced insulin secretion at high glucose levels *(53)*. The former allows the beta cells to release significantly more insulin at low blood glucose concentrations, resulting in an altered set point for insulin secretion and action during late pregnancy. PPARα is a potentially important regulator of the islet response to pregnancy where there is modified lipid handling to conserve glucose *(56)*.

Insulin Resistance in Obese Pregnancy

The extent of the decline in fasting glucose in early gestation was less with increasing maternal BMI, and there was no reduction in severely obese women *(45)*. In the third trimester of pregnancy obese women demonstrated both peripheral and hepatic insulin resistance manifest as reduced insulin-mediated glucose disposal, a large reduction in insulin-stimulated carbohydrate oxidation, and a reduction in insulin suppression of endogenous glucose production, which was reversed in the postpartum period *(57)*. Obese women show lower insulin sensitivity during pregnancy than the control group in both small longitudinal *(58)* and larger cross-sectional studies *(59)*. In lean women there is an inverse correlation between changes in insulin sensitivity and fat mass in early gestation *(18)*. In contrast, in obese women, there is no inverse correlation between changes in insulin sensitivity and fat mass in early gestation *(11)*. There was, however, a negative relationship between decrease in insulin sensitivity and accretion of fat mass from prepregnancy to late gestation. In obese subjects there was actually an increase in insulin sensitivity from prepregnancy to early gestation *(11)*.

Insulin Resistance in Glucose Intolerance and GDM Pregnancy

Abnormal glucose tolerance did not alter the insulin kinetics observed in healthy pregnancy *(49)*. In GDM, prepregnancy and early gestational insulin sensitivity are lower than in healthy controls. In the last trimester of pregnancy some groups find that insulin resistance is at the same level in control and GDM women *(60)*, whereas others find a significantly lower third trimester insulin sensitivity index in GDM *(61)*. Insulin sensitivity declines in both control and GDM women during pregnancy but the control women have higher insulin sensitivity at baseline. Women with NGT appear to have a greater flexibility to switch between insulin sensitivity in the nonpregnant state to insulin resistance in late pregnancy, whereas GDM women start from a position of compromised insulin sensitivity in the nonpregnant state. Both obese NGT and GDM women had an increase in endogenous glucose production during pregnancy *(11)*. Thus, although there are marked changes in insulin sensitivity within an individual during pregnancy these changes are relatively uniform in NGT. In women with GDM, there is generally lower insulin sensitivity than in control women throughout pregnancy but there is some discrepancy as to whether third trimester values are lower than or equivalent to those in control pregnancies. Perhaps the placental production of hormones helps to override the preexisting controls on insulin sensitivity during pregnancy.

LIPID METABOLISM IN PREGNANCY

There is no change in either basal carbohydrate oxidation or nonoxidizable carbohydrate metabolism but there is a significant 50–80% increase in fat oxidation during pregnancy both in the basal state and also during an euglycemic hyperinsulinemic clamp *(11)*. These data underline the importance of the switch from carbohydrate to fat metabolism in pregnancy that is potentially regulated by placenta-produced leptin. During fasting, pregnancy is a state of accelerated starvation with increased maternal reliance on lipids rather than on carbohydrate for energy demands *(62)*. These maternal responses to pregnancy have the result of sparing carbohydrates and amino acids for the fetus. Decreased PPARγ expression, and hence signaling through its target genes, has been suggested to be the mechanism by which fat catabolism is enabled *(63)*.

Lipid Changes in Normal Pregnancy

Pregnancy is marked by hyperlipidemia *(64, 65)*. There is a hypertriglyceridemia with very low density lipoprotein (VLDL) triglyceride concentrations increasing threefold from 14 weeks, gestation *(66)* to term. Postheparin hepatic lipase and lipoprotein lipase activities are decreased from the first and third trimesters, respectively *(64)*. The increase in plasma triglyceride concentration results in the appearance of small dense low density lipoprotein (LDL) particles in late pregnancy *(67)*. Plasma cholesterol levels rise to a lesser degree due to an early decrease in LDL followed by a modest continuous rise in high density lipoprotein (HDL) (particularly the HDL-2 subfraction) by over 40% after 14 weeks, gestation *(66)*. A fall in plasma HDL after the end of the second trimester has been observed by some researchers *(68)*. These changes in lipoprotein concentrations are associated with the progressive increases in the levels of the major pregnancy hormones estradiol, progesterone, and human placental lactogen, which may regulate their metabolism *(64, 68)*. For example, estrogens are known to enhance VLDL production and decrease hepatic lipase activity and may play a key role in the accumulation of triglycerides in lipoproteins of higher density than VLDL *(69)*. Resistance to the insulin-mediated suppression of lipolysis may also contribute to the hyperlipidemia *(70)*.

Lipid Changes in Obesity

Obese women demonstrated similar increases in fat oxidation, in the absence of changes to carbohydrate metabolism, to those observed in lean individuals *(11)*. In obese NGT and GDM women there was an inverse correlation between endogenous glucose production and fat oxidation from prepregnancy to early gestation *(11)*. Triglyceride oxidation, as assessed by recovery of exogenous ^{13}C Hiolein (a biosynthetic triglyceride) as exhaled $^{13}CO_2$ *(19)*, was significantly lower in GDM independent of obesity. The authors proposed that this could be due to decreased plasma triglyceride lipolysis, reduced nonesterified free fatty acid uptake and oxidation, or increased hepatic oxidation and esterification of nonesterified fatty acids to provide for increased gluconeogenesis and VLDL synthesis.

Maternal obesity is associated with increased total and VLDL triglycerides *(59, 71)*. Reduced levels of plasma HDL but similar levels of LDL were also observed *(59)*. A correlation between maternal BMI and susceptibility of LDL to become oxidized has been observed *(72)*. The pattern of dyslipidemia observed in obese pregnancy is similar therefore to those observed in nonpregnant obese individuals *(73)*.

Lipid Changes in Diabetes and GDM

Compared with healthy pregnancy, in pregnancy complicated by type 1 diabetes (DM1) some observers, using small sample sizes (<15), have found similar levels of plasma lipids including plasma triglyceride and HDL cholesterol levels *(74, 75)*. However, a large longitudinal case (n = 312) control (n = 356) comparison found a significantly lower plasma cholesterol throughout pregnancy and a significantly lower plasma triglyceride by the end of the third trimester in women with DM1 *(76)*. A more detailed investigation of the reduction in plasma cholesterol found that the lower total cholesterol in pregnancy complicated by DM1 was due to lower HDL, specifically the HDL-3 subfraction *(77)*. The main apolipoproteins (apo) associated with HDL, apoAI and apoAII, were also lower in DM1. Nonesterified fatty acids were lower in mothers with DM1 than in controls *(75)*. In GDM there was a higher total triglyceride and an increased triglyceride content of the lipoproteins (particularly VLDL and HDL) and elevated total cholesterol levels *(72, 78)*. Higher plasma triglyceride levels than control women were also observed in pregnant women with type 2 diabetes (DM2) throughout pregnancy *(79)*. Healthy control women showed a pattern whereby they have low plasma triglyceride levels in early pregnancy, which have been increased by later pregnancy demonstrating flexibility in their metabolic response to pregnancy. Women with GDM in contrast enter pregnancy with elevated plasma triglyceride levels, which have already reached maximal levels by the second trimester of pregnancy *(79)*. Women with GDM were found to have reduced insulin receptor substrate (IRS)-1 protein levels, which may contribute to a reduced insulin suppression of lipolysis *(63)*. In women with GDM, LDL had a greater susceptibility to oxidation *(72)*.

ENDOTHELIAL FUNCTION

Background

The vascular endothelium plays a key role in the maintenance of normal vascular function and is involved in the control of inflammation, vessel tone, flow dynamics, permeability, thrombosis, and platelet aggregation. Disturbances in its function have been associated with development of conditions including preeclampsia and atherosclerosis. Endothelial function can be assessed in a number of ways including venous occlusion plethysmography, brachial artery flow-mediated dilatation, iontophoresis with Laser Doppler imaging, and pulse wave analysis [recently reviewed in *(80)*]. Circulating levels of plasma markers of endothelial activation, such as soluble intercellular adhesion molecule 1 (sICAM 1), are often used as an indirect assessment of endothelial function. Unfortunately, these methods assess different vascular beds, and it is difficult to directly compare endothelial function assessed by different methods.

Change in Normal Pregnancy

Endothelial function improves progressively throughout pregnancy. This has been demonstrated most commonly using flow-mediated dilatation *(81–85)*. A late third trimester fall in flow-mediated dilatation has been observed after 30 weeks, gestation *(83, 85)* and after gestation of 36 plus weeks *(84)*. Assessment of endothelial function by pulse wave velocity (PWV) captures both physical and physiological aspects of vessel function. Aortic stiffness (i.e., PWV) was decreased from the first trimester and remained low throughout pregnancy *(86, 87)*. In a longitudinal study of a large population ($n = 167$) of healthy pregnant women it was observed that PWV significantly decreased between the first and second trimester. Thereafter, PWV began to increase slowly, eventually surpassing first trimester levels by delivery *(88)*. Similar data were obtained from a recent large cross-sectional study ($n = 193$) demonstrating a decrease in augmentation index (AIx) by the first trimester, reaching its lowest point mid-pregnancy and rising thereafter until term *(89)*, although this latter study noted no differences in PWV. Interestingly, these changes in stiffness somewhat parallel changes in blood pressure with an early fall to a nadir in mid-pregnancy before a rise back toward baseline levels in later pregnancy *(90)*.

Changes in Plasma Markers

Plasma markers of endothelial activation such as sICAM-1, soluble vascular cell adhesion molecule (sVCAM-1), and von Willebrand Factor (vWF) have been shown to increase longitudinally throughout pregnancy, reaching a peak in the third trimester of pregnancy *(91)*, although others have only observed a mild increase in endothelial activation markers in healthy pregnancy *(92)*. However, since pregnancy is associated with an inflammatory response, the pregnancy-related changes in adhesion molecules in particular may better reflect inflammation pathways than changes in vascular function.

Changes in Endothelial Function in Obese Pregnancy

None of the earlier studies considered obesity as a variable. However, a comparison of lean and obese women in the third trimester of pregnancy indicated that obese women had reduced endothelium-dependent and endothelium-independent microvascular function, as assessed by laser Doppler imaging with iontophoresis *(59)*. In the latter study, plasma C-reactive protein and fasting insulin were inversely correlated with endothelium-dependent microvascular function. More recent data using longitudinal assessment of microvascular function have shown that although lean and obese women show the same pattern of change in endothelial function throughout pregnancy, both endothelium-dependent and endothelium-independent vasodilation were significantly lower in obese women *(91)*.

Potential Mechanisms for Vascular Function Changes in Pregnancy

Investigations into the potential mechanisms for the vascular function changes during pregnancy are very few. Clearly, early circulating hormonal changes and a rise in HDL-cholesterol in the first half of pregnancy may beneficially influence vascular function at this stage. Beyond this, a recent study was unable to provide evidence that the increase in flow-mediated dilatation observed in pregnancy was related to changes in asymmetric dimethylarginine (ADMA) or L-arginine concentrations *(93)*. Flow-mediated dilatation in the third trimester of pregnancy was negatively correlated with the glucose response to a 100-g oral glucose load *(94)*. A positive relationship between flow-mediated dilatation and plasma triglyceride levels in multivariate analysis has also been observed *(95)*. This indicates that improvements in endothelial function can occur in the presence of hypertriglyceridemia. In a multivariate analysis of lean and obese pregnant women *(91)*, reduced endothelium-dependent vasodilation was associated with increased inflammatory cytokines such as interleukin 6 – data that are consistent with the suggestion that the endothelial dysfunction of preeclampsia is a result of an uncontrolled maternal inflammatory response *(96, 97)*. The links between insulin resistance, glycemia, inflammation, and endothelial function observed in pregnancy are consistent with the current understanding of the mechanism of endothelial dysfunction in nonpregnant women *(98)*.

Endothelial Function in Diabetic Pregnancy

Despite no difference in circulating levels of plasma markers of endothelial activation in pregnant women with DM1 *(99)*, pregnant women with DM1 have higher aortic stiffness during pregnancy than healthy control pregnant women *(100)*. Others confirmed that mothers with DM1 had impaired flow-mediated dilatation of the brachial artery during pregnancy and that the degree of impairment was associated with the duration of diabetes but not with levels of glycosylated hemoglobin *(101)*. A study of microvascular function in type 1 diabetic pregnant women showed that these women had impaired endothelium-dependent and -independent microvascular response compared with healthy pregnant women *(102)*, and this difference was attenuated by correcting for the degree of hyperglycemia. However, Ang et al. *(103)*, using a *ex vivo* wire myography model did not find any differences in subcutaneous fat artery endothelial or smooth muscle function between well-controlled pregnant women with DM1 and healthy pregnant controls. A higher plasma total nitrate/nitrite concentration was observed in pregnant women with type 1 diabetes than in pregnant controls suggesting that abnormalities in insulin-induced nitric oxide release might contribute to the vascular dysfunction observed in pregnancy complicated with DM1 *(104)*. Brachial artery flow-mediated dilatation was significantly lower in pregnant women with impaired glucose tolerance and with GDM than in pregnant healthy controls *(94)*. The degree of endothelial dysfunction was correlated to the level of glycemia.

SUMMARY

The energy costs of pregnancy show wide interindividual variation, but the measured energy intake during pregnancy does not account for the calculated increased energy requirements of pregnancy. It is likely that the mother makes adaptations in energy expenditure in response to pregnancy. The degree of obesity prior to pregnancy influences the maternal metabolic response to pregnancy possibly via a leptin-mediated mechanism. Glucose intolerance does not influence the adaptation of maternal energy metabolism to pregnancy. The large variability in energy costs makes compilation of guidelines for recommended energy intake during pregnancy very difficult *(16)*. Fat gain during pregnancy is highly variable, and there is neither consensus regarding the timing of fat deposition nor regarding whether it is accumulated in subcutaneous or visceral depots. Adipose tissue function *per se* is unaffected by pregnancy. There is no strong evidence that obese or glucose-intolerant pregnant women accumulate significantly more absolute amounts of fat than lean pregnant women.

Pregnancy is associated with increased maternal insulin resistance, which is further increased in obese and glucose-intolerant women. In pregnancy maternal fat metabolism is of increasing importance as gestation advances in order to spare carbohydrate for the fetus. The gestational hyperlipidemia is exaggerated in obese and glucose-intolerant pregnant women leading to the production of potentially harmful lipid fractions such as oxidized LDL. Endothelial function is improved in pregnancy but to a lesser extent in obese and glucose-intolerant mothers. The reduced endothelial function in obese and glucose-intolerant pregnant women may be linked to insulin resistance via inflammation and impaired nitric oxide production.

There are three aspects to the metabolic changes in pregnancy that are of relevance to their impact on endothelial function and adverse pregnancy outcomes. The first aspect is the absolute levels of change in metabolic parameters such as insulin sensitivity or plasma triglycerides, and these changes have been mostly described as outlined in this chapter. Second, there is the timing of these changes. It appears that in IGT, and perhaps also in obese pregnancy, women start from a baseline of greater insulin resistance and hypertriglyceridemia and reach a peak level in the second trimester rather than the third trimester as control women do. In other words, obese and IGT women are less flexible in their metabolic response to pregnancy, and the total exposure to adverse metabolic conditions is greater (Fig. 1). This aspect of metabolic change has attracted much less attention and is not yet fully described. The third aspect of the metabolic change in pregnancy is the quality of the metabolites to which the woman is exposed. For example, a description of the total levels of plasma lipids does not investigate whether the composition of these lipids is comparable between obese and IGT women on the one hand and in healthy women on the other. It is possible that there are higher levels of oxidized LDL, oxidized fatty acids, and less beneficial long-chain polyunsaturated fatty acids. This adverse metabolic environment may provoke or exacerbate the increased insulin resistance and impaired endothelial function observed in obese and IGT pregnancy. Much more research is required in this arena.

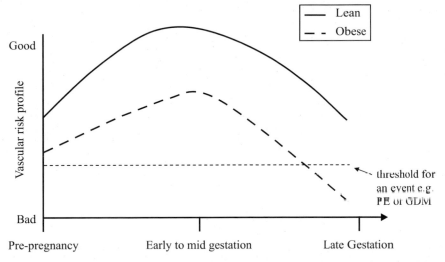

Fig. 1. Proposed model of vascular risk changes during pregnancy in lean and obese women. In lean women there is an initial general improvement in vascular risk profile in response to early pregnancy (i.e., increased endothelium-dependent function, increased HDL-cholesterol, and reduction in blood pressure), with many changes driven by early pregnancy-related hormonal changes. However, as pregnancy proceeds toward third trimester, metabolic and vascular stresses increase such that many of the early favorable changes start to reverse or attenuate back toward nonpregnant levels. In obese women, prepregnancy metabolic risk profile is less than optimal, and obese women may show either an attenuated initial improvement in metabolic response to pregnancy and/or a lower maximal improvement, such that in some women the increasing metabolic and vascular stresses in the second half of pregnancy vastly exceed early benefits or acquired buffering capacity. As a result, more overweight or obese women are at increased risk of developing gestational diabetes mellitus (GDM) or preeclampsia (PE).

Clearly there are many unanswered questions regarding changes in energy metabolism in healthy pregnancy and how these changes are influenced by maternal obesity and maternal diabetes. Maternal obesity is on the increase *(105, 106)*, and in the future clinicians will find increasing numbers of women of reproductive age presenting at antenatal clinics with type 2 diabetes. Both obesity and diabetes are associated with adverse pregnancy outcomes *(106, 107)*. It is imperative to understand how changes in maternal metabolism brought about by these conditions may contribute to the etiology of adverse pregnancy outcomes in order to inform sensible, evidence-based prevention strategies in pregnancy, perhaps via lifestyle measures *(106, 107)*.

REFERENCES

1. Prentice AM, Poppitt SD, Goldberg GR, Prentice A. Adaptive strategies regulating energy balance in human pregnancy. Hum Reprod Update 1995; 1(2):149–161.
2. Sparks JW, Girard JR, Battaglia FC. An estimate of the caloric requirements of the human fetus. Biol Neonate 1980; 38(3–4):113–119.
3. Baumann MU, Deborde S, Illsley NP. Placental glucose transfer and fetal growth. Endocrine 2002; 19(1):13–22.
4. Haggarty P. Placental regulation of fatty acid delivery and its effect on fetal growth – a review. Placenta 2002; 23(Suppl A):S28–S38.
5. Prentice AM, Goldberg GR. Energy adaptations in human pregnancy: limits and long-term consequences. Am J Clin Nutr 2000; 71(5 Suppl):1226S–1232S.
6. Poppitt SD, Prentice AM, Goldberg GR, Whitehead RG. Energy-sparing strategies to protect human fetal growth. Am J Obstet Gynecol 1994; 171(1):118 125.
7. Prentice AM, Coward WA, Davies HL, Murgatroyd PR, Black AE, Goldberg GR et al. Unexpectedly low levels of energy expenditure in healthy women. Lancet 1985; 1(8443):1419–1422.
8. Prentice AM, Goldberg GR, Davies HL, Murgatroyd PR, Scott W. Energy-sparing adaptations in human pregnancy assessed by whole-body calorimetry. Br J Nutr 1989; 62(1):5–22.
9. Goldberg GR, Prentice AM, Coward WA, Davies HL, Murgatroyd PR, Wensing C et al. Longitudinal assessment of energy expenditure in pregnancy by the doubly labeled water method. Am J Clin Nutr 1993; 57(4):494–505.
10. Lawrence M, Lawrence F, Coward WA, Cole TJ, Whitehead RG. Energy requirements of pregnancy in The Gambia. Lancet 1987; 2(8567):1072–1076.
11. Okereke NC, Huston-Presley L, Amini SB, Kalhan S, Catalano PM. Longitudinal changes in energy expenditure and body composition in obese women with normal and impaired glucose tolerance. Am J Physiol Endocrinol Metab 2004; 287(3):E472–E479.
12. Lof M, Olausson H, Bostrom K, Janerot-Sjoberg B, Sohlstrom A, Forsum E. Changes in basal metabolic rate during pregnancy in relation to changes in body weight and composition, cardiac output, insulin-like growth factor I, and thyroid hormones and in relation to fetal growth. Am J Clin Nutr 2005; 81(3):678–685.
13. Butte NF, Wong WW, Treuth MS, Ellis KJ, O'Brian SE. Energy requirements during pregnancy based on total energy expenditure and energy deposition. Am J Clin Nutr 2004; 79(6):1078–1087.
14. Illingworth PJ, Jung RT, Howie PW, Isles TE. Reduction in postprandial energy expenditure during pregnancy. Br Med J (Clin Res Ed) 1987; 294(6587):1573–1576.
15. Contaldo F, Scalfi L, Coltorti A, Di Palo MR, Martinelli P, Guerritore T. Reduced regulatory thermogenesis in pregnant and ovariectomized women. Int J Vitam Nutr Res 1987; 57(3):299–304.
16. Prentice AM, Whitehead RG, Coward WA, Goldberg GR, Davies HL, Murgatroyd PR. Reduction in postprandial energy expenditure during pregnancy. Br Med J (Clin Res Ed) 1987; 295(6592):266–267.
17. Forsum E. Energy requirements during pregnancy: old questions and new findings. Am J Clin Nutr 2004; 79(6):933–934.
18. Catalano PM, Roman-Drago NM, Amini SB, Sims EA. Longitudinal changes in body composition and energy balance in lean women with normal and abnormal glucose tolerance during pregnancy. Am J Obstet Gynecol 1998; 179(1):156–165.
19. Hsu HW, Butte NF, Wong WW, Moon JK, Ellis KJ, Klein PD et al. Oxidative metabolism in insulin-treated gestational diabetes mellitus. Am J Physiol 1997; 272(6 Pt 1):E1099–E1107.
20. Carmichael S, Abrams B, Selvin S. The pattern of maternal weight gain in women with good pregnancy outcomes. Am J Public Health 1997; 87(12):1984–1988.
21. Forsum E, Sadurskis A, Wager J. Estimation of body fat in healthy Swedish women during pregnancy and lactation. Am J Clin Nutr 1989; 50(3):465–473.

22. Lindsay CA, Huston L, Amini SB, Catalano PM. Longitudinal changes in the relationship between body mass index and percent body fat in pregnancy. Obstet Gynecol 1997; 89(3):377–382.

23. Kopp-Hoolihan LE, van Loan MD, Wong WW, King JC. Fat mass deposition during pregnancy using a four-component model. J Appl Physiol 1999; 87(1):196–202.

24. Larciprete G, Valensise H, Vasapollo B, Altomare F, Sorge R, Casalino B et al. Body composition during normal pregnancy: reference ranges. Acta Diabetol 2003; 40(Suppl 1):S225–S232.

25. Jaque-Fortunato SV, Khodiguian N, Artal R, Wiswell RA. Body composition in pregnancy. Semin Perinatol 1996; 20(4):340–342.

26. van Raaij JM, Peek ME, Vermaat-Miedema SH, Schonk CM, Hautvast JG. New equations for estimating body fat mass in pregnancy from body density or total body water. Am J Clin Nutr 1988; 48(1):24–29.

27. McCarthy EA, Strauss BJ, Walker SP, Permezel M. Determination of maternal body composition in pregnancy and its relevance to perinatal outcomes. Obstet Gynecol Surv 2004; 59(10):731–742.

28. Butte NF, King JC. Energy requirements during pregnancy and lactation. Public Health Nutr 2005; 8(7A):1010–1027.

29. Muscati SK, Gray-Donald K, Koski KG. Timing of weight gain during pregnancy: promoting fetal growth and minimizing maternal weight retention. Int J Obes Relat Metab Disord 1996; 20(6):526–532.

30. Forsum E, Sadurskis A, Wager J. Resting metabolic rate and body composition of healthy Swedish women during pregnancy. Am J Clin Nutr 1988; 47(6):942–947.

31. Highman TJ, Friedman JE, Huston LP, Wong WW, Catalano PM. Longitudinal changes in maternal serum leptin concentrations, body composition, and resting metabolic rate in pregnancy. Am J Obstet Gynecol 1998; 178(5):1010–1015.

32. Sohlstrom A, Forsum E. Changes in adipose tissue volume and distribution during reproduction in Swedish women as assessed by magnetic resonance imaging. Am J Clin Nutr 1995; 61(2):287–295.

33. Clapp JF, III, Seaward BL, Sleamaker RH, Hiser J. Maternal physiologic adaptations to early human pregnancy. Am J Obstet Gynecol 1988; 159(6):1456–1460.

34. Pipe NG, Smith T, Halliday D, Edmonds CJ, Williams C, Coltart TM. Changes in fat, fat-free mass and body water in human normal pregnancy. Br J Obstet Gynaecol 1979; 86(12):929–940.

35. Alam DS, van Raaij JM, Hautvast JG, Yunus M, Fuchs GJ. Energy stress during pregnancy and lactation: consequences for maternal nutrition in rural Bangladesh. Eur J Clin Nutr 2003; 57(1):151–156.

36. Ehrenberg HM, Huston-Presley L, Catalano PM. The influence of obesity and gestational diabetes mellitus on accretion and the distribution of adipose tissue in pregnancy. Am J Obstet Gynecol 2003; 189(4):944–948.

37. Kinoshita T, Itoh M. Longitudinal variance of fat mass deposition during pregnancy evaluated by ultrasonography: the ratio of visceral fat to subcutaneous fat in the abdomen. Gynecol Obstet Invest 2006; 61(2):115–118.

38. Zhang S, Folsom AR, Flack JM, Liu K. Body fat distribution before pregnancy and gestational diabetes: findings from coronary artery risk development in young adults (CARDIA) study. BMJ 1995; 311(7013):1139–1140.

39. Sattar N, Clark P, Holmes A, Lean ME, Walker I, Greer IA. Antenatal waist circumference and hypertension risk. Obstet Gynecol 2001; 97(2):268–271.

40. Ijuin H, Douchi T, Nakamura S, Oki T, Yamamoto S, Nagata Y. Possible association of body-fat distribution with preeclampsia. J Obstet Gynaecol Res 1997; 23(1):45–49.

41. Bartha JL, Marin-Segura P, Gonzalez-Gonzalez NL, Wagner F, Aguilar-Diosdado M, Hervias-Vivancos B. Ultrasound evaluation of visceral fat and metabolic risk factors during early pregnancy. Obesity (Silver Spring) 2007; 15(9):2233–2239.

42. Lindberg UB, Leibel RL, Silfverstolpe G, Hirsch J, Bjorntorp P, Rebuffe-Scrive M. Effects of early pregnancy on regional adipose tissue metabolism. Horm Metab Res 1991; 23(1):25–29.

43. Rebuffe-Scrive M, Enk L, Crona N, Lonnroth P, Abrahamsson L, Smith U et al. Fat cell metabolism in different regions in women. Effect of menstrual cycle, pregnancy, and lactation. J Clin Invest 1985; 75(6):1973–1976.

44. Thame M, Trotman H, Osmond C, Fletcher H, Antoine M. Body composition in pregnancies of adolescents and mature women and the relationship to birth anthropometry. Eur J Clin Nutr 2007; 61(1):47–53.

45. Mills JL, Jovanovic L, Knopp R, Aarons J, Conley M, Park E et al. Physiological reduction in fasting plasma glucose concentration in the first trimester of normal pregnancy: the diabetes in early pregnancy study. Metabolism 1998; 47(9):1140–1144.

46. Catalano PM, Tyzbir ED, Roman NM, Amini SB, Sims EA. Longitudinal changes in insulin release and insulin resistance in nonobese pregnant women. Am J Obstet Gynecol 1991; 165(6 Pt 1):1667–1672.

47. Catalano PM, Tyzbir ED, Wolfe RR, Roman NM, Amini SB, Sims EA. Longitudinal changes in basal hepatic glucose production and suppression during insulin infusion in normal pregnant women. Am J Obstet Gynecol 1992; 167(4 Pt 1): 913–919.

48. Agardh CD, Aberg A, Norden NE. Glucose levels and insulin secretion during a 75 g glucose challenge test in normal pregnancy. J Intern Med 1996; 240(5):303–309.

49. Catalano PM, Drago NM, Amini SB. Longitudinal changes in pancreatic beta-cell function and metabolic clearance rate of insulin in pregnant women with normal and abnormal glucose tolerance. Diabetes Care 1998; 21(3):403–408.

50. Catalano PM, Hoegh M, Minium J, Huston-Presley L, Bernard S, Kalhan S et al. Adiponectin in human pregnancy: implications for regulation of glucose and lipid metabolism. Diabetologia 2006; 49(7):1677–1685.

51. Sivan E, Homko CJ, Whittaker PG, Reece EA, Chen X, Boden G. Free fatty acids and insulin resistance during pregnancy. J Clin Endocrinol Metab 1998; 83(7):2338–2342.

52. Sivan E, Boden G. Free fatty acids, insulin resistance, and pregnancy. Curr Diab Rep 2003; 3(4):319–322.

53. Sorenson RL, Brelje TC. Adaptation of islets of Langerhans to pregnancy: beta-cell growth, enhanced insulin secretion and the role of lactogenic hormones. Horm Metab Res 1997; 29(6):301–307.

54. Weinhaus AJ, Stout LE, Bhagroo NV, Brelje TC, Sorenson RL. Regulation of glucokinase in pancreatic islets by prolactin: a mechanism for increasing glucose-stimulated insulin secretion during pregnancy. J Endocrinol 2007; 193(3):367–381.

55. Vasavada RC, Garcia-Ocana A, Zawalich WS, Sorenson RL, Dann P, Syed M et al. Targeted expression of placental lactogen in the beta cells of transgenic mice results in beta cell proliferation, islet mass augmentation, and hypoglycemia. J Biol Chem 2000; 275(20):15399–15406.

56. Holness MJ, Greenwood GK, Smith ND, Sugden MC. Peroxisome proliferator-activated receptor-alpha and glucocorticoids interactively regulate insulin secretion during pregnancy. Diabetes 2006; 55(12):3501–3508.

57. Sivan E, Chen X, Homko CJ, Reece EA, Boden G. Longitudinal study of carbohydrate metabolism in healthy obese pregnant women. Diabetes Care 1997; 20(9):1470–1475.

58. Catalano PM, Huston L, Amini SB, Kalhan SC. Longitudinal changes in glucose metabolism during pregnancy in obese women with normal glucose tolerance and gestational diabetes mellitus. Am J Obstet Gynecol 1999; 180(4):903–916.

59. Ramsay JE, Ferrell WR, Crawford L, Wallace AM, Greer IA, Sattar N. Maternal obesity is associated with dysregulation of metabolic, vascular, and inflammatory pathways. J Clin Endocrinol Metab 2002; 87(9):4231–4237.

60. Catalano PM, Tyzbir ED, Wolfe RR, Calles J, Roman NM, Amini SB et al. Carbohydrate metabolism during pregnancy in control subjects and women with gestational diabetes. Am J Physiol 1993; 264(1 Pt 1):E60–E67.

61. Homko C, Sivan E, Chen X, Reece EA, Boden G. Insulin secretion during and after pregnancy in patients with gestational diabetes mellitus. J Clin Endocrinol Metab 2001; 86(2):568–573.

62. Freinkel N. Banting Lecture 1980. Of pregnancy and progeny. Diabetes 1980; 29(12):1023–1035.

63. Catalano PM, Nizielski SE, Shao J, Preston L, Qiao L, Friedman JE. Downregulated IRS-1 and PPARgamma in obese women with gestational diabetes: relationship to FFA during pregnancy. Am J Physiol Endocrinol Metab 2002; 282(3):E522–E533.

64. Alvarez JJ, Montelongo A, Iglesias A, Lasuncion MA, Herrera E. Longitudinal study on lipoprotein profile, high density lipoprotein subclass, and postheparin lipases during gestation in women. J Lipid Res 1996; 37(2):299–308.

65. Knopp RH, Warth MR, Charles D, Childs M, Li JR, Mabuchi H et al. Lipoprotein metabolism in pregnancy, fat transport to the fetus, and the effects of diabetes. Biol Neonate 1986; 50(6):297–317.

66. Fahraeus L, Larsson-Cohn U, Wallentin L. Plasma lipoproteins including high density lipoprotein subfractions during normal pregnancy. Obstet Gynecol 1985; 66(4):468–472.

67. Sattar N, Greer IA, Louden J, Lindsay G, McConnell M, Shepherd J et al. Lipoprotein subfraction changes in normal pregnancy: threshold effect of plasma triglyceride on appearance of small, dense low density lipoprotein. J Clin Endocrinol Metab 1997; 82(8):2483–2491.

68. Desoye G, Schweditsch MO, Pfeiffer KP, Zechner R, Kostner GM. Correlation of hormones with lipid and lipoprotein levels during normal pregnancy and postpartum. J Clin Endocrinol Metab 1987; 64(4):704–712.

69. Sacks FM, Walsh BW. Sex hormones and lipoprotein metabolism. Curr Opin Lipidol 1994; 5(3):236–240.

70. Sivan E, Homko CJ, Chen X, Reece EA, Boden G. Effect of insulin on fat metabolism during and after normal pregnancy. Diabetes 1999; 48(4):834–838.

71. Merzouk H, Meghelli-Bouchenak M, Loukidi B, Prost J, Belleville J. Impaired serum lipids and lipoproteins in fetal macrosomia related to maternal obesity. Biol Neonate 2000; 77(1):17–24.

72. Sanchez-Vera I, Bonet B, Viana M, Quintanar A, Martin MD, Blanco P et al. Changes in plasma lipids and increased low-density lipoprotein susceptibility to oxidation in pregnancies complicated by gestational diabetes: consequences of obesity. Metabolism 2007; 56(11):1527–1533.

73. Sattar N, Tan CE, Han TS, Forster L, Lean ME, Shepherd J et al. Associations of indices of adiposity with atherogenic lipoprotein subfractions. Int J Obes Relat Metab Disord 1998; 22(5):432–439.

74. Montelongo A, Lasuncion MA, Pallardo LF, Herrera E. Longitudinal study of plasma lipoproteins and hormones during pregnancy in normal and diabetic women. Diabetes 1992; 41(12):1651–1659.

75. Kilby MD, Neary RH, Mackness MI, Durrington PN. Fetal and maternal lipoprotein metabolism in human pregnancy complicated by type I diabetes mellitus. J Clin Endocrinol Metab 1998; 83(5):1736–1741.

76. Peterson CM, Jovanovic-Peterson L, Mills JL, Conley MR, Knopp RH, Reed GF et al. The Diabetes in Early Pregnancy Study: changes in cholesterol, triglycerides, body weight, and blood pressure. The National Institute of Child Health and Human Development – the Diabetes in Early Pregnancy Study. Am J Obstet Gynecol 1992; 166(2):513–518.

77. Knopp RH, Van Allen MI, McNeely M, Walden CE, Plovie B, Shiota K et al. Effect of insulin-dependent diabetes on plasma lipoproteins in diabetic pregnancy. J Reprod Med 1993; 38(9):703–710.

78. Couch SC, Philipson EH, Bendel RB, Pujda LM, Milvae RA, Lammi-Keefe CJ. Elevated lipoprotein lipids and gestational hormones in women with diet-treated gestational diabetes mellitus compared to healthy pregnant controls. J Diabetes Complications 1998; 12(1):1–9.

79. Hollingsworth DR, Grundy SM. Pregnancy-associated hypertriglyceridemia in normal and diabetic women. Differences in insulin-dependent, non-insulin-dependent, and gestational diabetes. Diabetes 1982; 31(12):1092–1097.

80. Alam TA, Seifalian AM, Baker D. A review of methods currently used for assessment of in vivo endothelial function. Eur J Vasc Endovasc Surg 2005; 29(3):269–276.

81. Dorup I, Skajaa K, Sorensen KE. Normal pregnancy is associated with enhanced endothelium-dependent flow-mediated vasodilation. Am J Physiol 1999; 276(3 Pt 2):H821–H825.

82. Faber-Swensson AP, O'Callaghan SP, Walters WA. Endothelial cell function enhancement in a late normal human pregnancy. Aust N Z J Obstet Gynaecol 2004; 44(6):525–529.

83. Kinzler WL, Smulian JC, Ananth CV, Vintzileos AM. Noninvasive ultrasound assessment of maternal vascular reactivity during pregnancy: a longitudinal study. Obstet Gynecol 2004; 104(2):362–366.

84. Quinton AE, Cook CM, Peek MJ. A longitudinal study using ultrasound to assess flow-mediated dilatation in normal human pregnancy. Hypertens Pregnancy 2007; 26(3):273–281.

85. Savvidou MD, Kametas NA, Donald AE, Nicolaides KH. Non-invasive assessment of endothelial function in normal pregnancy. Ultrasound Obstet Gynecol 2000; 15(6):502–507.

86. Poppas A, Shroff SG, Korcarz CE, Hibbard JU, Berger DS, Lindheimer MD et al. Serial assessment of the cardiovascular system in normal pregnancy. Role of arterial compliance and pulsatile arterial load. Circulation 1997; 95(10):2407–2415.

87. Edouard DA, Pannier BM, London GM, Cuche JL, Safar ME. Venous and arterial behavior during normal pregnancy. Am J Physiol 1998; 274(5 Pt 2):H1605–H1612.

88. Oyama-Kato M, Ohmichi M, Takahashi K, Suzuki S, Henmi N, Yokoyama Y et al. Change in pulse wave velocity throughout normal pregnancy and its value in predicting pregnancy-induced hypertension: a longitudinal study. Am J Obstet Gynecol 2006; 195(2):464–469.

89. Macedo ML, Luminoso D, Savvidou MD, McEniery CM, Nicolaides KH. Maternal wave reflections and arterial stiffness in normal pregnancy as assessed by applanation tonometry. Hypertension 2008; 51(4):1047–1051.

90. Reiss RE, O'Shaughnessy RW, Quilligan TJ, Zuspan FP. Retrospective comparison of blood pressure course during preeclamptic and matched control pregnancies. Am J Obstet Gynecol 1987; 156(4):894–898.

91. Stewart FM, Freeman DJ, Ramsay JE, Greer IA, Caslake M, Ferrell WR. Longitudinal assessment of maternal endothelial function and markers of inflammation and placental function throughout pregnancy in lean and obese mothers. J Clin Endocrinol Metab 2007; 92(3):969–975.

92. Stone S, Hunt BJ, Seed PT, Parmar K, Khamashta MA, Poston L. Longitudinal evaluation of markers of endothelial cell dysfunction and hemostasis in treated antiphospholipid syndrome and in healthy pregnancy. Am J Obstet Gynecol 2003; 188(2):454–460.

93. Saarelainen H, Valtonen P, Punnonen K, Laitinen T, Raitakari OT, Juonala M et al. Subtle changes in ADMA and l-arginine concentrations in normal pregnancies are unlikely to account for pregnancy-related increased flow-mediated dilatation. Clin Physiol Funct Imaging 2008; 28(2):120–124.

94. Paradisi G, Biaggi A, Ferrazzani S, De Carolis S, Caruso A. Abnormal carbohydrate metabolism during pregnancy: association with endothelial dysfunction. Diabetes Care 2002; 25(3):560–564.

95. Saarelainen H, Laitinen T, Raitakari OT, Juonala M, Heiskanen N, Lyyra-Laitinen T et al. Pregnancy-related hyperlipidemia and endothelial function in healthy women. Circ J 2006; 70(6):768–772.

96. Redman CW, Sacks GP, Sargent IL. Preeclampsia: an excessive maternal inflammatory response to pregnancy. Am J Obstet Gynecol 1999; 180(2 Pt 1):499–506.

97. Greer IA, Lyall F, Perera T, Boswell F, Macara LM. Increased concentrations of cytokines interleukin-6 and interleukin-1 receptor antagonist in plasma of women with preeclampsia: a mechanism for endothelial dysfunction? Obstet Gynecol 1994; 84(6):937–940.

98. Kim JA, Montagnani M, Koh KK, Quon MJ. Reciprocal relationships between insulin resistance and endothelial dysfunction: molecular and pathophysiological mechanisms. Circulation 2006; 113(15):1888–1904.

99. Gibson JL, Lyall F, Boswell F, Young A, Maccuish AC, Greer IA. Circulating cell adhesion molecule concentrations in diabetic women during pregnancy. Obstet Gynecol 1997; 90(6):874–879.

100. Hu J, Bjorklund A, Nyman M, Gennser G. Mechanical Properties of Large Arteries in Mother and Fetus during Normal and Diabetic Pregnancy. J Matern Fetal Investig 1998; 8(4):185–193.

101. Savvidou MD, Geerts L, Nicolaides KH. Impaired vascular reactivity in pregnant women with insulin-dependent diabetes mellitus. Am J Obstet Gynecol 2002; 186(1):84–88.

102. Ramsay JE, Simms RJ, Ferrell WR, Crawford L, Greer IA, Lumsden MA et al. Enhancement of endothelial function by pregnancy: inadequate response in women with type 1 diabetes. Diabetes Care 2003; 26(2):475–479.

103. Ang C, Hillier C, Johnston F, Cameron A, Greer I, Lumsden MA. Endothelial function is preserved in pregnant women with well-controlled type 1 diabetes. BJOG 2002; 109(6):699–707.

104. Loukovaara MJ, Loukovaara S, Leinonen PJ, Teramo KA, Andersson SH. Endothelium-derived nitric oxide metabolites and soluble intercellular adhesion molecule-1 in diabetic and normal pregnancies. Eur J Obstet Gynecol Reprod Biol 2005; 118(2):160–165.

105. Kanagalingam MG, Forouhi NG, Greer IA, Sattar N. Changes in booking body mass index over a decade: retrospective analysis from a Glasgow Maternity Hospital. BJOG 2005; 112(10):1431–1433.

106. Ramsay JE, Greer I, Sattar N. ABC of obesity. Obesity and reproduction. BMJ 2006; 333(7579):1159–1162.

107. Guelinckx I, Devlieger R, Beckers K, Vansant G. Maternal obesity: pregnancy complications, gestational weight gain and nutrition. Obes Rev 2008; 9(2):140–150.

12

The Epidemiology of Diabetes in Women and the Looming Epidemic of GDM in the Third World

S.M. Sadikot

CONTENTS

ABSTRACT

The pandemic of diabetes and its related complications continues unabated despite strides in understanding its pathophysiology and the availability of new therapeutic interventions. Approximately 80% of people with diabetes live in poor and developing countries, and many of them, especially those living in rural areas and small towns, arc without access to adequate basic health care. Further as discussed in Chap. 6, the lack of access to adequate nutrition and the reduced opportunities for exercise in developing countries have created an obesity epidemic, which parallels the rising prevalence of diabetes and gestational diabetes (GDM). Unfortunately, there are scarce data regarding the short- and long-term health and socioeconomic consequences of gestational diabetes in these countries. On the basis of the experience of a diabetes health care provider in India, it is found that individuals and health care systems are unable to cope with the tremendous economic burden of this disease. It is essential that the health care planners in developing countries *(1)* make screening, diagnosis, and treatment of GDM and the preconception, antepartum, and

From: *Diabetes in Women: Pathophysiology and Therapy*
Edited by: A. Tsatsoulis et al. (eds.), DOI 10.1007/978-1-60327-250-6_12
© Humana Press, a part of Springer Science+Business Media, LLC 2009

postpartum care of women with type 2 diabetes (DM2) "available," "accessible," and, most importantly, "affordable" to their citizens. The aim of this chapter is to present what is known about the rising prevalence of diabetes and GDM in the developing countries of the "third world" and discuss the complex issues related to access to health care.

Key words: Gestational; Diabetes; Prevalence; Third world; Ethnicity; Screening; Management; Developing nations; Maternal; Fetus; Pregnancy; Postpartum; Economics; Health

THE PREVALENCE OF DIABETES IN WOMEN IN THIRD WORLD COUNTRIES

The prevalence of diabetes, especially type 2 diabetes mellitus (DM2) is increasing by leaps and bounds, and presently it is thought to be in the vicinity of 5.9% of the adult population (20–79 age group) or approximately 246 million people globally with the vast majority of diabetes affecting subjects living in developing countries (Table 1). T2DM is the most common form of diabetes and accounts for 85–95% of all diabetes in developed countries and an even higher proportion in developing countries *(2)*. Worldwide, diabetes has reached epidemic proportions *(3, 4)*. As seen in Table 1, the number is expected to reach some 380 million by 2025, representing 7.1% of the adult population *(2)*. For developing countries, there will be a projected increase of 170% of cases; for developed countries, there will be a projected rise of 40% *(2)*.

Since 1995, the top three countries estimated to have the highest numbers of people with diabetes have been India, China, and the USA. In 2000, Bangladesh, Brazil, Indonesia, Japan, and Pakistan also appeared in the top ten list along with the Russian Federation and Italy. The latter two are predicted to be replaced by the Philippines and Egypt in 2030, reflecting anticipated changes in the population size and prevalence in these countries between the two time periods *(4)*.

Seven out of the ten countries with the highest number of people living with diabetes are in the developing world *(2)* (Table 2), as are ten of ten with the highest prevalence (Table 3).

Table 1
Comparative Prevalence of Diabetes in the Years 2007 and 2025 (2)

Prevalence of diabetes (age 20–79 years)	2007	2025
Comparative prevalence (%)	5.9	7.1
Number of people with diabetes	246	380

Table 2
Top Ten Countries in Prevalence
of Diabetes (20–79 Age Group) 2007 (2)

Country	Prevalence (%)
Nauru	30.7
U.A.E.	19.5
Saudi Arabia	16.7
Bahrain	15.2
Kuwait	14.4
Oman	13.1
Tonga	12.9
Mauritius	11.1
Egypt	11.0
Mexico	10.6

Table 3
Top Ten Countries in Number of People with Diabetes
(20–79 Age Group) 2007 (2)

Country	Persons (million)
India	40.9
People's Republic of China	39.8
U.S.A.	19.2
Russia	9.6
Germany	7.4
Japan	7.0
Pakistan	6.9
Brazil	6.9
Mexico	6.1
Egypt	4.4

Most of the studies show that there is no significant difference in prevalence between men and women *(2–4)*. Moreover, the metabolic abnormalities that result in the development of DM2 appear to occur at a relatively younger (i.e., childbearing) age in people in developing countries and thus increases the percentage of people who are at risk for developing gestational diabetes also.

As with previous studies, these estimates of prevalence and total burden of disease are limited by a paucity of data, particularly for Eastern Europe and Southeast Asia, and by the assumptions required to generate the estimates. It is possible that individual studies are not representative of the whole country in which they were performed, and it is likely that extrapolation of results to neighboring countries may give inaccurate estimates of diabetes prevalence.

THE PREVALENCE OF GESTATIONAL DIABETES IN WOMEN IN THIRD WORLD COUNTRIES

Although gestational diabetes is estimated to complicate between 1 and 5% of pregnancies, there are only limited data on the role of race/ethnicity as well as other risk factors in the development of this disorder *(5)*. The prevalence of gestational diabetes mellitus (GDM) varies in direct proportion with the prevalence of DM2 in a given population or ethnic group *(6–10)*. In low-risk populations, such as those found in Sweden, the prevalence in population-based studies is lower than 2% even when universal testing is offered, whereas studies in high-risk populations report a much higher prevalence. Recent data show that GDM prevalence has increased by ~10–100% in several race/ethnicity groups during the past 20 years in US populations *(8)*, with Native Americans, Asians, Hispanics, and African-American women being at higher risk for GDM than non-Hispanic white women.

Epidemiologic characteristics of gestational diabetes were assessed in an ethnically diverse cohort of 10,187 women who had undergone standardized screening for glucose intolerance and who delivered a singleton infant at the Mount Sinai Medical Center in New York City between January 1987 and December 1989. The overall prevalence of gestational diabetes was 3.2%. Multiple logistic regression analysis showed excess risks for Oriental women, Hispanics born in Puerto Rico or elsewhere outside the USA, women from the Indian subcontinent and the Middle East, older mothers, heavier women, those with a positive family history of diabetes, women with a history of infertility, and those who delivered on the clinic service. These data suggest that, after controlling for traditional risk factors (maternal age, prepregnancy weight, and a family history of diabetes),

Orientals, first-generation Hispanics, women from the Indian subcontinent and the Middle East, those with a history of infertility, and women with low socioeconomic status are at an increased risk for gestational diabetes (5).

Green et al. (11) from the University of California, San Francisco showed that the incidence of gestational diabetes was significantly greater for Chinese (7.3%) and Hispanic (4.2%) women than for Black (1.7%) and non-Hispanic White (1.6%) women.

In a cross sectional study, Ferrara et al. (12) screened a total of 26,481 women using a 50-g, 1-h oral glucose tolerance test (GTT), and 4,190 of these women underwent a diagnostic 100-g, 3-h oral GTT after an abnormal screening. The age-adjusted GDM prevalence by NDDG and Carpenter and Coustan (C & C) criteria, respectively, was 5.0 and 7.4% in Asians, 3.9 and 5.6% in Hispanics, 3.0 and 4.0% in African-Americans, and 2.4 and 3.8% in whites.

Dabalea et al. (13) showed that the prevalence of GDM is increasing in a universally screened multiethnic population. The increasing GDM prevalence suggests that the vicious cycle prenatal exposure to maternal diabetes predisposing to DM2 initially described among Pima Indians may also be occurring among other US ethnic groups.

Engelgau et al. (14) report that while gestational diabetes complicates about 5% of all pregnancies, the rate of occurrence can range up to 14% depending on the population. Three other studies have also shown that gestational diabetes is more common in those ethnic groups who are at higher risk for diabetes per se – African Americans, Native Americans, Mexican Americans, Asian Americans, and Pacific Islanders (15–17).

Beischer et al. (18) reported in 1991 that in Australia, GDM prevalence was found to be higher in women whose country of birth was China or India than in women whose country of birth was Europe or Northern Africa, and Ishak et al. (19) reported that the prevalence of GDM is significantly higher in the Aboriginal population of Australia than in the country's non-Aboriginal population.

Cheung et al. (20) examined the records of 2,139 Asian women living in Australia. The overall incidence of GDM was 9.2%. Among women born in China, it was 8.6% – the Philippines 6.7%, Sri Lanka 10.5%, and Vietnam 10.6%. These incidences are comparable with those found in studies of Asian women in developed countries but are higher than those found in studies conducted in Asia.

In 1992, Dornhorst et al. (21) assessed 11,205 consecutive women attending a multiracial antenatal clinic in London, where all women were screened for gestational diabetes. Women from ethnic groups other than white had a higher frequency of gestational diabetes than white women (2.9% vs. 0.4%, P < 0.001). Compared with white women the relative risk (RR) of gestational diabetes in the other ethnic groups was as follows: Black 3.1 (95% confidence limits 1.8–5.5), South East Asian 7.6 (4.1–14.1), Indian 11.3 (6.8–18.8), and miscellaneous 5.9 (3.5–9.9).

It is apparent that most of the data relating to ethnic variations in the prevalence/incidence of gestational diabetes are typically based on US, UK, Canadian, or Australian statistics, which are then extrapolated to the country of origin. This extrapolation does not take into account any genetic, cultural, environmental, social, racial, or other differences across the various countries and regions.

At the same time, there a few studies that have been done in the developing countries themselves (Table 4) (22–39). These have been either population- or hospital-based studies.

Reported prevalence rates in population-based studies in Turkey, Iran, Bahrain, Ethiopia, and India ranged from 1.2% in Turkey by National Diabetes Data Group (NDDG) criteria following universal screening to 15.5% in Bahraini women by C & C criteria with a 3-h 75-g OGTT following universal screening. Reported prevalence rates in hospital-based studies in Turkey, Iran, Pakistan, India, and Sri Lanka are between 4.1 and 4.7%, with the exception of the study conducted in India, which used the 1999 World Health Organization (WHO) diagnostic criteria and reports a prevalence of 18.9%, as well as the study conducted in Turkey, which reports a prevalence of 6.6% using the C & C criteria.

Table 4
Community and Hospital-Based Gestational Diabetes Prevalence Studies Carried out in Third World Countries (22–39)

Country	Screening criteria	GDM criteria	Ethnic group	GDM prevalence
Iran				
Community based (22)	Universal screening at 24–28 weeks; 1-h 50-g GCT ≥ 130	NDDG	Urban Iranian, ethnicity non-specified	4.8%
Community based (23)	Universal screening at 24–28 weeks; 1-h 50-g GCT > 130	C & C and NDDG	Urban Iranian, ethnicity non-specified	6.3% NDDG; 8.9% C & C
Hospital based (24)	Universal screening high risk - initial visit and at 24–28 weeks; 1-h 50-g GCT ≥ 130	C & C	Urban Iranian, ethnicity non-specified	4.7%
Brazil				
Community based (25)	Universal testing at 24–28 weeks; 2-h 75-g OGTT	ADA post 1997 and WHO 1999 including 0 h ≥126	Mixed	2.4%, ADA; 7.2%, WHO
Ethiopia				
Community based (26)	Universal testing after 24 weeks	WHO 1999	Community based; ethnicity non-specified	3.7%
India				
Community based (27)	Universal screening second or third trimester; 1-h 50-g GCT ≥ 140	C & C and WHO 1999	Kashmiri Indian 6 districts	3.1% C & C; 4.4% WHO
Hospital based (28)	Universal screening second or third trimester; 1-h 50-g GCT ≥ 130	WHO, 1999 including 0 h ≥126	S. Indian urban, ethnicity non-specified	18.9%
Hospital based (29)	100-g, 3-h oral glucose tolerance test (GTT) at 30 ± 2 weeks gestation	C & C	S. Indian urban, ethnicity non-specified	6.2%
Turkey				
Community based (30)	Universal screening at 24–28 weeks; 1-h 50-g GCT ≥ 140	NDDG	Urban Turkish, ethnicity non-specified	1.2%
Hospital based (31)	Universal screening at 24–32 weeks; 1-h 50-g GCT ≥ 140	C & C	Urban Turkish	6.6%

(continued)

Table 4
(continued)

Country	Screening criteria	GDM criteria	Ethnic group	GDM prevalence
China				
Community based (32)	Universal screening at 26–30 weeks; 1-h 50-g GCT ≥ 140	WHO, 1999 including 0 h ≥126	Six urban districts	2.3%
Bahrain				
Community based (33)	Universal screening at 24–28 weeks; 1-h 50-g GCT ≥ 140	C & C with a 3 h 75 g OGTT	Mixed; Bahraini and expats	13.3% Total; 15.5% Bahraini; 7.5% expatriate
Mexico				
Hospital based (34)	Universal screening; 1-h 50-g GCT ≥ 140 (initial visit); WHO diagnostic (second visit)	NDDG; C & C; WHO 1999	Ethnicity non-specified	3.2%, NDDG; 4.1%, C & C; 8.7%, WHO
Pakistan				
Hospital based (35)	Universal screening at 24–36 weeks; 1-h 50-g GCT ≥ 130	NDDG	Urban Pakistani, ethnicity non-specified	4.3%
Hospital based (36)	2-h 75-g glucose challenge on initial visit; the test was repeated at 28–32 weeks of gestation	Modified O'Sullivan criteria	Urban Pakistani, ethnicity non-specified	3.2%
Hospital based (37)	50-g glucose load. 1-h 50-g GCT ≥ 130+ and followed by a 3-h oral GTT with a 100-g glucose load. Women with a negative result were retested at 24-weeks gestation	Modified O'Sullivan criteria	Urban Pakistani, ethnicity non-specified	3.45%
Sri Lanka				
Hospital based (38)	Universal testing at 24–28 weeks	WHO, 1985	Urban Sri Lankan, ethnicity nonspecified	4.1%
Hospital based (39)	Universal screening at 24–36 weeks; 1-h 50-g GCT ≥ 130	75-g oral GTT and WHO criteria	Urban Sri Lankan, ethnicity nonspecified	5.5%

SCREENING FOR GESTATIONAL DIABETES IN THIRD WORLD COUNTRIES: DO WE NEED ETHNIC AND NATIONAL SPECIFIC CRITERIA?

Defining the performance characteristics of screening strategies for GDM is complicated by the lack of a universally accepted "gold standard" for the diagnosis of GDM. As can be seen from Table 4, studies that have been carried out in developing countries have used differing screening and diagnostic criteria, mirroring the same lack of consensus in the developed world.

More work needs to be done to address a cost-effective diagnostic strategy for GDM that takes into account fetal outcomes rather than maternal risk of future diabetes and whether ethnicity alters these outcomes. The multicentered, multinational Hyperglycemia and Adverse Outcomes Study (HAPO) was designed to address this, and initial results have been reported *(40)*.

Ethnic differences in visceral fat distribution and percent body fat could theoretically impact optimal diagnostic criteria for gestational diabetes. This is the reason that ethnic and nation-specific criteria have been set forth by the International Diabetes Federation for waist circumference for the diagnosis of the metabolic syndrome *(41)* (Table 5).

This has been given all the more relevance as insulin resistance, which has been linked to gestational diabetes via maternal obesity, especially visceral obesity *(42–57)*. It has also been shown that the association of higher body fat, especially visceral fat with BMI is not universal but may be ethnically determined.

Obesity is a major contributor to insulin resistance, and amongst Caucasians, most people with DM2 are overweight or obese. However, the body mass index (BMI) defined that prevalence of obesity, an important risk factor in the development of type 2 diabetes, is significantly lower in Asian Indians than in Caucasians *(58)*. However, for any given BMI, the waist to hip ratio was higher among Indians than among other ethnic groups. Thus, they have a greater predisposition to visceral obesity and consequent increased visceral adipose tissue (VAT), which may explain their increased propensity to develop insulin resistance *(58, 59)*. Even when matched for body fat, Indians had greater insulin resistance than other ethnic groups. This and the metabolic abnormalities brought about by higher visceral fat mass relative to BMI are referred to as the "Asian Indian Phenotype" *(60)*.

With respect to optimum screening, Nahum et al. *(61)* categorized 921 women universally screened for the presence of GDM as white, Black, Asian, or Filipino. Using a 50-g, 1-h glucose load test, 17.5% of Blacks, 27.4% of whites, 31.3% of Filipinos, and 40.6% of Asians exceeded the 140-mg/dL threshold. The proportions with results above 140 mg/dL who also had an abnormal 3-h GTT also varied markedly by race: Blacks 42.9%, whites 17.3%, Filipinos 11.5%, and Asians 11.5%. Adjusted screening test thresholds, calculated for each race to establish consistency of the screening test, were

Table 5
Country/Ethnic Specific Criteria for Waist Circumference (W.C.)

Country/Ethnicity	W.C. Males (cm)	W.C. Females (cm)
Europids	≥94	≥80
USA	≥102	≥88
S. Asians	≥90	≥80
Chinese	≥90	≥80
Japanese	≥85	≥90

Note. For ethnic South and Central American populations, S. Asian criteria to be used until specific data become available; for ethnic sub-Saharan African, Eastern Mediterranean, and Middle Eastern (Arab) populations, European criteria to be used until specific data become available

130 mg/dL for Blacks, 140 mg/dL for whites, 145 mg/dL for Filipinos, and 150 mg/dL for Asians. They concluded that race-specific glucose screening test thresholds should be used to ensure consistency in properly identifying pregnant women at risk for GDM.

Esakoff et al. *(62)* also examined if the screening criteria should be modified depending on the ethnicity of the subject being tested. Values of the 50-g glucose-loading test were examined from 130 to 150 mg/dL. To achieve a false-positive rate of 10% for the glucose-loading test, the threshold value would be 133 mg/dL for African Americans, 140 mg/dL for whites, 143 mg/dL for Latinas, and 147 mg/dL for Asians. They concluded that to maximize the sensitivity and minimize the false-positive rate of the glucose-loading test, it may be reasonable to consider varying the threshold based on ethnicity with the caveat that further studies were necessary to determine if the different thresholds improved perinatal outcomes.

The ADA presently recommends that subjects be divided into high, average, and low-risk categories with high-risk patients undergoing screening at the initial antenatal visit *(63)*. The simplest method is a nonfasting 50-g oral glucose challenge test with a 1-h serum glucose concentration. If the glucose level exceeds the glucose threshold value on this test, the patient is further evaluated with the diagnostic OGTT described previously under diagnostic criteria. A 1-h glucose value >140 mg/dL identifies ~80% of women with GDM. A 1-h glucose value >130 mg/dL identifies ~90% of women with GDM, but it has a higher false-positive rate *(64)*. While a 130 mg/dL cutoff point increases the sensitivity of the test, the cost implications may be prohibitive in developing countries.

Yalcin et al. *(31)* aimed to determine a threshold value that perfectly demarcates women at high risk for GDM in the Turkish population. One thousand gravid women at 24–32 weeks of gestation were given 50-g, 1-h glucose screening tests. A 100-g, 3-h GTT was performed on all patients whose screening test plasma glucose value was 130 mg/dL or greater. The incidence of GDM was found to be 6.6%. The maximum specificity and sensitivity were met at 140 mg/dL. However, this value underestimated 12% of patients with GDM, and the lowest value for a positive GTT appeared to be 134 mg/dL. They recommend a 135 mg/dL threshold for the GTT since this threshold accurately diagnoses almost all women with GDM while eliminating unnecessary diagnostic testing.

de Sereday et al. *(65)* reported that based on the sensitivity and specificity for macrosomia, the 1-h, 50-g screening test had an optimal cutoff point of 137 mg/dL (vs. 140 mg/dL recommended by the ADA). The 2-h, 75-g OGTT value using a cutoff point of 119 mg/dL at 2 h had equivalent sensitivity, specificity, and positive predictive value as the 137 mg/dL cutoff at 1 h after the 50-g screening test.

In India, Seshiah et al. *(28)* reported that using a 2-h plasma glucose of [3]140 mg/dL after a 75-g oral glucose load as a one-step procedure is simple and economical, particularly for the countries ethnically more prone to a high prevalence of diabetes.

Vitoratos et al. *(66)* studied 602 pregnant women in Greece between 24 and 28 weeks of gestation, who received a 50-g glucose load followed by glucose determination 1 h later. They recommend 126 mg/dL threshold for the GLT since this threshold allows for the diagnosis of all women with carbohydrate intolerance during pregnancy.

Senanayake et al. *(67)* compared the fasting plasma glucose (FPG) with the 2-h postprandial plasma glucose (PPPG), following a carbohydrate meal, for screening of GDM in southern Asian women with one or more risk factors. The ability to predict GDM and to reduce the need for an OGTT was the main outcome measure. They reported that FPG is superior to the 2-h PPPG for screening high-risk women. A FPG above 126 mg/dL could reduce the number of OGTTs needed by 40.9%, compared with 20.6% by PPPG.

Screening, whether it is universal or selective, remains a controversial subject. Contradictory to the ADA recommendations described earlier, the United States Preventive Services Task Force *(68)* concluded that there was insufficient evidence to recommend for or against screening for GDM.

Although they found fair to good evidence that screening and treatment of GDM reduced the rate of fetal macrosomia, they found insufficient evidence that screening significantly reduced important adverse maternal or fetal outcomes, including outcomes related to macrosomia. In addition, they had concerns about the potential harms and costs of screening, especially given the high false-positive rate (>80%) of the 50-g glucose challenge test.

CHALLENGES TO HEATH CARE DELIVERY IN THIRD WORLD COUNTRIES

One can debate optimal ethnic-specific criteria for the diagnosis and treatment of GDM but the reality in many of the developing countries is that gestational diabetes is not even on the radar of the health concerns. The reasons for this are manifold, and although it is convenient to blame the health economics of many of these countries, one of the major reasons is lack of awareness, especially among the primary care physicians.

Medical Aspects

In the case of India, there is a broad network of family physicians, which must be mobilized to make diabetes care accessible to the people. More than 98–99% of all patients with diabetes in India are seen and managed by family practitioners. Even among the small percentage of patients who are seen by internists and diabetologists, the specialist's recommendations must be agreed to by the family physician before the patient will follow them.

This family physician network is hampered by the fact that many family physicians are trained primarily in the traditional systems of medicine, such as homeopathy, ayurveda, unani, and other ethnomedical traditions. The quality and amount of diabetes training they receive is highly variable. Even if they are trained in the allopathic branch of medicine, as India does not have a system of medical licensure mandating participation in accredited Continuing Medical Education programs, many of these doctors have outdated knowledge regarding DM and especially GDM diagnosis and management.

The family physicians usually carry out the day-to-day management of pregnant women as well. If women are referred to an obstetrician, it is quite late in the pregnancy. Thus, the diagnosis of gestational diabetes is often missed because it was not screened for or was screened for inadequately with a fasting glucose only.

Additional challenges to the health care in countries such as India relate to the vastness and ethnic diversity of its population and difference in access to medical care in large metros compared with smaller towns and especially rural areas where the majority of the population lives. The ethnic heterogeneity of India is manifested in significantly different religions, communities, castes, cultures, languages (>18 major languages and more than 200 dialects), food habits, lifestyles, and genetic endowment. Around 72% of the people live in rural areas and 28% in urban areas. The urban milieu is subdivided further into metros, larger cities, and small towns further complicating the diversity. This degree of diversity is often unrecognized by the academicians in the developed world who look at statistics from a large metropolitan hospital and extrapolate it to the whole country.

It has been estimated that many pregnant women especially in the rural areas do not even see a doctor and that more than a quarter of all deliveries take place at home in the absence of a midwife. Academic guidelines on gestational diabetes have little value if they are not widely disseminated and if patients do not have access to providers knowledgeable of them.

Access to screening for diabetes and impaired glucose tolerance (IGT) was inadequate throughout India as the "Prevalence of Diabetes in India Study (PODIS)" demonstrated *(69, 70)*. Four out of five people with diabetes in rural areas, two out of three in smaller urban towns, and one out of two in large cities and metros were undiagnosed with DM2.

Economic Aspects

Among the economic challenges to the delivery of comprehensive and acceptable diabetes care services are the cost of these programs and the capacity of the people to afford these services. Let us again take the case of India.

(a) India's per capita income, as per the revised estimates released by the Central Statistical Organization on May 31, 2006, has been estimated at Indian Rs. 23,222 annually at current prices during the year 2004–2005 (about $400) per annum. Considering the great disparity in income prevalent in India and the increasing gap between the well-off and the poor, most people would be earning significantly less than this *(71)*. Recent data have shown that around 40% of the population lives below the poverty line, which is usually defined as a per capita income of USD 1 per day *(72)*.

(b) The International Health Regulations (IHR) point out that the biggest problem with the Indian health system is the lack of government spending in the health sector (0.9–1.2% of GDP against an average of 2.2% by lower–middle-income countries) *(73)*. This works out to less than one US cent per day. The priorities of the health authorities focus on infectious diseases, mother and child care, and AIDS, which consume the major chunk of this meager amount.

(c) The health insurance industry is mostly government owned, although some private players are entering the market. An insurance policy is costly and does not cover those with diabetes. Moreover, the coverage is usually for in-hospital expenses, and ambulatory care for medical consultations and medicines is not usually covered.

(d) India does not have anything akin to the Social Security network or an antipoverty net.

Health is a federal subject in India and health care facilities are run by both the Central Government as well as by the various State Governments and the Municipalities. While the Central government runs a few major hospitals and University medical colleges with attached hospitals, these are few and usually restricted to what were at one time Union Government ruled areas, many of which have now become independent States. These hospitals bill people according to their economic circumstances with those who earn less than Rs. 200 per month allowed free treatment and others paying a nominal amount. These hospitals have been established in major cities and larger towns. In view of the constraints and priorities of the government, most of these hospitals specialize in the treatment of communicable diseases and provide general surgical procedures. Some of the larger hospitals do have specialty clinics, but even these are rarely fully equipped and staffed, and diabetes care does not seem to be a priority. Public hospitals that are well equipped and staffed are located in the major cities but are not affordable to the common people. In these hospitals, patients must buy their own medications and pay for costly investigations, although the cost may be less than that seen in private hospitals, which many people who can afford them go to.

The smaller towns and rural areas are serviced by what is on paper an organized health care system, comprising primary health centers (one for every 100,000 people), subcenters, and community health centers. These centers concentrate on managing communicable diseases, immunizations, maternal and child care. Here too, the treatment of noncommunicable diseases is not a priority. Many of these centers are understaffed, ill equipped, and often do not have basic medications or the capacity to treat noncommunicable diseases such as GDM. Since more than 90% of healthcare is out-of-pocket expense at these health centers, the system is set up to favor those who can pay *(74, 75)*.

There is an increasing trend to have "private" hospitals that again are found usually only in the metros and bigger towns. These are often called Clinical and Research Centers as having this moniker allows them to get tax relief as well as duty relief on any equipment and medications they import. These are usually very well equipped and some of these deliver world class care. Legally, they are supposed to treat 10% of the indoor patients and 40% of the outpatients for free but in reality this is not the case. Generally, most of these hospitals are beyond the affordability of a large part of the population.

MEDICAL IMPACT OF GDM IN THE THIRD WORLD

Short- and Long-Term Consequences of Fetal Complications

Fetal complications associated with the presence of gestational diabetes in the mother include macrosomia, neonatal hypoglycemia, perinatal mortality, congenital malformations (in the case of undiagnosed preexisting DM), hyperbilirubinemia, polycythemia, hypocalcemia, and respiratory distress syndrome, and associated complications of labor and delivery are the most frequent and serious types of morbidity. Macrosomia, defined as birth weight >4,000 g, occurs in ~20–30% of infants whose mothers have GDM. Maternal factors associated with an increased incidence of macrosomia include hyperglycemia, high BMI, older age, and multiparity. This excess in fetal growth can lead to increased fetal morbidity at delivery, such as shoulder dystocia, and an increased rate of cesarean deliveries.

Siribaddana et al. *(39)* showed that the mean birth weight was higher ($P < 0.05$) in GDM (3,615 g, SD ± 103) than in nondiabetic pregnancy (NDP) (2,898 g, SD ± 143.6). In a study in Iran, Keshavarz et al. *(22)* reported a higher rate of macrosomia in GDM pregnancies than in NDP (macrosomia $P < 0.05$; odds ratio 3.2, 95% CI = 1.2–8.6).

Kale et al. *(76)* in a study carried out in Pune, India reported that although 23% of GDM mothers delivered preterm (<37 weeks), despite the shorter gestation, infants of GDM pregnancies were heavier (BW 2,950.0 g vs. 2,824.0 g, $P < 0.001$, adjusted for gender), longer (48.9 cm vs. 48.0 cm, $P < 0.01$), and more adipose (sum of two skinfolds 10.5 mm vs. 8.5 mm) than infants of NDP. Only 5% of babies born to mothers with GDM weighed >4,000 g but 30% were >90th centile of birth weight of babies born to nondiabetic mothers. Infants of mothers with GDM suffered greater neonatal morbidity. In Bangalore, India, Hill et al. *(29)* reported that mothers with gestational diabetes had infants that were heavier (3,339 g vs. 2,956 g) and had greater fat, muscle, and skeletal measurements than infants of nondiabetic mothers. This shows the need to look for ethnic and nationality specific birthweight criteria, as possibly 4,000 g may be too high a weight to diagnose macrosomia in the Indian population.

There is epidemiologic evidence that persons exposed to maternal diabetes in utero have an increased risk of obesity and abnormal glucose tolerance as children and young adults. The associations have been reported even for offspring of women with gestational diabetes *(12, 17, 48, 77)*. While these consequences of gestational diabetes on fetal programing have been studied in the developed world, data evaluating this in third world countries are sparse.

Short- and Long-Term Consequences of Maternal Complications and Consequences

Maternal risks of GDM have been reported in developing nations. Siribaddana et al. *(39)* showed that GDM is associated with a higher risk of caesarean delivery ($P < 0.01$, RR 2.50, 95% CI = 1.56–3.95) in GDM pregnancies than in NDP. A higher incidence of hydramnios ($P < 0.01$, RR 3.41, 95% CI = 1.44–8.05) was recorded in GDM than in NDP. In a study in Iran, Keshavarz et al. *(22)* reported that women with GDM had a higher rate of stillbirth ($P < 0.001$; odds ratio 17.1, 95% CI = 4.5–65.5), hydramnios ($P < 0.001$; odds ratio 15.5, 95% CI = 4.8–50.5), gestational hypertension ($P < 0.001$; odds ratio 6, 95% CI = 2.3–15.3), and cesarean delivery ($P < 0.001$).

Kale et al. *(76)* compared clinical and metabolic features of mothers with GDM and their offspring with those in nondiabetic pregnancies in Pune, India. Sixty percent of mothers with GDM and 34% of nondiabetic mothers had cesarean delivery, and 23% of mothers with GDM delivered preterm (<37 weeks).

POSTPARTUM CONSEQUENCES OF GESTATIONAL DIABETES ON THE PREVALENCE OF SUBSEQUENT DIABETES

Medical Aspects

GDM substantially increases the risk of future DM2. Risk estimates of type 2 diabetes after GDM vary from 17 to 63% within 5–16 years after pregnancy, depending upon the ethnic background of the study population and the detection method for GDM and glucose intolerance *(78)*.

Coustan et al. studied former gestational diabetic women and found diabetes or IGT in 6% of those tested at 0–2 years, 13% at 3–4 years, 15% at 5–6 years, and 30% at 7–10 years postpartum *(79)*. Kim et al. analyzed 28 studies and showed that after the index pregnancy, the cumulative incidence of diabetes ranged from 2.6 to over 70% in studies that examined women 6 weeks postpartum to 28 years postpartum. Cumulative incidence of type 2 diabetes increased markedly in the first 5 years after delivery, with ~50% of women with GDM expected to develop type 2 diabetes within 5 years of the index pregnancy, and appeared to plateau after 10 years. An elevated fasting glucose level during pregnancy was the risk factor most commonly associated with future risk of type 2 diabetes. Differences in rates of progression between ethnic groups were reduced by adjustment for various lengths of follow-up and testing rates, so that women appeared to progress to type 2 diabetes at similar rates after a diagnosis of GDM *(80)*.

Catalano et al. *(81)* quoted the original studies by O'Sullivan that reported that the 15-year prevalence of type 2 diabetes in women with a history of gestational diabetes was approximately 60% in obese women during pregnancy and 30% in lean women at the time of diagnosis. The greatest risk factor for early-onset type 2 diabetes after pregnancy was early gestational age at the time of diagnosis and elevated fasting glucose. The greatest long-term risk factor was maternal obesity.

Peters et al. *(82)* found that episodes of insulin resistance due to additional pregnancies increased the rate of developing type 2 diabetes independent of pregnancy-associated weight gain. They also found that the RR for type 2 diabetes was 1.95 for each 10 pounds gained during follow-up after adjusting for the number of pregnancies and other risk factors.

Thus, one of the major long-term consequences of the increasing prevalence of gestational diabetes is an increase in the numbers of people affected with diabetes. As can be seen from Table 1, it is estimated that the numbers of people affected with diabetes in 2025 will be around 380 million. Unfortunately, the vast brunt of this will be borne by the third world countries, which would see an increase of almost 170% as compared with 40% for developed countries. Leaving aside the medical burden on the already overstretched health systems, the economics of managing this massive increase would be overwhelming, not only for governments but also for the individual patients *(2)*.

Economic Aspects

Global health expenditures to treat and prevent diabetes and its complications will total at least USD 232.0 billion in 2007. By 2025, this number will exceed USD 302.5 billion.

Expressed in international dollars (ID), which correct for differences in purchasing power, at least ID 286.1 billion of goods and services will be consumed for diabetes in 2007, and at least ID 381.1

billion in 2025. More than half of this will be spent in the USA. The European region will spend about half of the US amount (25%), and 12.5% of global spending will be spent in the Western Pacific Region, including Australia, China, Japan, and Korea. The remaining 9.2% of global spending will be divided among South-East Asia, the Eastern Mediterranean and Middle East, South and Central America, Africa, and the remainder of North America. India, the country with the largest population of persons living with diabetes, will spend an estimated USD 2.0 billion while the 47 countries in the African region will spend, in total, USD 0.7 billion for diabetes (2). Thus, more than 80% of expenditures for medical care for diabetes are made in the world's economically richest countries, not in the low- and middle-income countries where 80% of persons with diabetes will soon live. By 2025, if the resources devoted to diabetes in low- and middle-income countries are not increased, this disparity will widen (2).

The world suffers huge losses in the form of foregone economic growth as a result of diabetes. Lost economic growth may be a relatively greater problem in poorer countries. Between 2005 and 2015, the WHO predicts net losses in national income from diabetes and cardiovascular disease of ID 557.7 billion in China, ID 303.2 billion in the Russian Federation, ID 336.6 billion in India, ID 49.2 billion in Brazil, and ID 2.5 billion in the United Republic of Tanzania. These losses arise from the premature death and disability that untreated diabetes causes. Perhaps 25 million years of life are lost annually to mortality caused by diabetes. Reduced quality of life may reach a similar magnitude among the living (2).

CAN WE REDUCE THE FUTURE RISK OF DIABETES IN WOMEN WITH GESTATIONAL DIABETES?

Studies of diabetes prevention strategies (83–91) have shown what can be termed "mixed results." Lifestyle, acarbose, metformin, and thiazolinediones have all been studied. In the rosiglitazone arm of the DREAM trial, people from the Indian subcontinent, unlike others, showed the least benefit of drug compared with other ethnicities. Possibly this may have to do with the lesser degree of obesity or to genetic differences when compared with the subjects from developed countries (91). Ethnicity may need to be considered when designing diabetes prevention strategies that employ pharmaceuticals.

CONCLUSION

There are scarce data on the epidemiology and health and socioeconomic consequences of gestational diabetes and diabetes in the third world. One of the main reasons for this is that these diseases have not received adequate attention in terms of health planning and allocation of financial resources in many of the poor and transitional countries. It is essential that the health planners in the third world make diabetes diagnosis and treatment a health care priority. Guidelines for managing diabetes and GDM developed by international organizations must be disseminated to the level of the local health care provider. Cost-effective and timely diagnosis and treatment of GDM and postpartum DM2 must be widely "available," "accessible," and "affordable."

REFERENCES

1. Available at http://unpan1.un.org/intradoc/groups/public/documents/un/unpan008092.pdf Last accessed 12th August 2008
2. Diabetes Atlas, third edition © International Diabetes Federation, 2006
3. King H, Aubert R, Herman W. Global burden of diabetes, 1995–2025: prevalence, numerical estimates, and projections. Diabetes Care 1998;21:1414–1431

4. Wild S, Roglic G, Green A, et al. Global prevalence of diabetes: estimates for the year 2000 and projections for 2030. Diabetes Care 2004;27:1047–1053

5. Berkowitz G, Lapinski R, Wein R, et al. Race/ethnicity and other risk factors for gestational diabetes. Am J Epidemiol 1992;135:965–973

6. Coustan D. Gestational diabetes. In: Diabetes in America, 2nd edn. Harris MI (ed.) Bethesda, MD: National Institutes of Health, 1995, pp. 703–716

7. King H. Epidemiology of glucose intolerance and gestational diabetes in women of childbearing age. Diabetes Care 1998;21(Suppl. 2):B9–B13

8. Ferrara A. Increasing prevalence of gestational diabetes mellitus: a public health perspective. Diabetes Care 2007;30(Suppl. 2): S141–S146

9. King H. Epidemiology of glucose intolerance and gestational diabetes in women of childbearing age. Diabetes Care 1998;21:B9–B13

10. WHO Ad Hoc Diabetes Reporting Group. Diabetes and impaired glucose tolerance in women aged 20–39 years. World Health Stat Q 1992;45:321–327

11. Green J, Pawson I, Schumacher L, et al. Glucose tolerance in pregnancy: ethnic variation and influence of body habitus. Am J Obstet Gynecol 1990;163:86–92

12. Ferrara A, Hedderson MM, Quesenberry CP, et al. Prevalence of gestational diabetes mellitus detected by the National Diabetes Data Group or the Carpenter and Coustan plasma glucose thresholds. Diabetes Care 2002;25:1625–1630

13. Dabelea D, Snell-Bergeon J, Hartsfield C, et al. Increasing prevalence of gestational diabetes mellitus (GDM) over time and by birth cohort: Kaiser Permanente of Colorado GDM Screening Program. Diabetes Care 2005;28:579–584

14. Engelgau M, Herman W, Smith P, et al. The epidemiology of diabetes and pregnancy in the US, 1988. Diabetes Care 1995;18:1029–1033

15. Bloomgarden Z. Diabetes and pregnancy. Diabetes Care 2000;23:1699–1702

16. Lucas M, Lowe T, Bowe L, et al. Class A$_1$ gestational diabetes: a meaningful diagnosis? Obstet Gynecol 1993;82:250–265

17. Solomon C, Willett W, Carey V, et al. A prospective study of pregravid determinants of gestational diabetes mellitus. JAMA 1997;278:1078–1083

18. Beischer N, Oats J, Henry O, et al. Incidence and severity of gestational diabetes mellitus according to country of birth in women living in Australia. Diabetes 1991;40(Suppl. 2):35–38

19. Ishak M, Petocz P. Gestational diabetes among Aboriginal Australians: prevalence, time trend, and comparisons with non-Aboriginal Australians. Ethn Dis 2003;13:55–60

20. Cheung N, Wasmer G, Al-Ali J. Risk factors for gestational diabetes among Asian women. Diabetes Care 2001;24:955–956

21. Dornhorst A, Paterson C, Nicholls J, et al. High prevalence of gestational diabetes in women from ethnic minority groups. Diabet Med 1992;9:820–825

22. Keshavarz M, Cheung N, Babaee G, et al. Gestational diabetes in Iran: incidence, risk factors and pregnancy outcomes. Diabetes Res Clin Pract 2005;69:279–286

23. Hadaegh F., Tohidi M., Harati H., et al. Prevalence of gestational diabetes mellitus in southern Iran (Bandar Abbas City). Endocr Pract 2005;11:313–318

24. Larijani B, Hossein-Nezhad A, Rizvi S, et al. Cost analysis of different screening strategies for gestational diabetes mellitus. Endocr Pract 2003;9:504–509

25. Schmidt M, Duncan B, Reichelt A, et al. Gestational diabetes mellitus diagnosed with a 2-h 75-g oral glucose tolerance test and adverse pregnancy outcomes. Diabetes Care 2001;24:1151–1155

26. Seyoum B, Kiros K, Haileselase T, et al. Prevalence of gestational diabetes mellitus in rural pregnant mothers in northern Ethiopia. Diabetes Res Clin Pract 1999;46:247–251

27. Zargar A, Sheikh M, Bashir M, et al. Prevalence of gestational diabetes mellitus in Kashmiri women from the Indian subcontinent. Diabetes Res Clin Pract 2004;66:139–145

28. Seshiah V, Balaji V, Balaji M, et al. Gestational diabetes mellitus in India. J Assoc Physicians India 2004;52:707–711

29. Hill J, Krishnaveni G, Annama L, et al. Glucose tolerance in pregnancy in South India: relationships to neonatal anthropometry. Acta Obstet Gynecol Scand 2005;84(2):159–65

30. Erem C, Cihanyurdu N, Deger O, et al. Screening for gestational diabetes mellitus in northeastern Turkey (Trabzon City). Eur J Epidemiol 2003;18:39–43

31. Yalcin H, Zorlu G. Threshold value of glucose screening tests in pregnancy: could it be standardized for every population? Am J Perinatol 1996;13:317–320

32. Yang X, Hsu-Hage B, Zhang H, et al. Gestational diabetes mellitus in women of single gravidity in Tianjin City, China. Diabetes Care 2002;25:847–851

33. Al Mahroos S, Nagalla D, Yousif W, et al. A population-based screening for gestational diabetes mellitus in non-diabetic women in Bahrain. Ann Saudi Med 2005;25:129–133

34. Santos-Ayarzagoitia M, Salinas-Martinez A, Villarreal-Perez J. Gestational diabetes: validity of ADA and WHO diagnostic criteria using NDDG as the reference test. Diabetes Res Clin Pract 2006;74(3):322–328

35. Hassan A. Screening of pregnant women for gestational diabetes mellitus. J Ayub Med Coll Abbottabad 2005;17:54–58

36. Khan K. Gestational diabetes in a developing country; experience of screening at the Aga Khan University Medical Centre, Karachi. J Pak Med Assoc 1991;41:31–33

37. Jawad F, Irshaduddin P. Prevalence of gestational diabetes and pregnancy outcome in Pakistan. East Mediterr Health J 1996;2:268–273

38. Wagaarachchi P, Fernando L, Premachadra P, et al. Screening based on risk factors for gestational diabetes in an Asian population. J Obstet Gynaecol 2001;21:32–34

39. Sirihaddana S, Deshabandu R, Rajapakse D, et al. The prevalence of gestational diabetes in a Sri Lankan antenatal clinic. Ceylon Med J 1998;43(2):88–91

40. The HAPO Study Cooperative Research Group. Hyperglycemia and adverse pregnancy outcomes. N Engl J Med 2008;358:1991–2002

41. International Diabetes Federation. The IDF consensus worldwide definition of the metabolic syndrome, Available at http://www.idf.org/webdata/docs/IDF_Metasyndrome_definition.pdf Last Accessed 16th August 2006

42. Buchanan T, Xiang A. Gestational diabetes mellitus. J Clin Invest 2005;115:485–491

43. Di Cianni G, Miccoli R, Volpe L, et al. Intermediate metabolism in normal pregnancy and in gestational diabetes. Diabetes Metab Res Rev 2003;19:259–270

44. Perkins J, Dunn J, Jagasia S. Perspectives in gestational diabetes mellitus: a review of screening, diagnosis, and treatment. Clin Diabetes 2007;25:57–62

45. Chu S, Callaghan W, Kim S, et al. Maternal obesity and risk of gestational diabetes mellitus. Diabetes Care 2007;30(8):2070–2076

46. Barbour L, McCurdy C, Hernandez T, et al. Cellular mechanisms for insulin resistance in normal pregnancy and gestational diabetes. Diabetes Care 2007;30(Suppl. 2):S112–S119

47. Buchanan T, Xiang A, Kjos S, et al. What is gestational diabetes? Diabetes Care 2007;30(Suppl. 2):S105–S111

48. Setji T, Brown A, Feinglos M. Gestational diabetes mellitus. Clin Diabetes 2005;23(1):17–24

49. Retnakaran R, Hanley A, Connelly P et al. Ethnicity modifies the effect of obesity on insulin resistance in pregnancy: a comparison of Asian, South Asian, and Caucasian women. J Clin Endocrinol Metab 2006;91(1):93–97

50. Xiong X, Saunders L, Wang F, et al. Gestational diabetes mellitus: prevalence, risk factors, maternal and infant outcomes. Int J Gynaecol Obstet 2001;75:221–228

51. Wolf M, Sauk J, Shah A, et al. Inflammation and glucose intolerance: a prospective study of gestational diabetes mellitus. Diabetes Care 2004;27:21–27

52. Ategbo J, Grissa O, Yessoufou A, et al. Modulation of adipokines and cytokines in gestational diabetes and macrosomia. J Clin Endocrinol Metab 2006;91(10):4137–4143

53. Kahn S, Zinman B, Haffner S, et al. Obesity is a major determinant of the association of C-reactive protein levels and the metabolic syndrome in type 2 diabetes. Diabetes 2006;55(8):2357–2364

54. Retnakaran R., Hanley A, Raif N, et al. C-reactive protein and gestational diabetes: the central role of maternal obesity. J Clin Endocrinol Metab 2003;88:3507–3512

55. Retnakaran R., Hanley A, Raif N, et al. Reduced adiponectin concentration in women with gestational diabetes: a potential factor in progression to type 2 diabetes. Diabetes Care 2004;27:799–800

56. Richardson AC, Carpenter MW. Inflammatory mediators in gestational diabetes mellitus. Obstet Gynecol Clin North Am 2007;34:213–224

57. Desoye G, Hauguel-de Mouzon S. The human placenta in gestational diabetes mellitus. The insulin and cytokine network. Diabetes Care 2007;30:S120–S126

58. Abate N, Garg A, Peshock RM, Stray-Gundersen J, Grundy SM. Relationships of generalized and regional adiposity to insulin sensitivity in men. J Clin Invest 1995;96:88–98

59. Raji A, Seely EW, Arky RA, Simonson DC. Body fat distribution and insulin resistance in healthy Asian Indians and Caucasians. J Clin Endocrinol Metab 2001;86:5366–5371

60. Joshi R. Metabolic syndrome – emerging clusters of the Indian phenotype. J Assoc Physicians India 2003;51:445–446

61. Nahum G, Huffaker B. Racial differences in oral glucose screening test results: establishing race-specific criteria for abnormality in pregnancy. Obstet Gynecol 1993;81:517–522

62. Esakoff T, Cheng Y, Caughey A. Screening for gestational diabetes: different cut-offs for different ethnicities? Am J Obstet Gynecol 2005;193:1040–1044

63. ADA. Position statement: gestational diabetes mellitus. Diabetes Care 2004;27:S88–S90

64. Metzger B, Coustan D. Organizing Committee: summary and recommendations of the Fourth International Workshop-Conference on Gestational Diabetes Mellitus. Diabetes Care 1998;21(Suppl. 2):B161–B167

65. de Sereday M, Damiano M, Gonzalez C, et al. Diagnostic criteria for gestational diabetes in relation to pregnancy outcome. J Diabetes Complications 2003;17(3):115–119

66. Vitoratos N, Salamalekis E, Bettas P, et al. Which is the threshold glycose value for further investigation in pregnancy? Clin Exp Obstet Gynecol 1997;24(3):171–173

67. Senanayake H, Seneviratne S, Ariyaratne H, et al. Screening for gestational diabetes mellitus in southern Asian women. J Obstet Gynaecol Res 2006;32(3):286–291

68. Brody S, Harris R, Lohr K. Screening for gestational diabetes: a summary of the evidence for the U.S. Preventive Services Task Force. Obstet Gynecol 2003;101:380–392

69. Sadikot S, Nigam A, Das S, et al. The burden of diabetes and impaired glucose tolerance in India using the WHO 1999 criteria: prevalence of diabetes in India study (PODIS). Diabetes Res Clin Pract 2004;66(3):301–307

70. Sadikot S, Nigam A, Das S, et al. The burden of diabetes and impaired fasting glucose in India using the ADA 1997 criteria: prevalence of diabetes in India study (PODIS). Diabetes Res Clin Pract 2004;66(3):293–300

71. Available at http://www.rediff.com/money/2006/aug/10capita.htm Last accessed 12th March 2008

72. Available at http://www.indiatogether.org/2006/mar/ddz-povline.htm Last accessed 12th March 2008

73. Human Development Report 2006, United Nations. http://hdr.undp.org/hdr2006

74. Available at http://www.thehindubusinessline.com/2004/04/09/stories/2004040900090900.htm Last accessed 12th August 2008

75. Available at http://timesofindia.indiatimes.com/articleshow/1850075.cms Last accessed 12th August 2008

76. Kale S, Kulkarni S, Lubree H, et al. Characteristics of gestational diabetic mothers and their babies in an Indian diabetes clinic. J Assoc Physicians India 2005;53:857–63

77. Kjos A, Buchanan T. Gestational diabetes mellitus. N Engl J Med 1999;341:1749–1756

78. Löbner K, Knopff A, Baumgarten A, et al. Predictors of postpartum diabetes in women with gestational diabetes mellitus. Diabetes 2006;55:792–797

79. Coustan D, Carpenter M, O'Sullivan P, et al. Gestational diabetes mellitus: predictors of subsequent disordered glucose metabolism. Am J Obstet Gynecol 1993;168:1139–1145

80. Kim C, Newton K, Knopp R. Gestational diabetes and the incidence of type 2 diabetes. Diabetes Care 2002;25:1862–1868

81. Catalano P, Kirwan J, Haugel-de Mouzon S, et al. Gestational diabetes and insulin resistance: role in short- and long-term implications for mother and fetus. J Nutr 2003;133:1674S–1683S

82. Peters R, Kjos S, Xiang A, et al. Long-term diabetogenic effect of single pregnancy in women with previous gestational diabetes mellitus. Lancet 1996;347:227–230

83. Carr D, Gabbe S. Gestational diabetes: detection, management, and implications. Clin Diabetes 1998;16(1):4–13

84. Buchanan T, Xiang A, Kjos S, et al. Antepartum predictors of the development of type 2 diabetes in Latino women 11–26 months after pregnancies complicated by gestational diabetes. Diabetes 1999;48:2430–2436

85. Buchanan T, Xiang A, Peters R, et al. Preservation of pancreatic beta cell function and prevention of type 2 diabetes by pharmacological treatment of insulin resistance in high-risk Hispanic women. Diabetes 2002;51:2796–2803

86. Tuomilehto J, Lindstrom J, Eriksson J, et al. Prevention of type 2 diabetes mellitus by changes in lifestyle among subjects with impaired glucose tolerance. N Engl J Med 2001;344:1343–1350

87. Knowler W, Barrett-Conner E, Fowler S, et al. Diabetes Prevention Program Research Group.: Reduction in the incidence of type 2 diabetes with life style intervention or metformin. N Engl J Med 2002;346:393–403

88. Pan X, Li G, Hu Y, et al. Effects of diet and exercise in preventing NIDDM in people with impaired glucose tolerance. Diabetes Care 1997;20:537–544

89. Ramachandran A, Snehalatha C, Mary S, et al. The Indian Diabetes Prevention Programme shows that lifestyle modification and metformin prevent type 2 diabetes in Asian Indian subjects with impaired glucose tolerance (IDPP-1). Diabetologia 2006;49:289–297

90. Chiasson J, Josse R, Gomis R, et al. Acarbose for prevention of type 2 diabetes mellitus: the STOP-NIDDM randomised trial. Lancet 2002;359:2072–2077

91. DREAM Trial Investigators. DREAM: Effect of ramapril on the incidence of diabetes. N Engl J Med 2006;355:1551–1562

92. DREAM Trial Investigators. Effect of rosiglitazone on the frequency of diabetes in patients with impaired glucose tolerance or impaired fasting glucose: randomised controlled trial. Lancet 2006;368:1096–1105

13 Gestational Diabetes Mellitus: Diagnosis, Maternal and Fetal Outcomes, and Management

Assiamira Ferrara and Catherine Kim

CONTENTS

ABSTRACT

Gestational diabetes mellitus (GDM), or diabetes first recognized during pregnancy, is associated with increased risk of adverse perinatal outcomes. After GDM delivery, both mothers and offspring are at risk for long-term chronic disease. Clinical recognition and treatment of GDM may reduce peripartum risk, but there is a lack of consensus on how to define, screen and treat GDM. There is also a lack of information on how treatment affects long-term outcomes as well as precise information on the prevalence of long-term outcomes. Consensus regarding the definition of GDM may be achieved in the next several years with completion of the HAPO trial, but further study on the long-term effects of oral medications other than insulin is needed, and greater attention needs to be devoted to improving postpartum screening and to the follow-up and intervention for women and offspring to improve long-term outcomes.

Key words: Gestational diabetes mellitus; Pregnancy; Screening; Medication; Diabetes; Postpartum; Maternal; Fetal

Gestational diabetes mellitus (GDM), or diabetes first recognized during pregnancy, is associated with increased risk of adverse perinatal outcomes *(1, 2)*. While the risk is lower in GDM women than

From: *Diabetes in Women: Pathophysiology and Therapy*
Edited by: A. Tsatsoulis et al. (eds.), DOI 10.1007/978-1-60327-250-6_13
© Humana Press, a part of Springer Science+Business Media, LLC 2009

in women with preexisting diabetes, infants affected by GDM are at increased risk for peripartum complications such as macrosomia, hypoglycemia, hyperbilirubinemia, hypocalcemia, polyhydramnios, birth trauma and mortality. Women with GDM are also at increased risk for preeclampsia and Cesarean delivery *(3–5)*. After GDM delivery, offspring are at greater risk for obesity and diabetes *(6, 7)*, and mothers are at greater risk for diabetes and cardiovascular disease *(8, 9)*. Clinical recognition and treatment of GDM may reduce peripartum risks *(10)*. However, there is a lack of consensus on how to define, screen and treat GDM.

DIAGNOSTIC CRITERIA AND SCREENING PROCEDURES FOR GESTATIONAL DIABETES MELLITUS

Diagnostic Criteria

In several countries, the 100-g 3-h oral glucose tolerance test (OGTT) is used to diagnose GDM. The diagnostic glucose thresholds using the 100-g 3-h OGTT were first published by O'Sullivan and Mahan in 1964 *(11)* and were based on their ability to predict maternal diabetes subsequent to pregnancy. In this study, the medium assayed was whole blood, and the laboratory method used (Somogyi–Nelson) assayed for all reducing substances including glucose. In 1979, the National Diabetes Data Group (NDDG) *(12)* proposed glucose thresholds higher than those proposed by O'Sullivan and Mahan, based on a conversion from whole blood to plasma glucose, but not considering differences in the assay method. In 1982, Carpenter and Coustan *(13)* further modified the O'Sullivan and Mahan thresholds by including a correction to the assay for reducing substances to those specific for glucose. A study conducted by Sacks et al. *(14)* confirmed the validity of the correction proposed by Carpenter and Coustan. In 1998, the Fourth International Workshop Conference on GDM *(15)* noticed the need for more data linking pregnancy glycemia to perinatal adverse outcomes and proposed that until more data would be available, the Carpenter and Coustan thresholds be used for the interpretation of the 100-g, 3-h OGTT. In 2000, the American Diabetes Association (ADA) *(16)* endorsed the recommendations of the Fourth International Workshop Conference. The newly recommended ADA thresholds were lower than those of the NDDG (Table 1).

THREE-HOUR ORAL GLUCOSE TOLERANCE TEST THRESHOLDS

The rationale for revising the glucose thresholds downward included data suggesting that maternal glucose levels lower than the NDDG thresholds were associated with increased risk of adverse perinatal outcomes. Several studies *(17–20)* have examined the association between the ADA thresholds with perinatal complications among white women who did not meet the NDDG criteria. Magee et al. *(17)* reported that among 34 women who met only the ADA criteria, the average percentage incidence

Table 1
American Diabetes Association (ADA) and 1979 National Diabetes Data Group (NDDG) Gestational Diabetes Thresholds on the 3-h, 100-g Oral Glucose Tolerance Test

	ADA (mg/dl)	NDDG (mg/dl)	ADA (mmol/l)	NDDG (mmol/l)
Fasting	95	105	5.3	5.8
1 h	180	190	10	10.5
2 h	155	165	8.6	9.1
3 h	140	145	7.8	8

By both criteria, GDM is defined as at least two plasma glucose measurements during the diagnostic test at or higher than the reported cutoff of the composite measure of 33 possible perinatal complications was 41% higher than that in women with normal screening. The Toronto Tri-Hospital Gestational Diabetes project found that the proportion of infants with birth weight greater than 4,500 g was higher among 115 women who met only the ADA thresholds than among 2,940 women with otherwise normal test results (6.1% vs. 1.9%) *(19)*. Ricart et al. reported that after controlling for possible confounders, the risk of macrosomia (defined as birth weight greater than 4,000 g) was somewhat higher in 263 women who met only the ADA criteria than in 6,350 women with normal test results (OR 1.45; 95% CI 0.83–2.52) *(18)*. In 2006, Ferrara et al. *(20)* showed that in a multiethnic cohort (n = 45,245), women who did not meet the NDDG criteria, but who did exceed the Carpenter and Coustan plasma glucose thresholds, were at an increased risk of delivering an infant with macrosomia, hypoglycemia or hyperbilirubinemia. The risk of these complications appeared to increase with increasing number of glucose values exceeding the ADA thresholds.

Two-Hour Oral Glucose Tolerance Test Thresholds

In 1999, the need to lower the plasma glucose thresholds obtained during the 75-g, 2-h OGTT was addressed *(21)*. At this time, the World Health Organization (WHO) recommended diagnosing women formerly classified as having impaired glucose tolerance (IGT) with diabetes, by lowering the plasma glucose cutoff previously used *(22)*. The diagnostic cutoff were changed from a fasting plasma glucose of 7.8 to 7.0 mmol/l and a 2-h plasma glucose of 11.1 to 7.8 mmol/l. While the ADA recommended the 3-h 100-g OGTT for the diagnosis of GDM, it also stated that the 2-h 75-g OGTT was used for the diagnosis of GDM to apply the same glucose cutoffs recommended for the 3-h 100-g OGTT *(16)*. GDM was defined as at least two values exceeding the threshold values of a fasting glucose of 5.3 mmol/l, a 1-h glucose of 10 mmol/l, or a 2-h glucose of 8.6 mmol/l. In 2001, Schmidt et al. *(23)* reported that GDM diagnosed by either set of criteria predicted perinatal complications of macrosomia, preeclampsia and fetal death. Twenty-two women were diagnosed with GDM by the ADA criteria alone and 260 women were diagnosed by WHO criteria; the frequency of complications did not differ between groups. Of note, the population attributable fraction of any of these complications due to GDM was low, emphasizing that GDM was not the only factor contributing to poor outcomes *(24)*, although GDM is one factor that is treatable.

Screening Procedures

Universal vs. Selective Screening

In addition to the lack of consensus on the precise definition of GDM, there is a lack of consensus regarding who to screen, whether to use a one step vs. two step approach, and when to test. The American College of Obstetricians and Gynecologists (ACOG) notes that women at low risk for GDM do not necessarily have to be screened, but that universal screening may be a more practical approach *(25)*. The ADA recommends that women be screened if they have average or high-risk characteristics, including age greater than or equal to 25 years, overweight or obesity [defined as a body mass index (BMI) of greater than or equal to 25 kg/m^2], nonwhite race/ethnicity, a first degree relative with diabetes mellitus, history of abnormal glucose tolerance, or history of poor obstetric outcome *(26)*. Approximately 10% of women avoid testing using this approach while 97% cases of GDM detected by universal screening are found *(27)*. Naylor et al. *(28)* developed a risk calculator that assigned points to each specific risk factor. Women who scored one or no points were not screened, while other women underwent further testing; 35% of women were able to avoid further testing altogether. This approach had similar detection rates of GDM compared with universal screening, although race was categorized as white, black, Asian, and other, making application to mixed race-ethnic populations difficult.

ONE-STEP VS. TWO-STEP PROTOCOLS

There has also been considerable debate about the use of one-step vs. two-step protocols for the diagnosis of GDM *(29)*. One-step protocols, such as the 2-h 75-g OGTT, require all eligible women to be screened on a single day, whereas two-step protocols specify that eligible women undergo a 1-h 50-g screen. Women who exceed cutoff on the initial screen then proceed to a 3-h 100-g OGTT. The sensitivity of the 1-h 50-g screen is improved if the lower threshold is used. At the 130 mg/dl cutoff, the test is positive in 20–25% of women and detects 90% of women with GDM; at the 140 mg/dl cutoff, 14–18% of women will have positive tests and 80% of women with GDM will be detected *(13, 30)*.

The 50-g screen itself is influenced by testing procedures, such as gestational age at testing *(31)*. Watson et al. administered 1-h 50-g glucose screens to gravidas who were at 20, 28, and 34 weeks of gestational age *(31)*. Women had previously been demonstrated to have a glucose level less than 140 mg/dl. In cross-sectional analyses, the average increase in glucose levels was 1.1 mg/dl per week. A similar magnitude of change was observed in longitudinal analysis where women underwent 1-h 50-g glucose screens in the first and then again in the third trimester *(32)*. Therefore, women who had glucose levels less than 110 mg/dl in the first trimester were unlikely to exceed 135 mg/dl in the third trimester.

While only a single nonfasting blood draw is obtained during the 1-h 50-g screen, the test may also be influenced by the time of day. McElduff and Hitchman *(33)* found that women who had testing performed in the afternoon had elevated results compared with those found in the morning. Aparicio et al. *(34)* found that when the same cohort of women received the screen in the morning as well as the afternoon, the afternoon glucose levels were significantly elevated.

The 1-h 50-g screen may be influenced by the time since the last meal *(35)*. Sermer et al. *(35)* found that women had higher glucose levels associated with longer fasts. Coustan et al. *(30)* also found that a meal 1 h prior to testing was associated with lower glucose levels than an overnight fast, but only among women with GDM; women without dysglycemia did not have significant differences in their glucose levels whether fasting or fed. Presumably, this finding is attributable to the need for greater insulin secretion associated with increasing glucose levels, even in the absence of preconceptional diabetes *(36)*, although this association has not been replicated *(37)*.

The variation introduced by the 1-h 50-g screen may or may not be outweighed by its greater convenience compared with the 2-h 75-g OGTT. The one-step protocol requires women to be tested in the morning, after a 12-h fast, following 3 days of a diet with at least 150 g of carbohydrate per day. However, in the two-step procedure, only women with abnormal 1-h 50-g screens are required to go onto more intensive screening.

Guidelines recommend that screening be performed at 24–28 weeks of gestational age *(26)*. As noted earlier, women may have less insulin resistance earlier in pregnancy and may have false-negative screens, although screening earlier in pregnancy may detect undiagnosed type 2 diabetes, which would place the fetus at higher risk.

Hyperglycemia and Adverse Pregnancy Outcome (HAPO) Study

A primary aim of the HAPO Trial was to establish uniform GDM screening criteria based on maternal and fetal outcomes *(38)*. A total of 25,505 pregnant women at 15 centers in 9 countries underwent 2-h 75-g OGTTs between 24 and 32 weeks of gestation. Primary outcomes included macrosomia, Cesarean delivery and neonatal hypoglycemia. Secondary outcomes included delivery before 37 weeks, shoulder dystocia or other birth injury, hyperbilirubinemia and preeclampsia. While the risk of adverse pregnancy outcomes uniformly increased with greater glucose levels, no threshold existed, making the decision regarding cutoffs difficult. The risk of macrosomia increased approximately fivefold as fasting glucose increased above 75 mg/dl, 1-h glucose increased above 105 mg/dl, or 2-h glucose increased above 90 mg/dl. In other words, a fasting glucose greater than or equal to 100 mg/dl was associated with a risk of macrosomia five times that of a fasting glucose less than 75 mg/dl, with absolute macrosomia rates of 25% vs. 5%. Correlation with other outcomes was less marked, although still significant. HAPO excluded women with severe hyperglycemia from the analysis (fasting glucose greater than 105 mg/dl or 2-h glucose greater than 200 mg/dl), so the association actually underestimated the strength of the correlation by excluding women with extremely elevated glucose. An initial recommendation for screening cutoffs incorporating the HAPO results is expected later in 2009.

Following the publication of the consensus opinion, it is likely that medical organizations may eliminate the two-step procedure, as HAPO did not perform an initial screen. Whether the diagnostic test will include the measurement of fasting glucose only or the performance of a 75-g OGTT with measurements of fasting glucose and measurement of plasma glucose 1 h and 2 h after the 75-g oral glucose load still awaits determination as well. As HAPO focused on women with only mild hyperglycemia, women with preexisting diabetes would presumably be detected by these definitions as well.

MANAGEMENT OF GESTATIONAL DIABETES

Treatment of GDM is aimed at reducing the morbidity associated with elevated glycemic levels. In the Australian Carbohydrate Intolerance Study in Pregnant Women (ACHOIS) Trial, women with GDM were randomized between 24 and 34 weeks of gestational age to receive routine care or intervention (10). Intervention consisted of dietary advice, blood glucose monitoring and insulin therapy as needed. Outcomes of interest included macrosomia, perinatal complications as represented by a composite outcome including death, shoulder dystocia, bone fracture, nerve palsy and admission to the neonatal intensive care unit. Women in the intervention group had lower rates of macrosomia (10% vs. 21%) and perinatal complications (1% vs. 4%), a similar rate of Cesarean delivery, and a higher rate of induction and admission to the intensive care unit (71% vs. 61%) vs. women in routine care. Other outcomes, particularly hypoglycemia requiring therapy and jaundice, were not affected. Additionally, mood and quality of life scores were significantly better among women in the intervention group than among the control.

Medical Nutritional Therapy and Exercise

A mainstay of treatment is medical nutritional therapy and lifestyle intervention (39). Calorie allotment is based upon ideal body weight, with a suggested caloric intake based on BMI (40). Forty kilocalories per kg current weight per day is recommended in pregnant women with BMIs less than 22 kg/m², 30 kcal per kg current weight per day for women with BMIs of 22–25 kg/m², 24 kcal per kg current weight per day for women with BMIs of 26–29 kg/m², and 12 kcal per kg per current weight per day for women who have BMIs greater than or equal to 30 kg/m². Based on management of women with preconceptional diabetes, carbohydrate intake (ideally complex carbohydrates found in starches and vegetables) is restricted to 33–40% of calories, with the remainder divided between protein and fat (26).

Adherence to the regimen yields normoglycemia in four-fifths of women, with the remainder requiring more intensive therapy (26). However, normoglycemia may not lead to reduction of macrosomia or Cesarean delivery. In a Cochrane meta-analysis of 612 women, women treated with dietary therapy vs. no specific treatment had no differences in macrosomia rates (OR 0.78, 95% CI 0.45–1.35) or Cesarean deliveries (OR 0.97, 95% CI 0.65–1.44) *(41)*. As noted under diagnostic screening, the attributable risk of macrosomia to GDM was low, and other factors, particularly mother's body weight, contribute *(23)*.

Obesity is a risk factor for GDM, and in 1990 the Institute of Medicine issued the first weight-gain recommendations for pregnancy *(42)*. In addition to blood glucose levels, women with GDM need to be aware of optimal weight gain, as there is a strong correlation between infant birth weight and pregravid BMI, even after adjustment for insulin levels *(43)*. In addition, pregnancy weight gain, after adjustment for glucose levels, is also associated with neonatal hypoglycemia and hyper-bilirubinemia *(43)*. Women with normal BMI (19.8–26.0 kg/m^2) are recommended to gain a total of 25–35 lb or 11.4–15.9 kg. Women with BMIs between 26.1 and 29.0 kg/m^2 should gain between 15 and 25 lb or 6.8 and 11.4 kg. Obese women with BMI greater than 29 k/m^2 are supposed to gain 15 lb *(42)*.

Cardiovascular conditioning may improve peripheral insulin sensitivity and may reduce fasting and postprandial glucose concentrations *(44)* to the extent that insulin is not needed *(45)*. Jovanovic-Peterson et al. *(45)* found that women randomized to arm ergometry several times a week were able to decrease fasting glucose concentrations as well as postchallenge glucose levels, and Bung et al. *(46)* found that women randomized to bicycle exercise had similar mean glucose values and macro-somia rates as insulin-treated controls. No significant complications were observed in the exercise arms, although the numbers were small. Therefore, moderate exercise, in the absence of medical contraindications, is encouraged during pregnancy for GDM women.

Blood Glucose Monitoring

To monitor response to therapy, women with GDM are expected to measure their blood glucose concentration upon awakening and 1 h after each meal. Laird and McFarland *(47)* noted that among 52 pregnant women, fasting glucose did not predict who would need insulin. Among women with GDM who were using insulin, 1-h postprandial monitoring and consequent insulin adjustment was associated with better glycemic control, significantly reduced rates of macrosomia and lower rates of Cesarean delivery than fasting levels *(48)*. Of note, most blood glucose meters report glucose directly from whole blood, as opposed to plasma glucose, but some meters will multiply the whole blood result by a constant to obtain a plasma glucose equivalent. It is, therefore, important to know how the glucose concentration is measured by the patient's particular meter.

There is not a consensus on when insulin or other medications should be initiated. Reduction of macrosomia is a commonly used intermediate end point, and ACOG recommends initiating insulin when fasting glucose is greater than or equal to 5.3 mmol/l (95 mg/dl), 1-h glucose is greater than or equal to 7.2 mmol/l (130 mg/dl), or 2-h glucose is greater than or equal to 6.7 mmol/l (120 mg/dl) *(25)*. However, as indicated by the HAPO results, risks for macrosomia increase at lower levels of glucose continuously, so lower cutoffs could be justified *(5)*. Therefore, some advocate the use of lower cutoffs of approximately 5 mmol/l for fasting glucose (90 mg/dl) and 6.7 mmol/l for 1-h post-prandial glucose (120 mg/dl) *(49)*.

Medications

Women may have persistent hyperglycemia despite medical nutritional therapy and exercise. To improve macrosomia and morbidities, they may then initiate insulin or oral antihyperglycemic therapy. There is not a consensus on who should receive insulin therapy as opposed to other agents.

INSULIN

The dose of insulin is initiated in accord with fasting and postprandial glucose concentrations, although the dose eventually required varies with underlying insulin resistance. If fasting glucose levels are elevated, an intermediate-acting insulin such as NPH is given before bedtime at an initial dose of 0.2 U/kg body mass. If postprandial glucose concentrations are elevated, a short-acting insulin, such as insulin lispro at 1–1.5 U per 10 g carbohydrate, is also given. Women may undergo four injections per day if both occur. As insulin resistance increases as the pregnancy progresses, the dose will change over time, by as much as a total of 1.0 U/kg total between the first and third trimesters. Doses may need to be adjusted as much as 2.0 U/kg to overcome changes in weight, especially in women who are morbidly obese at baseline. Insulin is typically divided so that half is given as intermediate acting and half is given as three preprandial short-acting injections *(50)*. In the event of acute hypoglycemia, 10–20 g of carbohydrate addresses symptoms immediately, followed by a reduction in the amount of insulin, with each of unit of insulin lowering blood glucose by 25 mg/dl.

Instead of using glucose results to initiate or adjust insulin, as is commonly done, more direct evidence of fetal hyperinsulinemia has been used *(51)*. Targeting insulin administration to women with ultrasound evidence (greater than 75th percentile abdominal circumference early in the third trimester) may more accurately target treatment to macrosomia and avoid treatment of women at lower risk *(51)*. Kjos et al. *(51)* randomized women to intervention vs. insulin therapy, with the intervention women receiving insulin if fetal abdominal circumference was greater than or equal to 70th percentile of weight or if fasting plasma glucose measurements were greater than or equal to 120 mg/dl. Macrosomia was similar between groups, along with a broad range of neonatal outcomes including hypoglycemia requiring intravenous glucose, jaundice requiring phototherapy, birth trauma and transfusion. Thirty-eight percent of women in the experimental group avoided insulin. See Chap. 18 for more details.

ORAL ANTIHYPERGLYCEMIC AGENTS

Glyburide   While not endorsed by medical organizations in the USA, oral antihyperglycemic gents are commonly used in other countries for the treatment of hyperglycemia during GDM pregnancies. The two in common usage are glyburide, an insulin secretagogue, and metformin, an insulin sensitizer.

Langer et al. *(52)* randomized 404 women with GDM who required therapy beyond nutrition and exercise. Women were randomly assigned between 11 and 33 weeks of gestation to receive glyburide or insulin, with adjustments made as necessary to achieve normoglycemia. Secondary end points included maternal and neonatal complications. While 4% of women in the glyburide group eventually required insulin therapy, there were no significant differences between the glyburide and insulin groups in the percentage of infants who were large for gestational age (12 and 13%, respectively); who had macrosomia, defined as a birth weight of 4,000 g or more (7 and 4%); who had lung complications (8 and 6%); who had hypoglycemia (9 and 6%); who were admitted to a neonatal intensive care unit (6 and 7%); or who had fetal anomalies (2 and 2%). The cord-serum insulin concentrations were similar in the two groups, and glyburide was not detected in the cord serum of any infant in the glyburide group. However, the study was not necessarily powered to find significant differences between groups with these rates of complications.

Theoretical concerns about glyburide include the possible acceleration of postpartum incidence of maternal diabetes and the unknown effects on the long-term development of the offspring *(53)*. In a review of the trial and other retrospective studies of glyburide use, Moore *(53)* noted that the rate of glyburide failure may be higher, in the order of 20%, particularly if the initial fasting glucose level exceeded 115 mg/dl, rates of neonatal hyperbilirubinemia might be higher among glyburide users, and that glyburide users also achieved significantly lower fasting and postprandial glucose levels. It is likely that the controversy will not be settled until larger trials, stratified by therapy, are performed.

Metformin   Metformin has not been compared directly with glyburide, although both metformin and glyburide have been compared with insulin in randomized studies. In the MiG study, Rowan et al. *(54)* randomized 751 women with GDM at 20–33 weeks of gestation to open treatment with metformin (with supplemental insulin if required) or insulin. The primary outcome was a composite of neonatal hypoglycemia, respiratory distress, need for phototherapy, birth trauma, 5-min Apgar score less than 7 or prematurity. The trial was designed to rule out a 33% increase (from 30 to 40%) in this composite outcome in infants of women treated with metformin as compared with those treated with insulin. Secondary outcomes included neonatal anthropometric measurements, maternal glycemic control, maternal hypertensive complications, postpartum glucose tolerance, and acceptability of treatment. About half of the women (46%) randomized to metformin eventually required supplemental insulin during the trial in order to achieve glycemic goals. The rate of the primary composite outcome was similar in both groups (32.0% vs. 32.2%) as was the rate of secondary outcomes, although women in the metformin group greatly preferred their assignment compared with women in the insulin group (76.6% vs. 27.2%). In the Langer et al. *(52)* trial of glyburide vs. insulin, only 4% of women randomized to glyburide eventually required insulin.

In meta-analyses of metformin observational studies *(55)*, first trimester exposure to metformin did not increase risk of major malformations, and in the MiG study, second and third trimester exposure to metformin also was not associated with malformations *(54)*. Metformin may have the added benefit of reducing the incidence of recurrent GDM among women with polycystic ovary disease, although progression to GDM was not compared to a control group not using metformin *(56)*.

Treatment or observational trials examining the impact of treatment of therapy on other outcomes, particularly long-term outcomes, have not been conducted. While macrosomia is relatively easy to measure, it may not fully capture the fetal metabolic changes associated with GDM. Neonates of women with GDM have body composition different from that of women with normal glucose tolerance *(57)*. While infants have similar birth weight across groups, fat mass, percent body fat, and subcutaneous and abdominal measures of fat are greater in the infants of women with GDM. These differences persist regardless of whether infants were large or average for gestational age *(57)*.

POSTPARTUM CARE: POSTPARTUM DIABETES SCREENING AND DIABETES RISK

Maternal Diabetes and Cardiovascular Disease Risk

GDM confers a sixfold risk for future maternal diabetes, independent of other significant risk factors such as weight, visceral adiposity and physical activity *(58, 59)*. Up to a third of women with diabetes may have been affected by prior GDM *(60)*. Additionally, GDM is associated with vascular dysfunction and future cardiovascular disease. Heitritter et al. found that women with a GDM history had greater vascular resistance, lower stroke volume and lower cardiac output than women without a GDM history *(61)*. In a cross-sectional study, Carr et al. found that women with a GDM history were more likely to have metabolic syndrome and to experience cardiovascular events than women without a GDM history and, moreover, that these cardiovascular events occurred at a younger age *(8)*. Shah et al. found that this increased risk of cardiovascular events, although low, seemed to be primarily attributable to their greater risk of diabetes *(9)*. Contraception and breastfeeding are important aspects of postpartum care addressed in other chapters, so the subsequent section addresses postpartum diabetes screening and risk factors for diabetes among women with histories of GDM.

Diagnostic Criteria and Screening Procedures for Postpartum Diabetes Mellitus

As with criteria for the index diagnosis of GDM, criteria for postpartum glucose intolerance vary between medical organizations. The primary debate is whether screening should consist of performance of a postpartum fasting glucose alone vs. a 75-g oral glucose tolerance test (OGTT). The 2007 Fifth-International Workshop Conference on GDM recommends that a 75-g OGTT be performed greater than or equal to 6 weeks postpartum to screen for maternal glucose intolerance *(62)*. The Australasian Diabetes in Pregnancy Society also endorses the 75-g OGTT. The 2003 Canadian Diabetes Association guidelines prefer the 75-g OGTT but state that the fasting glucose is acceptable *(63)*. As of 2007, the United Kingdom-based National Institute for Health and Clinical Excellence (NICE) recommends a postpartum fasting glucose only, specifically without the OGTT *(64)*. The American College of Obstetricians and Gynecologists states that evidence to support the benefit of postpartum screening is minimal, but if performed, a 75-g OGTT should be used *(25)*.

The diabetes screening guidelines of other medical organizations adopt the guidelines for general at-risk populations. The 1999/2006 WHO guidelines recommend a 75-g OGTT *(21, 65)*. The 1997/2003 ADA guidelines recommend a fasting glucose in general practice, although the guidelines recognize the OGTT as a valid diagnostic method *(66, 67)*. The United States Preventive Services Task Force (USPSTF) does not make specific recommendations for postpartum screening among women with GDM, perhaps reflecting its lack of support for GDM screening during pregnancy *(68)*.

While organizations differ as to whether or not to obtain the 2-h glucose, the cutoffs for diabetes are similar across groups: fasting glucose of 7.0 mmol/l or 126 mg/dl and, if obtained, a 2-h glucose of 11.1 mmol/l or 200 mg/dl after a 75-g challenge. The fasting glucose value of 126 mg/dl was chosen due to its threshold association with retinopathy *(69)*. The 2-h criterion of 200 mg/dl corresponded with both all-cause and cardiovascular disease mortality, as well as providing roughly the same risk as a fasting glucose of 126 mg/dl *(69)*. More sensitive criteria result in greater estimates of postpartum diabetes risk. In general, the OGTT is more sensitive than the fasting glucose alone, because the fasting glucose and 2-h glucose capture overlapping but not identical populations *(70, 71)*. However, the OGTT has greater initial cost and inconvenience, which are the drawbacks cited by the ADA and NICE *(64, 66, 67)*.

The debate over which diabetes screening test is optimal extends to postpartum women with a GDM history. Among these women, as in the general population, the fasting glucose and 2-h glucose identify distinct groups. Pallardo et al. found that among 588 postpartum GDM women, 5.8% had IFG only, 10.4% had IGT only, and only 3.7% had both *(72)*. Kitzmiller et al. found that among 527 postpartum GDM women, 6.3% had IFG only, 13.5% had elevated 2-h glucose values only, and 11.5% had abnormalities of both *(73)*. Hunt and Conway found that one-third of postpartum GDM women had an isolated 2-h value only *(74)*. Ferrara et al. found that among 600 postpartum GDM women, 16 had diabetes and 188 had IFG and/or IGT *(75)*. Only four women were diagnosed with diabetes by fasting glucose alone. Seventy-four women (39%) would have been classified as having normal glucose tolerance based on the fasting glucose value alone. Other studies also have found limited sensitivity of fasting glucose for impaired fasting glucose, impaired glucose tolerance, or DM in postpartum GDM women *(76, 77)*, particularly for IFG or IGT *(77)*.

The value of intervention for IGT women with a GDM history is assumed to be similar to that in the general population but has not been independently established. Among women with a GDM history, no cohort study documents the morbidity associated with abnormalities in the fasting value vs. the 2-h value. Similarly, among women with a GDM history, the intraindividual variation in the fasting vs. the 2-h value has not been examined. In statistical models, the postpartum OGTT is generally more advantageous among women with recent GDM *(78)*.

Performance of Postpartum Screening

Regardless of the screening criteria used, multiple reports demonstrate that performance of postpartum screening for those with a GDM history has been the exception, rather than the rule *(72, 74, 75, 79–81)*. While performance of screening has improved over the past decade, almost half of women with a GDM history do not undergo screening of any kind or undergo screening with tests such as glycosylated hemoglobins *(75, 82)*. The latter tests are not recommended as screening tests due to relatively decreased sensitivity and specificity *(69)*.

Reasons why women forego screening are speculative but include women's low perception of diabetes risk *(83)*, lack of healthcare provider perception of risk *(84, 85)*, and lack of other steps necessary for screening such as lab slip distribution or test ordering *(84, 86)*. The reasons why women forego screening may also differ between study populations. Russell et al. found that screened and unscreened women had similar glucose levels during pregnancy *(80)*, but screened women were more likely to attend the postpartum visit, suggesting that barriers to the postpartum visit also presented barriers to screening. In contrast, Smirnakis et al. found that screened women had more favorable fasting and 1-h glucose values from the index GDM diagnosis *(79)*. Even though many women were not screened, greater than 90% attended a postpartum visit, suggesting that lower risk during pregnancy influenced rates of return after pregnancy rather than postpartum visit barriers in that health system.

Quality improvement studies on this topic are few. Hunt and Conway noted that screening performance improved with nurse case-management *(74)*, including mailed reminders, telephone calls and home visits. We are not aware of other interventions aimed at improving postpartum screening. Infrequent postpartum screening leads to missed diagnoses of postpartum glucose intolerance. In addition, low performance of postpartum screening could bias estimates of future diabetes risk if screened women were different than unscreened women. In a systematic review of studies examining conversion to type 2 diabetes, Nicholson et al. found that 75% of studies included reported a loss to follow-up greater than 20% *(87)*.

In particular, retrospective cohorts including only women who have undergone the postpartum test might misrepresent risk. If women who were not screened were at lower or higher risk than women who were screened, this would overestimate and underestimate diabetes risk estimates, respectively. Indeed, women who are not screened may have greater prevalence of risk factors for diabetes, including elevated glucose levels *(74, 79)*, prior macrosomia *(72)*, poorer education *(75)*, obesity *(75)* and macrosomia with the current pregnancy*(75)*.

Risk Factors for Maternal Postpartum Diabetes Among Women with GDM

Glucose intolerance during the index GDM pregnancy, reflected by the glucose values on the 50-g glucose challenge screening test as well as the diagnostic prenatal OGTT, is associated with postpartum hyperglycemia and diabetes *(88–93)*. Because of variation in diagnostic testing procedures for GDM, as well as the continuous relationship between glucose values and future risk, no single glucose value consistently identifies women at risk for future diabetes *(88)*.

As discussed earlier in the chapter, the 50-g glucose challenge is often, but not always, performed during pregnancy as the baseline screening test for GDM. The glucose value from this screen is independently associated with postpartum hyperglycemia (88), even after adjustment for women's prenatal OGTT values (93).

The glucose values on the diagnostic prenatal OGTT, whether measured as area under the curve or as tertiles for individual values, and whether measured as part of a 75- or 100-g OGTT, predict greater maternal postpartum glucose intolerance (72, 89–99). As fasting and postchallenge glucose values detect different populations at risk for glucose intolerance in nonpregnant adults, fasting and postchallenge values on the prenatal OGTT are associated with postpartum hyperglycemia to different degrees and in different groups of pregnant women. Women with a greater number of abnormal tests, that is, elevated fasting or postchallenge values, are at greater risk for diabetes (72). The prenatal glucose area under the curve reflects an average of all of the prenatal OGTT values and reflects any abnormality in glucose metabolism, although the area under the curve does not distinguish between specific defects in insulin sensitivity or secretion.

Treatment required during the index GDM pregnancy may also reflect underlying glucose intolerance. Pregnancies requiring sulfonylureas (75) or insulin (89, 90, 92, 93, 100–104) may reflect greater glucose intolerance than pregnancies requiring lifestyle management only. Class A-2 GDM is GDM requiring insulin therapy because of fasting levels greater than or equal to 105 mg/dl; this particular category of GDM is associated with postpartum diabetes even after adjustment for the actual fasting glucose level as well as other prenatal OGTT levels (93). Women eventually placed on insulin or a sulfonylurea may still be at higher risk for future diabetes after adjustment for A2 class (75, 89, 90, 100). Treatment status may provide additional predictive value, because treatment may reflect progression of insulin resistance and/or beta-cell dysfunction later in the pregnancy, whereas prenatal OGTT levels reflect glucose metabolism at the time of diagnosis. However, treatment may reflect other health-care delivery factors such as greater likelihood of follow-up, compliance with medication and compliance with a postpartum OGTT (75).

Earlier gestational age at the time of GDM diagnosis, indicating earlier onset of glucose intolerance, has been associated with greater risk of postpartum diabetes (91–93, 96, 101, 102, 105, 106), even after consideration of the degree of elevation in glucose levels (92–94). This association is driven by pregnancies diagnosed at extremes of gestational age, as this risk was not significantly elevated when women in the middle of the gestational age distribution were included (91–93, 96, 107).

Anthropometric factors reflect adiposity, a step in the causal pathway of insulin resistance (108). While adiposity is generally associated with future glucose intolerance, different anthropometric measures reflect different types of adiposity, which in turn are associated with future diabetes to differing degrees. Greater central or visceral adiposity, as reflected by waist circumference and waist hip ratio, has stronger risk for GDM than subcutaneous adiposity or traditional measures of body mass (109).

CONCLUSIONS

GDM burdens both the fetus and mother with perinatal and long-term morbidity. While medical care has traditionally treated prenatal and postpartum care as separate conditions, glucose tolerance does not respect this boundary. Consensus regarding the definition of GDM may be achieved in the next several years with further analyses of the HAPO trial. Further study on the long-term effects of metformin and glyburide compared with insulin is needed to determine the safety of these agents and their long-term effects on glucose tolerance in the offspring and mother. Greater attention needs to be devoted to improving postpartum screening and consensus on screening guidelines.

Interventions for women with recent GDM need to be developed, in order to improve postpartum screening and maternal chronic disease prevention. Such interventions also need to be evaluated for their long-term effects on offspring. Successful interventions would leverage the tight interrelationship between maternal and child health during the unique condition of pregnancy, and in doing so, avert disease in an efficient and cost-effective manner.

REFERENCES

1. Kjos S, Buchanan T. Gestational diabetes mellitus. N Engl J Med 1999;341(23):1749–56.
2. Jovanovic L, Pettitt D. Gestational diabetes mellitus. JAMA 2001;286(20):2516–9.
3. Dodd J, Crowther C, Antoniou G, Baghurst P, Robinson J. Screening for gestational diabetes: the effect of varying blood glucose definitions in the prediction of adverse maternal and infant health outcomes. Aust N Z J Obstet Gynaecol 2007;47(4):307–12.
4. Saydah S, Chandra A, Eberhardt M. Pregnancy experience among women with and without gestational diabetes in the U.S. 1995 National Survey of Family Growth. Diabetes Care 2005;28:1035–40.
5. HAPO Study Cooperative Research Group. The hyperglycemia and adverse pregnancy outcome (HAPO) study. Int J Gynaecol Obstet 2002;78(1):69–77.
6. Dabelea D. The predisposition to obesity and diabetes in offspring of diabetic mothers. Diabetes Care 2007;30(Suppl 2):S169–74.
7. Dabelea D, Hanson R, Lindsay R, et al. Intrauterine exposure to diabetes conveys risks for type 2 diabetes and obesity: a study of discordant sibships. Diabetes 2000;49(12):2208–11.
8. Carr D, Utzschneider K, Hull R, et al. Gestational diabetes mellitus increases the risk of cardiovascular disease in women with a family history of type 2 diabetes. Diabetes Care 2006;29:2078–83.
9. Shah B, Retnakaran R, Booth G. Increased risk of cardiovascular disease in young women following gestational diabetes. Diabetes Care 2008;31(8):1668–9.
10. Crowther C, Hiller J, Moss J, et al. Effect of treatment of gestational diabetes mellitus on pregnancy outcomes. N Engl J Med 2005;352:2477–86.'
11. O'Sullivan J, Mahan C. Criteria for the oral glucose tolerance test in pregnancy. Diabetes 1964;13:278–85.
12. National Diabetes Data Group. Classification and diagnosis of diabetes mellitus and other categories of glucose intolerance. Diabetes 1979;18:1039–57.
13. Carpenter M, Coustan D. Criteria for screening tests for gestational diabetes. Am J Obstet Gynecol 1982;144(7):768–73.
14. Sacks D, Abu-Fadil S, Greenspoon J, Fotheringham N. Do the current standards for glucose tolerance testing in pregnancy represent a valid conversion of O'Sullivan's original criteria? Am J Obstet Gynecol 1989;161(3):638–41.
15. Metzger B, Coustan D. Summary and recommendations of the Fourth International Workshop-Conference on Gestational Diabetes Mellitus: the Organizing Committee. Diabetes Care 1998;21:B161–7.
16. American Diabetes Association. Clinical practice recommendations 2000. Gestational diabetes mellitus. Diabetes Care 2000;23:S77–9.
17. Magee M, Walden C, Benedetti T, Knopp R. Influence of diagnostic criteria on the incidence of gestational diabetes and perinatal morbidity. JAMA 1993;269(5):609–15.
18. Ricart W, Lopez J, Mozas J, et al. Potential impact of the American Diabetes Association (2000) criteria for the diagnosis of gestational diabetes mellitus in Spain. Diabetologia 2005;48(6):1135–41.
19. Sermer M, Naylor C, Gare D, et al. Impact of increasing carbohydrate intolerance on maternal-fetal outcomes in 3637 women without gestational diabetes. The Toronto Tri-Hospital Gestational Diabetes Project. Am J Obstet Gynecol 1995;173(1): 146–56.
20. Ferrara A, Weiss N, Hedderson M, et al. Pregnancy plasma glucose levels exceeding the American Diabetes Association thresholds, but below the National Diabetes Data Group thresholds for gestational diabetes mellitus, are related to the risk of neonatal macrosomia, hypoglycaemia, and hyperbilirubinaemia. Diabetologia 2007;50(2):298–306.
21. World Health Organization. Definition, diagnosis, and classification of diabetes mellitus and its complications: report of a WHO consultation, Part 1: Diagnosis and classification of diabetes mellitus. Geneva: World Health Organization; 1999.
22. World Health Organization. World Health Expert Committee on diabetes mellitus: second report. Geneva: World Health Organization; 1980.
23. Schmidt M, Duncan B, Reichelt A, et al. Gestational diabetes mellitus diagnosed with a 2-h 75-g oral glucose tolerance test and adverse pregnancy outcomes. Diabetes Care 2001;24(7):1151–5.
24. Pettitt D. The 75-g oral glucose tolerance test in pregnancy. Diabetes Care 2001;24(7):1129.
25. ACOG Practice Bulletin. Clinical management guidelines for obstetrician-gynecologists. Number 30, September 2001 (replaces Technical Bulletin Number 200, December 1994). Obstet Gynecol 2001;98(3):525–38.
26. American Diabetes Association. Gestational diabetes mellitus. Diabetes Care 2004;27(Suppl 1):S88–90.

27. Danilenko-Dixon D, Van Winter J, Nelson R, Ogburn P. Jr. Universal versus selective gestational diabetes screening: application of 1997 American Diabetes Association recommendations. Am J Obstet Gynecol 1999;181(4):798–802.

28. Naylor C, Sermer M, Chen E, Farine D. Selective screening for gestational diabetes mellitus: Toronto Trihospital Gestational Diabetes Project Investigators. N Engl J Med 1997;337(22):1591–6.

29. Carr S. Screening for gestational diabetes mellitus. A perspective in 1998. Diabetes Care 1998;21(Suppl 2):B14–8.

30. Coustan D, Widness J, Carpenter M, Rotondo L, Pratt D, Oh W. Should the fifty-gram, one-hour plasma glucose screening test for gestational diabetes be administered in the fasting or fed state? Am J Obstet Gynecol 1986;154(5):1031–5.

31. Watson W. Serial changes in the 50-g oral glucose test in pregnancy: implications for screening. Obstet Gynecol 1989;74(1): 40–3.

32. Nahum G, Huffaker B. Correlation between first- and early third-trimester glucose screening test results. Obstet Gynecol 1990;76(4):709–13.

33. McElduff A, Hitchman R. Screening for gestational diabetes: the time of day is important. Med J Aust 2002;176(3):136.

34. Aparicio N, Joao M, Cortelezzi M, et al. Pregnant women with impaired glucose tolerance to an oral glucose load in the afternoon. Am J Obstet Gynecol 1998;178(5):1059–66.

35. Sermer M, Naylor C, Gare D, et al. Impact of time since last meal on the gestational glucose challenge test. The Toronto Tri-Hospital Gestational Diabetes Project. Am J Obstet Gynecol 1994;171(3):607–16.

36. Berkus M, Stern M, Mitchell B, Abashawl A, Langer O. Relationships between glucose levels and insulin secretion during a glucose challenge test. Am J Obstet Gynecol 1990;163(6 Pt 1):1818–22.

37. Lewis G, McNally C, Blackman J, Polonsky K, Barron W. Prior feeding alters the response to the 50-g glucose challenge test in pregnancy. The Staub-Traugott effect revisited. Diabetes Care 1993;16(12):1551–6.

38. HAPO Study Cooperative Research Group. Hyperglycemia and adverse pregnancy outcomes. N Engl J Med 2008;358(19): 1991–2002.

39. Reader D. Medical nutrition therapy and lifestyle interventions. Diabetes Care 2007;30(Suppl 2):S188–93.

40. Jovanovic-Peterson L, Peterson C. Nutritional management of the obese gestational diabetic pregnant woman. J Am Coll Nutr 1992;3:246–50.

41. Walkinshaw S. Dietary regulation for gestational diabetes. Cochrane Database Syst Rev 2000;(4)CD000070.

42. Food and Nutrition Board. Nutrition during pregnancy, Part 1: weight gain, Part 2: nutrition supplements. Washington, DC: Institute of Medicine, National Academy of Sciences; 1990.

43. Hedderson M, Weiss N, Sacks D, et al. Pregnancy weight gain and risk of neonatal complications: macrosomia, hypoglycemia, and hyperbilirubinemia. Obstet Gynecol 2006;108(5):1153–61.

44. Horton E. Exercise in the treatment of NIDDK. Applications for GDM? Diabetes 1991;40(Suppl 2):175–8.

45. Jovanovic-Peterson L, Durak E, Peterson C. Randomized trial of diet versus diet plus cardiovascular conditioning on glucose levels in gestational diabetes. Am J Obstet Gynecol 1989;161:415–9.

46. Bung P, Artal R, Khodiguian N, Kjos S. Exercise in gestational diabetes. An optional therapeutic approach? Diabetes 1991;40(Suppl 2):182–5.

47. Laird J, McFarland K. Fasting blood glucose levels and initiation of insulin therapy in gestational diabetes. Endocr Pract 1996;2:330–2.

48. de Veciana M, Major C, Morgan M, et al. Postprandial versus preprandial blood glucose monitoring in women with gestational diabetes mellitus requiring insulin therapy. N Engl J Med 1995;333(19):1237–41.

49. Jovanovic-Peterson L, Peterson C, Reed G, et al. Maternal postprandial glucose levels and infant birth weight: the Diabetes in Early Pregnancy Study. The National Institute of Child Health and Human Development - Diabetes in Early Pregnancy Study. Am J Obstet Gynecol 1991;164(1 Pt 1):103–11.

50. Nachum Z, Ben-Shlomo I, Weiner E, Shalev E. Twice daily vs. four times daily insulin dose regimens for diabetes in pregnancy: randomised controlled trial. BMJ 1999;319:1223–7.

51. Kjos S, Schaefer-Graf U, Sardesi S, et al. A randomized controlled trial using glycemic plus fetal ultrasound parameters versus glycemic parameters to determine insulin therapy in gestational diabetes with fasting hyperglycemia. Diabetes Care 2001;24(11):1904–10.

52. Langer O, Conway D, Berkus M, Xenakis E, Gonzales O. A comparison of glyburide and insulin in women with gestational diabetes mellitus. N Engl J Med 2000;343(16):1134–8.

53. Moore T. Glyburide for the treatment of gestational diabetes: a critical appraisal. Diabetes Care 2007;30:S209–13.

54. Rowan J, Hague W, Gao W, Battin M, Moore M, MiG Trial Investigators. Metformin versus insulin for the treatment of gestational diabetes. N Engl J Med 2008;358(19):2003–15.

55. Gilbert C, Valois M, Koren G. Pregnancy outcome after first-trimester exposure to metformin; a meta-analysis. Fertil Steril 2006;86:658–63.

56. Glueck C, Pranikoff J, Aregawi D, Wang P. Prevention of gestational diabetes by metformin plus diet in patients with polycystic ovary syndrome. Fertil Steril 2008;89:625–34.

57. Catalano P, Thomas A, Huston-Presley L, Amini S. Increased fetal adiposity: a very sensitive marker of abnormal in-utero development. Am J Obstet Gynecol 2003;189:1698–704.

58. Heikes K, Eddy D, Arondekar B, Schlessinger L. Diabetes Risk Calculator: a simple tool for detecting undiagnosed diabetes and pre-diabetes. Diabetes Care 2008;31(5):1040–5.

59. Gunderson E, Lewis C, Tsai A, et al. A 20-year prospective study of childbearing and incidence of diabetes in young women, controlling for glycemia before conception: the Coronary Artery Risk Development in Young Adults (CARDIA) Study. Diabetes 2007;56(12):2990–6.

60. Cheung N, Byth K. Population health significance of gestational diabetes. Diabetes Care 2003;26:2005–9.

61. Heitritter S, Solomon C, Mitchell G, Skali-Ounis N, Seely E. Subclinical inflammation and vascular dysfunction in women with previous gestational diabetes mellitus. J Clin Endocrinol Metab 2005;90:3983–88.

62. Metzger B, Buchanan T, Coustan D, et al. Summary and recommendations of the Fifth International Workshop-Conference on Gestational Diabetes Mellitus. Diabetes Care 2007;30(2):S251–60.

63. Canadian Diabetes Association. Gestational diabetes mellitus.Clinical Practice Guidelines Expert Committee. 2003 Practice Guidelines. Toronto, ON: Canadian Diabetes Association; 2003 (accessed August 1, 2008, at http://www.diabetes.ca/cpg2003/downloads/gdm.pdf).

64. National Institute for Health and Clinical Excellence (NICE). Diabetes in pregnancy: management of diabetes and its complications from preconception to the postnatal period. London: National Collaborating Centre for Women's and Children's Health; 2008.

65. World Health Organization. Definition and diagnosis of diabetes mellitus and intermediate hyperglycemia: a report of WHO/IDF consultation. Geneva: World Health Organization; 2006.

66. American Diabetes Association. Diagnosis and classification of diabetes mellitus. Diabetes Care 2008;31(Suppl1):S55–60.

67. The Expert Committee on the Diagnosis and Classification of Diabetes Mellitus. Follow-up report on the diagnosis of diabetes mellitus. Diabetes Care 2003;26:3160–7.

68. United States Preventive Services Task Force. Screening for gestational diabetes mellitus: U.S. Preventive Services Task Force recommendation statement. Ann Intern Med 2008;148(10):759–65.

69. The Expert Committee on the Diagnosis and Classification of Diabetes Mellitus. Report of the expert committee on the diagnosis and classification of diabetes mellitus. Diabetes Care 1997;20:1183–97.

70. Harris M, Eastman R, Cowie C, Flegal K, Eberhardt M. Comparison of diabetes diagnostic categories in the U.S. population according to 1997 American Diabetes Association and 1980–1985 World Health Organization diagnostic criteria. Diabetes Care 1997;20:1859–62.

71. DECODE Study Group. Will new diagnostic criteria for diabetes mellitus change phenotype of patients with diabetes? BMJ 1998;317:371–5.

72. Pallardo F, Herranz L, Garcia-Ingelmo T, et al. Early postpartum metabolic assessment in women with prior gestational diabetes. Diabetes Care 1999;22:1053–8.

73. Kitzmiller J, Dang-Kilduff L, Taslimi M. Gestational diabetes after delivery: short-term management and long-term risks. Diabetes Care 2007;30(Suppl2):S225–35.

74. Hunt K, Conway D. Who returns for postpartum glucose screening following gestational diabetes mellitus? Am J Obstet Gynecol 2008;198(4):404.e1–6.

75. Ferrara A, Peng T, Kim C. Trends in postpartum diabetes screening and subsequent diabetes and impaired fasting glucose among women with histories of gestational diabetes mellitus: a report from the Translating Research Into Action for Diabetes (TRIAD) Study. Diabetes Care 2009;32:269–74.

76. Reinblatt S, Morin L, Meltzer S. The importance of a postpartum 75 gram oral glucose tolerance test in women with gestational diabetes. J Obstet Gynaecol Can 2006;28(8):690–4.

77. Agarwal M, Punnose J, Dhatt G. Gestational diabetes: implications of variation in post-partum follow-up criteria. Eur J Obstet Gynecol Reprod Biol 2004;113(2):149–53.

78. Kim C, Herman W, Vijan S. Efficacy and cost of postpartum screening strategies for diabetes among women with histories of gestational diabetes mellitus. Diabetes Care 2007;30:1102–6.

79. Smirnakis K, Chasan-Taber L, Wolf M, Markenson G, Ecker J, Thadhani R. Postpartum diabetes screening in women with a history of gestational diabetes. Obstet Gynecol 2005;106(6):1297–303.

80. Russell M, Phipps M, Olson C, Welch H, Carpenter M. Rates of postpartum glucose testing after gestational diabetes mellitus. Obstet Gynecol 2006;108(6):1456–62.

81. Kim C, Tabaei B, Burke R, et al. Missed opportunities for diabetes screening among women with a history of gestational diabetes. Am J Public Health 2006;96:1–9.

82. Clark H, van Walraven C, Code C, Karovitch A, Keely E. Did publication of a clinical practice guideline recommendation to screen for type 2 diabetes in women with gestational diabetes change practice? Diabetes Care 2003;26:265–8.

83. Kim C, McEwen L, Piette J, Goewey J, Ferrara A, Walker E. Risk perception for diabetes among women with histories of gestational diabetes mellitus. Diabetes Care 2007;30(9):2281–6.

84. Gabbe S, Gregory R, Power M, Williams S, Schulkin J. Management of diabetes mellitus by obstetrician-gynecologists. Obstet Gynecol 2004;103(6):1229–34.

85. Gabbe S, Hill L, Schmidt L, Schulkin J. Management of diabetes by obstetrician-gynecologists. Obstet Gynecol 1998;91(5 Pt 1):643–7.

86. Kim C, McEwen L, Kerr E, et al. Preventive counseling among women with histories of gestational diabetes mellitus. Diabetes Care 2007;30(10):2489–95.

87. Nicholson W, Wilson L, Witkop C, et al. Therapeutic management, delivery, and postpartum risk assessment and screening in gestational diabetes. Evid Rep Technol Assess (Full Rep) 2008;162:1–96.

88. Retnakaran R, Qi Y, Sermer M, Connelly P, Zinman B, Hanley A. Isolated hyperglycemia at 1-hour on oral glucose tolerance test in pregnancy resembles gestational diabetes in predicting postpartum metabolic dysfunction. Diabetes Care 2008;31(7):1275–81.

89. Cheung N, Helmink D. Gestational diabetes: the significant of persistent fasting hyperglycemia for the subsequent development of diabetes mellitus. J Diabetes Complications 2006;20(1):21–5.

90. Steinhart J, Sugarman J, Connell F. Gestational diabetes is a herald of NIDDM in Navajo women. Diabetes Care 1997;20(6):943–7.

91. Cho N, Lim S, Jang H, Park H, Metzger B. Elevated homocysteine as a risk factor for the development of diabetes in women with a previous history of gestational diabetes mellitus: a 4-year prospective study. Diabetes Care 2005;28(11):2750–5.

92. Kjos S, Peters R, Xiang A, Henry O, Montoro M, Buchanan T. Predicting future diabetes in Latino women with gestational diabetes. Diabetes 1995;44:586–91.

93. Schaefer-Graf U, Buchanan T, Xiang A, Peters R, Kjos S. Clinical predictors for a high risk for the development of diabetes mellitus in the early puerperium in women with recent gestational diabetes mellitus. Am J Obstet Gynecol 2002;186:751–6.

94. Catalano P, Vargo K, Bernstein I, Amini S. Incidence and risk factors associated with abnormal postpartum glucose tolerance in women with gestational diabetes. Am J Obstet Gynecol 1991;165(4 Pt 1):914–9.

95. Buchanan T, Xiang A, Kjos S, Trigo E, Lee W, Peters R. Antepartum predictors of the development of type 2 diabetes in Latino women 11–26 months after pregnancies complicated by gestational diabetes. Diabetes 1999;48:2430–6.

96. Jang H, Yim C, Han K, et al. Gestational diabetes mellitus in Korea: prevalence and prediction of glucose intolerance at early postpartum. Diabetes Res Clin Pract 2003;61(2):117–24.

97. Metzger B, Cho N, Roston S, Radvany R. Prepregnancy weight and antepartum insulin secretion predict glucose tolerance five years after gestational diabetes mellitus. Diabetes Care 1993;16:1598–605.

98. Peters R, Kjos S, Xiang A, Buchanan T. Long-term diabetogenic effect of a single pregnancy in women with prior gestational diabetes mellitus. Lancet 1996;347:227–30.

99. Buchanan T, et al. Gestational diabetes: antepartum characteristics that predict postpartum glucose intolerance and type 2 diabetes in Latino women. Diabetes 1998;47(8):1302–10.

100. Lobner K, Knopff A, Baumgarten A, et al. Predictors of postpartum diabetes in women with gestational diabetes mellitus. Diabetes 2006;55(3):792–7.

101. Greenberg L, Moore T, Murphy H. Gestational diabetes mellitus: antenatal variables as predictors of postpartum glucose intolerance. Obstet Gynecol 1995;86(1):97–101.

102. Dalfra M, Lapolla A, Masin M. Antepartum and early postpartum predictors of type 2 diabetes development in women with gestational diabetes mellitus. Diabetes Metab 2001;27(6):675–80.

103. Henry O, Beischer N. Long-term implications of gestational diabetes for the mother. Baillieres Clin Obstet Gynaecol 1991; 5(2):461–83.

104. Catalano P, Vargo K, Bernstein I, Amini S. Incidence and risk factors associated with abnormal postpartum glucose tolerance in women with gestational diabetes. Am J Obstet Gynecol 1991;163:93–8.

105. Bartha J, Martinez-del-Fresno P, Comino-Delgado R. Postpartum metabolism and autoantibody markers in women with gestational diabetes mellitus diagnosed in early pregnancy. Am J Obstet Gynecol 2001;184(5):965–70.

106. Persson B, Hanson U, Hartling S, Binder C. Follow-up of women with previous GDM: insulin, C-peptide, and proinsulin responses to oral glucose load. Diabetes 1991;40(Suppl2):136–41.

107. Dacus J, Meyer N, Muram D, Stilson R, Phipps P, Sibai B. Gestational diabetes: postpartum glucose tolerance testing. Am J Obstet Gynecol 1994;171(4):927–31.

108. Shuldiner A, Yang R, Gong D. Resistin, obesity, and insulin resistance - the emerging role of the adipocyte as an endocrine organ. N Engl J Med 2001;345(18):1345–6.

109. Branchtein L, Schmidt M, Mengue S, Reichelt A, Matos M, Duncan B. Waist circumference and waist-to-hip ratio are related to gestational glucose tolerance. Diabetes Care 1997;20(4):509–11.

14   Nutrition and Pregnancy

Jo-Anne M. Rizzotto, Judy Giusti, and Laurie Higgins

CONTENTS

From: *Diabetes in Women: Pathophysiology and Therapy*
Edited by: A. Tsatsoulis et al. (eds.), DOI 10.1007/978-1-60327-250-6_14
© Humana Press, a part of Springer Science+Business Media, LLC 2009

ABSTRACT

Pregnancy complicated by diabetes presents unique challenges for women with preexisting diabetes and those with gestational diabetes. All women with preexisting diabetes, who are of childbearing years, should receive preconception counseling to prepare for pregnancy. Prenatal counseling and care should include a team consisting of healthcare providers who are well versed in the care of diabetes and pregnancy. Women with diabetes should receive Medical Nutrition Therapy (MNT) counseling prior to and throughout pregnancy. The goals of MNT and meal planning are (1) to provide adequate calories and nutrients to achieve target pregnancy weight gain and glycemic control and (2) to promote lifelong healthy lifestyle behaviors. These goals will optimize maternal, fetal, and perinatal outcomes and minimize pregnancy complications. They require balancing food and activity with insulin to meet glucose goals.

Key words: preconception counseling; diabetes and pregnancy; meal planning; weight gain; breast-feeding; celiac diaease

INTRODUCTION

This chapter will cover the current nutrition recommendations for women with preexisting diabetes and gestational diabetes. Optimal glycemic control reduces morbidity and mortality in pregnancies complicated by diabetes *(1)*. Appropriate nutrition therapy is essential to achieve optimal glycemic control. Medical Nutrition Therapy (MNT) must be included in the preconception and prenatal management of all women with diabetes to achieve this goal.

PRECONCEPTION COUNSELING

All women of reproductive age with diabetes should receive preconception counseling, as reviewed in Chap. 15. Both preconception counseling and prenatal care entail a team approach including an obstetrician, endocrinologist, nurse educator, dietitian, and social worker. Education should focus on the rationale for good blood glucose control, blood glucose goals for preconception and pregnancy, MNT, exercise, insulin, and effects of diabetes on pregnancy and of pregnancy on diabetes with an assessment of social support.

During preconception nutrition counseling, the registered dietitian should assess current eating habits, nutritional adequacy and knowledge as well as cultural and ethnic preferences, work schedules, and financial considerations. A meal plan with sufficient calories and nutrients for optimal blood glucose control should be provided prior to pregnancy with a focus on carbohydrate counting. Nutrition requirements for preconception planning are individually determined based on the woman's weight, height, age, and activity.

NUTRITION REQUIREMENTS AND MEAL PLANNING WITH PREGNANCY AND PREEXISTING DIABETES

The focus of this chapter is MNT in pregnancy complicated by preexisting diabetes. However, the value of preconception counseling in women with preexisting diabetes cannot be ignored. All women with diabetes should receive MNT counseling prior to and throughout pregnancy, ideally provided by a registered dietitian who is well versed in diabetes and pregnancy. The role of the dietitian is to assess nutrition knowledge and determine a meal plan approach based on individual preferences to meet MNT goals of (1) providing adequate calories and nutrients that are important for optimal maternal and fetal outcomes and good glycemic control to minimize pregnancy complications, (2) balancing food, activity, and insulin doses to achieve adequate weight gain and to meet glucose goals to maximize perinatal outcomes, and (3) promoting healthy lifestyle behaviors that will contribute to lifelong health.

CALORIES FOR PREGNANCY

The new weight gain guidelines for pregnancy are based on the World Health Organization (WHO) BMI categories. The new Institute of Medicine (IOM) guidelines cover a specific range of recommended weight gains for each category of prepregnancy BMI. (Table 1). Estimated energy requirements (EER) can also be used to determine calorie needs for pregnancy. EER is based on age, height, weight, and activity level *(3)*.

Calorie recommendations for pregnancy are based on prepregnancy BMI (4). Recommendations for women in the underweight category are 36-40 kcals/kg;normal weight 30 kcals/kg;overweight 24 kcals/kg; obese moderate calorie restriction not <1800 kcals/day. Recommendations for multiple fetuses add an additional 150 kcals/day per fetus. All women need an additional 150-300 kcals/day in the second and third trimester *(4)*. Urine ketones, food intake, and maternal body weight should be monitored to ensure that calories are not being overrestricted. Dietary recommendations are individualized and should provide enough calories without causing undue weight gain or hyperglycemia.

WEIGHT GAIN

Women should be weighed at each prenatal visit. Weight gain goals should be made for each trimester to optimize maternal and fetal outcomes. During the first trimester, a weight gain of 2–5 pounds occurs as a result of maternal blood volume expansion and hypertrophy of breast and uterine tissue. Excessive weight gain during the first 20 weeks increases the risk of weight retention postpartum *(5)*. See Table 1 for recommendations for total pregnancy weight gain and weight gain recommendations for the second and third trimester. Weight gain recommendations for women with normal BMI pregnant with twins is 37-54 pounds; overweight women, 31-50 pounds; and obese women, 25-42 pounds *(4)*. Gradual weight gain over the entire pregnancy is expected. Excessive weight gain increases the risk of fetal macrosomia, cesarean section, birth trauma, and postpartum weight retention. Any weight loss during pregnancy calls for immediate evaluation and intervention. Underweight women who fail to gain adequate weight are at risk for premature birth and low-birth weight infants *(7)*.

Table 1

New Recommendations for Total and Rate of Weight Gain During Pregnancy, by Prepregnancy BMI

Prepregnancy BMI	BMI+ (kg/m²) (WHO)	Total Weight Gain Range(lbs)	Rates of Weight Gain* 2nd and 3rd Trimester (Mean Range in lbs/wk)
Underweight	<18.5	28-40	1 (1-1.3)
Normal Weight	18.5-24.9	25-35	1 (0.8-1)
Overweight	25.0-29.9	15-25	0.6 (0.5-0.7)
Obese (includes all classes)	≥30.0	11-20	0.5 (0.4-0.6)

+ *To calculate BMI go to www.nhlbisupport.com/bmi/*

Committee to Reexamine IOM Pregnancy Weight Guidelines Institute of Medicine; National Research Council. *Weight Gain During Pregnancy: Reexamining the Guidelines.* Rasmussen, KM. and Yaktine AL, eds. 2009: The National Academies Press, Washington D.C. in press

MEAL PLAN RECOMMENDATIONS

It is important to establish a meal plan to help meet calorie and macronutrient recommendations for pregnancy. A macronutrient balance of 45–55% of carbohydrate, 20–25% protein, and 30–40% fat is essential in meeting the nutrient needs of both mom and baby *(6)*. The timing of meals and snacks is important to optimize blood glucose control and to provide the fetus with glucose needs for growth. Planning a daily food intake of three meals and two to four snacks, including a bedtime snack, will help meet these goals.

Women should consume a variety of foods according to the Dietary Guidelines *(8)* with cultural food practices considered to meet energy and nutrient needs appropriate for adequate weight gain.

PHYSICAL ACTIVITY

Regular physical activity is recommended during pregnancy. However, medical clearance by a healthcare provider is needed before an exercise program is begun. Modifications in physical activity may need to be made in women with preexisting diabetes who have diabetes complications, such as retinopathy, nephropathy, neuropathy, or cardiovascular disease.

If there are no contraindications to physical activity, it is recommended that pregnant women include 30 min of moderate physical activity on most days of the week. The 30 min may be divided into three 10-min sessions. Vigorous activity should be avoided during peak insulin action time *(9)*. Activities, such as walking, that do not have a risk of abdominal trauma or high risk of falling should be chosen. The benefits of physical activity are many; including reduced insulin resistance, better blood glucose control, a better tolerance of labor, minimized excessive weight gain, and an overall feeling of well-being *(10)*.

Activity guidelines are the same for preexisting and gestational diabetes. In gestational diabetes walking after eating may meet postprandial blood glucose goals without the addition of insulin *(10)*.

CAUTIONS DURING PHYSICAL ACTIVITY

Exercise-induced hypoglycemia may worsen during pregnancy. Blood glucose should be checked before and after exercise. Carbohydrate snacks before, during, and after physical activity may help prevent hypoglycemia. If there is poor maternal weight gain or fetal growth retardation, exercise should be modified or discontinued.

CARBOHYDRATES

Carbohydrates are converted into glucose and have the biggest impact on postprandial blood glucose results. Therefore, it is important to control carbohydrate intake throughout the day. Appropriate distribution of carbohydrates over the day helps attain optimal glycemic control and can prevent hypoglycemia and ketonemia in pregnant women.

The IOM recommends 130 g of carbohydrate per day for women of childbearing years based on the minimum of carbohydrate utilized by the brain and red blood cell function. For pregnancy, the RDA is a minimum of 175 g of carbohydrate per day *(11)* (Table 2).

The pregnant woman with diabetes needs to be educated on the amounts and types of carbohydrate that will promote postprandial blood glucose control with individualized recommendations that pertain to her food preferences. It is important to tailor information to the learning level of the individual particularly when choosing a carbohydrate counting method.

The first step in learning how to count carbohydrates is learning which foods are rich in "carbs." Many foods contain carbohydrate, for example, whole grains, beans, fruit, milk, and some vegetables. So, when developing a healthy meal plan, it is important to have a variety to optimize nutrient intake.

Table 2

Distribution of Macronutrients for Pregnancy (Reprinted with Permission from Joslin Diabetes Center and Joslin Clinic Guideline for the Detection and Management of Diabetes in Pregnancy (http://www.joslin.org). Copyright © by Joslin Diabetes Center. All rights reserved)

Macronutrient	Gestational diabetes mellitus	Preexisting diabetes
Carbohydrate[a]	40–45% total calories	45–55% total calories
Breakfast	15–30 g[a,b]	Individualize as per usual intake and premeal BG levels
HS Snack	15–30 g carb	15–30 g carb
Fiber	25–35 g	25–35 g
Protein	1.1 g protein/kg DBW or 25 g of extra protein/day	
Fat	<40% total calories	30–35% total calories
	<10% from saturated fat	<10% from saturated fat

[a] Pregnant women should consume a minimum of 175 g carb/day
[b] May be increased if insulin is added

Table 3

Nutrition Resources for Carbohydrate Counting and Meal Planning

Free nutrition Web sites

http://www.dietfacts.com
http://www.calorie-count.com
http://www.nutritiondata.com
http://www.diabetes.org/my-food-advisor.jsp
http://www.calorieking.com/foods/
http://www.nal.usda.gov/fnic/foodcomp/search/

Carbohydrate counting books

The CalorieKing Calorie, Fat & Carbohydrate Counter. 2008 Edition
The Diabetes Carbohydrate and Fat Gram Guide, 3rd Edition. Lea Ann Holzmeister, 2006
Fast Fact Series: Carb Counting Made Easy. Marie McCarren, 2002
The ADA's Complete Guide to Carb Counting. Hope Warshaw, MMSc, RD, CDE and K. Kulkarni, MS, RD, C.D.E. 2004
Practical Carbohydrate Counting, 2nd Edition. A How-to-Teach Guide for Health Professionals. Hope S. Warshaw, MMSc, RD, CDE and Karen M. Bolderman, RD, LD, CDE. 2008
Ultimate Guide to Accurate Carb Counting. Gary Scheiner, 2006

Label reading is important when trying to estimate the amount of carbohydrate in a portion and is an essential concept of nutrition education. Labels can be tricky. The total carbohydrate and fiber content of a food is based on a single serving size that is listed on the package. In addition to label reading, there are many carbohydrate resources available; reference books, as well as Internet and software programs, help identify the carbohydrate content of a food (see Table 3).

DIETARY FIBER

Dietary fiber is the nondigestible carbohydrate and lignin that are found in plants. Fiber is an important part of a pregnant woman's diet as constipation is a common symptom during pregnancy. Fiber promotes bowel regularity and may help with postprandial blood glucose excursions by slowing down digestion and absorption of nutrients. Optimal fiber intake is 28 g per day *(2)* in pregnancy. (See Table 2) Good sources of fiber are whole grains, fruits, legumes, peas, nuts and vegetables. Sources of fiber are divided into two categories: soluble and insoluble fiber.

Insoluble fiber does not dissolve in water. It reduces constipation by adding bulk to the stool and decreasing stool transit time. Good food sources of insoluble fiber are whole wheat, bran, nuts, and vegetables. Soluble fiber such as pectin and guar gum dissolve in water and form a gel-like substance, which slows gastric emptying and increases satiety and may reduce peak postprandial blood glucose *(12)*. Good food sources of soluble fiber are oats, peas, beans, barley, vegetables, and some fruits (apples, citrus) and pysllium (found in bran cereals and Metamucil). It is important to consume fiber with plenty of fluids and to increase the quantity of fiber slowly to avoid cramping, gas, and diarrhea. Healthcare providers may recommend a fiber supplement to women who are unable to eat enough fiber each day.

CARBOHYDRATE COUNTING

Either basic or advanced carbohydrate counting can be used, depending on the needs of the patient. Basic carbohydrate counting makes use of a carbohydrate allowance for meals and snacks and provides education on portion sizes. Skills are taught that help identify carbohydrate foods, quantify the amount of carbohydrate in a food serving, and determine the actual portion size eaten. Patients are taught how food, insulin, and physical activity affect blood glucoses.

A portion size of each serving of food is equal to 15 g of carbohydrate (see Table 4 for common food portions).

Advanced carbohydrate counting is taught, once basic carbohydrate counting has been mastered, for the individual who intends to use a continuous subcutaneous insulin infusion (CSII) or a basal

Table 4
Common Carbohydrate Foods and Portion Sizes Equal to 15 g of "Carb"

Carbohydrate foods	*Portion size for 15 g of carbohydrate*
Breads, cereal, rice, and pasta	½ C. cooked cereal
	⅓ C. cooked rice, couscous
	⅓ C. cooked pasta
Beans, peas, and lentils	½ C. cooked beans, peas
	½ C. lima beans
	½ C. cooked lentils
Fruit	1 C. canned fruit (unsweetened)
	1 small to medium fresh fruit
	¼ C. dried fruit
	½ C. orange juice
Milk	1 C. (8 oz) milk
	½ C. chocolate milk
Starchy vegetables	½ C. corn
	½ C. mashed potato
	1 C. winter squash
Sweets, snacks	⅟₁₂ angel food cake
	2 in. sq. brownie
	½ C. ice cream
Combination foods	¾ C. casserole dish
30 g of carb	⅛ of 12 in. pie Cheese pizza, hand tossed

bolus regime with multiple daily injections (MDI). This is a sophisticated approach that matches premeal insulin doses to carbohydrate consumption at meals. It requires learning to use an insulin-to-carbohydrate ratio (ICR). The ICR indicates the amount of carbohydrate utilized by one unit of rapid-acting insulin. For an example a 1:10 ratio means that one unit of insulin covers 10 g of carbohydrate. The ICR varies depending on the individual's insulin needs and insulin sensitivity. There are a variety of ways to calculate the ICR *(12)*. One method is to use the 500 rule. Calculate the total daily dose (TDD) of insulin when blood glucose is in good control. The TDD includes rapid acting and the basal insulin over 24 h. Five hundred divided by the TDD will give the ICR. For example, someone who takes a TDD of 40 units will need an ICR of approximately 1:12 to cover mealtime carbohydrate. Detailed blood glucose, insulin, and food records can help refine the ICR *(13)*.

The ICR is often combined with a correction dose of insulin. This is known as the insulin sensitivity factor (ISF). The ISF tells how many mg/dl one unit of insulin will lower blood glucose. Additional insulin can be added to a meal bolus to correct high premeal blood glucose. One method to determine the ISF is the 1800 rule. Eighteen hundred divided by the TDD determines the ISF. For example, someone who takes a TDD of 60 units will have an ISF of 30 which means that one unit of insulin will lower blood glucose by 30 mg/dl. Together the ICR and the ISF constitute the premeal insulin dose. Advanced carbohydrate counting is based on the ability of the individual to understand intensive insulin therapy, target blood glucose levels, keep detailed food records, and be willing to make daily self-care decisions. Record keeping is crucial to fine-tuning the ICR and ISF to achieve target range postprandial blood glucose goals. Education by a diabetes educator is invaluable to the success of using the advanced carbohydrate counting method. This highly accepted method of meal planning presents challenges, as record keeping can be burdensome; still its advantages are many. It focuses on one nutrient and allows for variation in carbohydrate consumption and flexibility in food selection.

GLYCEMIC RESPONSE TO FOODS

Carbohydrate foods can have a varied response in postprandial blood glucose results. Therefore, it is helpful to include glycemic response in the meal planning discussion. Glycemic response is defined as either glycemic index (GI) or as glycemic load (GL) *(3)*.

GI is a measurement of the increase of blood glucose within 2 h after eating a given amount of carbohydrate, 50 g compared to its response to a reference carb (glucose or white bread). The GI is a meal planning tool that ranks carbohydrates according to their effect on blood glucose when foods of equivalent carbohydrate are compared. Foods that ranked high on the scale cause a quick rise in blood glucose after eating, whereas foods that ranked low cause a gradual rise in blood glucose *(3)*.

GL takes into account the GI and the carbohydrate content of the amount of food eaten. The use of the GI and GL may be of some benefit for glycemic control but can be a cumbersome approach to use. Simplifying things by evaluating food records and identifying an individual's response to favorite carbohydrate foods may be more beneficial. Individuals may do best with simple guideline instructions like limiting high glycemic carbohydrate foods such as white bread, white rice, pastries, and sugar-sweetened foods. They should be encouraged to eat lower glycemic, less processed carbohydrates; such as whole-wheat pasta and breads, brown rice, steel cut oats, dried beans, fresh fruits, soy products, and most vegetables.

Because of the effect of pregnancy on early morning blood glucose levels, meeting postprandial blood glucose goals can be challenging. To assist with glycemic control, women may benefit from choosing whole grain foods with the addition of a serving of protein and fat for breakfast. Protein and fat contribute calories and also can increase satiety. Food selections such as fresh fruit and dairy can produce a higher postprandial glycemic response; thus, these may be better choices for use later in the day *(10)*.

PROTEIN

The Recommended Dietary Allowance (RDA) for protein in the first trimester is 0.88 g/kg daily, and in the second half of pregnancy it increases to 1.1 gm/kg of desirable body weight or 20–25% total daily calories for a singleton pregnancy (Table 2). Twin pregnancies require an additional 50 g of protein a day beginning in the second trimester. Protein is needed for growth, maintenance, and repair of tissues and during pregnancy to meet the high rate of protein turnover in the second and third trimesters *(3)*.

The type of protein one consumes during pregnancy is important. Foods that contain all nine essential amino acids are called complete proteins. Sources of complete protein include lean cuts of meat, chicken, eggs, fish, cheese, and yogurt *(3)*. Incomplete proteins are lacking in one or more essential amino acids. Some examples of incomplete proteins are dried beans, peas, lentils, and soy products, such as, tofu, tempeh, low-fat soymilk, soy burgers, and nuts and seeds. While vegetarian diets using complementary mixtures of plant proteins provide the same protein quality as animal products, special attention should be paid to vegetarian meal planning during pregnancy *(14)*.

FAT

Fat provides a major source of calories and aids in the absorption of fat-soluble vitamins, A, D, E, and K. Fat intake should be between 20 and 35% of total calories to prevent undue maternal weight gain, promote long-term maternal health, and still allow for adequate fetal growth (Table 2). Saturated and trans fats should be as low as possible and no more than 7–10% of total fat intake *(3)*. Primary sources of saturated fats are meat, dairy, and baked goods. Monounsaturated fat can be made in the body and is found in canola oil, olive oil, and some animal products.

HEART HEALTHY FATS

Fat is also a source of essential fatty acids (EFA). EFA are not made by the body but must be ingested from food. There are two types of EFA, omega 6 and omega 3 polyunsaturated fatty acids (PUFA) *(3)*. Omega 6 PUFA are formed from linoleic acid (LA). LA is a precursor for arachidonic acid, which is important for maternal and fetal cell signaling pathways *(15)*. Omega 6 FAs are the predominant fat found in the typical American diet. Commonly consumed foods such as corn and soybean oil, eggs, poultry, and trans fat-free margarines are rich in Omega 6 PUFAs. Adequate intake for omega 6 (PUFA) LA is 13 g/day, and for omega 3 (PUFA) alpha-linolenic acid (ALA) it is 1.4 g/day *(3)*.

Long chain Omega 3 FAs are lacking in the American diet. There are three types of omega 3 FAs: ALA, eicosapentaenoic acid (EPA), and docosahexaenoic acid (DHA) *(3)*. Good sources of ALA are walnuts, canola and walnut oil, and green leafy vegetables. The body can convert ALA to EPA and DHA. Direct sources of EPA and DHA are fish, fish oil supplements, flax seed, and flaxseed oil *(3)*.

Both omega 3 and omega 6 PUFAs are needed in cell membranes and also in the brain and retina. They are needed for neurons in the brain and nervous system to function properly.

During pregnancy a deficiency in omega 3s can cause problems in fetal nervous and visual system development. DHA is necessary for brain, eye development, and cognitive, motor, and behavioral skills *(15)*. DHA may also decrease preterm birth and aid in preventing postpartum depression *(16)*. It is also found in breast milk and is now added to infant formulas.

SEAFOOD RECOMMENDATIONS DURING PREGNANCY

During rapid fetal growth, postpartum and breastfeeding, long chain omega 3s cannot be made fast enough to meet maternal and fetal needs and must be consumed in the maternal diet *(17)*.

A controversy has existed in regard to the risk-benefit of eating fish during pregnancy because of the possible harmful effects of methyl mercury present in ocean fish. Present recommendations for pregnancy, however, are to eat 12 oz of fish per week, which can include shrimp, canned light tuna, salmon, pollock, and catfish *(18)*. Six oz may be consumed from white albacore tuna. Another good source of omega 3s is DHA fortified eggs. Fish oil capsules may be of benefit but more research is needed. Pregnant women are still cautioned against eating swordfish, shark, king mackerel, and tile fish because of unsafe levels of methyl mercury *(19)*.

Current thought is that the nutritional benefits of fish far outweigh the risks. Deficiencies of long chain omega 3s are common while toxicity from methyl mercury is very rare. Oily ocean fish, such as salmon, tuna, sardines, and mackerel are lean proteins that meet the needs of DHA and EPA in pregnancy. They also contain vitamins B, D, zinc, iodine, and selenium, which are all important in pregnancy. Selenium is needed for thyroid function and may counteract the effects of methyl mercury *(20)*.

FOOD-BORNE ILLNESS

Pregnant women and their unborn babies are susceptible to food-borne illnesses. Specific concerns include *Listeria monocytogenes*, *Salmonella*, and *Toxoplasma gondii*. Infections from these food-borne illnesses can be passed to the fetus and have the potential for causing a miscarriage, stillbirth, or serious health problems for the newborn. Pregnant women are advised to avoid hot dogs, cold cuts, soft cheeses such as Feta, Brie, Camembert, blue-veined cheeses, or Mexican style cheeses, and all unpasteurized milk, milk products, and cheese. Other foods to avoid are pates, meat spreads, and refrigerated smoked seafood. Women are advised to avoid cleaning cat litter boxes and to avoid touching pets during food preparation *(20)*.

SWEETENERS

Sweeteners are classified as nutritive or nonnutritive. Nutritive sweeteners are glucose, sucrose, lactose, and fructose. Nutritive sweeteners are acceptable in pregnancy; however, one needs to pay attention to the glycemic effect on postprandial blood glucose levels. Nonnutritive sweeteners (listed in Table 5) such as saccharin, aspartame, acesulfame-K and sucralose have been shown to be safe for consumption in pregnancy. Some concern has been raised about saccharin, thus women had been cautioned in the past to avoid its use. Since saccharin has now been removed from the list of potential carcinogens, it is considered safe in pregnancy *(21)*. Nonnutritive sweeteners approved by the FDA are considered safe for use in pregnancy when they are used within the acceptable daily intake (ADI) recommendations (see Table 5). Stevia a nonnutritive sweetener from a South American shrub has not been approved for use in the USA by the FDA. The use of Stevia by pregnant or lactating women is not recommended since its safety is unknown.

Another class of sweeteners, the polyols, also known as sugar alcohols, is considered low-calorie sweeteners. Examples of low-calorie sweeteners are sorbitol, mannitol, xylitol, and maltitol, which are acceptable in pregnancy but in excessive amounts these can have a laxative effect.

Table 5
Approved Nonnutritive Sweeteners [Adapted from (21)]

Type	kcal/g	Regulatory status/ADI	Other names	Description
Saccharin	0	Approved as a sweetener for beverages and as a tabletop sweetener in foods with specific maximum amounts allowed ADI: 0–5 mg/kgbw/day[a]	Sweet'N Low, Sugar Twin®, Sweet'N Low Brown	200–700 Times sweeter than sucrose, noncarcinogenic, and produces no glycemic response; synergizes the sweetening power of nutritive and nonnutritive sweeteners; sweetening power is not reduced with heating
Aspartame	0	Approved as a general-purpose sweetener ADI: 50 mg/kg bw/day	NutraSweet®, Equal®	160–220 Times sweeter than sucrose; noncarcinogenic, and produces limited glycemic response
Acesulfame-K	0	Approved as a general-purpose sweetener ADI: 15 mg/kg bw/day	Sunette®, Sweet One®	200 Times sweeter than sucrose; noncarcinogenic, and produces no glycemic response; synergizes the sweetening power of nutritive and nonnutritive sweeteners; sweetening power is not reduced with heating
Sucralose	0	Approved as a general-purpose sweetener ADI: 5 mg/kg bw/day	Splenda®	600 Times sweeter than sucrose; noncarcinogenic, and produces no glycemic response; synergizes the sweetening power of nutritive and nonnutritive sweeteners; sweetening power is not reduced with heating

[a]Joint FAO/WHO Expert Committee on Food Additives (JECFA): http://www.who.int/ipcs/food/jecfa/en

MICRONUTRIENTS

The 2006 Dietary Reference Intake of micronutrients for pregnant women, lactating women, and adult women is listed in Table 6 (22). While following a nutritionally balanced meal plan is important, nutrients of particular importance are iron, folic acid, calcium, and vitamin D.

Iron

Women should consume 27 mg of iron per day through food sources. A supplement may be needed if there is a first or third trimester hemoglobin less than 11.0 mg/dl or a second trimester hemoglobin less than 10.5 mg/dl (2). Iron can interfere with the absorption of zinc and copper. Women taking greater than 30 mg of iron a day as a supplement should also take 15 mg of zinc and 2 mg of copper as supplements (23).

Folic Acid

All women planning to conceive should receive 400 µg of folic acid per day. Pregnant women should consume 600 µg of folic acid per day, in addition to folate from foods to reduce the risk of

Table 6
Dietary Reference Intakes for Women[a] [Data from (22)(Institute of Medicine. Dietary Reference Intakes: The Essential Guide to Nutrient Requirements Washington, DC: National Academies Press, 2006)]

Nutrient	Adult woman	Pregnancy	Lactation (0–6 months)
Energy (kcal)	2,403	2,743[b], 2,855[c]	2,698
Protein (g/kg/d)	0.8	1.1	1.1
Carbohydrate (g/d)	130	175	210
Total fiber (g/d)	25	28	29
Linoleic acid (g/d)	12	13	13
α-Linolenic acid (g/d)	12	13	13
Vitamin A (µg RAE)	700	770	1,300
Vitamin D (µg)	5	5	5
Vitamin E (mg α-tocopherol)	15	15	19
Vitamin K (µg)	90	90	90
Vitamin C (mg)	75	85	120
Thiamin (mg)	1.1	1.4	1.4
Riboflavin (mg)	1.1	1.4	1.6
Vitamin B-6 (mg)	1.3	1.9	2.0
Niacin (mg NE)	14	18	17
Folate (µg dietary folate equivalents)	400	600	500
Vitamin B-12 (µg)	2.4	2.6	2.8
Pantothenic acid (mg)	5	6	7
Biotin (µg)	30	30	35
Choline (mg)	425	450	550
Calcium (mg)	1,000	1,000	1,000
Phosphorus (mg)	700	700	700
Magnesium (mg)	320	350	310
Iron (mg)	8	27	9
Zinc (mg)	8	11	12
Iodine (µg)	150	220	290
Selenium (µg)	55	60	70
Fluoride (mg)	3	3	3
Manganese (mg)	1.8	2.0	2.6
Molybdenum (µg)	45	50	50
Chromium (µg)	25	30	45
Copper (µg)	900	1,000	1,300
Sodium (mg)	2,300	2,300	2,300
Potassium (mg)	4,700	4,700	5,100

RAE retinol activity equivalents, NE niacin equivalents

[a] Values are recommended dietary allowances except for energy (estimated energy requirement) and total fiber, linoteic acid, α linotenic acid, vitamin D, vitamin K, pantothenic acid, biotin, choline, calcium, manganese, chromium, sodium, and potassium (adequate intakes)

[b] Second trimester for women of age 19–50 years

[c] Third trimester for women of age 19–50 years

neural tube defects (20). Vegetarian women may need B12 and vitamin D supplementation (2). High doses of folic acid may mask a B12 deficiency. B12 status should be checked when folic acid intake is greater than the RDA (3).

Calcium and Vitamin D

Vitamin D aids in the absorption of calcium and is either ingested from food or synthesized by sunlight on the skin. During pregnancy calcium is absorbed more efficiently. Adequate intakes of calcium are 1,000 mg/day in women of age 19 through 50 and 1,300 mg in women of age 14 through 18 *(3)*. For women who are unable to consume milk products, calcium and vitamin D supplementation is needed. The daily recommended intake of vitamin D for pregnant women is 200 IU/day. In populations where exposure to sunlight is limited and in people with high levels of melanin, or those who use sunscreen, sunlight is not sufficient to make enough vitamin D. Therefore, vitamin D supplementation is important *(24)*. Most prenatal vitamins contain 400 IUs of vitamin D.

Women with preexisting diabetes may not have optimal levels of copper, magnesium, zinc, vitamin C, and vitamin E; therefore, a prenatal vitamin and mineral supplement may be needed. Women who smoke, abuse alcohol, and have a suboptimal nutrient intake may also benefit from taking a prenatal supplement.

RECORD KEEPING

Keeping a food diary may be beneficial as it reveals the nutrient balance and carbohydrate intake to help with healthy eating and blood glucose control.

ALCOHOL

Alcohol is not recommended during pregnancy. The US Surgeon General advises pregnant women to abstain from consuming alcohol to prevent birth defects and avoid developmental delays brought about by prenatal alcohol exposure.

CAFFEINE

Recommendations for caffeine consumption in pregnant women are less than 200 mg per day. Two recent published studies have produced conflicting results regarding the consumption of caffeine and miscarriage in pregnant women *(25;26)*. Until more is known the March of Dimes recommends a cautious approach that pregnant women limit their daily caffeine consumption to 200 mg per day. Caffeine is found in coffee, some soda, tea, chocolate, and some medications *(27)*.

BREASTFEEDING

The benefits of breastfeeding are discussed in Chap. 22 and include improved bonding, reduced maternal anxiety, monetary savings, decreased risk for postmenopausal hip fractures, and decreased infant illness with improved cognitive function of the newborn *(28)*. Breastfeeding may lower the child's risk of developing diabetes and helps to prevent many infant and childhood illnesses such as otitis media, gastroenteritis, asthma, respiratory tract infection, obesity, and sudden infant death syndrome (SIDS) *(28)*. Maternal weight loss is also a benefit. Calorie requirements are increased during lactation and are the same as calories needed in the third trimester with a recommended carbohydrate intake of 210 g per day *(11)*. The estimated calorie expended in milk production is ~500 kcal per day during the first 6 months and 400 kcal per day during the second 6 months of breastfeeding.

Breastfeeding women with diabetes may experience erratic blood glucose patterns. Frequent episodes of hypoglycemia are common, especially within 1 h of feeding and nocturnally. Women should snack prior to and after breastfeeding to prevent hypoglycemia *(29)*. Frequent self-monitoring of blood glucose is important with close attention to insulin therapy as insulin requirements are decreased during this time. Women are encouraged to drink about eight cups of water per day and a cup of water with each breastfeeding *(30)*. Successful breastfeeding, which can be achieved with proper education and planning, should be encouraged *(28)*.

NUTRITION AND MEAL PLANNING IN GESTATIONAL DIABETES

MNT is the cornerstone of treatment for gestational diabetes (GDM). Within 48 h of diagnosis, a woman should see a diabetes educator, preferably a registered dietitian for meal planning to assist with blood glucose control *(31)*. Education can be conducted in a class or an individual counseling session. The ideal amount of carbohydrate is unknown but is generally limited to 40–45% of the total calories needed for the day *(32)*. For obese women one can reduce the amount of carbohydrate to 35–40% *(23)*. The meal plan needs to be individualized to a woman's eating style and food preferences. Forty percent of an average 2,000 calorie meal plan would yield 200 g of carbohydrate per day, which is well above the recommended 175 g. Focusing on one nutrient, carbohydrate helps control postprandial blood glucose and aids in making the meal plan. Basic carbohydrate counting is used to achieve a consistent carbohydrate meal plan with three meals and four to five snacks per day.

Distribution of carbohydrates is important at meals and snacks (Table 2). As pregnancy progresses, hormone levels continue to rise causing insulin resistance and making carbohydrates less tolerable in the morning. Women may need to limit their carbohydrate intake at breakfast to 15–30 g and divide the rest of the carbohydrates throughout the day. Fruit juice and sweetened beverages should be discouraged as portion sizes are limited, and they can have a profound glycemic effect on postprandial blood glucose.

We recommend checking urine ketones each morning. The presence of ketones may suggest insufficient caloric intake. To minimize the presence of morning ketones, a bedtime snack of 15–30 g of carbohydrate with a protein and fatty food source is recommended. Women should be taught self-monitoring of blood glucose. Detailed food and blood glucose record keeping is essential to evaluate blood glucose and meal plan adequacy. If blood glucose goals are not achieved through meal plan adjustment and the addition of moderate physical activity, insulin therapy may be initiated. A persistent fasting BG above target indicates a need for bedtime intermediate-acting insulin. The insulin regimen should be based on glycemic patterns and fetal growth characteristics (see Chap. 17).

FOLLOW-UP

Regular visits to the healthcare team are recommended. Educator appointments are scheduled as needed for self-monitoring of blood glucose review, preferably with a certified diabetes educator

The Nutrition Guidelines for GDM *(31)* establish a minimum of three nutrition visits with preferably an RD, CDE. Additional communications may be needed by fax, phone, or e-mail.

POSTPARTUM CARE/CLINICAL IMPLICATIONS

GDM is associated with a high lifetime risk of diabetes. Women who had gestational diabetes should receive counseling on the prevention of type 2 diabetes. They should have a 2-h, 75-g oral glucose tolerance test (OGTT) at 6 weeks postpartum and yearly fasting glucose or OGTT screening thereafter. Women who have a history of GDM should be screened for diabetes before conception when planning another pregnancy.

Maternal postpartum follow-up care is recommended to prevent or delay the development of type 2 diabetes. The National Diabetes Education Program (NDEP), "Small Steps. Big Rewards Prevent

Type 2 Diabetes" campaign recommends breastfeeding and achieving prepregnancy weight within 12 months after delivery. If BMI is still ≥25 kg/m², then an additional 5–7% of body weight should be reduced slowly over time through healthy food choices and increasing physical activity to at least 30 min 5 days per week (33).

CELIAC DISEASE

Celiac disease (CD) is an immune-mediated enteropathy that results from the exposure to gluten found in wheat, barley, and rye. The gluten causes an immune response that causes an inflammatory reaction in the upper small intestine leading to villous atrophy. CD occurs in about 1% of the population in the USA, and it is estimated that 97% of those people are not diagnosed (34). Approximately 6–10% of individuals with type 1 diabetes have CD (35).

Clinical symptoms vary dramatically according to the individual and the age. Young children often present with diarrhea, abdominal pain, and poor growth, though vomiting, irritability, anorexia, and even constipation are common. Older children and adolescents sometimes present with short stature, neurological symptoms, and anemia (36). The classic presentation among adults is diarrhea, abdominal distention or discomfort though only about 50% of new cases in the last 10 years have presented with diarrhea (37). Many people have silent symptoms such as chronic anemia, osteoporosis, gastroesophageal reflux, unrecognized weight loss, and elevated liver enzymes. Erratic blood glucoses from untreated CD in individuals with type 1 diabetes are sometimes exacerbated by concomitant gastroparesis.

Recognizing the disease can be difficult because of the variety of nonspecific symptoms. (See Table 7) Current guidelines for screening recommend a tissue transglutaminase-IgA (tTG-IgA) or endomysial IgA antibody (EMA IgA). In addition, the physician should draw a total IgA, as approximately 2–3% of people with CD are IgA deficient and neither of the IgA antibody tests will be valid. Many celiac screening panels will include the tissue tranglutaminase-IgG, which is less specific but is useful in those individuals who are IgA antibody deficient (38).

Patients with a positive screening test are referred to a gastroenterologist for the definitive diagnostic procedure, an upper endoscopy with small bowel biopsy. Once the diagnosis is confirmed in an individual with type 1 diabetes, it is important for them to follow up with their healthcare team, which should include an endocrinologist, diabetes nurse educator, social worker/psychology support, and a dietitian with expertise in both diabetes and CD. As the individuals' small bowel heals and their absorption improves, they will need to work closely with their team to adjust their insulin needs.

The autoimmune response is directed to the prolamin storage proteins in some grains: wheat (gliadin), rye (secalin), and barley (horedin). The treatment for CD is to remove all foods from the diet that contain wheat, rye, and barley. This is referred to as a gluten-free diet (GFD). All sources of gluten-containing grains should be avoided and some of those ingredients are as follows: bulgur, cracked wheat, durum flour, enriched flour, farina flour, gluten flour, graham flour, self-rising flours, semolina, spelt, and triticale. Many gluten-free grains are more refined and lower in fiber, have a higher GI then their gluten-containing counterparts, and may warrant additional insulin to provide the same blood glucose control. The GFD can be well balanced but traditionally many of the flours used to make the commercially prepared GF foods are not fortified or enriched, and thus they are much lower in the B vitamins, iron, and fiber. Patients should be encouraged to use products made with whole GF grains (amaranth, buckwheat, quinoa, Montina®, bean flours, millet, corn, nut flours), which are better sources of iron, fiber, and some B vitamins (39).

Table 7
Signs and Symptoms of Celiac Disease

Abdominal distention
Abdominal pain
Anemia
Anorexia (poor appetite)
Bloating
Bone and joint pain
Constipation
Cramping (abdominal and/or muscle)
Dental hypoplasia (enamel missing on teeth)
Dermatitis herpetiformis (rash)
Diarrhea
Elevated liver enzymes
Failure to grow (children)
Fatigue (tired, no energy)
Folate deficiency
Foul-smelling stools pale in color
Inability to concentrate
Infertility in women
Irritability
Iron deficiency anemia
Muscle cramps
Osteopenia and osteoporosis (bone loss)
Short stature
Sleep disturbance
Sores in the mouth called aphthous ulcers (canker sores)
Weakness
Weight loss
Vomiting

GLUTEN-FREE DIET

Grains and Grain Products

- Gluten-free breads and bread products are made with gluten free grains such as amaranth, arrowroot, buckwheat, corn, corn bran, corn flour, cornmeal, cornstarch, flax, Job's tears, legumes flours [bean, garbanzo (chickpea), garfava, lentil, pea], millet, Montina®flour (Indian rice grass), potato flour, potato starch, sweet potato, quinoa, rice bran, rice flours (white, brown, sweet), sago, sorghum, soy, tapioca, and teff.
- Oats are gluten-free but most commercial brands available on the market are contaminated with gluten. There are a few sources in the USA that are certified gluten-free and are listed at the Gluten-Free Certification Organization (http://www.GFCO.org). They should only be used with the advice of the medical team.
- Hot Cereal: amaranth, cornmeal, cream of corn, cream of rice, hominy grits, rice flakes, quinoa flakes, soy flakes, and soy grits.
- Cold cereals are made from the aforementioned allowed grains in a designated gluten-free facility.
- Pastas are made from beans, corn, peas, potato, quinoa, rice, soy, and wild rice.
- Miscellaneous: corn tortillas, corn chips, and mochi.

Milk and Milk Products

Milk, cream, most ice creams, buttermilk, plain yogurt, cheese, cream cheese, processed cheese, processed cheese foods, and cottage cheese.

Meat and Meat Alternatives

- All fresh meat, poultry, and fish
- Eggs
- Meat alternatives: chickpeas, lentils, beans, nuts, seeds, and soy (tofu)

Fruits and Vegetables

- All fresh, frozen, and canned or bottled fruits and fruit juices
- All fresh, frozen, and canned vegetable and vegetables juices

Soups

- Homemade broths and soups made with gluten-free bouillon cubes and allowed ingredients

Fats

- Butter, margarine, lard, vegetables oil, cream, shortening, and homemade salad dressing made with allowed ingredients

Desserts

- Most ice creams, sherbets, whipped topping custards, or pudding
- Baked cookies, cakes, or pastries made with the allowed ingredients.

Miscellaneous

- Beverages: tea instant or ground coffee (regular or decaffeinated) cocoa, soft drinks, cider, distilled alcohol beverages such as rum, gin, whiskey, vodka, wines, and pure liqueurs, and some soy, rice, or nut beverages.
- Sweets: honey, jam, jelly, marmalade, corn syrup, maple syrup, molasses, sugar (brown and white), icing
- Snack foods: plain popcorn, nuts, seeds, soy nuts, and corn chips
- Condiments: pickles, relish, olives, ketchup, mustard, tomato paste, pure herbs, spices, pure black pepper, vinegars (apple, distilled, white, grape or wine, spirit), gluten-free soy, or steak sauce
- Other: sauces and gravies made with the allowed ingredients, pure cocoa, pure baking chocolate, carob chips and powder, chocolate chips, monosodium glutamate (MSG), cream or tarter, baking soda, yeast, brewer's yeast, aspartame, coconut, vanilla, and gluten-free communion wafers

RESOURCES FOR CELIAC DISEASE AND THE GLUTEN-FREE DIET

Celiac Medical Centers in the USA

- Celiac Center at Beth Israel Deaconess Medical Center, Boston, MA - http://www.bidmc.harvard.edu/celiaccenter
- Celiac Disease Center at Columbia University, New York, New York - http://www.celiacdiseasecenter.columbia.edu/CF-HOME.htm

- Celiac Disease Clinic Mayo Clinic, Rochester, MN - http://www.mayoclinic.org/celiac-disease/rsttreatment.html
- Celiac Center, Department of Internal Medicine, University of Iowa Hospitals and Clinics, Iowa City, IA – http://www.uihealthcare.com
- Celiac Clinic, Digestive Center of Excellence, University of Virginia Health System, Charlottesville, VA – http://www.healthsystem.virginia.edu/uvahealth/adult_digest/celiac.cfm
- Celiac Sprue Research Foundation, Palo Alto, CA – http://www.celiacsprue.org
- Celiac Disease Program, University of Chicago, Chicago, IL – http://www.uchospitals.edu/specialties/celiac
- Center for Celiac Research, University of Maryland Celiac Research Center, Baltimore, MD - http://www.celiaccenter.org
- Wm. K. Warren Medical Research Center for Celiac Disease, University of California, San Diego, CA - http://celiaccenter.ucsd.edu/index.shtml

Associations and Organizations

- American Celiac Society – http://www.americanceliacsociety.org
- American Celiac Disease Alliance – http://www.americanceliac.org/home.htm
- American Dietetic Association (ADA) – http://www.eatright.org
- Celiac Disease Foundation, Studio City, CA – http://www.celiac.org
- Celiac Sprue Association of the United States of America (CSA/USA, Inc), Omaha, NE – http://www.csaceliacs.org
- Gluten Intolerance Group, Seattle WA – http://www.gluten.net
- Canadian Celiac Association/L'association Canadienne de la Maladic Cocliaquc, Toronto, Canada – http://www.celiac.ca

REFERENCES

1. Jovanovic L. Medical nutritional therapy in pregnant women with pregestational diabetes mellitus. J Matern Fetal Med 2000;9(1):21–28
2. Kitzmiller JL, Block JM, Brown FM, Catalano PM, Conway DL, Coustan DR, et al. Managing preexisting diabetes for pregnancy: summary of evidence and consensus recommendations for care. Diabetes Care 2008;31(5):1060–1079
3. Institute of Medicine of the National Academies. Dietary DRI Reference Intakes: The Essential Guide to Nutrient Requirements. Washington, DC: The National Academies Press, 2006
4. Committee to Reexamine IOM Pregnancy Weight Guidelines Institute of Medicine; National Research Council. Weight Gain During Pregnancy: Reexamining the Guidelines. Rasmussen, KM. and Yaktine AL, eds. 2009: The National Academies Press, Washington D.C. in press
5. Muscati SK, Gray-Donald K, Koski KG. Timing of weight gain during pregnancy: promoting fetal growth and minimizing maternal weight retention. Int J Obes Relat Metab Disord 1996;20(6):526–532
6. Centers for Disease Control and Prevention. Pregnancy Nutrition Surveillance Survey. Atlanta, GA: Centers for Disease Control and Prevention, 2008, 8-28-2008
7. USDA. Nutrition and Your Health: Dietary Guidelines for Americans. US Department of Agriculture and Health and Human Services. http://www.health.gov/dietaryguidelines/, accessed 5-17-2008
8. American Association of Diabetes Educators. Pregnancy with Preexisting Diabetes. The Art and Science of Diabetes Self Management Education. Chicago, IL: AADE, 2006, pp. 233–257
9. Thomas AM, Gutierrez YM. American Dietetic Association Guide to Gestational Diabetes Mellitus. Chicago, IL: American Dietetic Association, 2005
10. Institute of Medicine of the National Academies. Dietary Carbohydrates: Sugars and Starches. Dietary Reference Intakes: The Eessential Guide to Nutrient Requirements. Washington, DC: The National Academies Press, 2006, pp. 102–109
11. American Association of Diabetes Educators. Intensifying Insulin Therapy. The Art and Science of Diabetes Self Management Education. Chicago, IL: AADE, 2006

12. Warshaw H, Kulkarni K. Complete Guide to Carbohydrate Counting, 2nd edn. Alexandria, VA: American Diabetes Association, 2004

13. Position of the American Dietetic Association and Dietitians of Canada. Vegetarian diets. J Am Diet Assoc 2003;103(6):748–765

14. Innis SM. Fatty acids and early human development. Early Hum Dev 2007;83(12):761–766

15. Cheatham CL, Colombo J, Carlson SE. N-3 fatty acids and cognitive and visual acuity development: methodologic and conceptual considerations. Am J Clin Nutr 2006;83(6 Suppl):1458S–1466S

16. Koletzko B, Cetin I, Brenna JT. Dietary fat intakes for pregnant and lactating women. Br J Nutr 2007;98(5):873–877

17. Kris-Etherton PM, Innis S, Ammerican DA. Dietitians of Canada. Position of the American Dietetic Association and Dietitians of Canada: dietary fatty acids. J Am Diet Assoc 2007;107(9):1599–1611

18. U.S. Food and Drug Administration. Fresh and Frozen Seafood: Selecting and Serving it Safely. Center Food Safety and Applied Nutrition. 8-29-2008 http://www.fda.gov/Food/ResourcesForYou/Consumers/ucm077331.htm, accessed 8-29-2008

19. Kaiser L, Allen LH. Position of the American Dietetic Association: nutrition and lifestyle for a healthy pregnancy outcome. J Am Diet Assoc 2008;108(3):553–561

20. American Dietetic Association. Position of the American Dietetic Association: use of nutritive and nonnutritive sweeteners. J Am Diet Assoc 2004;104(2):255–275

21. US Department of Agriculture. MyPyramid for Pregnancy and Breastfeeding. USDA, 2008. 7-17-2008

22. Kaiser LL, Allen L. Position of the American Dietetic Association: nutrition and lifestyle for a healthy pregnancy outcome. J Am Diet Assoc 2002;102(10):1479–1490

23. Hollis BW, Wagner CL. Assessment of dietary vitamin D requirements during pregnancy and lactation. Am J Clin Nutr 2004;79(5):717–726

24. Weng X, Odouli R, Li DK. Maternal caffeine consumption during pregnancy and the risk of miscarriage: a prospective cohort study. Am J Obstet Gynecol 2008;198(3):279.e1–e8

25. Savitz DA, Chan RL, Herring AH, Howards PP, Hartmann KE. Caffeine and miscarriage risk. Epidemiology 2008;19(1):55–62

26. USDA National Nutrient Database for Standard Reference. 2008 http://www.nal.usda.gov/fnic/foodcomp/, accessed 7-17-2008

27. James DC, Dobson B. Position of the American Dietetic Association: promoting and supporting breastfeeding. J Am Diet Assoc 2005;105(5):810–818.

28. Slocum J, Barcio L, Darany J, Friedley K, Homko C, Mills JJ, et al. Preconception to postpartum: management of pregnancy complicated by diabetes. Diabetes Educ 2004;30(5):740, 742–740, 753

29. Evert A, Vande-Hei K. Gestational diabetes education and diabetes prevention strategies. Diabetes Spectr 2006;19(3):135–139

30. American Dietetic Association. Medical Nutrition Therapy Evidence-Based Guides for Practice. Nutrition Practice Guidelines for GDM. Chicago, IL: American Dietetic Association, 2001

31. Marcason W. What is the appropriate amount and distribution of carbohydrates for a woman diagnosed with gestational diabetes mellitus? J Am Diet Assoc 2005;105(10):1673

32. National Diabetes Education Program. It's Never Too Early to Prevent Diabetes. A Lifetime of Small Steps for a Healthy Family. Tip Sheet. NIH, 2008. 7-19-2008

33. Fasano A, Berti I, Gerarduzzi T, Not T, Colletti RB, Drago S, et al. Prevalence of celiac disease in at-risk and not-at-risk groups in the United States: a large multicenter study. Arch Intern Med 2003;163(3):286–292

34. Not T, Tommasini A, Tonini G, Buratti E, Pocecco M, Tortul C, et al. Undiagnosed coeliac disease and risk of autoimmune disorders in subjects with Type I diabetes mellitus. Diabetologia 2001;44(2):151–155

35. D'Amico MA, Holmes J, Stavropoulos SN, Frederick M, Levy J, DeFelice AR, et al. Presentation of pediatric celiac disease in the United States: prominent effect of breastfeeding. Clin Pediatr (Phila) 2005;44(3):249–258

36. Rampertab SD, Pooran N, Brar P, Singh P, Green PH. Trends in the presentation of celiac disease. Am J Med 2006;119(4):355.e9–355.e14

37. Cataldo F, Marino V, Ventura A, Bottaro G, Corazza GR. Prevalence and clinical features of selective immunoglobulin A deficiency in coeliac disease: an Italian multicentre study. Italian Society of Pediatric Gastroenterology and Hepatology (SIGEP) and "Club del Tenue" Working Groups on Coeliac Disease. Gut 1998;42(3):362–365

38. Thompson T, Dennis M, Higgins LA, Lee AR, Sharrett MK. Gluten-free diet survey: are Americans with coeliac disease consuming recommended amounts of fibre, iron, calcium and grain foods? J Hum Nutr Diet 2005;18(3):163–169

15

Preconception Care for Women with Diabetes Mellitus

Howard Blank and Jennifer Wyckoff

CONTENTS

ABSTRACT

Established preexisting diabetes affects over 1% of pregnancies, and that number is expected to rise. Hyperglycemia during the first few weeks of pregnancy can result in congenital malformations or miscarriage. Preexisting diabetes increases the risk of developing both fetal and maternal complications in pregnancy; some of which can be devastating. Through careful attention to *contraception*, preconception *counseling* and preconception medical *care*, many of these complications can be avoided. Preconception care (PCC) programs have been shown to be efficacious at reducing complications and perinatal mortality as well as cost effective. Wider adoption of PCC programs is needed.

Key words: Diabetes; Pregnancy; Women; Preconception; Congenital malformations; Miscarriage

INTRODUCTION: WHAT IS PRECONCEPTION CARE?

Diabetes diagnosed prior to pregnancy, whether type 1 (DM1) or type 2 (DM2), is defined as preexisting diabetes (preexisting DM). Preexisting DM was previously estimated to complicate 0.48–0.72% of pregnancies each year in the US *(1, 2)*. However, there is clear evidence that the prevalence is rising. A recent study from a single Health Maintenance Organization (HMO) system

From: *Diabetes in Women: Pathophysiology and Therapy*
Edited by: A. Tsatsoulis et al. (eds.), DOI 10.1007/978-1-60327-250-6_15
© Humana Press, a part of Springer Science+Business Media, LLC 2009

in southern California reported that in 1999 the age and race/ethnicity adjusted prevalence of preexisting diabetes was 0.81/100 cases, and by 2005 it had increased to 1.82/100 cases *(3)*. Preexisting diabetes is associated with a substantial increase in perinatal mortality as well as other maternal and fetal complications *(4–8)*. Approximately half the excess perinatal mortality is attributed to congenital malformations *(5)*. Preconception care (PCC) has been shown to markedly reduce the rate of congenital malformations *(9)*. Given the increasing prevalence of preexisting diabetes, there is an urgent need for increased emphasis on PCC. PCC is defined as "specialized care that focuses on issues not typically addressed during a routine exam which are specific to ensuring an optimal pregnancy outcome" *(10)*. The three key components (the three Cs) of PCC for women with diabetes are outlined in Table 1. All women with diabetes who are planning pregnancies should receive PCC consisting of (1) advice on effective *contraception* to be used until optimal glycemic control is documented, (2) *counseling* regarding the maternal and fetal risks associated with diabetes and strategies to minimize these risks during pregnancy, and (3) comprehensive medical *care* designed to optimize glycemic control and treat diabetic complications, hypertension, and hyperlipidemia in preparation for pregnancy.

EFFICACY OF PRECONCEPTION CARE AT REDUCING PREGNANCY COMPLICATIONS: WHY DO I NEED PRECONCEPTION CARE?

PCC reduces the risk of congenital malformations and perinatal mortality. In 1949, Dr. Priscilla White published a landmark case series on 439 pregnancies in patients with preexisting diabetes, which highlighted the association of congenital malformations, preeclampsia and prematurity with excess perinatal mortality in infants of mothers with diabetes *(11)*. Since that time, numerous studies have demonstrated an association between glycemic control and the occurrence of congenital malformations *(12–16)*. Further studies have shown that PCC programs that optimize glycemic control can substantially reduce the risk of congenital malformations *(17–23)*.

The cornerstone of PCC is the concept that hyperglycemia during organogenesis causes congenital malformations and that by avoiding hyperglycemia, congenital malformations can be prevented. Therefore, the goal of glycemic management in PCC is for the patient to attain as close to euglycemia, defined as a normal hemoglobin A1c (HbA1c), as possible while avoiding hypoglycemia *(24)*.

One recent study demonstrating the relationship between glycemic control and outcomes was a population-based study in the Netherlands, which investigated 573 pregnancies in 301 women with preexisting diabetes between 1985 and 2003 *(15)*. First trimester HbA1c values were identified in 474 (83%) of pregnancies. Those pregnancies in which a first trimester HbA1c was not identified were more likely to end with an adverse outcome [RR 3.3 (95% CI 2.6–4.1)]. Mean first trimester HbA1c was 7.4% (95% CI 7.3–7.5) in pregnancies terminating in good outcome as opposed to 8.5% (95% CI 8.2–8.9) in those with an adverse outcome. The investigators found a consistently positive and almost continually linear relationship between adverse outcome and first trimester HbA1c values >7%. Importantly, there was no lower threshold of HbA1c, with respect to the increased risk of malformation.

Table 1
The Three Cs of Preconception Care (PCC)

Contraception
Counseling
Care

A meta-analysis of seven older previously published studies found that for each 0.7% increase in the HbA1c, the associated risk of a congenital anomaly increased by an odds ratio of 1.2 (95% CI 1.1–1.4) *(14)* (see Fig. 1).

Despite the ominous relationship between hyperglycemia and pregnancy outcomes, it is clear that much of the excess risk can be avoided by attaining optimal glycemic control prior to pregnancy utilizing appropriate PCC. Kitzmiller's influential 1991 JAMA article demonstrated a greatly reduced rate of major congenital anomalies with PCC *(22)*. In his study, 10.9% of pregnancies presenting after conception were complicated by congenital anomalies compared with only 1.2% of pregnancies that had received PCC. The success was attributed largely to early glycemic control.

The Maine Diabetes in Pregnancy Project went a step further to demonstrate a reduction in perinatal mortality through PCC *(23)*. This study included women with preexisting diabetes and focused on good diabetes control before conception, the benefits of preconception counseling and appropriate antepartum and postpartum care. The effort resulted in significant improvements in fetal and neonatal death rates in offspring of women with DM1 and DM2, even though the women who received PCC were older and had diabetes for a longer period of time.

The Diabetes Control and Complications Trial (DCCT) had less dramatic but still consistent results *(21)*. It reviewed 270 pregnancies in 180 women with DM1 from 1983 to 1993. The women had been placed in one of two groups - an intensive therapy group or a conventional therapy group. At conception, the intensive therapy group had significantly lower HbA1c than the conventional therapy group (7.4 ± 1.3% vs. 8.1 ± 1.7%, respectively), and there was a trend toward reduced congenital malformations (*P* = 0.06). The intensive insulin group had a very low 1% incidence of congenital anomalies, comparable to the rates noted for the general population. Another evaluation of pregnancies in women with DM1 found that only women with a normal early pregnancy HbA1c (<5.6%) had a rate of congenital malformation comparable to the general population *(20)*.

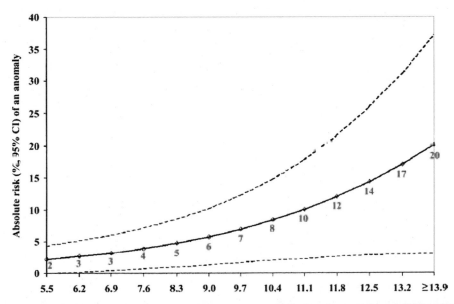

Fig. 1. Preconception hemoglobin A1c vs. absolute risk of congenital anomaly (solid) and 95% CI *(14)*. (Copyright © 2007 American Diabetes Association. From Diabetes Care®, Vol. 30, 2007; 1920–1925. Reprinted with permission from *The American Diabetes Association.*).

Another study analyzed the efficacy of PCC in a single center throughout time from before a program for PCC planning was in place until after funding for the center expired. They found that perinatal mortality in women with type 1 diabetes fell to zero occurrences by the end of the funding period and that congenital malformations also declined *(18)* (see Fig. 2).

The efficacy of PCC was analyzed in a 2001 metaanalysis, which found that patients undergoing PCC had lower early first trimester glycated hemoglobin. Pooled results indicate a marked reduction in major and minor congenital anomalies [2.4% (PCC) vs. 7.7% (no PCC)] even though PCC patients were older. When prospective studies were analyzed separately, the relative risk of congenital anomalies was 0.42 (95% CI 0.22–0.60) in those who received PCC *(9)*.

More recently, the Scottish Diabetes in Pregnancy Study found that the lowest rates of adverse pregnancy outcomes in women with DM1 occurred in those who had attained optimal HgbA1c (<7.0%) before discontinuing contraception *(25)*.

A 2006 prospective cohort study of women with DM1 identified that a PCC program that advocated education and attainment of preprandial blood glucose <6 mmol/l, postprandial blood glucose <8 mmol/l, and HbA1c <7.5% prior to conception led to significantly fewer adverse outcomes of pregnancy (malformations, stillbirths and neonatal deaths) *(19)*. There was a 2.9% adverse event rate in women receiving PCC compared with a 10.2% rate in those who did not receive PCC ($P = 0.03$), and the occurrence of premature delivery was also significantly lower.

An interesting comparison of congenital anomaly rates among different types of diabetes found that patients with "gestational diabetes" who were found after pregnancy from testing to actually have DM2 had a similar rate of congenital malformation as those with preexisting DM2 *(26)*.

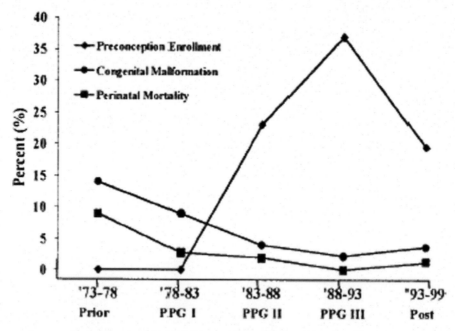

Fig. 2. Preconception enrollment, perinatal mortality, and congenital malformation rates for periods before, during, and after diabetes in Pregnancy Program Project Grant (PPG) at the University of Cincinnati from 1973 to 1999 *(18)*. (Reprinted (with permission) from Sherrie S. McElvy. A focused preconceptional and early pregnancy program in women with type 1 diabetes reduces perinatal mortality and malformation rates to general population levels. The Journal of Maternal-Fetal Medicine 2000;9:14–20.).

While all PCC programs stress the importance of good glycemic control, there are additional benefits of PCC, including counseling women about the importance of taking a prenatal multivitamin, which can reduce neural tube defects as just one example *(27)*. The efficacy of PCC programs at reducing congenital malformations and perinatal mortality is clearly well established.

Recommendation. All women with preexisting diabetes should receive PCC from a multidisciplinary team familiar with the area of diabetes and pregnancy.

THE THREE Cs: CONTRACEPTION, COUNSELING AND CARE

Contraception: Why Should I Use Contraception if I Want to Get Pregnant?

It is essential to optimize glycemic control before conception to prevent congenital anomalies. Given this fact, one can not overemphasize the importance of prepregnancy planning.

Despite this, close to 60% of women with diabetes do not plan their pregnancies. One highly concerning fact is that more than 80% of those who had one unplanned pregnancy had a second unplanned pregnancy *(28)*. Each and every reproductive age woman with diabetes should be counseled on contraception and the importance of PCC. Contraceptive choices should be tailored to the individual's needs and preferences and are discussed in detail in Chap. 9. Contraception should be continued until the glycemic control is optimal, preconception counseling has occurred, and the medical management of diabetes complications and comorbidities has been addressed.

Recommendation. All reproductive age women should be counseled on contraception and contraceptive choices and be advised that contraception should be continued until glycemic control is optimal.

Counseling and Preconception Care Recommendations to Reduce Maternal and Fetal Risks of Preexisting Diabetes: What Are the Risks of Diabetes in Pregnancy?

Women with diabetes and their families need a clear understanding of the risks of diabetes in pregnancy, as the women themselves must play the key role in preventing many of these complications. Diabetes education, both general and specific to pregnancy, is essential, as is a clear, straightforward discussion of risks and strategies to prevent complications.

Table 2 provides a checklist for some of the specific components of preconception counseling and care. Structuring preconception counseling is complex, both due to the complexity of the disease and due to the emotional impact that this information can have. Various complications are entangled with other complications [i.e., nephropathy with preeclampsia, and prematurity, diabetic ketoacidosis (DKA) with intrauterine fetal demise (IUFD), making counseling even more difficult].

Recommendation. All women with diabetes who are planning a pregnancy should be advised of the risks of diabetes and pregnancy and ways to minimize those risks.

FERTILITY: WILL WE HAVE TROUBLE GETTING PREGNANT?

Few data exist regarding the fertility of women with DM1. A Swedish population-based study examined the Standardized Fertility Ratio (ratio of observed to expected number of live births) as a proxy for fertility in which one would equal that of the general population *(29)*. The ratio was 0.77 (95% CI 0.60–0.98) in women with DM1 and macrovascular and microvascular complications such as retinopathy, nephropathy, and neuropathy. This suggests some decrease in fertility, though more data is needed on the relative impact of DM1, hyperglycemia and diabetes complications on fertility.

Fertility in women with DM2 is an even more complex issue. Obesity and polycystic ovarian syndrome (PCOS), both known to effect fertility, often occur with DM2. One review found that

Table 2
Checklist for Preconception Counseling and Care

Initial visit

Establish near euglycemia as preconception goal

Initiate insulin and discontinue oral hypoglycemic agents (except possibly metformin).
    Diabetes education for insulin dosing to improve glycemic control

Develop plan for contraception until euglycemia is achieved

Counsel on the natural history of insulin resistance in pregnancy

Counsel on risks to pregnancy including spontaneous abortion, congenital malformations, macrosomia,
    neonatal hypoglycemia, IUFD, etc.

Counsel on management of significant hyperglycemia. (For patients with DM1, review DKA prevention with
    special consideration for pregnancy's impact on risk for DKA and DKA's potential impact on pregnancy).

Counsel on hypoglycemia safety, including driving safety and the use of glucagon

Genetic counseling for diabetes

Counsel on the risk of retinopathy

Initiate preconception ophthalmologic evaluation

Obtain lipid profile, if not previously performed

Medical nutrition therapy (MNT)

Consider need for cardiac evaluation in high-risk patients

Counsel on smoking cessation strategies and set this as a preconception goal, if applicable

Obtain a baseline measure of urine albumin excretion

Counsel on the risks of preeclampsia and preterm delivery

Counsel on the risk of progressive renal disease

Counsel on maternal fertility, and if applicable, PCOS

Obtain baseline TSH, if no previous one available

Subsequent hyperglycemic visits

Evaluation of and counseling on insulin dosing to improve glycemic control

MNT for improving glycemic control

Reinforcement of smoking cessation if applicable

Initial euglycemic visit

Once glycemic goal is achieved, discontinue contraception and reevaluate medication list with special atten-
    tion to lipid-lowering and antihypertensive medications

Begin prenatal vitamin

Refer to reproductive endocrinology, if needed

women with a BMI greater than 30 kg/m^2 have a much higher risk of infertility and a higher risk of miscarriage *(30)*. A more detailed discussion of fertility in these settings is provided in Chap. 10.

Recommendation. Some women with preexisting diabetes may have trouble conceiving, but most will not. Clinicians should maintain a high index of suspicion for PCOS, and if clinical criteria are met, further investigation for PCOS and possibly, congenital adrenal hyperplasia may be warranted. If infertility is documented or there are other clinical concerns, referral to a reproductive endocrinologist may be indicated.

Maternal Hypoglycemia: Will Low Blood Sugars Hurt My Baby?

Hypoglycemia can be a serious problem, endangering maternal safety, especially during the first trimester of pregnancy. Careful attention should be paid to patient education, including the correct treatment of mild hypoglycemia, family education on the use of glucagon, and a thorough discussion of safe driving practices. To investigate the effect of hypoglycemia during organogenesis, an analysis of major congenital anomalies in offspring from a prepregnancy clinic was performed. One of the 12 women who had abnormal babies experienced hypoglycemia during organogenesis; 45 other women with severe hypoglycemia had normal babies. In fact, women who attended the prepregnancy clinic, as opposed to those who did not, had lower first trimester HbA1c and significantly lower rates of congenital malformations *(31)*. This was consistent with earlier findings showing no increased rate of malformations in women with hypoglycemia *(22)*.

Recommendations. Careful education on hypoglycemia treatment and safety precautions are important for maternal safety. However, hypoglycemia does not appear to increase the risk of congenital malformations.

Diabetic Ketoacidosis and Intrauterine Fetal Demise (IUFD): How High Is Dangerous?

In contrast to the fetus' relative tolerance of hypoglycemia, the fetus does not tolerate severe hyperglycemia or DKA well. To make matters worse, pregnant women are more likely to go into DKA at lower levels of hyperglycemia than women who are not pregnant *(32)*. As a result, the diagnosis of DKA may be delayed. Fetal mortality may occur in 9–35% of cases in which DKA occurs in the mother *(33, 34)*.

IUFD is more common in pregnancies complicated by diabetes. Not all cases are found to have a clear cause. Peripheral vascular disease and placental factors are thought to play a role in some cases. Extreme hyperglycemia may play a role also, as Priscilla White's original article showed a now well-recognized association between DKA and IUFD *(11)*.

Recommendation. All women with DM1 should be counseled on appropriate measures to prevent, recognize, and treat DKA.

Hypertension/Nephropathy/Preeclampsia and Prematurity

The relationship between hypertension, diabetic nephropathy and preeclampsia is complex, the increased rate of preterm birth seen in women with diabetes is influenced by multiple factors including the higher rate of preeclampsia.

Hypertension: How Does Hypertension Effect a Pregnancy? Are My Blood Pressure Medications Safe in Pregnancy? Hypertension is a risk factor for preeclampsia, which is discussed in more detail in the section "Preeclampsia: What is the danger of preeclampsia?" and in Chaps. 16 and 19. The main focus of PCC, one study found that hypertension is selecting appropriate medications. Antihypertensive medications considered unsafe in pregnancy include ACE inhibitors *(35)* and ARBs *(36)*. These should be discontinued prior to conception, and if necessary, replaced with antihypertensives commonly used in pregnancy. Calcium channel blockers (nifedipine), certain beta blockers (metoprolol or labetalol), and methyl dopa are commonly used.

Recommendations. The antihypertensive medication regimen should be reviewed and modified prior to conception to include only those antihypertensives considered safe in pregnancy.

Nephropathy: Does Pregnancy Increase My Risk of Kidney Disease? Does My Kidney Disease Affect My Pregnancy? For most women with diabetes, pregnancy does not increase the risk for renal disease. Even though the urine albumin excretion rate naturally increases in pregnancy, it usually returns to baseline after pregnancy, even in patients with diabetes *(37)*. The EURODIAB trial showed that pregnancy was not a factor in the development of microalbuminuria *(38)*, and the DCCT found no important long-term effects of pregnancy on the development of renal disease or nephropathy *(39)*. A 2002 study found that in women with microalbuminuria and normal baseline renal function, pregnancy had no prolonged impact on renal function *(40)*. Studies in women with other forms of mild renal impairment have shown similar results *(41)*.

However, some women with diabetes will have progression of renal disease during pregnancy. Gordon et al. found that women with an initial creatinine clearance less than 90 ml/min or proteinuria greater than 1 g/day had a significantly increased risk for progression of renal disease during pregnancy *(42)*. In women with moderate renal impairment (serum creatinine 1.4–1.9 mg/dl), 40% demonstrated a decline in renal function during pregnancy *(41)*. In women with severe renal impairment (serum creatinine greater than 2.0 mg/dl) 13 out of 20 had a decline in renal function, which persisted and resulted in end-stage renal failure in 7 out of 13 *(41)*.

Severity of nephropathy is a risk factor for preeclampsia and increased perinatal mortality. For women with serum creatinine greater than 2.0 mg/dl the risk of preterm delivery is greater then 90%; the risk of preeclampsia is 60%, and the risk of perinatal death is 10% *(43)*.

Recommendations. A serum creatinine and an assessment of urinary protein excretion to assess risk are needed in all women with preexisting diabetes. In women with renal disease, a clear discussion of the maternal and fetal risks related to renal disease, preeclampsia and pre term delivery is important.

Preeclampsia: What Is the Danger of Preeclampsia?   Preeclampsia is the onset of hypertension and proteinuria during pregnancy after the 20th week of gestation. It can lead to maternal acute renal failure, cerebrovascular and cardiovascular events, and death *(44)*. It occurs in 5–7% of the general population during pregnancy, and significant risk factors for the development of preeclampsia include nulliparity [RR 2.91 (95% CI 1.28–6.61)], preexisting diabetes [RR 3.56 (95% CI 2.54–4.99)], and previous preeclampsia in pregnancy [RR 7.91 (95% CI 5.85–8.83)]. Additional risk factors include advanced maternal age (greater than 40 years old), BMI greater than 35 kg/m^2, and hypertension *(45)*.

Multiple studies have recognized the increased risk of developing preeclampsia in pregnancies specifically complicated by diabetes *(7, 46)*. A nationwide Dutch study prospectively compared pregnant women with type 1 diabetes with the nondiabetic pregnant population and found a 12-fold increase in the risk of developing preeclampsia (95% CI 9–16.1) *(46)*. In Denmark 18.1% of women with DM1 developed preeclampsia compared with 2.6% of the background population *(7)*.

The level of glycemic control has also been shown to be an independent risk factor for the development of preeclampsia. One study found that for each 1% increment in first trimester HbA1c, the risk for development of preeclampsia rose by a factor of 1.6; each 1% decrement in baseline HbA1c lowered the risk by 0.6-fold *(47)*.

In studies that compared pregnancies affected by DM1 to those with DM2, no significant difference was found in rates of preeclampsia and pregnancy-induced hypertension between the populations *(4, 48)*. While the occurrence of hypertension in pregnancy appears similar in women with type 1 and type 2 diabetes, women with type 2 diabetes more often had chronic prepregnancy hypertension. Prepregnancy microalbuminuria and diabetic nephropathy are significant risk factors for preeclampsia *(49)*. One metaanalysis demonstrated that women with macroalbuminuria have a 41% incidence of preeclampsia *(50)*.

Recommendations. All women with preexisting DM should be counseled on the risk and the signs and symptoms of preeclampsia. Careful monitoring in the third trimester for the development of preeclampsia is warranted.

Prematurity/Preterm Delivery: Will I Deliver Full Term? A year 2000 prospective multicenter observational study compared the rates of preterm delivery between patients with preexisting diabetes and healthy controls. The total rate (38%) of preterm delivery [both indicated (21.9%) and spontaneous (16.1%)] among healthy singleton pregnancies in women with preexisting DM was found to be elevated compared with that among pregnancies in women with normal controls (overall rate 13.9%; indicated 3.4% and spontaneous 10.5%) *(51)*.

A year 2004 study looking consecutively at 168 deliveries in patients with DM1 found that factors associated with spontaneous preterm delivery (which occurred in 9% of women with DM1) included age less than 25 years old, polyhydramnios, and elevated HbA1c at delivery time. Factors associated with indicated preterm delivery (which occurred in 15%) were nulliparity, chronic hypertension, worsened nephropathy or retinopathy, elevated HbA1c at delivery, and preeclampsia when compared with those associated with diabetic women who had full-term pregnancies *(52)*.

In a large observational study, pregnant hypertensive women with DM1 more often had preterm delivery and cesarean deliveries, and their babies went to the special care unit with higher frequency than hypertensive women with DM2 *(53)*.

Recommendations. Women need to be counseled as to the risks of preterm delivery and should consider delivering at a hospital with a neonatal intensive care unit.

RETINOPATHY: WHY DO I HAVE TO HAVE AN EYE EXAM?

Accelerated retinopathy leading to visual loss during pregnancy or the peripartum period can occur *(54)*. Several studies, including the Diabetes in Early Pregnancy Study (DIEP) *(55)*, the DCCT *(39)*, and the EURODIAB trial *(38)*, have investigated the relationship between preexisting diabetes and the development or progression of diabetic retinopathy.

The DCCT showed an overall twofold increased risk for worsened diabetic retinopathy during pregnancy compared with nonpregnant women. Generally the effect was transient but it was sustained during the first postpartum year. Three out of 183 women who had no retinopathy or minimal nonproliferative baseline retinopathy progressed to severe retinopathy during the study. Although this study is one of the "gold standard" studies of DM1, the overall number of pregnancies was low, and HbA1c values generally were low at baseline, likely decreasing the magnitude of effect seen *(39)*.

The presence and severity of baseline diabetic retinopathy has been shown to be an important risk factor for progression *(55–57)*. In one observational study, progression was defined as "development of retinopathy de novo or upgrading of retinopathy from the first trimester to later trimesters or postpartum or development or progression of new vessels requiring laser photocoagulation in one or both eyes" *(56)*. This study noted that 9.1% of patients with no baseline retinopathy progressed during pregnancy and 38.3% of those with PDR progressed *(56)*. These findings were remarkably similar to those of the DIEP, which reported that 10.3% of patients with no baseline retinopathy, 18.8% of those with mild nonproliferative retinopathy, and 54.8% of those with moderate to severe nonproliferative retinopathy progressed *(55)*.

Other risk factors for the development or progression of retinopathy include level of glycemic control *(38, 39, 55)*, the duration of diabetes *(57)*, rapidly improving glucose control in the first trimester *(55)*, and smoking *(57)*. It appeared that performing laser photocoagulation on women with proliferative disease before pregnancy helped to abate progression *(56, 58)*.

Recommendations. All women with preexisting diabetes should have a dilated retinal exam to assess retinopathy prior to conception. If active proliferative diabetic retinopathy is present, some practitioners recommend delaying conception until retinopathy has become quiescent.

Hyperlipidemia: When Should I Stop My Cholesterol Medication?

During preconception, standard monitoring and management of lipid disorders should be maintained until discontinuation of birth control methods. Once a woman is trying to conceive, HMG Co reductase inhibitors, fibric acid derivatives and most other lipid lowering agents should be discontinued. Medical Nutrition Therapy remains the mainstay of lipid management during pregnancy.

Pregnancy is known to increase triglyceride levels markedly in the second and third trimesters (59). One dangerous complication of hyperlipidemia in pregnancy occurs in severe familial hypertriglyceridemia, where pancreatitis has been known to complicate pregnancies with devastating results. Therefore, it is important that during preconception women are screened for lipid disorders and that women with severe hypertriglyceridemia have sequential measurements of triglycerides during pregnancy (60).

Recommendations. All lipid-lowering medications should be discontinued at the time that contraception is discontinued.

Macrovascular Disease: Should I Have a Stress Test Before Becoming Pregnant?

There are relatively few cases of myocardial infarction during pregnancy. However, diabetes is clearly a risk factor for this rare event. In Roth's review of all cases reported prior to 1996, 5% of the cases of MI in pregnancy were in patients with preexisting diabetes. Risk factors for acute myocardial infarction in pregnancy or peripartum are similar to those in the general population: family history, familial hyperlipoproteinemia, low concentration of high-density lipoprotein, high concentration of low-density lipoprotein, diabetes, smoking, and previous use of oral contraceptives. Most events occurred in the third trimester or in the postpartum period. Interestingly less than half were associated with atherosclerotic disease (61).

Smoking is an important risk factor not only for macrovascular disease but also for intrauterine growth retardation. Smoking cessation should be urged for all women in the preconception period.

Recommendations. Exercise echocardiograms may be considered for women with diabetes over the age of 35. Duration of diabetes, presence of diabetes complications, and other CAD risk factors should be included in this decision. Provide all women who smoke with counseling on smoking cessation prior to conception.

IUGR: Why Do I Have to Worry About Small Babies Too?

In a manner similar to preterm birth, there are many factors that affect the rate of IUGR. Smoking and vascular disease are thought to be two of the predominant factors. Pregnancies in women with nephropathy more frequently result in intrauterine growth restriction (49).

Recommendations. Women with preexisting diabetes should be aware of their risk for IUGR and the risk factors for it. Again smoking cessation is advised.

Thyroid Disease: Does My Thyroid Disease Affect My Pregnancy?

Thyroid disease is a common problem for women with both DM1 and DM2. All women with diabetes should be screened with a TSH for thyroid abnormalities in the preconception period. Women with hypothyroidism on stable replacement hormone doses should be advised to increase their thyroid hormone dose by 30% once pregnancy is confirmed (62). It is beyond the scope of this chapter to discuss the management of hyper or hypothyroidism in detail.

Recommendations. All women with diabetes should be screened with a TSH for thyroid dysfunction in the preconception period.

Congenital Malformations: What Congenital Malformations Are Associated with Diabetes?

Because perinatal mortality is closely related to the congenital anomaly rate, an analysis of types of anomalies is vital to understanding adverse pregnancy outcomes in diabetes. In 1971, Kucera identified rates of anomalies observed in infants of mothers with diabetes *(63)*. These included caudal regression, situs inversus, arthrogryposis, spinal anomalies, ureter duplex, hydronephrosis, pseudo-hermaphroditism, gross skeletal anomalies and anencephaly.

Since then numerous articles have been published, reporting congenital malformations, including cardiac (atrio- and ventriculoseptal defects, great artery abnormalities, Tetralogy of Fallot), genitourinary (hypospadias, ureter duplex, hydronephrosis), musculoskeletal (hemivertebra), central nervous system (neural tube defects, caudal regression, anencephaly), upper respiratory tract (cleft palate), and gastroschisis *(13, 46)*. In a separate study, more than a third of all anomalies reported were cardiac in origin *(14)*. Neural tube defects were generally found to be the second most common defect. One hypothesis of "diabetic embryopathy" suggests that the anomalies may be due to mesodermal and neural crest defects *(64)*.

Multiple studies have investigated the link between diabetes control and congenital malformations *(12–16)* and further established that preconception interventions aimed at reducing the HbA1c at conception can reduce the rate of congenital malformations *(17–23)*.

Recommendations. Glycemic control should be a goal prior to discontinuation of contraception.

SPONTANEOUS ABORTION: AM I AT RISK FOR MISCARRIAGE?

Spontaneous abortion occurs at a higher rate in pregnancies complicated by diabetes. A Danish study of women with type 1 diabetes showed a 17.5% miscarriage rate compared with 10–12% in the general population, with a longer duration of disease and older age as risk factors *(65)*. Other studies found similar rates of early pregnancy loss (EPL) ranging from 13.5 to 16.5% *(25, 66)*. The rate of EPL is related to the level of glycated serum protein levels *(67)* and HbA1c *(68, 69)*.

Recommendations. Women should be counseled on the higher rate or EPL and its relationship to glycemic control.

MACROSOMIA: WHAT IS WRONG WITH HAVING A BIG BABY?

Macrosomia is defined as a birth weight at the 90th percentile. It is a factor in many cases of shoulder dystocia, which occurs when the infant's shoulders fail to pass through the pubic bones spontaneously and can result in birth injury. Macrosomia is also a risk factor for both cesarean delivery (see section "Cesarean Delivery: Will I Have to Have a Cesarean Delivery?") and a risk factor for "metabolic imprinting" (see Chap. 20).

There are several risk factors for macrosomia other than maternal glycemia including maternal obesity, previous maternal delivery of a macrosomic infant and family history. However, the main modifiable risk factor for macrosomia is maternal glycemia. While HbA1c at conception is a risk factor for macrosomia, macrosomia is associated most closely with postprandial glucose values between 29 and 32 weeks of pregnancy *(70)*.

Metabolic imprinting refers to metabolic changes in the neonate caused by exposure to metabolic factors that increase the neonate's risk component for metabolic syndrome later in life. This is discussed in more detail in Chap. 20.

CESAREAN DELIVERY: WILL I HAVE TO HAVE A CESAREAN DELIVERY?

The rate of cesarean delivery is much higher in women with diabetes than in women without diabetes. In fact, findings indicate a relative risk 1.78–4.5 times higher for women with DM1 than in the general population *(7, 46, 71)*. Women with DM1 have a greater risk for cesarean delivery than women with DM2 *(4, 48)* these findings. The increased rate in cesarean delivery is due in part to the higher rate of macrosomia, but other factors also play a role.

Recommendations. Women with diabetes should be aware of their increased risk for cesarean delivery.

Neonatal Hypoglycemia: Will My Baby Need a NICU?

Neonatal hypoglycemia is defined as neonatal blood glucose <40 mg/dl; this can result in further adverse events, such as neonatal seizures.. One study found that 7.8% of infants born to mothers with preexisting diabetes experienced neonatal hypoglycemia (72).

Recommendations. Women with diabetes should be aware of this potential complication.

Genetic Risk: Will My Baby Have Diabetes?

Offspring of parents with DM1 have an increased risk of developing diabetes later in life. Children have a 3.5% and 7.6% cumulative risk of developing diabetes if their mothers or fathers have type 1 diabetes, respectively (73). The Framingham study evaluated the prevalence of DM2 in offspring and found that maternal DM2 diagnosed earlier than 50 years of age conferred an odds ratio of 9.7 (95% CI 4.3–22) and paternal DM2 diagnosed earlier than 50 years of age conferred an odds ratio of 5.3 (95% CI 2.1–13.6) when compared with offspring without parental diabetes (74).

Recommendations. Women with diabetes should be aware of their offsprings risk for diabetes.

Perinatal Mortality and Morbidity: What Is the Chance My Baby Will Die?

The perinatal mortality rate for infants of mothers with preexisting diabetes remains several times that of the general population, yet there have been marked improvements in the last 60 years. Priscilla White's case series found an 18% fetal fatality rate (11). Between the 1940s and 1988, the perinatal mortality rate due to complications from DM1 in pregnancy fell from 250–300/1,000 live births down to 30–50/1,000 live births in the US; while this represents a marked improvement in the care of women with preexisting diabetes, the background perinatal mortality rate in cases not complicated by diabetes fell from 60/1,000 live births down to 15/1,000 live births (75). Another study found a decline in perinatal mortality between 1940 and 1990 in pregnancies of women with DM1 from greater than 30% to 4% approaching (76).

Despite these dramatic gains, increased perinatal mortality remains a significant problem. A Danish study found that DM2 is associated with higher perinatal mortality [RR 4 (95% CI 1.0–15.5)] than DM1 and the general population [RR 8.9 (95% CI 3.4–23)], and the frequency of perinatal mortality along with major congenital anomalies is actually increasing since the 1980s and early 1990s, possibly due to older maternal age, more complicated diabetes and higher body weight (4). Another study found a perinatal mortality rate for infants of mothers with DM2 of 39.1/1,000 live births, which was higher than either that for gestational diabetes (16.2/1,000) or the general population (12.5/1,000) (8).

Perhaps one reason that there may be an increased risk for mothers with DM2 is that obesity itself is a significant risk factor for stillbirth or neonatal death, doubling the risk compared with nonobese mothers (77). A body mass index less than 20 kg/m^2 is also significantly associated with late fetal death (78). Although data looking at patients with preexisting DM are lacking, surgical interventions aimed at controlling prepregnancy obesity have been analyzed. Patients with prior gestational diabetes who have had gastric banding procedures before pregnancy do not incur increased risk of adverse perinatal outcomes compared with the general population, and there does not seem to be increased risk of postsurgical complications (79, 80).

While the causes of IUFD in women are not always identifiable, it is believed that uncontrolled hyperglycemia may account for half of stillbirth occurrences while congenital malformations and infection may cause a significant portion as well (81). While the frequency of pregnancy loss has been found to be similar within different types of preexisting DM, death in DM1 pregnancies is most often due to congenital anomalies and prematurity, and death in DM2 pregnancies is most often due to IUFD significantly later in pregnancy (5) (see Fig. 3).

A Scottish study showed a more than threefold higher risk of stillbirth and perinatal mortality in pregnancies of mothers with diabetes than in the background population (6). A Danish national study

Fig. 3. Rates and causes of pregnancy loss in type 1 and type 2 diabetics (including newly recognized diabetes). The scale indicates percentage of the total number of fetuses. (Reprinted with permission from (5).)

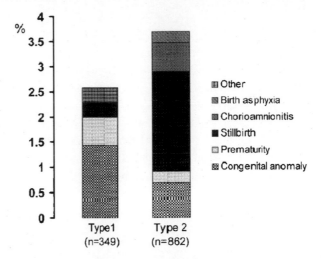

prospectively compared pregnancies in women with type 1 diabetes with the nondiabetic pregnant population from 1993 to 1999. The perinatal mortality rate was much higher in pregnancies complicated by DM1 [RR 4.1 (95% CI 2.9–5.6)]; babies were delivered earlier and had higher rates of cesarean delivery and macrosomia (7).

Perinatal morbidity for infants of mothers with diabetes includes not just macrosomia and neonatal hypoglycemia, but also rarer complications including hypocalcemia and hypomagnesemia, polycythemia, iron deficiency, respiratory distress, hyperbilirubinemia, cardiomyopathy and perinatal asphyxia (82).

Nutrition: What Should I Eat?

A universal question among women with diabetes who are planning pregnancies is "What should I eat?" Nutrition counseling is an integral part of any diabetes PCC program as it is necessary to ensure both glycemic control and nutritional adequacy before, during and after pregnancy. Individual recommendations will vary depending on insulin-dosing plan and patient characteristics and preferences. This requires a team approach with the dietitian working in concert with the endocrinologist, obstetrician, nurse and other health care providers. The patient must have a firm understanding of carbohydrates and their relation to blood glucose measurement and insulin dosing. In addition, it is recommended that folic acid supplementation be started prior to conception. This topic is reviewed in detail and recommendations are outlined in Chap. 14: Nutrition in Pregnancy.

Glycemic Control: What Do I Have to Do?

PCC has been successful in improving pregnancy outcomes for women with preexisting diabetes. PCC should involve a multidisciplinary approach with participation by endocrinologists, primary care physicians, obstetricians familiar with high-risk care, diabetes educators and an actively engaged patient. The ADA states that preconception and early pregnancy care need to include (1) education about the interaction of diabetes with pregnancy, (2) education in diabetes self-management skills, (3) physician-directed care and laboratory diagnosis and (4) engaging mental health professionals to reduce stress and improve adherence (60).

Preconception glycemic goals should target fasting glucose levels between 66 and 99 mg/dl and peak postprandial goals between 100 and 129 mg/dl. The goal HbA1c prior to pregnancy is "as close to normal as possible without significant hypoglycemia" (60). Basal/bolus insulin regimens are recommended. Given the increase in insulin resistance that occurs progressively during the later half of pregnancy, almost every women with preexisting diabetes will require insulin therapy during a pregnancy. Oral hypoglycemic medications, including sulfonylureas and thiazolidinediones, should be discontinued and insulin started in the preconception period. One may consider continuing metformin in women with PCOS as discussed in more detail in Chapter 10. Basal insulin can be supplied either through the use of NPH insulin or through CSII. Lispro and aspart have been studied in pregnancy and can be used for bolus therapy. Glargine has not been studied in randomized controlled trials in pregnancy *(60)*. A large study of insulin detemir in pregnancy is underway. Results of this study have not been published at the time of submission of this chapter.

General recommendations for monitoring are to check fasting glucoses levels and glucoses levels before and after each meal and at bedtime. The frequency of return visits and glucose log reviews during the PCC period needs to be individualized in order to ensure optimal glycemic control at the time of conception. Some patients need ongoing support on a weekly basis, while others need less intensive support. It is our recommendation to check the HbA1c every 4 weeks during the preconception period.

ADOPTION OF PRECONCEPTION CARE PROGRAMS: WHY DID I NOT KNOW ABOUT THIS WITH MY LAST PREGNANCY?

PCC has been shown to be highly effective in increasing the success of pregnancy in women with preexisting DM, yet only about a third of women attend PCC programs *(19)*. One study found that women who received PCC were older, more likely to be white, married, living with their partners, and had higher education and income than those who did not receive PCC. PCC patients were also more likely to have DM1. Importantly, the patients' health providers were more likely to have encouraged PCC with patients before pregnancy *(83)*. Similar findings were seen in a study published in 1998 *(28)*. A multicenter study found that about one-half of women recall receiving preconception glucose counseling and one-third recall receiving preconception family planning counseling from their primary care physicians. Male physicians were significantly more likely to provide counseling than female physicians while older, heavier patients were less likely to have been counseled by their primary care physicians *(84)*. One study found that documentation of PCC was quite low, occurring in only 25% of records of patients with DM1; close to one-half of patients were currently taking potentially teratogenic agents without comment about the effects to future pregnancies in the charts *(85)*.

The barriers to receiving appropriate PCC include lack of health insurance or a relationship with a physician, lack of adoption of established guidelines for PCC by individual physicians and medical centers, lack of education about the importance of PCC among women of childbearing age, and lack of nonmedical economic means, such as reliable transportation *(86)*. Sixty five percent of teenage women with DM1 were unfamiliar with the term "preconception counseling." Among the many misconceptions present in the patients in the study pool was that birth control was "dangerous" for patients with DM1. One-third did not know where PCC was available to them. Highlighting the need to perform "awareness counseling," which is the first phase of PCC aimed at women who are not imminently planning a pregnancy, is the fact that 43% of these teens had already engaged in intercourse and only 85% reported using some form of contraception *(87)*.

Although there are numerous studies showing the medical success of PCC, few studies have examined the economic benefits of PCC. When evaluating economic success it is important to understand that businesses want short-term financial rewards but most efforts to improve health care quality pay off economically in the long term. The dearth of data limited a review of this subject to three studies and all showed short-term benefit but did not expand their reach beyond this *(10)*.

SUMMARY

Preexisting diabetes increases the risk of pregnancy complications for both the mother and the infant. Many of these risks can be reduced by tight glycemic control at the time of conception; this requires effective preconception education and management. Numerous studies have shown that a reduction in congenital malformations and perinatal mortality can be achieved with such interventions. Components of PCC programs should include comprehensive diabetes education, specific education regarding the risks related to diabetes and pregnancy and ways to minimize them, advice regarding contraceptive options, supportive care designed to optimize glycemic control, careful consideration of management of comorbidities and complications in anticipation of pregnancy, comprehensive obstetric assessment, and initiation of folic acid supplementation and smoking cessation. This type of care is best delivered by a health care team skilled in the management of diabetes in the pregnant woman, including obstetrics, endocrinology, nursing, and nutrition support.

REFERENCES

1. Engelgau MM, Herman WH, Smith PJ, German RR, Aubert RE. The epidemiology of diabetes and pregnancy in the U.S., 1988. Diabetes Care 1995;18:1029–33.
2. Martin JA, Hamilton BE, Sutton PD, Ventura SJ, Manacker F, Kirmeyer S, Munson ML, Division of vital statistics. Births: final data for 2005. Natl Vital Stat Rep 2007;56:1–103.
3. Lawrence JM, Contreras R, Chen W, Sacks DA. Trends in the prevalence of preexisting diabetes and gestational diabetes mellitus among a racially/ethnically diverse population of pregnant women, 1999–2005. Diabetes Care 2008;31:899–904.
4. Clausen TD, Mathiesen E, Ekbom P, Hellmuth E, Mandrup-Poulsen T, Damm P. Poor pregnancy outcome in women with type 2 diabetes. Diabetes Care 2005;28:323–8.
5. Cundy T, Gamble G, Neale L, et al. Differing causes of pregnancy loss in type 1 and type 2 diabetes. (Pathophysiology/Complications) (Clinical report). Diabetes Care 2007;30:2603–7.
6. Penney GC, Mair G, Pearson DW, Scottish Diabetes in Pregnancy Group. Outcomes of pregnancies in women with type 1 diabetes in Scotland: a national population-based study. BJOG 2003;110:315–8.
7. Jensen DM, Damm P, Moelsted-Pedersen L, et al. Outcomes in type 1 diabetic pregnancies: a nationwide, population-based study. Diabetes Care 2004;27:2819–23.
8. Cundy T, Gamble G, Townend K, Henley PG, MacPherson P, Roberts AB Perinatal mortality in type 2 diabetes mellitus. Diabet Med 2000;17:33–9.
9. Ray JG, O'Brien TE, Chan WS. Preconception care and the risk of congenital anomalies in the offspring of women with diabetes mellitus: a meta-analysis. Q J Med 2001;94:435–44.
10. Grosse S, Sotnikov S, Leatherman S, Curtis M. The business case for preconception care: methods and issues. Matern Child Health J 2006;10:93–9.
11. White P. Pregnancy complicating diabetes. Am J Med 1949:609–17.
12. Miller E, Hare JW, Cloherty JP, Dunn PJ, Gleason RE, Soeldner JS, Kitzmiller JL. Elevated maternal hemoglobin A1c in early pregnancy and major congenital anomalies in infants of diabetic mothers. N Engl J Med 1981;304:1331–4.
13. Galindo A, Burguillo AG, Azriel S, Fuente Pde L. Outcome of fetuses in women with pregestational diabetes mellitus. J Perinat Med 2006;34:323.
14. Guerin A, Nisenbaum R, Ray JG. Use of maternal GHb concentration to estimate the risk of congenital anomalies in the offspring of women with prepregnancy diabetes. Diabetes Care 2007;30:1920–5.
15. Nielsen GL, Moller M, Sorensen HT. HbA1c in early diabetic pregnancy and pregnancy outcomes: a Danish population-based cohort study of 573 pregnancies in women with type 1 diabetes. Diabetes Care 2006;29:2612–6.
16. Greene MF, Hare JW, Cloherty JP, Benacerraf BR, Soeldner JS. First-trimester hemoglobin A1 and risk for major malformation and spontaneous abortion in diabetic pregnancy. Teratology 1989;39:225–31.
17. Dunne FP, Brydon P, Smith T, Essex M, Nicholson H, Dunn J. Pre-conception diabetes care in insulin-dependent diabetes mellitus. Q J Med 1999;92:175–6.
18. McElvy SS, Miodovnik M, Rosenn B, Khoury JC, Siddiqi T, Dignan PS, Tsang RC. A focused preconceptional and early pregnancy program in women with Type 1 diabetes reduces perinatal mortality and malformation rates to general population levels. J Matern Fetal Med 2000;9:14–20.
19. Temple RC, Aldridge VJ, Murphy HR. Prepregnancy care and pregnancy outcomes in women with type 1 diabetes. Diabetes Care 2006;29:1744–9.
20. Suhonen L, Hiilesmaa V, Teramo K. Glycaemic control during early pregnancy and fetal malformations in women with Type I diabetes mellitus. Diabetologia 2000;43:79–82.
21. Pregnancy outcomes in the Diabetes Control and Complications Trial. Am J Obstet Gynecol 1996;174:1343–53.

22. Kitzmiller JL, Gavin LA, Gin GD, Jovanovic-Peterson L, Main EK, Zigrang WD. Preconception care of diabetes. Glycemic control prevents congenital anomalies. JAMA 1991;265:731–6.

23. Willhoite MB, Bennert HW Jr, Palomaki GE, Zaremba MM, Herman WH, Williams JR, Spear NH. The impact of preconception counseling on pregnancy outcomes. The experience of the Maine diabetes in pregnancy program. Diabetes Care 1993;16:450–5.

24. Kitzmiller J BJ. Glycemic control and perinatal outcome. In: Kitzmiller J, Jovanovic L, Brown F, Coustan D, Reader D., ed. Managing Preexisting Diabetes and Pregnancy. Alexandria, VA: American Diabetes Association, 2008, p. 9.

25. Pearson DW, Kernaghan D, Lee R, Penney GC, Scottish Diabetes in Pregnancy Study Group The relationship between pre-pregnancy care and early pregnancy loss, major congenital anomaly or perinatal death in type I diabetes mellitus. BJOG 2007;114:104–7.

26. Farrell T, Neale L, Cundy T. Congenital anomalies in the offspring of women with type 1, type 2 and gestational diabetes. Diabet Med 2002;19:322–6.

27. Correa A, Botto L, Liu Y, Mulinare J, Erickson JD. Do multivitamin supplements attenuate the risk for diabetes-associated birth defects? Pediatrics 2003;111:1146–51.

28. Holing EV, Beyer CS, Brown ZA, Connell FA. Why don't women with diabetes plan their pregnancies? Diabetes Care 1998;21:889–95.

29. Jonasson JM, Brismar K, Sparen P, et al. Fertility in women with type 1 diabetes: a population-based cohort study in Sweden. Diabetes Care 2007;30:2271–6.

30. Linné Y. Effects of obesity on women's reproduction and complications during pregnancy. Obes Rev 2004;5:137–43.

31. Steel JM, Johnstone FD, Hepburn DA, Smith AF. Can prepregnancy care of diabetic women reduce the risk of abnormal babies? Br Med J 1990;301:1070–4.

32. Guo RX, Yang LZ, Li LX, Zhao XP. Diabetic ketoacidosis in pregnancy tends to occur at lower blood glucose levels: case-control study and a case report of euglycemic diabetic ketoacidosis in pregnancy. J Obstet Gynaecol Res 2008;34:324–30.

33. Kamalakannan D, Baskar V, Barton DM, Abdu TAM. Diabetic ketoacidosis in pregnancy. Postgrad Med J 2003;79:454–7.

34. Montoro MN, Myers VP, Mestman JH, Xu Y, Anderson BG, Golde SH. Outcome of pregnancy in diabetic ketoacidosis. Am J Perinatol 1993;10:17–20.

35. Cooper WO, Hernandez-Diaz S, Arbogast PG, et al. Major congenital malformations after first-trimester exposure to ACE inhibitors. N Engl J Med 2006;354:2443–51.

36. Bos-Thompson M-A, Hillaire-Buys D, Muller F, et al. Fetal toxic effects of angiotensin II receptor antagonists: case report and followup after birth. Ann Pharmacother 2005;39:157–61.

37. McCance DR, Traub AI, Harley JMG, Madden DR, Kennedy L. Urinary albumin excretion in diabetic pregnancy. Diabetologia 1989;32:236–9.

38. Vérier-Mine O, Chaturvedi N, Webb D, Fuller JH Is pregnancy a risk factor for microvascular complications? The EURODIAB Prospective Complications Study. Diabet Med 2005;22:1503–9.

39. Effect of pregnancy on microvascular complications in the diabetes control and complications trial. The diabetes control and complications trial research group. Diabetes Care 2000;23:1084–91.

40. Rossing K, Jacobsen P, Hommel E, et al. Pregnancy and progression of diabetic nephropathy. Diabetologia 2002;45:36–41.

41. Jones DC, Hayslett JP. Outcome of pregnancy in women with moderate or severe renal insufficiency. N Engl J Med 1996;335:226–32.

42. Gordon M, Landon MB, Samuels P, Hissrich S, Gabbe SG. Perinatal outcome and long-term follow-up associated with modern management of diabetic nephropathy. Obstet Gynecol 1996;87:401–9.

43. Williams D, Davison J. Chronic kidney disease in pregnancy. Br Med J 2008;336:211–5.

44. Wagner LK. Diagnosis and management of preeclampsia. Am Fam Physician 2004;70:2317–24.

45. Duckitt K, Harrington D. Risk factors for pre-eclampsia at antenatal booking: systematic review of controlled studies. Br Med J 2005;330:565.

46. Evers IM, de Valk HW, Visser GH. Risk of complications of pregnancy in women with type 1 diabetes: nationwide prospective study in the Netherlands. Br Med J 2004;328:915.

47. Hiilesmaa V, Suhonen L, Teramo K. Glycaemic control is associated with pre-eclampsia but not with pregnancy-induced hypertension in women with type 1 diabetes mellitus. Diabetologia 2000;43:1534–9.

48. Hillman N, Herranz L, Vaquero PM, Villarroel A, Fernandez A, Pallardo LF. Is pregnancy outcome worse in type 2 than in type 1 diabetic women? Diabetes Care 2006;29:2557–8.

49. Ekbom P, Damm P, Feldt-Rasmussen B, Feldt-Rasmussen U, Molvig J, Mathiesen ER. Pregnancy outcome in type 1 diabetic women with microalbuminuria. Diabetes Care 2001;24:1739–44.

50. Reece EA, Leguizamon G, Homko C. Pregnancy performance and outcomes associated with diabetic nephropathy. Am J Perinatol 1998;15:413–21.

51. Sibai BM, Caritis SN, Hauth JC, et al. Preterm delivery in women with pregestational diabetes mellitus or chronic hypertension relative to women with uncomplicated pregnancies. Am J Obstet Gynecol 2000;183:1520–4.

52. Lepercq J, Coste J, Theau A, Dubois-Laforgue D, Timsit J. Factors associated with preterm delivery in women with type 1 diabetes: a cohort study. Diabetes Care 2004;27:2824–8.

53. Cundy T, Slee F, Gamble G, Neale L. Hypertensive disorders of pregnancy in women with type 1 and type 2 diabetes. Diabet Med 2002;19:482–9.

54. Bastion ML, Barkeh HJ, Muhaya M. Accelerated diabetic retinopathy in pregnancy - a real and present danger. Med J Malaysia 2005;60:502–4.

55. Chew EY, Mills JL, Metzger BE, Remaley NA, Jovanovic-Peterson L, Knopp RH, Conley M, Rand L, Simpson JL, Holmes LB, et al. Metabolic control and progression of retinopathy. The Diabetes in Early Pregnancy Study. National Institute of Child Health and Human Development Diabetes in Early Pregnancy Study. Diabetes Care 1995;18:631–7.

56. Rahman W, Rahman FZ, Yassin S, Al-Suleiman SA, Rahman J. Progression of retinopathy during pregnancy in type 1 diabetes mellitus. Clin Experiment Ophthalmol 2007;35:231–6.

57. Temple RC, Aldridge VA, Sampson MJ, Greenwood RH, Heyburn PJ, Glenn A. Impact of pregnancy on the progression of diabetic retinopathy in type 1 diabetes. Diabet Med 2001;18:573–7.

58. Lapolla A, Cardone C, Negrin P, et al. Pregnancy does not induce or worsen retinal and peripheral nerve dysfunction in insulin-dependent diabetic women. J Diabetes Complications 1998;12:74–80.

59. Crisan LS, Steidl ET, Rivera-Alsina ME. Acute hyperlipidemic pancreatitis in pregnancy. Am J Obstet Gynecol 2008;198:e57–9.

60. Kitzmiller JL, Block JM, Brown FM, et al. Managing preexisting diabetes for pregnancy: summary of evidence and consensus recommendations for care. Diabetes Care 2008;31:1060–79.

61. Roth A, Elkayam U. Acute myocardial infarction associated with pregnancy. Ann Int Med 1996;125:751–62.

62. Alexander EK, Marqusee E, Lawrence J, Jarolim P, Fischer GA, Larsen PR. Timing and magnitude of increases in levothyroxine requirements during pregnancy in women with hypothyroidism. N Engl J Med 2004;351:241–9.

63. Kucera J. Rate and type of congenital anomalies among offspring of diabetic women. J Reprod Med 1971;7:73–82.

64. Sadler LS, Robinson LK, Msall ME. Diabetic embryopathy: possible pathogenesis. Am J Med Genet 1995;55:363–6.

65. Lorenzen T, Pociot F, Johannesen J, Kristiansen OP, Nerup J. A population-based survey of frequencies of self-reported spontaneous and induced abortions in Danish women with type 1 diabetes mellitus. Diabet Med 1999;16:472–6.

66. Casson IF, Clarke CA, Howard CV, et al. Outcomes of pregnancy in insulin dependent diabetic women: results of a five year population cohort study. Br Med J 1997;315:275–8.

67. Jovanovic L, Knopp RH, Kim H, et al. Elevated pregnancy losses at high and low extremes of maternal glucose in early normal and diabetic pregnancy: evidence for a protective adaptation in diabetes. Diabetes Care 2005;28:1113–7.

68. Key TC, Giuffrida R, Moore TR. Predictive value of early pregnancy glycohemoglobin in the insulin-treated diabetic patient. Am J Obstet Gynecol 1987;156:1096–100.

69. Rosenn B, Miodovnik M, Combs CA, Khoury J, Siddiqi TA. Glycemic thresholds for spontaneous abortion and congenital malformations in insulin-dependent diabetes mellitus. Obstet Gynecol 1994;84:515–20.

70. Combs CA, Gunderson E, Kitzmiller JL, Gavin LA, Main EK. Relationship of fetal macrosomia to maternal postprandial glucose control during pregnancy. Diabetes Care 1992;15:1251–7.

71. Feig DS, Razzaq A, Sykora K, Hux JE, Anderson GM. Trends in deliveries, prenatal care, and obstetrical complications in women with pregestational diabetes: a population-based study in Ontario, Canada, 1996–2001. Diabetes Care 2006;29:232–5.

72. Weintrob N, Karp M, Hod M. Short- and long-range complications in offspring of diabetic mothers. J Diabetes Complications 1996;10:294–301.

73. Tuomilehto J, Podar T, Tuomilehto-Wolf E, Virtala E. Evidence for importance of gender and birth cohort for risk of IDDM in offspring of IDDM parents. Diabetologia 1995;38:975–82.

74. Meigs JB, Cupples LA, Wilson PW. Parental transmission of type 2 diabetes: The Framingham Offspring Study. Diabetes 2000;49:2201–7.

75. Centers for Disease Control. Perinatal mortality and congenital malformations in infants born to women with insulin-dependent diabetes mellitus - United States, Canada, and Europe, 1940–1988. MMWR Morb Mortal Wkly Rep 1990;39:363–5.

76. Hadden DR, McCance DR. Advances in management of type 1 diabetes and pregnancy. Curr Opin Obstet Gynecol 1999;11:557–62.

77. Kristensen J, Vestergaard M, Wisborg K, Kesmodel U, Secher NJ. Pre-pregnancy weight and the risk of stillbirth and neonatal death. BJOG 2005;112:403–8.

78. Cnattingius S, Bergstrom R, Lipworth L, Kramer MS. Prepregnancy weight and the risk of adverse pregnancy outcomes. N Engl J Med 1998;338:147–52.

79. Dixon JB, Dixon ME, O'Brien PE. Birth outcomes in obese women after laparoscopic adjustable gastric banding. Obstet Gynecol 2005;106:965–72.

80. Sheiner E, Menes TS, Silverberg D, et al. Pregnancy outcome of patients with gestational diabetes mellitus following bariatric surgery. Am J Obstet Gynecol 2006;194:431–5.

81. Dudley DJ. Diabetic-associated stillbirth: incidence, pathophysiology, and prevention. Clin Perinatol 2007;34:611–26.

82. Nold JL, Georgieff MK. Infants of diabetic mothers. Pediatr Clin North Am 2004;51:619–37.

83. Janz NK, Herman WH, Becker MP, et al. Diabetes and pregnancy: factors associated with seeking pre-conception care. Diabetes Care 1995;18:157–65.

84. Kim C, Ferrara A, McEwen LN, et al. Preconception care in managed care: the translating research into action for diabetes study. Am J Obstet Gynecol 2005;192:227–32.

85. Varughese GI, Chowdhury SR, Warner DP, Barton DM. Preconception care of women attending adult general diabetes clinics - are we doing enough? Diabetes Res Clin Pract 2007;76:142–5.

86. Owens M, Kieffer E, Chowdhury F. Preconception care and women with or at risk for diabetes: implications for community intervention. Matern Child Health J 2006;10:137–41.

87. Charron-Prochownik D, Sereika SM, Wang S-L, et al. Reproductive health and preconception counseling awareness in adolescents with diabetes: what they don't know can hurt them. Diabetes Edu 2006;32:235–42.

16

Obstetric Care of the Woman with Diabetes

Tamara C. Takoudes M.D.

CONTENTS

ABSTRACT

Diabetes increases the risk of complications during pregnancy. Starting in the preconception period and continuing throughout pregnancy and postpartum, heightened surveillance is necessary in order to achieve a healthy outcome for both mother and neonate. This chapter will outline the complications that may arise during pregnancies complicated by diabetes and suggest a management scheme for the gravid woman with diabetes.

Specific concerns in the first trimester include an increased risk of miscarriage and careful evaluation of the maternal risks specific to the patient's cardiovascular, renal, thyroid, and ophthalmologic status. In the early second trimester, fetal testing for congenital birth defects and other diagnostic procedures are recommended. This trimester is complicated by increasing insulin requirements that usually continue into the third trimester. In late pregnancy, concern shifts to fetal size, preeclampsia, stillbirth, and deciding delivery timing and route.

Labor and delivery is a unique time for the gravid woman with diabetes, as there are specific challenges with changing insulin requirements related to labor, mode of delivery, and type of diabetes. This chapter will give a brief overview of the use of insulin during pregnancy, intrapartum as well as postpartum, but please refer to Chap. 17 for a more complete discussion. Postpartum concerns in women with diabetes include an increased risk of endometritis and wound infection, postpartum thyroiditis, decreased insulin requirements, and contraception challenges.

Key words: Hemoglobin A1c; Congenital anomalies; Miscarriage; Preeclampsia; Stillbirth; Insulin; Macrosomia.

From: *Diabetes in Women: Pathophysiology and Therapy*
Edited by: A. Tsatsoulis et al. (eds.), DOI 10.1007/978-1-60327-250-6_16
© Humana Press, a part of Springer Science+Business Media, LLC 2009

FIRST TRIMESTER (0–12 WEEKS)

The first prenatal visit may be the first time a patient with diabetes is seen. Ideally baseline evaluation and education take place before preconception as outlined in Chap. 15, but in many cases, pregnancies are unplanned. In the case of the unplanned pregnancy, this evaluation and education should take place as soon as the pregnancy is diagnosed. For patients who have had the benefit of preconception care, the first prenatal visit is usually scheduled between 6 and 8 weeks of gestation. This first visit should include a comprehensive medical assessment, including an assessment of the patient's diabetes control, renal, cardiac, thyroid, and ophthalmologic status, and counseling about diabetes management during pregnancy. A second visit in a short time frame may help prevent the patient from being overwhelmed as well as accomplish all these goals. A visit for the gravid patient who has not had preconception counseling or who may not be under excellent glycemic control is scheduled as soon as possible.

The White classification (Table 1) can be used to determine the level of risk for pregnancy and has correlation with pregnancy outcomes (Table 2). The early groups of White's class B and C do not have

Table 1
White's Classification of Diabetes in Pregnancy [Adapted from (1)]

White's class	Age at onset (years)	Duration (years)	Complications
A	Any	Any	No vascular disease
B	≥20 or	<10	No vascular disease
C	10–19 or	10–19	No vascular disease
D	<10 or	≥20	Background retinopathy only or HTN
E			Calcification of pelvic arteries (no longer used)
F			Nephropathy (>500 mg protein/day)
H			Arteriosclerotic heart disease
R			Proliferative retinopathy or vitreous hemorrhage
T			After renal transplantation

Table 2
Maternal Morbidity Associated with Diabetic Pregnancy by White's Classification
[Adapted from (2)]

Complication	GDMA or A_2 (%)	B, C (%)	D, F, R (%)	Total (%)
Preeclampsia	10	8	16	12
Chronic hypertension	10	8	17	10
All hypertension	15	15	31	18
Ketoacidosis	8	7	9	–
Hydramnios	5	–	18	18
Preterm labor	8	5	10	–
Cesarean delivery	12	44	57	–

vascular complications but D and beyond are associated with vascular disease. Vascular disease in a gravid woman with diabetes is associated with higher risks of placenta-related complications such as preterm delivery, preeclampsia, and growth restriction in the fetus *(1–3)*.

A team approach with joint management by the obstetrician, endocrinologist, nurse educator, and dietician is recommended as early as possible to maintain strict euglycemia, avoid ketonuria, and achieve the lowest glucose values while avoiding frequent hypoglycemia. Hyperemesis gravidarum is routinely addressed and aggressively treated to avoid hyper- or hypoglycemia and ketosis.

Baseline testing for the woman with diabetes should include a hemoglobin A1c (HbA1c), routine prenatal screens including pap smear if needed, complete blood count, serum creatinine, liver functions tests (ALT, AST), uric acid, thyrotropin (TSH), electrocardiogram (EKG), and a comprehensive dilated eye exam. In addition, if the physician suspects vascular disease or there are abnormalities on the EKG, a maternal echocardiogram or exercise echocardiogram may be indicated without exposing the pregnant gravida to radiation. Urinary protein excretion should be measured with a spot check protein/creatinine or albumin/creatinine ratio, which are both highly correlated with 24-h urine protein excretion *(4, 5)*. The advantage of a spot check is the ease of collection as more than 20% of 24-h collections are incomplete *(4, 5)*. We recommend a baseline 24-h urine collection in the first trimester on any patient with preexisting renal disease, history of preeclampsia, or an abnormal spot urine protein/creatinine ratio (≥ 0.2) or microalbumin (≥ 30 μg/mg). In the second and third trimesters, there can be fluctuating amounts of protein in each random sample, thus the 24-h urine remains the gold standard. For the immediate office and triage evaluation, there has been shown to be high correlation between random protein/creatinine ratios and the 24-h urine collection *(6–10)*.

The first trimester HbA1c is used to counsel patients about the risks of miscarriage and congenital birth defects. Higher HbA1c levels are associated with higher risks of birth defects. The pathophysiology of this association is not known. There are likely many variables in the pathway for embryopathy that may be synergistic with or resulting from hyperglycemia including disruption of regulatory genes (Pax3 that controls embryo development), oxidative stress interrupting prostaglandin metabolism, inhibition of somatomedin activity, deficiency in myoinosotol, accumulation of sorbitol, ketonuria, and other genes responsible for cell proliferation as well as apoptosis *(11–18)*. Table 3 lists the associated percentages of major and minor fetal malformations based on the HbA1c. The summary of all the studies shows that HgA1c's in the moderate range [standard deviation (SD) from the mean < + 7] pose barely elevated risks of congenital anomalies over the baseline risk in the general population about 2.2%, whereas a HbA$_1$c's in the high range (SD +7–10) is associated with at least 8.6% risk and in the highest range (>SD +10) have a risk of 26.6% or more of major and minor malformations (Table 3). The HbA1c's goal preconception pregnancy should be as close to the upper range of normal as possible without incurring severe maternal hypoglycemia *(19)*. Screening for congenital malformations is done routinely in all gravidas with diabetes [see the section "Second Trimester (13–24 weeks)"].

A first trimester ultrasound (USG) examination is performed on all patients to evaluate for spontaneous miscarriage *(20)*. USG also ensures the most accurate dating of the pregnancy, as either growth restriction or macrosomia can be issues in the third trimester. In addition, in the patients with a high a HbA1c, an increased nuchal translucency in the first trimester may represent the earliest sign of congenital cardiac disease, even though it has a poor screening sensitivity when used in this fashion *(21–23)*.

All current medication usage must be reviewed to assess safety and benefit in pregnancy. Angiotensin-converting enzyme (ACE) inhibitors, angiotensin receptor blockers (ARBs), and cholesterol lowering agents are discontinued if the patient is still taking these medications due to increased risks for teratogenicity and fetal toxicity *(24, 25)*.

Table 3
Association of Major Malformations in IDM with Initial Maternal Glycohemoglobin Level. Degree of Elevation of Glycohemoglobin (Malformations/Infants) [Adapted from Kitzmiller JL et al. Diabetes Care 1996; 19(5)]

Author (date)	N	Moderate	High	Highest
Miller et al. (1981)	106	<7 [2/48 (4.2)]	7–9.8 [8/35 (22.9)]	≥10 [5/23(21.7)]
Ylinen et al. (1984)	142	<6 [2/63 (3.2)]	6–9.8 [5/62 (8.1)]	≥10 [4/17 (23.5)]
Reid et al. (1984)	127	<6 [2/58 (3.4)]	6–9.9 [5/44 (11.4)]	≥10 [6/25(24)]
Key et al. (1987)	61	<5.8 [2/45(4.4)]	5.8–9.4 [4/13(30.8)]	≥9.5 [3/3 (100)]
Greene et al. (1989)	250	<6 [3/99 (3.0)]	6–12 [6/123(4.9)]	≥12 [11/28(39.3)]
Hanson et al. (1990)	491	<6 [3/429(0.7)]	6–7.9 [2/31 (6.5)]	≥8 [5/31(16.1)]
Rosenn et al. (1994)	228	<4 [4/95 (4.2)]	4–9.9 [7/121 (5.8)]	≥ 10 [3/12(25.0)]
Total	1,405	[18/837(2.2)]	[37/429(8.6)]	[37/139(26.6)]

Data are SD above normal mean [n/n (%)]

Coincident thyroid disease is very common in type 1 diabetes, up to 40% (26). In addition, women who are euthyroid but have thyroid autoimmunity (TAI) are at risk of developing hypothyroidism during pregnancy and should be monitored. The thyroxine dose often will require increased dosing of 30–50% by 4–6 weeks of gestation. Women who do not require increased amounts of replacement in the first trimester may still require increased dosing later in gestation, and therefore a serum TSH should be measured every 30–40 days. The TSH goal is less than 2.5 mLU/L if hypothyroidism is diagnosed prior to pregnancy in the first trimester and 3.0 mLU/L in the second and third trimesters (27).

Blood pressure control is important in the patient with known micro or macrovascular disease or chronic hypertension. Blood pressure goals are 110–129/65–79 mm Hg based on nonpregnant women with diabetes, as no data exist for pregnancy (28). In contrast, mild gestational hypertension is not routinely treated (29). The most commonly used antihypertensives in pregnancy are nifedipine, aldomet, or labetolol. Beta blockers may mask hypoglycemic symptoms and should be used with caution in these patients in whom we are aiming for very tight glycemic control. Atenolol has been associated with fetal growth restriction and should be avoided. Blood pressure trends lower in almost all women after the first trimester and then start to rise again in the third trimester when surveillance for preeclampsia intensifies (30–32).

Preeclampsia is a disease of the later gestation but prevention strategies have been evaluated. Low-dose aspirin (81 mg/day) has not been shown to prevent preeclampsia in patients with diabetes when they were not stratified by risk (33, 34). However, in the largest meta-analysis to date, the relative risk of preeclampsia was 0.85 (CI 0.78–0.92) when low-dose aspirin was started prior to 12-weeks gestation in a high-risk population. Data from this study that included 15,000 patients with diabetes, hypertension, renal disease, or a history of severe preeclampsia thus supports the use of low-dose aspirin in high-risk individuals (33, 34). Research in the area of preeclampsia is rapidly growing, and the future holds great potential for better diagnostic strategies with the discovery of antiangiogenic factors such as sflt-1 (35). This is covered in greater detail in Chap. 19.

SECOND TRIMESTER (13–24 WEEKS)

The frequency of prenatal visits depends on the level of compliance, comorbid diseases, and fetal complications but is usually every 2–4 weeks in the second trimester in gravidas with diabetes.

Routine testing such as serum screening for neural tube defects as well as aneuploidy is offered to all patients. Diabetes does not increase the risk of aneuploidy. However, the serum markers (especially alpha fetal protein and unconjugated estriol) are lowered in diabetic pregnancies, which can mimic a serum profile of Down's syndrome. Therefore, the provider must report the presence of diabetes in order to factor this into the final report *(36)*. Some institutions will add to the final report that "*a precise estimate of Down's syndrome cannot be estimated in diabetes due to lack of sufficient data in this area.*" Further, in order to improve sensitivity for detection of neural tube defects given the high prevalence of neural tube defects in pregnancies complicated by diabetes, a lower cutoff in serum alpha fetal protein must be used *(37)*.

USG in the second trimester is utilized to help diagnose fetal congenital anomalies. The risk was reviewed in the section "First Trimester (0–12 Weeks)," but again it is directly related to the HgA1c at conception *(37)*. USG should be performed by sonographers and physicians trained and experienced in fetal anatomy in order to diagnose congenital abnormalities. The best timing of this sonogram is unclear and is usually related to maternal body habitus as well as fetal position at the time of the study *(38)*. For patients with well-controlled diabetes, this ultrasound is usually done around the 18th week of gestation. In poorly controlled patients, first trimester USG can detect up to 80% of central nervous system abnormalities *(39)*. Repeat second trimester studies are always done but earlier detection allows parents to prepare for the challenges of a fetus with an anomaly and also allows for more options if a patient wishes to terminate the pregnancy. Studies in patients with diabetes have reaffirmed the utility of ultrasound with a high positive predictive value (90%) when done prior to 24 weeks for the detection of fetal anomalies *(40)*. Despite the high detection rates, the most common defects missed were ventriculoseptal defects, limb abnormalities, unilateral renal abnormalities, and cleft palate without cleft lip.

Fetal echocardiography is routinely recommended and is usually done at approximately 20–22 weeks of gestation by a perinatologist or pediatric cardiologist. Congenital heart disease accounts for almost half of the anomalies in diabetic pregnancies, and there is an increased risk of fetal cardiac hypertrophy and asymmetric septal hypertrophy (ASH) sometimes related to poor glycemic control and also in well-controlled patients *(41)*. Cardiac hypertrophy in the poorly controlled patient is thought to be secondary to fetal hyperinsulinemia that increases synthesis and deposition of fat and glycogen in the myocardial cells. This can also occur in the offspring of women whose diabetes are well controlled and are due to increased muscle mass. The cardiac hypertrophy may contribute to 22% of the stillbirth rate seen in poorly controlled diabetic gravidas *(42)*. Likewise, it is more prevalent in large for gestational age infants of diabetic mothers than in gestational age-matched, nondiabetic controls (39% vs. 7%) *(43)*. Overall, cardiac hypertrophy may be present in up to 30–50% of infants born to diabetic mothers, but only 5–10% are symptomatic *(44)*. Fetal echocardiography is repeated in the third trimester if fetal cardiac hypertrophy was detected earlier to help manage the neonate after delivery *(45)*.

THIRD TRIMESTER (25–40 WEEKS)

The third trimester is characterized by a significant rise in insulin requirements and care is focused on continuing glycemic control and monitoring for complications such as macrosomia, preeclampsia, stillbirth, and preterm labor.

Macrosomia is defined as an absolute estimated fetal weight (EFW) of >4,500 g or >90% EFW for the gestational age and intrauterine growth restriction (IUGR) and as EFW < 10% for the gestational age. Macrosomia is suspected in about 9–28%, and IUGR is suspected in 2–8% of pregnancies complicated by pregestational diabetes *(44)*. IUGR is more common in pregnant women with vascular disease which is why there is a wide range of prevalence data. In addition, the IUGR may predate the onset of preeclampsia. Fetal growth abnormalities are typically detected on routine ultrasounds done every 3–4 weeks after 24-weeks gestation (46).

Macrosomia is of particular concern as it increases the length of the second stage of labor and the risks of shoulder dystocia, operative delivery, birth trauma, such as brachial plexus injury, and perinatal death (47). Diabetes during pregnancy significantly increases the risk of shoulder dystocia for any given birth weight when compared with nondiabetic patients (see Table 5) (49, 50). Unfortunately, these tables are based on birth weight, not ultrasound weight estimates that are fraught with error and hence not able to predict exact risk. The sensitivity and specificity of ultrasound is poor, but it is currently the only validated modality commonly used to predict macrosomia. In one review of EFW calculation by ultrasound by Chauhan et al., the range for prediction was wider in the general patient population than in the diabetic patients (i.e., ability to predict an infant >4,000 g had a sensitivity of 15–79% in all patients and 60% in diabetic patients) (51). The larger the infant and the closer to term, the less accurate USG becomes. Alternatively, USG of fetal peripheral fat at the level of the mid-humerus, shoulder, abdominal wall, and thigh have not been found to be reliably reproducible and have not been validated in any large studies. MRI measurement at the level of the fetal shoulder as well as similar USG-derived calculations in EFW have not been shown to have higher sensitivity yet either. Furthermore, MRI is an expensive modality (52–55). Please see Chap. 18 for a discussion of the use of ultrasound in determining the need for intensive management of hyperglycemia in pregnancies that are at risk for accelerated fetal growth.

Cesarean delivery is recommended for gravidas with diabetes, when the EFW is >4,500 g, given the high risk of shoulder dystocia and neurologic injury as recommended by the American College of Obstetrics and Gynecologists (ACOG) (56, 57). Induction of labor for the suspected macrosomic infant is not recommended as two systematic reviews concluded that this did not result in a lower rate of shoulder dystocia or cesarean delivery than expectant management (30, 32, 58, 59).

Fetal surveillance with nonstress tests and biophysical profiles is usually started by 32 weeks, in all patients with diabetes, as the risk of intrauterine fetal demise or still birth is significantly increased. ACOG recommends antepartum surveillance for all pregnancies complicated by pregestational diabetes (56). Table 4 is an outline developed for fetal testing at our institution and is based on the literature available, although there are no large randomized studies on which to make an evidence-based recommendation about timing, frequency, type of testing, or gestational age at which to start surveillance (60–70). Diabetes is a unique condition, because if fetal testing is not reassuring in the setting of ketosis or significant hyperglycemia, the hyperglycemic state should be treated prior to taking action

Table 4
Pregestational Diabetes Testing Guidelines at Beth Israel Deaconess Medical Center [Adapted from (33, 35–44)]

1. Start testing at 32 weeks with weekly NST&BPP or NST&AFI and 2× week at 36 weeks
2. EFW every 4 weeks after 24 weeks
3. If under poor control, IUGR, HTN, or Class D or higher diabetes, start at 28 weeks with weekly BPP (with an NST at provider discretion)
4. Change to 2× week testing if there is any abnormal testing or if new condition such as hypertension arises
5. Add umbilical artery Doppler studies and contraction stress testing when other conditions such as IUGR or abnormal testing arise

IUGR intrauterine growth restriction; *HTN* hypertension; *NST* nonstress testing; *BPP* biophysical profile testing; *EFW* estimated fetal weight; AFI amniotic fluid index

Table 5
Rates of Indicated and Spontaneous Preterm Delivery in Pregestational DM Treated with Insulin Group and Control Group [Adapted from (48)]

	Pregestational DM treated with insulin (n = 461)		Control (n = 2738)		Odds ratio	
	No.	%	No.	%	Value	95% CI
Delivery at <37 weeks	175	38	380	13.9	2.7	2.3–3.2
Indicated	101	21.9	92	3.4	8.1	6.0–10.9
Spontaneous	74	16.1	288	10.5	1.6	1.2–2.2
Delivery at <35 weeks	75	16.3	167	6.1	2.7	2.1 3.4
Indicated	34	7.4	45	1.6	4.8	3.0–7.5
Spontaneous	41	8.9	122	4.5	2.1	1.4–3.0

on the abnormal fetal testing (71). This is in stark contrast to nonreassuring testing in a nonreversible condition, such as preeclampsia, where optimal management would be to administer steroids for fetal lung maturity, if there is time, and/or deliver.

The administration of steroids in diabetes is a predictable dilemma. A common maternal steroid regimen for fetal lung maturity is two doses of 12-mg betamethasone 24 h apart. Steroids given to the mother will start to increase the maternal glucose within 12 h of administration and persist until about 5 days after the last dose (72). In one study the increase in insulin requirements were 6, 38, 36, 27 and 17% above baseline for the 5 days after steroid administration. If subcutaneous insulin cannot be adjusted or if severe hyperglycemia occurs, the patient is managed with an intravenous insulin infusion during the period of time of glucose elevation in the hospital.

Another third trimester concern is preeclampsia. This complication is increased in diabetic pregnancies, with the highest risk occurring in patients who have longstanding diabetes with preexisting nephropathy, retinopathy, or hypertension. In one review by the National Institutes of Health evaluating 462 women with diabetes, the rate of preeclampsia was 11, 22, 21, and 36% in Class B, C, D, R, and F diabetes, respectively.(73) The baseline risk of preeclampsia in nondiabetic patients varies between 5 and 8% (74, 75). Preeclampsia is unique to pregnancy and usually occurs after 20-weeks gestation in a previously normotensive patient. Elevations in the systolic blood pressure of 140 mmHg or greater and diastolic blood pressure of 90 mmHg or greater may occur in combination with more than 300-mg protein in a 24-h urine collection. Risk factors for preeclampsia are previous pregnancy affected by preeclampsia, first pregnancy, family history of preeclampsia, preexisting diabetes, multiple gestations, obesity, underlying hypertension, renal disease, vascular disease, anticardiolipin antibody syndrome, and advanced maternal age. Preeclampsia can involve changes to the central nervous, hematopoietic, renal, cardiovascular, and pulmonary systems as well as the feto-placenta unit. Laboratory tests typically ordered are a complete blood count, serum creatinine, liver function tests, uric acid, and a 24-h urine protein collection. All cases of preeclampsia in a diabetic gravida should be delivered when the gestational age is after 37 weeks. Patients with mild cases of preeclampsia who have blood pressures less than 160/110 and do not show evidence of systemic disease listed earlier can be managed expectantly without delivery if the gravida is less than 37 weeks. In the patient with severe disease, which is defined as hypertension >160/110 and/or more than 5 g of protein on a 24 h urine collection and/or evidence of changes to any of the earlier listed systems either in laboratory findings or symptoms of the mother/fetus, delivery is usually indicated especially after 32–34 weeks. Betamethasone is usually indicated for any patient less than 34 weeks with preeclampsia. Once the decision to deliver is made, magnesium sulfate is typically used as a continuous intravenous infusion in order to decrease the risk for maternal seizure. The diagnosis of preeclampsia in patients with diabetes who have preexisting hypertension or proteinuria is difficult but can be suspected if there are low platelets less than 100,000, increased liver transaminases, and fetal compromise such as IUGR or oligohydramnios. In these patients, the typical worsening of hypertension or proteinuria, which may occur in the third trimester, cannot be distinguished from preeclampsia. So, in hospital surveillance is usually needed. Overall, the management of preeclampsia in women with diabetes is similar to that in nondiabetic patients *(76)*. Please see Chap. 19 that discusses the pathophysiology and new developments in this area. Recurrence rates of preeclampsia in a diabetic gravida are extremely variable but are somewhat dependent on underlying vascular disease, gestational age at onset in the previous pregnancy, and the presence of multiple gestations.

Preterm delivery (less than 35–37 weeks) is increased in the diabetic pregnancy than in the nondiabetic pregnancy. More deliveries are medically indicated due to suspected preeclampsia or nonreassuring fetal testing (22 vs. 3%), but a small percentage is due to spontaneous preterm labor as well (16 vs. 11%) (see Table 5) *(48)*. This higher risk of spontaneous preterm birth may be due to poor glycemic control leading to polyhydramnios, infection, and fetal stress *(77, 78)*. Preterm labor can be managed with tocolytic therapy such as magnesium sulfate, nifedipine, and indocin. One tocolytic, terbutaline, a beta adrenergic drug should be used with caution in patients with diabetes as it can increase the serum glucose, lower the potassium concentration, and precipitate cardiac arrhythmias. Since there are other acceptable medications available, terbutaline should only be used in patients with well-controlled diabetes in the setting of close monitoring of glucose and potassium levels. In addition, betamethasone can worsen the effect of beta adrenergic drugs.

Diabetic ketoacidosis (DKA) is a complication that can occur more easily and at lower glucose levels in pregnancy than in a nonpregnant state in any trimester. Common precipitants in pregnancy include hyperemesis, infection (especially genitourinary infections), and noncompliance. Hyperglycemia in pregnancy causes a more significant volume depletion that puts both the mother and the fetus at risk with decreased uterine perfusion that can lead to fetal death in 10–35% of patients with DKA in pregnancy *(79)*. The prompt recognition of ketosis, search for the precipitant, and treatment can help avoid these serious complications. The treatment of DKA is the same as in nonpregnant patients with volume replacement, intravenous insulin, careful attention to electrolyte imbalances and reversal, or treatment of the underlying cause. The fetus is at risk for stillbirth with severe acid–base imbalances. Prompt diagnosis and correction is important with admission to either an obstetric or intensive care unit with continuous fetal monitoring. Immediate attention is given to simultaneously correct the fluid deficits (goal is to correct ¾ volume depletion approximately 100 cc/kg body weight in 24 h with normal saline), start insulin therapy (0.1 unit/kg IV bolus followed by 0.1 unit/kg/h infusion), replete electrolytes (potassium and phosphate are usually depleted, even if initial measurements are normal), and give bicarbonate if the arterial pH is <7.1 or bicarbonate is less than 5 mEq/L while monitoring hourly glucose and electrolytes *(80)*. As stated earlier, if there is nonreassuring fetal testing, the primary goal is to correct the acid-base imbalance, and if the nonreassuring fetal testing persists, then delivery may be required *(71)*.

Assessment of fetal lung maturity by amniocentesis is not routinely done if delivery is after 39 weeks. The assessment of fetal lung maturity is recommended if delivery is contemplated prior to 39 weeks, in the absence of a medical indication to deliver immediately such as severe preeclampsia. We most commonly use the fluorescence polarization test (TDx-FLM) from amniotic fluid obtained by amniocentesis. This test uses polarized light to quantitate the amount of binding of a probe to both albumin and surfactant in amniotic fluid. A mature index is considered to be 55 mg of surfactant per gram of albumin. Tests such as the lecithin/sphingomyelin ratios (L/S ratio) and phosphatidylglycerol (PG) use thin layer chromatography to measure other components of amniotic fluid. These tests have been limited by their technical difficulty and by their limited supply from manufacturers. Thus, the TDx-FLM has come into favor. The ability to predict respiratory distress syndrome is based on gestational age and other risk factors. For example, fetuses of mothers with DM have less mature lungs due to high fetal insulin levels, which cause cellular hypertrophy/hyperplasia at the expense of cellular maturation, although this risk is not apparent after 38.5 weeks of gestation (59, 81). The FLM assay has been reviewed in pregnant women with diabetes and performs well with similar cutoffs as in nondiabetic patients, but glycemic control was not rigorously assessed (82–85).

LABOR AND DELIVERY

Thirty-eight percent of deliveries for diabetic gravidas are less than 37 weeks due to preeclampsia, premature labor, nonreassuring fetal testing, and suspected growth restriction [(48); Table 5]. However, even if all testing is reassuring, elective delivery between 39 and 40 weeks has been advocated to reduce the risk of unexplained stillbirth (especially after 40 weeks), delivery complications, and neonatal injury, even though this has not been rigorously studied (81). There is one randomized trial of 200 women (most had insulin-requiring gestational diabetes and some had class B diabetes) with appropriately grown infants who were randomized to expectant management vs. induction of labor in the 38th week. The induction group had less macrosomia (10% vs. 23%, $p < 0.0001$) and fewer cases of shoulder dystocia (0% vs. 3%) with a similar rate of cesarean delivery (25% vs. 31%). More than half of the expectantly managed group required induction at some point after study entry (86). If the cervix is unfavorable, the uncomplicated pregnancy may continue if there is normal fetal growth, reassuring fetal testing, good compliance with diabetes self-management, and prenatal follow-up.

The route of delivery is usually vaginal with cesarean delivery reserved for those with obstetric indications such as nonreassuring fetal heart rate, arrest of dilation, arrest of descent, breech presentation, and/or an EFW > 4,500 g as discussed in the section "Third Trimester (25–40 Weeks)" (87, 88) (Table 6).

During labor and delivery, the fetus and the mother should be continuously monitored. Continuous fetal monitoring is necessary as abnormal fetal heart rate patterns are more likely (87, 88). Maternal glucose levels should be checked at least every hour. The maternal glucose goals are between 80 and 110 mg/dL in order to achieve the lowest rate of neonatal hypoglycemia (89–91). Insulin requirements are higher in latent labor and can be given by subcutaneous injections, insulin pump, or insulin infusions. Insulin infusions usually consist of 15 units of regular insulin in 150 cc (mL) of normal saline and can be infused intravenously in increments of 0.5 units/h, as needed. Patients can usually drink fluids in the early stages of labor but once they are unable, intravenous dextrose is used in conjunction with

Table 6
Rate of Shoulder Dystocia by Birth Weight in Nondiabetic and Diabetic Women

Birth weight (g)	Nondiabetic women (%)	Diabetic women (%)
≤4,000	0.1–1.1	0.6–3.7
4,000–4,449	1.1–10.0	4.9–23.1
≥4,500	2.7–22.6	20.0–50.0

Adapted from ACOG Practice Pattern No 7, Oct 1997

insulin (see Table 7). As the pregnancy progresses to active labor, insulin requirements drop, and the insulin infusion will need to be lowered and/or a dextrose infusion started or increased.

Insulin drip protocols are safe ways to manage expected and unexpected fluctuations. Insulin pumps can be used successfully in the setting of well-educated patients and medical personnel, but if the patient becomes temporarily unable to manage the pump, most medical personnel are not adequately trained to use the pump safely. Therefore, we recommend an insulin drip for most patients in active labor.

In patients with gestational and type 2 diabetes, it is important to avoid infusing dextrose without insulin given either IV or subcutaneously, as this usually leads to hyperglycemia. Some of these

Table 7

OPTIONAL

INSULIN INFUSION ALGORITHM FOR LOWER GLUCOSE TARGETS
(Target BG 80 – 110 mg/dl)

Insulin dose adjustments using this algorithm do not replace sound medical judgment.

Some evidence suggests a higher incidence of hypoglycemia using these lower glucose targets. There is disagreement among experts about the degree of glycemic control needed to decrease morbidity and mortality while avoiding severe hypoglycemia. The following meets the AACE recommendations.

*Whichever is greater change   Previous Blood Glucose (mg/dl)

Current Blood Glucose (mg/dl)	<60	60-80	81-110	111-150	151-200	201-250	251-300	301-400	>400
<60	Hold drip and give 1 amp 50% glucose and check BG every 30 minutes until >100 mg/dl and then re-initiate drip at 50% previous rate								
60-80	Hold drip and check BG every 30 minutes until >100 mg/dl and then re-initiate drip at 50% previous rate								
81-110	No change				↓rate by 0.5 units/hr	↓rate by 50% or 2 units/hr*		↓ rate by 75% or 2 units/hr*	
111-150	↑ rate by 1 unit/hr	↑ rate by 0.5 units/hr			No change		↓ rate by 50% or 2 units/hr*		
151-200	↑rate by 1 unit/hr		↑rate by 0.5 units/hr	↑ rate by 1 unit/hr		No Change	↓ rate by 25% or 2 units/hr*		
201-250	↑ rate by 25% or 2 units/hr*			↑ rate by 25% or 1 unit/hr*				↑rate by 1 unit/hr	No Change
251-300	↑rate by 33% or 2.5 units/hr*		↑rate by 25% or 1.5 units/hr*	↑rate by 25% or 1 unit/hr*	↑rate by 1 unit/hr	↑ rate by 1.5 units/hr	↑rate by 25% or 2 units/hr*	No Change	
301-400	↑ rate by 40% or 3 units/hr*								
>400	↑ rate by 50% or 4 units/hr*								

↓

This algorithm assumes hourly BG checks during insulin dose titration.

↓

If BG in desirable range (81-110 mg/dl) for 2-3 hours can decrease frequency of BG checks to every 2 hours while BG stays in target.
If experiencing unexplained hypoglycemia or hyperglycemia, investigate and correct causative factors.
If there is any significant change in glycemic source (i.e., parenteral, enteral or oral intake), expect to make insulin adjustment.

↓

Common reasons to discontinue insulin infusion:
Patient tolerating at least 50% of normal oral intake or enteral feedings
Clinically appropriate to transfer patient to a unit that does not do insulin infusions
Patient on stable regimen of TPN with most of insulin already in TPN solution

↓

patients may not need insulin or dextrose during labor and delivery. Careful monitoring of glucose is essential. Patients with type 1 diabetes always require insulin, and intravenous insulin drip protocols are helpful in maintaining euglycemia, avoiding severe glucose fluctuations and reducing the rate of neonatal hypoglycemia.

POSTPARTUM

Immediately postpartum there is a rapid decline in insulin requirements, once the fetus and placenta are delivered. For the first 24–72 h after delivery, most women with type 1 diabetes require very small doses of insulin (approximately 1/3 to ½ of the preconception dose), and some women with type 2 diabetes require no insulin at all. Breastfeeding is encouraged in all patients and contributes to the reduced insulin requirements. Breastfeeding will be discussed in greater detail in Chap. 22.

Careful attention is made to patients with cesarean deliveries as women with preexisting diabetes have at least a 2.5-fold increased risk of wound complications, even after adjusting for maternal obesity and labor prior to cesarean delivery vs. the nondiabetic patient (92). One mechanism for this increased risk may be due to hyperglycemia, which may inhibit the immune response to infection. Wound care should be aggressive, and seromas, cellulitis, hematomas, and purulence should be drained and packed, and antibiotics should be given if infection is suspected. Daily wound care should be provided by visiting nurses, and weekly visits to the obstetrician are recommended to monitor wound healing.

Chronic autoimmune or lymphocytic thyroiditis (or TPO antibodies) is present in 18–25% of patients with type 1 diabetes (26). If there is already known hypothyroidism, levothyroxine doses are reduced to the preconception dose. Women with type 1 diabetes who have TPO antibodies without hypothyroidism are at increased risk of postpartum thyroiditis (25%) (26).

Final Postpartum Visit

The final postpartum visit, which is usually done 6 weeks after delivery, is comprehensive and covers a wide range of systems from general well-being, coping with changes since delivery, and breastfeeding support. The visit focuses on questions pertaining to diabetes care, insulin requirements, blood pressure control (especially if preeclampsia occurred), eye health, maternal weight loss, a thorough physical exam, and contraception. Please see Chap. 9 for a more comprehensive review of fertility control.

SUMMARY

Most women with pregestational diabetes can deliver healthy babies with careful counseling, management, and surveillance. This care requires a careful team approach, frequent visits, extra testing, and delivery prior to 40 weeks of gestation. Complications such as miscarriage, congenital anomalies, preeclampsia, macrosomia, stillbirth, birth injury as well as cesarean delivery are more common in gravidas with diabetes but are even higher in those with poor glycemic control.

REFERENCES

1. Hare JW, White P. Gestational diabetes and the White classification. Diabetes Care 1980; 3:394
2. Cousins L. Pregnancy complications among diabetic women: review. Obstet Gynecol 1987; 42:140

3. Hare JW, White P. Pregnancy in diabetes complicated by vascular disease. Diabetes 1977; 26(10):953–5

4. Eknoyan G, Hostetter T, Bakris GL, Hebert L, Levey AS, Parving HH, Steffes MW, Toto R. Proteinuria and other markers of chronic kidney disease: a position statement of the national kidney foundation (NKF) and the national institute of diabetes and digestive and kidney diseases (NIDDK). Am J Kidney Dis 2003; 42(4):617–22

5. National Kidney Foundation. K/DOQI clinical practice guidelines for chronic kidney disease: evaluation, classification and stratification. Am J Kidney Dis 2002; 39(Suppl 1):S1

6. Kyle PM, Fielder JN, Pullar B, Horwood LJ, Moore MP. Comparison of methods to identify significant proteinuria in pregnancy in the outpatient setting. BJOG 2008; 115(4):523–7

7. Rodriguez-Thompson D, Lieberman ES. Use of random urinary protein-to-creatinine ratio for the diagnosis of significant proteinuria during pregnancy. Am J Obstet Gynecol 2001; 185(4):808–11

8. Haas DM, Sabi F, McNamara M, Rivera Alsina M. Comparing ambulatory spot urine protein/creatinine ratios and 24-h urine protein measurements in normal pregnancies. J Matern Fetal Neonatal Med 2003; 14(4):233–6

9. Wheeler TL, II, Blackhurst DW, Dellinger EH, Ramsey PS. Am J Obstet Gynecol 2007; 196(5):465

10. Durnwald C, Mercer B. A prospective comparison of total protein/creatinine ratio versus 24hours urine protein in women with suspected preeclampsia. Am J Obstet Gynecol 2003; 189(3):848–52

11. Moley KH, Chi MM, Knudson CM, et al. Hyperglycemia-induces apoptosis in pre-implantation embryos through cell death effector pathways. Nat Med 1998; 4:1421

12. Keim AL, Chi MM, Moley KH. Hyperglycemia-induced apoptotic cell death in the mouse blastocyst is dependent on expression of p53. Mol Reprod Dev 2001; 60:214

13. Pani L, Horal M, Loeken MR. Rescue of neural tube defects in Pax-3-deficient embryos by p53 loss of function: implications for Pax-3 dependent development and tumorigenesis. Genes Dev 2002; 16:676

14. Loeken MR. Current perspectives on the causes of neural tube defects resulting from diabetic pregnancy. Am J Med Genet C Semin Med Genet 2005; 135:77

15. Wentzel P, Welsh N, Eriksson UJ. Developmental damage, increased lipid peroxidation, diminished cyclooxygenase-2 gene expression, and lowered prostaglandin E2 levels in rat embryos exposed to a diabetic environment. Diabetes 1999; 48:813

16. Wentzel P, Erikkson UJ. Antioxidants diminish developmental damage induced by high glucose and cyclooxygenase inhibitors in rat embryos in vitro. Diabetes 1998; 47:677

17. Li R, Chase M, Jung SK, et al. Hypoxic stress in diabetic pregnancy contributes to impaired embryo gene expression and defective development by inducing oxidative stress. Am J Physiol Endocrinol Metab 2005; 289:E591

18. Fu J, Tay SS, Ling EA, Dheen ST. Glucose alters the expression of genes involved in proliferation and cell-fate specification of embryonic neural stem cells. Diabetologia 2006; 5(49):1027–38

19. Kitzmiller JL, Block JM, Brown FM, Catalano PM, Conway DL, Coustan DR, Gunderson EP, Herman WH, Hoffman LD, Inturrisi M, Jovanovic LB, Kjos SI, Knopp RH, Montoro MN, Ogata ES, Paramsothy P, Reader DM, Rosenn BM, Thomas AM, Kirkman MS. Managing preexisting diabetes for pregnancy: summary of evidence and consensus recommendations for care. Diabetes Care 2008; 31:1060–79

20. Sutherland HW, Pritchard CW. Increased incidence of spontaneous abortion in pregnancies complicated by maternal diabetes mellitus. Am J Obstet Gynecol 1986; 155:135

21. Johnson B, Simpson LL. Screening for congenital heart disease: a move toward earlier echocardiography. Am J Perinatol 2007; 24(8):449–56

22. Weiner Z, Goldstein I, Bombard A, Applewhite L, Itzkovits-Eldor J. Screening for structural fetal anomalies during the nuchal translucency ultrasound examination. Am J Obstet Gynecol 2007; 197(2):e1–5

23. Simpson LL, Malone FD, Bianci DW, Ball RH, Nyberg DA, Comstock CH, Saade G, Eddleman K, Gross SJ, Dugoff L, Craigo SD, Timor-Tritsch IE, Carr SR, Wolfe HM, Tripp T, D'Alton ME. Nuchal translucency and the risk of congenital heart disease. Obstet Gynecol 2007; 109:376–83

24. American Diabetes Association. Standards of medical care for patients with diabetes mellitus. Diabetes Care 2003; 26(Suppl 1):S33

25. Cooper WO, Hernandez-Diaz S, Arbogast PG, et al. Major congenital malformations after first trimester exposure to ACE inhibitors. N Engl J Med 2006; 354:2443

26. Umpierrez GE, Latif KA, Murphy MB, et al. Thyroid dysfunction in patients with type 1 diabetes: a longitudinal study. Diabetes Care 2003; 26 (4):1181–5

27. Abalovich M, et al. Clinical practice guideline management of thyroid dysfunction during pregnancy and postpartum: an endocrine society clinical practice guideline. J Clin Endocrinol Metab 2007; 92:S1–47

28. American Diabetes Association. Standards of medical care for patients with diabetes mellitus. Diabetes Care 2006; 29:Suppl 1:S4

29. Sibai BM. Chronic hypertension in pregnancy. Obstet Gynecol 2002; 100(2):367

30. Magee LA, von Dadelszen P, Bohun CM, Rey E, El-Zibdeh M, Stalker S, Ross S, Hewson S, Logan AG, Ohlsson A, Naeem T, Thornton JG, Abdalla M, Walkinshaw S, Brown M, Davis G, Hannah ME. Serious perinatal complications of non-proteinuric hypertension: an international, multi-center, retrospective cohort study. J Obstet Gynecol Can 2003; 25:372–82

31. Butters L, Kennedy S, Rubin PC. Atenolol in essential hypertension during pregnancy. BMJ 1990 301:587–589

32. Abalos E, Duley L, Steyn DW, Henderson-Smart DJ. Antihypertensive drug therapy for mild to moderate hypertension during pregnancy (Cochrane Review). In: The Cochrane Library, Issue 2. Chichester, UK: Wiley, 2004

33. Duley L, Henderson-Smart D, Knight M, King J. Antiplatelet drugs for prevention of preeclampsia and its consequences: systematic review. BMJ 2001; 322:329

34. Sibai BM. Risk factors, pregnancy complications and prevention of hypertensive disorders in women with pregravid diabetes mellitus. J Matern Fetal Med 2000; 9:62

35. Levine RJ, Maynard SE, Qian C, Lim KH, England LJ, Yu KF, Schisterman EF, Thadhani R, Sachs BP, Epstein FH, Sibai BM, Sukhatme VP, Karumanchi SA. Circulating angiogenic factors and the risk of preeclampsia. N Engl J Med 2004; 350 (7):672–83

36. Milunsky A. Prenatal diagnosis of neural tube defects. VIII The importance of serum alpha fetoprotein screening in diabetic pregnant women. Am J Obstet Gynecol 1982; 142:1030

37. Ylinen K, AuLa P, Stenman UH, et al. risk of minor and major malformations in diabetics with high haemoglobin A1c values in early pregnancy. Br Med J 1984; 289:345

38. National Institutes of Health publication 1984; 64–667, and American College of Radiology 2003

39. Ndumbe FM, Navti O, Chilaka VN, Konje JC. Prenatal diagnosis in the first trimester of pregnancy. Obstet Gynecol Surv 2008; 63:317–28

40. Greene MF, Benacerraf BR. Prenatal diagnosis in diabetic gravidas: utility of ultrasound and maternal serum alpha-fetoprotein screening. Obstet Gynecol 1991; 17:311

41. Langer O. Ultrasound biometry evolves in the management of diabetes in pregnancy. Ultrasound Obstet Gynecol 2005; 26:585

42. Russell NE, Holloway P, Quinn S, Foley M, et al. Cardiomyopathy and cardiomegaly in stillborn infants of diabetic mothers. Pediatr Dev Pathol 2008; 11(1):10–14

43. Vela-Huerta MM, Vargas-Origel A, Olvera-Lopez A. Asymmetrical septal hypertrophy in newborn infants of diabetic mothers. Am J Perinatol 2000; 17(2):89–94

44. Riskin A, Garcia-Prats JA. Infant of a diabetic mother from UpToDate version 16.2, 2008

45. Jaeggi ET, Fouron JC, Proulx F. Fetal cardiac performance in uncomplicated and well-controlled maternal type I diabetes. Ultrasound Obstet Gynecol 2001; 17:311

46. Lampl M, Jeanty P. Exposure to maternal diabetes is associated with altered fetal growth patterns: a hypothesis regarding metabolic allocation to growth under hyperglycemic-hypoxemic conditions. Am J Hum Biol 2004; 16:237

47. Benedetti TJ, Gabbe SG. Shoulder dystocia: a complication of fetal macrosomia and prolonged second stage of labor with mid-pelvic delivery. Obstet Gynecol 1978; 52:526

48. Sibai BM, Caritas SN, Hauth JC, et al. Preterm delivery in women with pregestational diabetes mellitus or chronic hypertension relative to women with uncomplicated pregnancies. The National Institute of Child Health and Human Development Network of Maternal-Fetal Medicine Units. Am J Obstet Gynecol 2000; 183:1520

49. Dildy GA, Clark SL. Shoulder dystocia: risk identification. Clin Obstet Gynecol 2000; 43:265

50. Ecker JL, Greenberg JA, Norwitz ER, et al. Birth weight as a predictor of brachial plexus injury Obstet Gynecol 1997; 89:643

51. Chauhan SP, Grobman WA, Gherman RA, et al. Suspicion and treatment of macrosomic fetus: a review. Am J Obstet Gynecol 2005; 193(2):332–46

52. Chauhan SP, Lynn NN, Sanderson M, Humphries J, Cole JH, Scardo JA. A scoring system for detection of macrosomia and prediction of shoulder dystocia: a disappointment. J Matern Fetal Neonatal Med 2006; 19(11):699–705

53. Tukeva TA, Salmi H, Poutanen VP, Karjalainen PT, Hytinantti T, Paavonen J, Teramo KA, Aronen HJ. Fetal shoulder measurements by fast and ultrafast MRI techniques. J Magn Reson Imaging 2001; 13 (6):938–42

54. Jovanovic-Peterson L, Crues J, Durak E, Peterson CM. Magnetic resonance imaging in pregnancies complicated by gestational diabetes predicts infant birth weight ratio and neonatal morbidity. Am J Perinatol 1993; 10(6):432–37

55. Baker PN, Johnson IR, Gowland PA, et al. Fetal weight estimation by echo-planar magnetic resonance imaging. Lancet 1994; 343(8898):644–5

56. ACOG Practice Bulletin #60. Pregestational diabetes mellitus. Obstet Gynecol 2005; 105:675

57. Rouse DJ, Owen J, Goldenberg RL, et al. The effectiveness and costs of elective cesarean delivery for fetal macrosomia diagnosed by ultrasound. JAMA 1996; 276:1480

58. Irion O, Boulvain M. Induction of labor for suspected fetal macrosomia. Cochrane Database Syst Rev 2000;(2):CD000938
59. Sanchez-Ramos L, Bernstein S, Kaunitz AM. Expectant management versus labor induction for suspected fetal macrosomia: a systematic review. Obstet Gynecol 2002; 100:997
60. American College of Obstetricians and Gynecologists (ACOG), Committee on Practice Bulletins - Obstetrics. Antepartum Fetal Surveillance. ACOG Practice Bulletin No. 9. Washington, DC: ACOG; October 1999
61. ACOG Practice Bulletin. Gestational Diabetes. Number 30, September 2001. Obstet Gynecol 2001; 98(3):525–38
62. Guidelines for Preconception Care, California Diabetes and Pregnancy Program, 1998
63. Creasy R, Resnick R. Maternal Fetal-Medicine; Principles and Practice. Chapter 49, Diabetes in pregnancy, 5th edn. Philadelphia, PA: Saunders, 2004
64. Gabbe SG. Obstetrics: normal and problem pregnancies. In: Gabbe SG, Neibyl JR, Simpson JL (eds.), Diabetes Mellitus, Chapter 32 and Antepartum Fetal Evaluation, Chapter 12, 4th edn. New York: Churchill Livingstone, 2002, pp. 1081–1116
65. Miller DA, et al. The modified BPP: AP testing in the 1990s. Am J Obstet Gynecol 1995; 38:3–10
66. Manning FA, et al. Fetal assessment based on BPP scoring: experience in 12,620 referred high-risk pregnancies. Am J Obstet Gynecol 1985; 151:343–50
67. Manning FA, et al. Fetal breathing movements and the NST: selective use of the NST. Am J Obstet Gynecol 1987; 156:709–12
68. Nageotte MP, et al. Perinatal outcome with the modified BPP. Am J Obstet Gynecol 1994; 170:1672–76
69. Devoe LD, et al. NST: evidence based use in high risk pregnancy. Clin Obstet Gynecol 2002; 45:986–92
70. Boehm FH, et al. Improved outcome of twice weekly non-stress testing. Obstet Gynecol 1986; 67:566
71. Hughes AB. Fetal heart rate changes during ketosis. Acta Obstet Gynceol Scand 1987; 66:71
72. Mathiesen ER, Christiansen AB, Hellmuth E, et al. Insulin dose during glucocorticoid treatment for fetal lung maturation in diabetic pregnancy: test of an algorithm (correction of analgorithm). Acta Obstet Gynecol Scand 2002; 81:835
73. Sibai BM, Caritas S, Hauth J, et al. Risks of preeclampsia and adverse neonatal outcomes among women with pregestational diabetes mellitus. National Institute of Child Health and Human Development Network of Maternal-Fetal Medicine Units. Am J Obstet Gynecol 2000; 182:364
74. Sibai BM. Diagnosis, prevention and management of eclampsia. Obstet Gynecol 2005; 105(2):402
75. Wagner LK. Diagnosis and management of preeclampsia. Am Fam Physician 2004; 70 (12):2317–24
76. ACOG Committee on Obstetric Practice. Diagnosis and management of preeclampsia-eclampsia, ACOG Practice Bulletin. Int J Gynaecol Obstet 2002; 77(1):67–75
77. Mimouni F, Miodovnik M, Siddiqi TA, et al. High spontaneous premature labor rate in insulin-dependent diabetic pregnant women: an association with poor glycemic control and urogenital infection. Obstet Gynecol 1988; 72:175
78. Reece EA, Sivan E, Francis G, Homko CJ. Pregnancy outcomes among women with and without diabetic microvascular disease (White's classes B to RF) versus non-diabetic controls. Am J Perinatol 1998; 15:549
79. Ramin KD. Diabetic ketoacidosis in pregnancy. Obstet Gynecol Clin North Am 1999; 26:481
80. Foley MR, Story TH. Obstetric Intensive Care; DKA in pregnancy, Philadelphia, PA: Saunders, ed 1997, pp. 158–170
81. Kjos, SL Henry OA, Montoro M, et al. Insulin-requiring diabetes in pregnancy: a randomized trial of active induction of labor and expectant management. Am J Obstet Gynecol 1993; 169:611
82. Livingston EG, Herbert WN, Hage ML, et al. Use of the TDx-FLM assay in evaluating fetal lung maturity in an insulin-dependent diabetic population. The Diabetes and Fetal Maturity Study Group. Obstet Gynecol 1995; 86:826
83. Tanasijevic MJ, Winkelman JW, Wybenga DR, et al. Prediction of fetal lung maturity in infants of diabetic mothers using the FLM S/A and disaturated phosphatidylcholine tests. Am J Clin Pathol 1996; 105:17
84. Robert MF, Neff RK, Hubbell JP, et al. Association between maternal diabetes and the respiratory-distress syndrome in the newborn. N Engl J Med 1976; 294(7):357–60
85. Piper JM, Xenakis EM, Langer O. Delayed appearance of pulmonary maturation markers is associated with poor glucose control in diabetic pregnancies. J Matern Fetal Med 1998; 7(3):148–53
86. Molsted-Pederson L, Kuhl C. Obstetrical management in diabetic pregnancy: the Copenhagen experience. Diabetologia 1986; 29:13
87. Gabbe SG, Mestman JH, Freeman RK, et al. Management and outcome of pregnancy in diabetes mellitus, classes B to R. Am J Obstet Gynecol 1977; 129:723
88. Olofsson P, Ingemarsson I, Solum T. Fetal distress during labour in diabetic pregnancy. Br J Obstet Gynaecol 1986; 93:1067
89. Jovanovic L, Peterson CM. Insulin and glucose requirements during the first stage of labor in insulin-dependent diabetic women. Am J Med 1983; 75:607

90. Grylack LJ, Chu SS, Scanlon JW, et al. Use of intravenous fluids before cesarean section: effects on perinatal glucose, insulin and sodium hemostasis. Obstet Gynecol 1984; 63:654

91. Kenepp NB, Kumar S, Shelley WC, et al. Fetal and neonatal hazards of maternal hydration with 5% dextrose before cesarean section. Lancet 1982; 1:1150

92. Takoudes TC, Weitzen S, Slocum J, et al. Risk of cesarean wound infections in diabetic gestation. Am J Obstet Gynecol 2004; 191(3):95

17

Medical Management of Preexisting Diabetes in Pregnancy

Angelina L. Trujillo, Lorena Wright, and Lois Jovanovic

CONTENTS

ABSTRACT

Approximately 1.3% of pregnancies in the USA occur in women with preexisting diabetes mellitus. Women with pregestational diabetes mellitus who are in poor glycemic control during the first 7 weeks of pregnancy when fetal organogenesis is occurring have an increased incidence of spontaneous abortion and fetuses with congenital anomalies. Prepregnancy care of women with either type 1 diabetes mellitus (DM1) or type 2 diabetes mellitus (DM2) must include achievement of glucose control prior to conception to reduce the risk of maternal and fetal complications. Retinopathy, nephropathy, hypertension, and neuropathy each have an impact on the success of the pregnancy. Medical treatment of diabetes during pregnancy and treatment of coexisting diabetic complications will improve maternal and fetal outcome of pregnancies complicated by preexisting diabetes mellitus.

Key words: Pregestational; Diabetes; Pregnancy

From: *Diabetes in Women: Pathophysiology and Therapy*
Edited by: A. Tsatsoulis et al. (eds.), DOI 10.1007/978-1-60327-250-6_17
© Humana Press, a part of Springer Science+Business Media, LLC 2009

Pregnancy complicated by preexisting diabetes mellitus has been estimated to occur in approximately 1.3% of pregnancies in the USA *(1)*. Pregestational diabetes is a major risk factor for spontaneous abortions, congenital malformations, macrosomia, neonatal hypoglycemia, intrauterine death, and cesarean delivery *(2, 3)*. Appropriate intensive therapy and maintenance of glucose levels to achieve a lowering of glycosylated hemoglobin (A1C), as close to the normal range, as possible without significant hypoglycemia before and throughout pregnancy can result in reducing the rate of fetal and maternal complications to a similar rate to that observed among nondiabetic pregnancies *(4)*.

NUTRITION

Intrauterine growth and development are dependent upon adequate maternal nutrition throughout pregnancy. Low birth weight infants born to mothers with inadequate nutrition during pregnancy are at risk for cardiovascular and metabolic disease as adults *(5)*. While the amount of weight to be gained during pregnancy may still be controversial, several studies have demonstrated that maternal and fetal outcomes are improved when total weight gain is within the ranges recommended by the Institute of Medicine (IOM) in 1990 that were based on prepregnancy body mass index (BMI) (Table 1) *(6)*. However, it has been noted that these guidelines may not be appropriate for pregnant women of Chinese or other ethnic cultures *(7)*. In addition, the IOM guidelines do not establish an upper limit of weight gain for obese women during pregnancy. The Diabetes Endocrine Pregnancy Outcome Study in Toronto (DEPOSIT) Study reported that maternal obesity and excessive weight gain are independent risk factors for adverse maternal and neonatal outcomes among women with any type of diabetes *(8)*. A recent observational study by Kiel et al. evaluated 120,251 women who were categorized as obese by their prepregnancy BMI being greater than or equal to 30 kg/m^2 *(9)*. This study concluded that limited or no weight gain in women during pregnancy is associated with favorable maternal and neonatal outcomes.

Maternal obesity that frequently accompanies DM2 increases the risk of maternal and fetal complications including cesarean delivery, macrosomia, and congenital defects *(10)*. Therefore, the optimal diet recommended during pregnancy in diabetic women must contain adequate calories and micronutrients sufficient to sustain the pregnancy without causing starvation ketosis, postprandial hyperglycemia, or excessive weight gain. We recommend that the calories be distributed among three meals and three snacks except in overweight and obese women in whom the snacks can be eliminated. The calories should be allocated 10% to breakfast, 30% to lunch, and 30% to dinner, and the remainder should be distributed among the three snacks. This is discussed in more detail in Chap. 14.

Table 1
Pregnancy Total Weight Gain Based on Prepregnancy Body Mass Index (Women Whose Height is <62 in. (157 cm) Should Be in the Lower Weight Gain Range) (Adapted from Institute of Medicine Executive Summary, 1990 *(6)*)

Prepregnancy BMI	Weight gain (lb)	Weight gain (Kg)
<19.8	28–40	12.5–18
19.8–26.0	25–35	11.5–16
>26.0–29.0	15–25	7–11.5

Women who are obese (BMI > 29) should gain at least 15 lb (6.8 kg)

EXERCISE

Physical activity or exercise can improve insulin sensitivity and increase insulin-stimulated muscle glucose uptake in diabetes mellitus. There are no increases in adverse maternal or neonatal outcomes associated with exercise in pregnancy when activities are undertaken that minimize the risk of falls or fetal trauma *(11)*. As pregnancy progresses, nonweight-bearing exercise may be more efficient than weight-bearing exercise *(12)*. Serum creatinine levels and urinary microalbumin can be transiently increased after exercise; therefore, assessment of these parameters should not be undertaken following exercise. There is also an increased risk of underlying cardiovascular disease when nephropathy is present, or when the duration of diabetes mellitus has been long-standing such that modification of exercise will need to be made to accommodate the cardiovascular status *(13)*. An exercise prescription during diabetic pregnancy must be individualized taking into consideration the woman's prepregnancy fitness status as well as the assessment of her renal and cardiovascular status.

INSULIN THERAPY

Intensive insulin therapy during preconception and during pregnancy of women with DM1 can significantly reduce the risk of adverse pregnancy outcomes to a level similar to the risk among women with normal pregnancies *(14)*. Good glycemic control in DM2 should also be achieved prior to pregnancy; however, women who are being treated with oral hypoglycemic agents must discontinue the oral agents when they become pregnant. In addition, it may be possible for some women with diet-controlled DM2 to achieve good glycemic control with diet and exercise alone during pregnancy. When these interventions fail, then insulin treatment is required for pregnant women with DM2.

Among pregnant women with preexisting diabetes mellitus, during the first trimester of pregnancy, insulin requirements will be similar to those who are treated with insulin in the nonpregnant state with a decline in the insulin requirement occurring in the late first trimester *(15)*. As pregnancy progresses, the insulin requirements will increase, with the increase being proportionately larger among pregnant women with DM2 than among pregnant women with DM1.

Human insulin will only cross the placenta when it becomes bound to immunoglobulin antibody. Recombinant DNA-human insulin is the least immunogenic insulin along with the insulin analogs that also have low immunogenicity. Figure 1 shows that maternal insulin does not cross the placenta

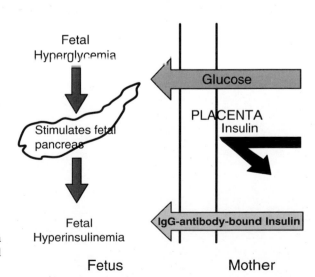

Fig. 1 Antibody bound insulin can cross the placenta resulting in increased fetal hyperinsulinemia (Adapted from Pedersen, 1954) *(16)*.

except when exogenously injected insulin creates an IgG antibody response, and then the IgG-bound insulin will cross the placenta *(16, 17)*.

Human insulin and the rapid-acting insulin analogs have been adequately studied to demonstrate not only efficacy, but also to have acceptable safety profiles with minimal placental transfer and no evidence of teratogenesis *(18)*. Human regular insulin has been approved for use during pregnancy; however, its longer delay to onset of action of 30–60 min requires that it be administered up 30 min prior to a meal. The rapid-acting insulin analogs, insulin lispro and insulin aspart, have been classified in the same category risk (category B) as human insulin for use in pregnancy *(18, 19)*. With a more rapid onset of 5–15 min, the insulin analogs can be administered at the time of the meal. Insulin glulisine (category C) has not been adequately studied in human pregnancy, and long-term clinical studies are needed. Therefore, during pregnancy we recommend only the rapid-acting insulins, insulin lispro or insulin aspart, as part of a multiple-injection regimen or for use in an insulin pump for women who have preexisting diabetes mellitus. Regular insulin is an alternative short-acting insulin that has been used successfully for insulin pump therapy.

The long-acting insulin analogs including detemir and glargine have also not been adequately studied during pregnancy. Insulin glargine has been shown to have a high affinity for the IGF-1 receptor, which has been proposed as a potential source for development of fetal macrosomia *(19)*. Currently, we recommend only human NPH insulin during pregnancy including discontinuation of glargine and changing to NPH insulin for the basal insulin requirements.

Table 2 demonstrates the usual insulin requirements during pregnancy, although a greater increase in insulin will be required with significant maternal weight gain. We recommend calculating the daily insulin dosage referred to as "Big I," which is equal to the units multiplied by kilogram of weight based on trimester of pregnancy in which "Big I" is the total daily units of insulin required. For women who are using multiple injections, one-half of the total requirement consists of NPH divided into three daily doses approximately 8 h apart (breakfast, 4 p.m., and midnight) and one-half consists of insulin lispro or insulin aspart divided into three premeal doses (breakfast, lunch, and dinner).

Frequently, women with DM1 who use an insulin pump prior to pregnancy will continue to use an insulin pump to achieve improved glycemic control during pregnancy *(20)*. The pregnant patient who is using an insulin pump will require a minimum of three basal rates over a daily 24-h period. An increased early morning basal infusion is often required to counteract the anti-insulin effect of the early morning physiologic release of cortisol and growth hormone, which has been reported in both DM1 and DM2 and potentiated in pregnancy *(21)*.

Table 2
Insulin Calculation for Diabetic Pregnancy

Trimester	*Weeks*	*Dosage (U/Kg)*
1st	1–12	0.7
2nd	13–28	0.8
23rd	29–34	0.9
	35–40	1.0

Example: 20-weeks gestation, weight = 75 kg
Big I = 0.8 × 75 = 60 units total daily requirement
NPH = 30 units (10 units 8 a.m., 10 units 4 p.m., and 10 units mid-night)
Rapid acting = 10 units prebreakfast, prelunch, and preevening meal

The goal of medical therapy for diabetes mellitus during pregnancy is to maintain fasting and premeal glucose levels between 60 and 99 mg/dL (3.3–5.5 mmol/L) and peak (usually 1–1½ h) postprandial glucose levels less than 130 mg/dL (7.2 mmol/L) *(4)*. We suggest self-monitoring of blood glucose (SMBG) fasting, before each meal and 1 h after the start of each meal.

Insulin therapy is the standard treatment of preexisting diabetes during pregnancy. Oral glucose-lowering agents are not recommended during pregnancy for women with DM2 because these agents cannot achieve the postprandial glycemic goals recommended during pregnancy. In addition, the oral agents cross the placenta, which can impact on fetal development. The sulfonyurea agents (glimiperide, glyburide, glipizide) and the meglitinide analogs (nateglinide, repaglinide) are risk-classified for pregnancy as category C. Metformin (a biguanide) and the α-glucosidase inhibitors (acarbose, miglitol) are classified as category B. Long-term studies with the oral agents are required to adequately evaluate the safety of these oral agents during pregnancy.

GLUCOSE MONITORING

Self-Monitoring of Blood Glucose

Prior to 1975, routine patient glucose monitoring consisted of urine glucose and ketone determinations. The primary purpose of monitoring was to provide information to the patient's health care provider to guide changes in therapy to relieve symptoms due to hyperglycemia – polyuria, polydipsia, and nocturia - rather than to achieve specific glycemic goals *(22–24)*.

It was not until 1978 that Skyler et al. first reported a study on 32 insulin-dependent patients, including nine pregnant women, who monitored home blood glucose and demonstrated that monitoring of blood glucose by ambulatory patients at home was feasible *(25)*. Many studies agreed on the potential of SMBG to increase the likelihood for achieving a degree of control approximating euglycemia *(26, 27)*. In 1980, Jovanovic et al. established an intensive program in insulin-dependent pregnant women that consisted of normalizing blood glucose while in the hospital and instructing them in the technique of SMBG *(28)*. In this study, patients were also taught how to titrate insulin according to blood glucose levels and diet/exchange lists to achieve glycemic control. The mean fasting blood glucose for the first ten patients accepted to the program was 169 mg/dL (9.3 mmol/L) at the start of the program, with a mean A1C by monoclonal antibody of 9.4% for the group (normal < 5.5%). After discharge, mean fasting glucose was 91 mg/dL (5.1 mmol/L). The A1C levels fell into the normal assay range of 3.4% within 5 weeks after normoglycemia was reached and were maintained in the outpatient setting. Mean glucose at delivery was 87 mg/dL (4.8 mmol/L) and A1C was 3% (normal < 5.5%). This study demonstrated that with SMBG, achievement of glycemic control in insulin-dependent pregnant women was feasible in the outpatient setting *(29)*. By the mid-1980s, patient monitoring of capillary blood glucose had replaced urine glucose testing as the recommended method of day-to-day testing *(30)*. The process requires intermittent capillary blood sampling and the use of a glucose monitor, with various frequency of testing indicated for DM1, DM2, and pregnancy complicated by diabetes *(31, 32)*.

Self-management skills are essential for attaining an optimal level of glycemic control. When used properly, SMBG gives an acceptably accurate reflection of immediate plasma glucose levels. It is possible that treatments may be inappropriately added, omitted, or doses altered on the basis of an inaccurate test result. The importance of the accuracy of blood glucose testing is paramount especially as the benefits of tighter control regimens have become evident. The use of SMBG for metabolic regulation during pregnancy should be monitored carefully for accuracy and in conjunction with an A1C. The glucose meter should be checked against standard values periodically, and the patient should receive education and assessment of the technique to maintain accuracy.

Dramatic changes continue to take place in the methods and goals of glucose monitoring. These changes are driven by technical advances in testing and steadily increasing evidence that the chronic complications of diabetes are the result of chronic hyperglycemia (33). Devices to sample glucose continuously from subcutaneous fluid are now available, with ongoing development in progress. Availability of real-time, continuously measured glucose levels can significantly improve glycemic excursions by reducing exposure to hyperglycemia without increasing the risk of hypoglycemia (34).

CONTINUOUS GLUCOSE MONITORING

SMBG is, without question, one of the most important advances in the field of diabetes and pregnancy, since the discovery of insulin in 1921.

To achieve glucose control, it is important to know the target blood glucose levels, and frequent glucose measurements allow a more precise understanding of daily glucose fluctuations. A recent study by Kerssen, which included 43 women with DM1, demonstrated that the detection rate of hyper- and hypoglycemic episodes was significantly higher in patients with ten or more SMBG determinations daily than in patients with less than ten determinations (35). Unfortunately, it is not practical to perform self-monitoring frequently enough throughout the day to identify every blood glucose excursion accurately. Glucose excursions may reach their maximum at varying times, based on the size and number of meals ingested. Therefore, intermittent blood glucose monitoring may underestimate the number of hyperglycemic events (36). Continuous glucose monitoring systems (CGMS) can facilitate the detection of all postprandial peaks, including those due to unscheduled meals, and could provide an opportunity for intervention by providing the complete glucose profile. CGMS is a better monitoring method than SMBG for detecting hypoglycemic events as well, which are usually asymptomatic and frequently occur at night (37).

The CGMS measures glucose levels in subcutaneous interstitial tissue. CGMS were originally composed of disposable subcutaneous glucose-sensing devices with electrodes impregnated with glucose oxidase connected by a cable to a lightweight monitor, which is worn over the clothing or on a belt. Current CGMS are wireless devices that send information via a transmitter to the monitor that is worn. The system takes a glucose measurement every 10 s, based on the electrochemical detection of glucose by its reaction with glucose oxidase, and stores an average value every 5 min, for a total of 288 measurements each day. A communication device enables the data stored in the monitor to be downloaded and reviewed on a personal computer (33, 38). In contrast with a static picture (six to eight blood glucose measurements a day), a more complete profile by CGMS may help physicians individualize the treatment of pregnant patients with diabetes. This personalized treatment can reduce the frequency of hyperglycemia that contributes to the risk of fetal malformations and macrosomia.

The first trial of CGMS use in pregnancy was reported in 2000 by Jovanovic et al. The study evaluated ten women with GDM and identified that an average of 5.5 h per day was spent in hyperglycemia that was undetected by SMBG (39). In addition, an average of 1 h per day was spent with glucose levels exceeding 140 mg/dL (7.8 mmol/L). The data obtained from this study helped to educate the patients about their behavior and improved compliance to treatment (39).

In 2003, Yogev et al. evaluated 34 pregnant DM1 women who were between 16 and 32 weeks of gestation (40). Seventy-two hours of CGMS data were compared with six to eight capillary glucose measurements obtained daily. The patients documented the time of food intake, insulin injections, and hypoglycemic events. A glucose level greater than 140 mg/dL (7.8 mmol/L) was undetected by the finger stick method for a mean total time of 192 ±28 min per day. In 26 of the patients, glucose levels less than 50 mg/dL (2.8 mmol/L) were recorded, but there was an interval of 1–4 h before clinical manifestations appeared or the event was documented by random blood glucose testing (40).

With the information obtained by CGMS, insulin therapy was adjusted in 24 of the patients in this particular study *(40)*.

Similar results have been obtained in other studies that also included women with gestational diabetes *(41, 42)*. One study monitored eight patients with diabetic pregnancy, six with prepregnancy DM1, and two with GDM treated with insulin, at 24–32 weeks of gestation *(37)*. Patients were monitored with CGMS for 72 h, and the results were compared with SMBG taken 6–8 times daily. Adjustments in insulin therapy were made in all patients based on the CGMS results. The patients were reevaluated after adjustment of therapy. The mean total time of hyperglycemia undetected by the finger stick method was reduced from 152 ±33 min/day before insulin adjustment to 89 ± 17 min/day after the insulin regimen was changed based on the data obtained by CGMS. The number of patients with nocturnal hypoglycemic events decreased from 7 patients to 1 patient *(37)*.

By 2006, four CGMS had been approved by the Food and Drug Administration (FDA) for use in the USA. These monitoring systems included the CGMS® Gold (Medtronic MiniMed, Northridge, CA), the GlucoWatch® G2 Biographer (developed by Cygnus, Redwood City, CA), the Guardian® Telemetered Glucose Monitoring System (Medtronic MiniMed, Northridge, CA), and the DexCom–STS– CGMS (DexCom, San Diego, CA). In 2006, the safety and efficacy of a 7-day transcutaneous CGMS (DexCom–STS-7–, San Diego, CA) was evaluated in 86 insulin-requiring patients by Garg et al. *(40)*. This 7-day system received FDA approval in 2007. The Paradigm® REAL-Time Insulin Pump combined with the Guardian® REAL-Time CGMS (Medtronic MiniMed, Northridge, CA) was also FDA approved in 2007. In 2008, the FreeStyle Navigator® (Abbott Diabetes Care, Alameda, CA) was also approved for continuous glucose monitoring. Each of these CGMS is defined as minimally invasive because they compromise the skin barrier but do not puncture blood vessels. Every manufacturer of a continuous glucose monitor produces at least one model that sounds an alarm if the glucose level falls beyond a preset euglycemia range.

In Europe, the GlucoDay (A. Menarini Diagnostics, Florence, Italy) and the Pendra (Pendragon Medical, Zurich, Switzerland) CGMS systems are approved but have not yet been approved for use in the USA.

To create a normoglycemic profile to help pregnant diabetic women achieve target glycemic values similar to those of normal nondiabetic pregnancy, nondiabetic women have also been monitored using CGMS. Yogev et al. studied 57 nondiabetic pregnant women (obese and normal weight) in the second half of pregnancy *(43)*. Fasting blood glucose level was 75 ± 12 mg/dL (4.2 ± 0.7 mmol/L) with a postprandial peak glucose level of 110 ± 16 mg/dL (6.1 ± 0.9 mmol/L). The time interval that was needed to reach peak postprandial glucose (PPG) level was 70 ± 13 min. Postprandial glycemic profiles were similar after breakfast, lunch, and dinner meals. As a result of this observational study and other studies, the ADA now recommends lower targets as noted previously *(4)*.

A topic of continuing controversy has been identification of the most appropriate timing for blood glucose monitoring in the diabetic pregnancy. On the basis of data using CGMS in a study of 65 women (26 treated by diet alone, 19 receiving insulin therapy, and 20 with T1DM), Ben-Haroush et al. concluded that 90 min postprandial was the appropriate time interval for testing *(44)*. During this study, for each meal, the first postprandial 240 min was analyzed. The time interval was approximately 90 min from meal to peak PPG levels in all the evaluated types of diabetic pregnancies independent of level of control. Bühling et al. has also recommended that the optimal time for testing is between 45 and 120 min postprandial *(45)*. This recommendation was based on the results of a trial with 53 women (13 with GDM, 4 pregnant women with DM1, and 36 nondiabetic pregnant women), who wore a CGMS for 72 h. The group was divided into three clinical outcome parameters: mode of delivery, birth weight percentile, and diabetes-associated complications. The pre- and postprandial glucose levels were documented at 15-min intervals for 3 h from the beginning of each meal.

The time to PPG peak was not statistically significant between the groups (82 ± 18 min in the nondiabetics compared with 74 ± 23 min in the pregnancy complicated by diabetes group). However, when the subjects were divided into clinical outcome parameters, there was a significant difference between the postprandial time intervals of 75 and 105 min ($P < 0.05$). The time interval of 120 min was too long and did not have a high correlation to clinical outcome parameters. Bühling et al. recommended a 60-min timing interval, since patients could calculate this time easily and have more freedom to eat the recommended number of snacks (45).

Alternative Site Testing

The validity and similarity of Alternative Site Testing (*AST) relative to fingertip testing have been debated. Reliability and reproducibility of postprandial blood glucose results have been reported to show significant differences between samples obtained at the forearm, thigh, and fingertip, even when samples were collected simultaneously.

In a study by Jungheim et al. capillary blood glucose samples were collected from the fingertip and the forearm of 17 insulin-treated diabetic patients every 15 min for 3–5 h (46). A rapid increase in blood glucose was induced by oral administration of glucose, and subsequently, a rapid decrease in glucose was induced by intravenous administration of insulin. In the fasting state, the glucose values at the fingertip and the forearm were similar (7.8 ± 2.4 vs. 7.2 ± 2.3 mmol/L). However, during rapid increases in blood glucose, the values at the fingertip were consistently higher than at the forearm (maximal difference 4.6 ± 1.2 mmol/L). During a rapid decrease in blood glucose, lower values were recorded at the fingertip (maximal difference to forearm 5.0 ± 1.0 mmol/L). In addition, forearm blood glucose was significantly delayed by a median time of 35 min in relation to the fingertip. On the basis of observations in this trial Jungheim et al. recommended that blood glucose monitoring from the arm site should be limited to situations in which ongoing rapid changes of blood glucose can be excluded (46).

A study by Ellison et al. compared capillary blood glucose concentrations from the finger, forearm, and thigh, measuring premeal and approximately 60, 90, 120, 150, and 180 min postprandial (47). Fingertip results were accurate at all time points relative to venous readings. Again, alternate sites tended to produce lower glucose readings than fingertip readings at times when glucose was increasing rapidly (60 and 90 min postmeal). They concluded that although changes in blood glucose immediately after a meal may be identified at finger sites before detection at forearm or thigh sites, alternate site testing appeared to be a useful option for routine self-monitoring *before* meals (47). Bina et al. studied alternative site testing (AST) and the impact of prandial state and exercise in 86 patients with DM2 (48). Fasting blood glucose was measured at the fingertip, palm, thigh, and each forearm. After consuming a 40-g carbohydrate meal, the blood glucose was again measured from each site at 60, 90, and 120 min postmeal. Patients then exercised for 15 min after which blood glucose was again measured at each site. Significant differences in blood glucose between fingertip and at alternative sites were found at 60 min postmeal and postexercise. These findings further confirmed that there are clinically relevant differences in AST compared with fingertip testing when testing occurs during periods of rapid blood glucose changes (48).

Other factors, such as subject age, BMI, diabetes type, and insulin dependence do not seem to have a significant impact on site differences in nonpregnant diabetes mellitus (47). Because of the variability in PPG measurements with AST, we currently do not recommend alternate site testing during pregnancy for women with diabetes mellitus.

Optimal Timing and Frequency

For most patients with DM1 SMBG before and after meals (and exercise) will provide useful information for adjusting insulin and carbohydrate intake. The ADA suggests that there are no data to support that postmeal glucose monitoring has a specific role in preconception diabetes care beyond what is needed to achieve the target for A1C (30). However, there is increasing evidence that elevated PPG levels exert a more deleterious effect than elevation of fasting plasma glucose (49). Many studies advocate the introduction of PPG measurements in the monitoring of preexisting diabetes, as well as in individuals with normal fasting plasma glucose but impaired glucose tolerance (50–53). On the basis of our own experience regarding the frequency of postprandial hyperglycemia even in patients who have reached the goal A1C, we recommend that in addition to A1C and fasting blood glucose PPG be monitored and targeted in all pregnant women with diabetes beginning in the preconception period to achieve maximum glycemic control. Ideally, with this approach euglycemia can be achieved before conception and maintained throughout pregnancy and through the postpartum period (54–56).

Frequent measurements of blood glucose during pregnancy are advised for women with either DM1 or DM2 to help prevent or treat both hyper and hypoglycemia, as intensive therapy regimens and the establishment of maternal euglycemia have dramatically improved fetal outcomes in these patients (57, 58).Optimal SMBG evaluation of capillary blood glucose consists of testing before and after meals, at bedtime, and occasionally during the night if nocturnal hypoglycemia is suspected. Glucose excursions may reach their maximum at varying times, based on the size and number of meals; therefore, SMBG alone may not capture the full extent of total daily postprandial hyperglycemia. The same rationale applies to nocturnal hypoglycemic events, which may also go unrecognized by intermittent blood glucose monitoring (38, 40, 59). Pregnancy is associated with an exaggerated rebound from hypoglycemia such that an elevation in morning blood glucose values may reflect hypoglycemia at night. Normalization of glycemia is the main therapeutic goal at all times.

Studies in pregnancy indicate that the most important glucose concentration is the peak postprandial response since it is the highest blood glucose of the day and is the most important variable associated with overgrowth of the fetus (55–58). One hour after the start of the meal has been shown to be the time of peak postprandial response in 90% of pregnant woman (45); therefore, 1 h after the meal is the primary target for attaining glycemic control during pregnancy.

The Diabetes in Early Pregnancy (DIEP) study was a multicenter case controlled trial of women with DM1 compared with normal control women throughout pregnancy with the primary objective to relate maternal glucose to risk of spontaneous abortions and malformations (14). Also studied was the relationship between maternal PPG concentrations and the risk of neonatal macrosomia. The DIEP study identified 28.5% of infants from diabetic mothers who were greater than the 90th percentile infant birth weight. The birth weight correlated positively with the first trimester maternal fasting blood glucose and A1C. When adjusted for fasting blood glucose concentration and A1C, the 1 h postprandial maternal blood glucose in the third trimester was an even stronger predictor of infant birth weight and fetal macrosomia (14).

Manderson et al. compared a preprandial monitoring group with a PPG monitoring group in 61 pregnant women with DM1 who were randomly assigned at 16-weeks gestation to using memory-based glucose reflectance meters throughout pregnancy (58). Maternal age, parity, age of onset of diabetes, number of prior miscarriages, smoking status, social class, weight gain in pregnancy, and compliance with therapy were similar in the two groups. However, the postprandial monitoring group had greater success in achieving glycemic control targets than the preprandial monitoring group (55% vs. 30%) (58).

Although controversy remains relative to the most appropriate timing of the postprandial blood glucose measurement, in our experience the risk of macrosomia appears to increase with increasing PPG levels exceeding 120 mg/dL (6.7 mmol/L) *(14)*. On the basis of these observations, we recommend women to maintain their blood glucose levels at the levels of nondiabetic pregnant women, not exceeding a preprandial value of 99 mg/dL (5.0 mmol/L) and a 1-h postprandial value of 129 mg/dL (6.7 mmol/L). Other studies have reported that keeping 1-h postprandial blood glucose levels between 120 and 140 mg/dL (6.7–7.8 mmol/L) minimizes the risk of macrosomia *(55, 56)*. Until the time when CGMS replaces SMBG and optimal timing is confirmed, the most effective manner in which patients can currently accomplish control of their glucose is to perform SMBG both before and 1 h after meals.

HEMOGLOBIN A1C

The A1C assay provides information about the degree of long-term glucose control that is not otherwise obtainable in the usual clinical setting. Therefore, the A1C goal prior to pregnancy is to achieve the lowest A1C value as close to normal as possible without increasing hypoglycemia. Poorly controlled pregnant women with high A1C levels early in pregnancy have an increased risk of spontaneous abortion and major fetal congenital malformations *(59–61)*. Many studies have demonstrated that adverse fetal outcomes are related to hyperglycemia in early pregnancy as measured by an elevated A1C reflecting hyperglycemia in the early weeks of pregnancy when organogenesis is occurring. To reduce the incidence of fetal complications, women with preexisting diabetes who are planning to have children should receive early counseling for family planning and intensified metabolic control prior to pregnancy.

The American Diabetes Association (ADA) recommends an A1C value <1% above the upper limit of normal *(30)*. An A1C level of 6% correlates with an average glucose concentration of 110–120 mg/dL (6.1–6.7 mmol/L) (Table 3). Therefore, in pregnant women, an A1C level as near to normal as

Table 3
Correlation Between A1C Level and Mean Plasma Glucose Levels (Adapted from http://www.diagnostics.siemens/com*(62)*)

HbA1C (%)	Average blood glucose	
	mg/dL	mmol/L
14	360	20.0
13	330	18.3
12	300	16.7
11	270	15.0
10	240	13.3
9	210	11.7
8	180	10.0
7	150	8.3
6	120	6.7
5	90	5.0
4	60	3.3

possible is the optimal goal. The rationale for choosing this target is that observational studies have shown that A1C values up to 1% above normal (reference range 4–6%; 5.0% is the nondiabetic mean) are associated with rates of congenital anomalies and miscarriages similar to the rates in the general population (63). During pregnancy the red blood cell (RBC) has a shortened life span due to increased RBC production stimulated by increased erythropoietin levels (64). Several studies have demonstrated that the reference range for A1C during pregnancy should be lower than that for nonpregnant patients (65, 66). Therefore, our recommended goal during diabetic pregnancy is an A1C as near to normal as possible without inducing hypoglycemia. In our practice, the A1C is measured every 2–4 weeks with a goal of A1C 5.0%.

MEDICAL MANAGEMENT OF COMPLICATIONS DURING DIABETIC PREGNANCY

Diabetic Retinopathy in Pregnancy

Pregnancy per se is a risk factor for progression of diabetic retinopathy (DR). Achieving good glucose control prior to pregnancy can decrease the risk of development and/or progression of DR (14). The classification of retinopathy during pregnancy is the same as the classification in nonpregnant diabetic patients. DR progresses from mild nonproliferative abnormalities with increased vascular permeability, to moderate and severe nonproliferative diabetic retinopathy (NPDR), characterized by vascular closure, to proliferative diabetic retinopathy (PDR), characterized by the growth of new blood vessels on the retina and posterior surface of the vitreous (67, 68).

The gestational effect on progression of DR is not completely understood. Many of the hormonal factors of pregnancy have been considered to increase the risk of development and progression of DR by several biochemical mechanisms that are not yet completely understood. Studies in vitro suggest that the growth factors, insulin-like growth factor-1 (IGF-1) and vascular endothelial growth factor (VEGF), as well as placental growth hormone (pGH) that are produced by the placenta may contribute to retinopathy during pregnancy (62, 69, 70). An early clinical report of four nonpregnant patients with upregulation of IGF-1 prior to onset of retinal deterioration suggested that IGF-1 is a contributor to acceleration of DR (71). However, in a clinical study comparing pregnant diabetic women with nondiabetic pregnant women, it was reported that serum levels of IGF-1 and insulin-like growth factor binding protein-3 (IGFBP-3) were lower among pregnant diabetic women than among nondiabetic pregnant controls and/or postpartum indicating that there is not a clear connection between the IGF system and progression of DR during pregnancy (72). It has also been suggested that as blood levels of hormones such as estrogen, progesterone, and human placental lactogen (hPL) increase dramatically in pregnancy, they too may accelerate retinopathy (73).

It has been considered that inflammation during pregnancy contributes to retinopathy. Loukovaara et al. reported that CRP levels are higher among diabetic women with progression of retinopathy and also among those women with poor glycemic control; however, inflammatory markers such as interleukin-6 (IL-6) and vascular cell adhesion molecule-1 (VCAM-1) were similar in women with DM1 and nondiabetic women (74).

When retinopathy is present prior to pregnancy, the progression of retinopathy during pregnancy to PDR or within NPDR is common. Several factors have been identified that increase the risk for progression during pregnancy (Table 4).

The severity of retinopathy at the onset of pregnancy is an independent risk factor. In a recent study of pregnant patients with DM1, it was observed that among patients with PDR who had not received laser treatment before pregnancy, 75% showed progression of retinopathy, compared with

Table 4
Factors that Increase the Risk for Progression of
Retinopathy during Pregnancy (Adapted from
Rahman, 2007 *(76)*)

Retinal status at conception
Early onset of diabetes
Duration of diabetes
Elevated first trimester A1C or poor glycemic control
Rapid normalization of blood glucose
Hypertension

only 25% of the patients who had PDR and had laser treatment prior to pregnancy *(76)*. These results provide further support for careful preconception evaluation and treatment of women with diabetes mellitus *(77)*.

A retrospective study by Lovestam-Adrian in 1997 addressed the issue whether the short-term risk of progression of DR in pregnant women with DM1 is increased than in nonpregnant women with DM1 and similar diabetes characteristics matched for age and duration of diabetes *(78)*. The patients had been followed for 12 months before, during, and 6 months after pregnancy. The results indicated that progression of retinopathy to potential loss of sight was similar between the pregnancy group and the control group, and pregestational elevated A1C and a rapid decrease in A1C were each significant risk factors for progression of preexisting retinopathy in the groups *(78)*.

The duration of diabetes mellitus is also a significant risk factor for DR. When DM1 has been present more than 5 years, there is a 14% risk for a greater than two-step progression of DR that continues to increase until the risk peaks at approximately 46% between 16 and 20 years duration of DM1 *(79, 80)*. This suggests that women with DM1 onset in childhood and teens have an increased risk for retinopathy during their reproductive years.

During the DCCT it had been observed that in the first year of intensified diabetes management in nonpregnant women with DM1, there was a transient increase of retinopathy, known as "early worsening" that was characterized as development of soft exudates, dilated tortuous intraretinal vessels, or clinically important retinopathy that were noted at the 6- or 12-month follow-up visits *(81, 82)*. In the intensively treated group, the frequency of early worsening was somewhat greater when moderate/severe NPDR was present at the baseline visit *(75, 81, 82)*. In a study comparing Conti-nuous Subcutaneous Insulin Infusion therapy (CSII) to Conventional Insulin Therapy (CIT), the proportion of patients whose retinopathy progressed did not differ significantly between the CSII and CIT groups, and in the majority the deterioration was mild *(83)*. However, two patients in the CSII group who had the highest and most rapidly decreased A1C developed acute ischemic retinopathy that progressed to the proliferative stage in spite of laser treatment *(83)*. Other investigators have also reported that during pregnancy, elevated first trimester A1C followed by rapid improvement of maternal blood glucose increases progression of DR during pregnancy *(77, 80)*. Many investigators have concluded that initial poor glycemic control and rapid institution of strict control during pregnancy are associated with the progression of retinopathy *(78, 84, 85)*. One prospective study with the least progression of retinopathy reported the lowest A1C levels at conception and also the least decrease of A1C during pregnancy *(80)*. Therefore, optimal glycemic control should be achieved prior to conception with planning of pregnancy to allow normalization of blood glucose before conception.

Evaluation of the retina is essential during preconception care of women with preexisting diabetes mellitus. An adequate examination requires the appropriate equipment by an experienced ophthalmologist who understands the risk for progression of retinopathy during pregnancy. A dilated eye exam and baseline retinal photographs are necessary since direct ophthalmoscopic examination alone may not identify DR (86). The frequency of eye examinations during pregnancy should be determined by the initial baseline evaluation of retinopathy and the risk factors associated with pregnancy. Currently, it is recommended that ophthalmologic follow-up continues throughout pregnancy and the postpartum period with photocoagulation initiated for significant neovascularization (67, 87).

Although there are no controlled studies evaluating the risk of retinal hemorrhage during different modes of delivery, it may be recommended to use assisted second-stage labor during vaginal delivery or a cesarean section in order to avoid the valsalva maneuver associated with maternal pushing during labor if the woman has significant retinopathy or risk for retinal hemorrhage.

NEPHROPATHY

The prevalence of diabetic nephropathy among patients with DM1 has been reported to rapidly increase after diabetes has been present for 10 years (88). This suggests that in some women with DM2 and early onset of diabetes, renal insufficiency may be present during the reproductive years. With the increase in diagnosis of DM2 among teenagers there is an increase in the potential risk for development of nephropathy in young adults during their reproductive years. Currently, nephropathy complicates between 5 and 10% of pregnancies among women with preexisting diabetes mellitus (89–91). The presence of nephropathy during pregnancy not only increased risks to the mother (preeclampsia, anemia, renal failure), but there are significant risks to the fetus including intrauterine growth restriction, stillbirth, and preterm delivery (92, 93).

Pregnancy and parity do not appear to increase the risk for development of diabetic nephropathy nor do they increase the progression of established diabetic nephropathy (94). Rossing et al. have reported an observational study of 93 diabetic women who were followed over a range of 3–28 years during which 26 of the women became pregnant after developing nephropathy (95). The study demonstrated that pregnancy did not have any long-term effect on renal function or survival, comparing the pregnant diabetic women with those women who did not become pregnant (95). Other studies have demonstrated that among pregnant women with decreased renal function due to either diabetic or nondiabetic causes, there is an increased risk of end-stage renal disease within months to a few years after delivery (96, 97). Although the rates of maternal complications are increased when moderate or severe renal insufficiency is present among pregnant diabetic women, the fetal survival rate remains high (97). Aggressive medical management of renal complications preconception and during pregnancy can reduce both maternal and fetal morbidities and mortality (98–100).

In nonpregnant diabetes mellitus, nephropathy is characterized by albumin excretion in a spot or 24-h urine collection (Table 5).

Table 5
Nephropathy in Nonpregnant Patients with Diabetes Mellitus (Adapted from ADA (29))

Albumin excretion	Spot urine collection[a](mg/mg creatinine)	24-h urine collection[a](mg/24 h)
Normal	<30	<30
Microalbuminuria	30–299	30–299
Clinical albuminuria	³300	³300

[a]Two of three collections over 3–6 months are abnormal

During pregnancy, urinary albumin excretion increases in both nondiabetic and diabetic women; however, the effect among pregnant women with diabetes has been shown to be an exaggeration of the normal pattern that is observed in nondiabetic women and returns to prepregnancy levels after delivery (101). An assessment of serum creatinine and urinary excretion of total protein and/or albumin (albumin-to-creatinine ratio or 24-h excretion rate) should be measured not only prior to pregnancy or in the first trimester but also at intervals during pregnancy, particularly if there is preexisting elevated albumin excretion or an increase with urine dipstick testing or increasing blood pressure (31). No specific nephropathy treatment is recommended, but the patient should be counseled regarding the possible transient decline in renal function during pregnancy.

Hypertension

Chronic hypertension should be treated to decrease the progression of nephropathy and retinopathy. However, treatment of hypertension during pregnancy must be adjusted such that uteroplacental blood flow is not compromised (102). ACE inhibitors must be discontinued prior to conception. Fetal exposure to ACE inhibitors during the first trimester of pregnancy is associated with an increased risk of major congenital malformations including malformations of the cardiovascular system and central nervous system (103). When used in the second half of pregnancy ACE inhibitors have been associated with fetal growth retardation, oligohydramnios, hypocalvaria, neonatal renal failure, hypotension, and death (104). Angiotensin receptor blockers (ARB) also interfere with the renin-angiotensin system and are contraindicated during pregnancy. The effects of ARBs on the fetus appear to be similar to the fetal complications resulting from ACE inhibitor use (105).

Currently, methyldopa is the preferred antihypertensive medication for use in pregnancy because it has been well studied with long-term follow-up of infants of mothers treated with methyldopa during pregnancy (106). Table 6 lists the medications currently available to treat hypertension during pregnancy (102, 108).

NEUROPATHY

The prevalence of diabetic neuropathy during pregnancy is not well documented. Although female gender is an independent risk factor for autonomic neuropathy in DM1, pregnancy has not been shown to add to the risk (109). Autonomic neuropathic gastrointestinal symptoms such as nausea and

Table 6   Medical Therapy of Hypertension during Pregnancy and Lactation (Adapted from AAP 2001 (107))

Medication	Pregnancy classification	Compatible with breastfeeding
First-line therapy		
Methyldopa	B	Yes
Labetalol	C	Yes
Nifedipine	C	Yes
Second-line therapy		
Hydralazine	C	Yes
Hydrochlorothiazide	B	Yes
Metoprolol	C	Yes
Clonidine	C	Not recommended
Calcium channel blockers diltiazem	C	Yes

emesis associated with diabetic gastroparesis may be exacerbated when hyperemesis of pregnancy occurs. Severe hyperemesis in nondiabetic pregnancies has been reported to result in fetal demise with one case of fetal demise reported in a diabetic pregnancy complicated by autonomic neuropathy *(110, 111)*. The treatment for exacerbations of gastroparesis during pregnancy will require modification of diet to include multiple small meals distributed throughout the day and many times the addition of erythromycin or metoclopramide, which are prokinetic agents, to decrease the delay in gastric emptying. In severe cases, total parenteral nutrition may be required.

Peripheral neuropathy during pregnancy was studied by Lapolla et al. during which 14 pregnant nondiabetic women were monitored and compared with 16 pregnant women with DM1 and 12 non-pregnant women with DM1 *(109)*. Peripheral neuropathy endpoints including motor conduction velocities were not significantly different for pregnant women with DM1 compared with pregnant women without DM in the third trimester *(109)*. At the start of the study, none of the pregnant women with DM1 had signs of autonomic neuropathy. At the end of pregnancy, all of the pregnant women (both nondiabetic and DM1) had a reduced cardiovascular autonomic test of deep breathing that was considered to be a result of the decreased ventilatory excursion due to the pregnancy. Overall, pregnancy did not worsen autonomic neuropathy in this small study.

Treatment of peripheral neuropathic pain symptoms during pregnancy is limited. When pain is associated with peripheral neuropathy, topical capsaicin is considered safe. However, medications such as tricyclic antidepressants (TCA) or antiepileptics that are used for neuropathic pain in nonpregnant diabetics are not recommended due to the increased risk to the fetus during pregnancy. In a prospective, controlled study by Maschi et al. comparing 200 neonates exposed to various antidepressants with 1,200 control neonates, there was not a statistically significant difference in the rate of adverse fetal or neonatal events between the two groups *(112)*. However, the prematurity rate was significantly greater in the group with antidepressant exposure. The newer antidepressants including selective serotonin reuptake inhibitors (SSRIs) are not considered major teratogens, although there are limited data evaluating their impact on fetal demise or spontaneous abortion *(112)*.

The antiepileptic drugs (AEDs) carbamazepine and gabapentin have been used extensively for neuropathic pain relief for nonpregnant diabetic neuropathy. The Gabapentin Pregnancy Registry retrospectively reported on 39 women with 59 fetuses of which 44 were live births and had been exposed to gabapentin during pregnancy *(113)*. The results indicated that there was no increased risk for adverse maternal or fetal outcomes; however, specific conclusions regarding safety of gabapentin during pregnancy are limited due to the small size of this study. Other studies of AED exposure during pregnancy have demonstrated that the risk for congenital malformations may be reduced but not eliminated with the addition of folic acid supplements during pregnancy *(114)*.

At the present time, it is our recommendation to use topical capsaicin for neuropathic pain symptoms during pregnancy. When more severe pain is present, judicious use of an antidepressant at the lowest effective dosage may be indicated.

LIPID CHANGES DURING PREGNANCY AND PREEXISTING DIABETES

Cholesterol levels and LDL-C levels increased up to 50% during normal pregnancy *(107)*. Triglycerides may increase threefold during normal pregnancy *(115, 116)*. Especially among women with DM2 who have increased triglycerides prepregnancy, the risk of progressive elevation in triglycerides to >2,000 mg/dL increases the risk for pancreatitis during pregnancy *(117, 118)*. The goals of managing dyslipidemia during pregnancy are similar to those of nondiabetic patients with cardiometabolic risk, since diabetes is considered a cardiometabolic risk *(119)*. Management includes dietary recommended limits of saturated fat <7% of calories, cholesterol <200 mg/day, and eliminating trans-fatty acid-containing foods *(119, 120)*.

Although specific exercise recommendations for lipid lowering during pregnancy with preexisting diabetes have not been established, postprandial walking among pregnant women with and without DM1 has been reported to significantly reduce triglyceride and cholesterol levels *(121)*.

Medical treatment of dyslipidemia is limited. Statins are contraindicated during pregnancy because of their teratogenic effects in animal studies. Instituting medical treatment for severe hypertriglyceridemia (triglycerides > 1,000 mg/dL) is clinically important to avoid the development of pancreatitis. Fish oil is the drug of choice *(4)*. Fibric acids such as gemfibrozil and fenofibrate are both category C for use in pregnancy. Low-dose niacin is not as effective as fibrates but is a possible treatment alternative. There has been limited research on the use of niacin during pregnancy. One caution with niacin is its potential to increase plasma glucose; therefore, monitoring glycemic control is recommended after starting niacin treatment, and adjustment in glucose lowering treatment may be required *(122)*.

THYROID DISEASE IN PREEXISTING DIABETIC PREGNANCY

During pregnancy, thyroid levels are altered by several mechanisms: hCG stimulation of the TSH receptor increases the free T4 during early pregnancy, and increased thyroid-binding globulin related to estrogen stimulation later in pregnancy results in lowering of free T4. Currently, there is not a consensus regarding routine screening of TSH during pregnancy. However, 10–12% of women of reproductive age have thyroid antibodies *(123)*. Prepregnancy screening of women with DM1 or DM2 seems warranted since early treatment may improve pregnancy outcome. For women with preexisting hypothyroidism, levothyroxine dose should be titrated every 4–6 weeks to target TSH not higher than 2.5 microunits/mL preconception and in the first trimester and 3.0 microunits/mL in the second and third trimesters *(124)*.

MANAGEMENT OF DIABETIC KETOACIDOSIS DURING PREGNANCY

Diabetic ketoacidosis (DKA) is an acute complication that has an impact on neonatal outcome. Although the prevalence of DKA during pregnancy has decreased over the past 20 years, it is still an a medical emergency, which, untreated, can result in fetal demise *(125, 126)*. A frequent cause of DKA during pregnancy is inappropriate decrease or cessation of insulin treatment *(126)*. Other causes include underlying infection, or the use of obstetric interventions such as tocolytic agents or corticosteroids *(127, 128)*. The common symptoms of DKA in nonpregnant women with diabetes including emesis, dehydration, and ketosis are also characteristic of DKA during pregnancy. Significant hyperglycemia may not always be present *(129)*. However, the osmotic diuresis and resulting decrease in circulating volume can reduce uterine perfusion, thereby placing the fetus at risk. Management of DKA during pregnancy is similar to the treatment of DKA in nonpregnant women with diabetes. The patient will require careful monitoring in the intensive care setting, while intravenous volume and electrolyte replacement in addition to continuous insulin infusion are administered *(130)*. Initial volume replacement with isotonic saline will effectively correct the dehydration and circulating fluid volume as well as decrease glucose concentration. Short-acting or rapid-acting insulin are each appropriate for intravenous insulin treatment. Successful management of DKA also includes identification and treatment of the underlying cause of DKA while carefully monitoring the pregnancy patient.

SUMMARY

In summary, normoglycemia is the goal for all pregnant women. The glucose targets may be still debated after 30 years of use of self-monitored glucose systems for pregnant diabetic women, but the first order of priority is to have a normal infant. While the consensus groups debate the mean and standard deviations of blood glucose that should be the goals for the treatment of pregnant diabetic women, mimicking glucose concentrations of nondiabetic pregnant women who have normal pregnancies and infant outcome is optimal. Thus, normoglycemia should be achieved before pregnancy and sustained during, and after all pregnancies (labeled as "diabetic" or not). There must be an increased awareness of the chronic and acute complications of diabetes mellitus that may be present or become manifest during pregnancy. Instituting timely and appropriate management of these complications during pregnancy will reduce the risk of a poor maternal and fetal outcome.

REFERENCES

1. Lawrence JM, Contreras R, Chen W, Sacks DA. Trends in the prevalence of preexisting diabetes and gestational diabetes mellitus among a racially/ethnically diverse population of pregnant women, 1999–2005. Diabetes Care 2008;31:899–204

2. Kitzmiller JL, Gavin LA, Gin GD, et al. Preconception care of diabetes. Glycemic control prevents congenital anomalies. JAMA 1991;265:731–736

3. Walkinshaw SA. Pregnancy in women with pre-existing diabetes: management issues. Semin Fetal Neonatal Med 2005;10:307–315

4. Kitzmiller JL, Block JM, Brown FM, et al. Managing preexisting diabetes for pregnancy. Summary of evidence and consensus recommendations for care. Diabetes Care 2008;31:1060–1079

5. Godfrey KM, Barker DJP. Fetal nutrition and adult disease. Am J Clin Nutr 2000;71:1344S–1352S

6. Institute of Medicine. Nutrition during pregnancy, weight gain and nutrient supplements. Report of the subcommittee on Nutritional Status and Weight Gain during pregnancy, Subcommittee on dietary Intake and Nutrient Supplements during pregnancy, Committee on Nutritional Status during Pregnancy and Lactation, Food and Nutrition Board. Washington DC: National Academy Press, 1990, pp. 1–233

7. Wong W, Tang NLS, Lau TK, Wong TW. A new recommendation for maternal weight gain in Chinese women. J Am Diet Assoc 2000;100:791–796

8. Ray JG, Vermeulen MJ, Shapiro JL, Kenshole AB. Maternal and neonatal outcomes in pregestational and gestational diabetes mellitus, and the influence of maternal obesity and weight gain: the DEPOSIT study. Q J Med 2001;94:347–356

9. Galtier-Dereure F, Boegner C, Bringer J. Obesity and pregnancy: complications and cost. Am J Clin Nutr 2000;71:1242S–1238S

10. Kiel DW, Dodson EA, Artal R, et al. Gestational weight gain and pregnancy outcomes in obese women how much is enough? Obstet Gynecol 2007;100:752–758

11. Davies GA, Wolfe LA, Mottola MF, MacKinnon C, SOGC Clinical Practice Obstetrics Committee, Canadian Society for Exercise Physiology Board of Directors. Exercise in pregnancy and the postpartum period. J Obstet Gynaecol Can 2003;25:516–529

12. Artal R, Masaki DI, Khodiguian N, et al. Exercise prescription in pregnancy: weight-bearing versus non-weight-bearing exercise. Am J Obstet Gynecol 1989;151:1464–1469

13. American Diabetes Association. Standards of medical care in diabetes. Diabetes Care 2005;28(Suppl 1):S4–S36

14. Jovanovic-Peterson L, Peterson CM, Reed GF, et al. Maternal postprandial glucose levels and infant birth weight: the Diabetes in Early Pregnancy Study. The National Institute of Child Health and Human Development - Diabetes in Early Pregnancy Study. Am J Obstet Gynecol 1991;164(1 Pt 1):103–111

15. Mills JL, Jovanovic L, Knopp R, et al. Physiological reduction in fasting plasma glucose concentration in the first trimester of normal pregnancy: the diabetes in early pregnancy study. Metabolism 1998;47:1140–1144

16. Pedersen J. Weight and length of infants of diabetic mothers. Acta Endocrinol 1954;12:330–342

17. Pettitt DJ. Ospina P, Howard C, et al. Efficacy, safety and lack of immunogenicity of insulin aspart compared with regular human insulin for women with gestational diabetes mellitus. Diabet Med 2007;24:1129–1135

18. Hirsch IB. Drug therapy insulin analogues. N Engl J Med 2005;352:174–183

19. Olausson H, Lof M, Brismar K, et al. Longitudinal study of the maternal insulin-like growth factor system before, during and after pregnancy in relation to fetal and infant weight. Horm Res 2007;69:99–106

20. Rudolf MC, Coustan DR, Sherwin RS, et al. Efficacy of the insulin pump in the home treatment of pregnant diabetics. Diabetes 1981;30:891–895

21. Bolli GB, Gerich JE. The "dawn phenomenon" – a common occurrence in both non-insulin-dependent and insulin-dependent diabetes mellitus. N Engl J Med 1984;310:746–750

22. Berger W. [Self-testing of urine in insulin treatment (author's transl)] MMW Munch Med Wochenschr 1975 117:1671–1676

23. Moffitt PS. Interpretation of glycosuria in the teenage diabetic patient. Diabetes Care 1980;3:112–116

24. Rubin AL, Bernstein RI. Self-monitoring of blood glucose by diabetic patients. West J Med 1981;135:244

25. Skyler JS, Lasky IA, Skyler DL, et al. Home blood glucose monitoring as an aid in diabetes management. Diabetes Care 1978;1:150–157

26. Sönksen PH, Judd SL, Lowy C. Home monitoring of blood-glucose. Method for improving diabetic control. Lancet 1978;1(8067):729–732
27. Walford S, Gale EA, Allison SP, Tattersall RB. Self-monitoring of blood-glucose. Improvement of diabetic control. Lancet 1978;1(8067):732–735
28. Jovanovic L, Peterson CM. Management of the pregnant, insulin-dependent diabetic woman. Diabetes Care 1980;3:63–68
29. Peterson CM, Forhan SE, Jones RL. Self-management: an approach to patients with insulin-dependent diabetes mellitus. Diabetes Care 1980;3:82–87
30. American Diabetes Association. Standards of medical care in diabetes. Diabetes Care 2004;27(Suppl 1):S15–S35
31. Diabetes Association. Position Statement Preconception care of women with diabetes. Diabetes Care 2004;27(Suppl 1): S76–S78
32. Prospective Diabetes Study (UKPDS) Group. Intensive blood-glucose control with sulphonylureas or insulin compared with conventional treatment and risk of complications in patients with type 2 diabetes (UKPDS 33). Lancet 1998 352(9131):837–853
33. Kerssen A, De Valk HW, Visser GHA. Validation of the continuous glucose monitoring system (CGMS) by the use of two cgms simultaneously in pregnant women with type 1 diabetes mellitus. Diabetes Technol Ther 2005;7:699–706
34. Garg S, Jovanovic L. Relationship of fasting and hourly blood glucose levels to HbA1C values: safety, accuracy, and improvements in glucose profiles obtained using a 7-day continuous glucose sensor. Diabetes Care 2006;29:2644–2649
35. Kerssen A, de Valk HW, Visser GH. Do HbA1C levels and the self-monitoring of blood glucose levels adequately reflect glycaemic control during pregnancy in women with type 1 diabetes mellitus? Diabetologia 2006;49:25–28
36. Jovanovic L. Continuous glucose monitoring during pregnancy complicated by gestational diabetes mellitus. Curr Diab Rep 2001;1(1):82–85
37. Yogev Y, Ben-Haroush A, Chen R, et al. Continuous glucose monitoring for treatment adjustment in diabetic pregnancies - a pilot study. Diabet Med 2003;20:558–562
38. Mastrototaro JJ. The MiniMed continuous glucose monitoring system. Diabetes Technol Ther 2000;2(Suppl):S13–S18
39. Jovanovic L. The role of continuous glucose monitoring in gestational diabetes mellitus. Diabetes Technol Ther 2000;2 (Suppl 1):S67–S71
40. Yogev Y, Chen R, Ben-Haroush A, et al. Continuous glucose monitoring for the evaluation of gravid women with type 1 diabetes mellitus. Obstet Gynecol 2003;101:633–638
41. Chen R, Yogev Y, Ben-Haroush A, et al. Continuous glucose monitoring for the evaluation and improved control of gestational diabetes mellitus. J Matern Fetal Neonatal Med 2003;14:256–260
42. Klonoff DC. Continuous glucose monitoring. Roadmap for 21st century diabetes therapy. Diabetes Care 2005;28:1231–1239
43. Yogev Y, Ben-Haroush A, Chen R, et al. Diurnal glycemic profile in obese and normal weight nondiabetic pregnant women. Am J Obstet Gynecol 2004;191:949–953
44. Ben-Haroush A, Yogev Y, Chen R, et al. The postprandial glucose profile in the diabetic pregnancy. Am J Obstet Gynecol 2004;191:576–581
45. Bühling KJ, Winkel T, Wolf C, et al. Optimal timing for postprandial glucose measurement in pregnant women with diabetes and a non-diabetic pregnant population evaluated by the continuous glucose monitoring system (CGMS). J Perinat Med 2005;33:125–131
46. Jungheim K, Koschinsky T. Glucose monitoring at the arm: risky delays of hypoglycemia and hyperglycemia detection. Diabetes Care 2002;25:956–960
47. Ellison JM, Stegmann JM, Colner SL, et al. Rapid changes in postprandial blood glucose produce concentration differences at finger, forearm, and thigh sampling sites. Diabetes Care 2002;25:961–964
48. Bina DM, Anderson RL, Johnson ML, et al. Clinical impact of prandial state, exercise, and site preparation on the equivalence of alternative-site blood glucose testing. Diabetes Care 2003;26:981–985
49. Avignon A, Radauceanu A,, Monnier L Nonfasting plasma glucose is a better marker of diabetic control than fasting plasma glucose in type 2 diabetes. Diabetes Care 1997;20:1822–1826
50. Monnier L. Is postprandial glucose a neglected cardiovascular risk factor in type 2 diabetes? Eur J Clin Invest 2000;30 (Suppl 2):3–11
51. Avignon A, Monnier L. Specific effect of postprandial glycemic peaks on HBA1C and angiopathy. Diabetes Metab 2000;26(Suppl 2):12–15
52. Ceriello A, Davidson J, Hanefeld M, et al. Postprandial hyperglycaemia and cardiovascular complications of diabetes: an update. Nutr Metab Cardiovasc Dis 2006;16:453–456
53. Jovanovic R, Jovanovic L. Obstetric management when normoglycemia is maintained in diabetic pregnant women with vascular compromise. Am J Obstet Gynecol 1984;149:617
54. Rendell MS, Jovanovic L. Targeting postprandial hyperglycemia. Metabolism 2006 Sep;55:1263–1281
55. Combs CA, Gunderson E, Kitzmiller JL, et al. Relationship of fetal macrosomia to maternal postprandial glucose control during pregnancy. Diabetes Care 1992;15:1251–1257
56. De Veciana M, Major CA, Morgan MA, et al. Postprandial versus preprandial blood glucose monitoring in women with gestational diabetes mellitus requiring insulin therapy. N Engl J Med 1995;333:1237–1241
57. Jovanovic L. The importance of postprandial glucose concentration: lessons learned from diabetes and pregnancy. Drug Dev Res 2006;67:591–594

58. Manderson JG, Patterson CC, Hadden DR, et al. Preprandial versus postprandial blood glucose monitoring in type 1 diabetic pregnancy: a randomized controlled clinical trial. Am J Obstet Gynecol 2003;189:507–512

59. Miodovnik M, Skillman C, Holroyde JC, et al. Elevated maternal glycohemoglobin in early pregnancy and spontaneous abortion among insulin-dependent diabetic women. Am J Obstet Gynecol 1985;153:439–442

60. Ylinen K, Aula P, Stenman UH, et al. Risk of minor and major fetal malformations in diabetics with high haemoglobin A1C values in early pregnancy. Br Med J (Clin Res Ed) 1984;289:345–346

61. Wender-Ozeqowska E, Wroblewska K, Zawiejska A, et al. Threshold values of maternal blood glucose in early diabetic pregnancy-prediction of fetal malformations. Acta Obstet Gynecol Scand 2005;84:17–25

62. Khaliq A, Foreman D, Ahmed A, et al. Increased expression of placenta growth factor in proliferative diabetic retinopathy. Lab Invest 1998;78:109–116

63. Miller JM, Crenshaw MC Jr, Welt SI. Hemoglobin A1C in normal and diabetic pregnancy. JAMA 1979;242:2785–2787

64. Lurie S, Mamet Y. Red blood cell survival and kinetics during pregnancy. Euro J Obstet Gynecol Reprod Biol 2000;93:185–192

65. Mosca A, Paleari A, Dalfra M, et al. Reference intervals for hemoglobin A1C in pregnant women: data from an Italian multi-center study. Clin Chem 2006;52:1128–1143

66. O'Kane MJ, Lynch PLM, Moles KW, Magee SE. Determination of a diabetes control and complications trial-aligned HbA1C reference range in pregnancy. Clin Chim Acta 2001;311:157–159

67. Fong DS, Aiello LP, Gardner TW, et al. Retinopathy in diabetes. Diabetes Care 2004a;27(Suppl 1):S84–S87

68. Fong DS, Aiello LP, Ferris FL III, Klein R. Diabetic retinopathy. Diabetes Care 2004b;27:2540–2553

69. Desalvo J, Conn G, Trivedi PG, et al. Purification and characterization of a naturally occurring vascular endothelial growth factor – placenta growth factor heterodimer. J Biol Chem 1995;270:7717–7723

70. Lauszus FF, Klebe JG, Bek T, Flyvbjerg A. Increased serum IGF-1 during pregnancy is associated with progression of diabetic retinopathy. Diabetes 2003;52:852–856

71. Chantelau E. Evidence that upregulation of serum IGF-1 concentration can trigger acceleration of diabetic retinopathy. Br J Ophthalmol 1998;812:725–730

72. Loukovaara S, Immonen IJ, Koistenen R, Rutanen EM, Hiilesmaa V, Loukoaara M, et al. The insulin-like growth factor system and type 1 diabetic retinopathy during pregnancy. J Diabetes Complications 2005;19:297–304

73. Larinkari J, Laatikainen L, Ranta T, et al. Metabolic control and serum hormone levels in relation to retinopathy in diabetic pregnancy. Diabetologia 1982;22:327–332

74. Loukovaara S, Immonen I, Koistinen R, et al. Inflammatory markers and retinopathy in pregnancies complicated with type I diabetes. Eye 2005;19:422–430

75. Early worsening of diabetic retinopathy in the diabetes control and complications trial. Arch Ophthalmol 1998;116:874–876

76. Rahman W, Rahman FZ, Yassin S, et al. Progression of retinopathy during pregnancy in type 1 diabetes mellitus. Clin Experiment Ophthalmol 2007;35:231–236

77. Axer-Siegel R, Hod M, Fink-Cohen S, et al. Diabetic retinopathy during pregnancy. Ophthalmology 1996;103:1815–1819

78. Lovestam-Adrian M, Agardh C-D, Aberg A, Agardh E. Pre-eclampsia is a potent risk factor for deterioration of retinopathy during pregnancy in type 1 diabetic patients. Diabet Med 1997;14:1059–1065

79. Chew EY, Mills JL, Metzger BE, et al. Metabolic control and progression of retinopathy. The Diabetes in Early Pregnancy Study. National Institute of Child Health and Human Development Diabetes in Early Pregnancy Study. Diabetes Care 1995;18:631–637

80. Temple RC, Aldridge VA, Sampson MJ, et al. Impact of pregnancy on the progression of diabetic retinopathy in type 1 diabetes. Diabet Med 2001;18:573–577

81. Chantelau E, Kohner EM. Why some cases of retinopathy worsen when diabetic control improves. BMJ 1997;315:1105–1106

82. Henricsson M, Nilsson A, Janzon L, Groop L. The effect of glycaemic control and the introduction of insulin therapy on retinopathy in non-insulin-dependent diabetes mellitus. Diabet Med 1997;14:123–131

83. Laatikainen L, Teramo K, Hieta-Heikurainen H, et al. A controlled study of the influence of continuous subcutaneous insulin infusion treatment on diabetic retinopathy during pregnancy. Acta Med Scand 1987;221:367–376

84. Rosenn BM, Miodovnik M. Medical complications of diabetes mellitus in pregnancy. Clin Obstet Gynecol 2000;43:17–31

85. Dinn RB, Harris A, Marcus PS. Ocular changes in pregnancy. Obstet Gynecol Surv 2003;58:137–144

86. Moss SE, Klein R, Klein BE. Factors associated with having eye examinations in persons with diabetes. Arch Fam Med 1995;4:529–534

87. Kohner EM, Hamilton AM, Tunbridge WM. Diabetic retinopathy managed through a pregnancy. Proc R Soc Med 1973;66:442–444

88. Andersen AR, Christeansen JS, Andersen JK, et al. Diabetic nephropathy in type 1 (insulin-dependent) diabetes: an epidemiological study. Diabetologia 1983;25:496–501

89. Kitzmiller JL, Brown ER, Phillippe M, et al. Diabetic nephropathy and perinatal outcome. Am J Obstet Gynecol 1981;141:741–751

90. Reece EA, Coustan DR, Hayslett JP, et al. Diabetic nephropathy: pregnancy performance and fetomaternal outcome. Am J Obstet Gynecol 1988;159:56–66

91. Khoury JC, Miodovnik M, LeMasters G, Sibai BM. Pregnancy outcome and progression of diabetic nephropathy. What's next? J Matern Fetal Neonatal Med 2002;11:238–244

92. Holley JL, Bernardini J, Quadri KH, et al. Pregnancy outcomes in a prospective matched control of pregnancy and renal disease. Clin Nephrol 1996;45:77–82

93. Rosenn B, Miodovnik M, Combs CA, Khoury J, Siddiqi TA. Preconception management of insulin-dependent diabetes: improvement of pregnancy outcome. Obstet Gynecol 1991;77:846–849

94. Miodovnik M, Rosenn BM, Khoury JC, et al. Does pregnancy increase the risk for development and progression of diabetic nephropathy? Am J Obstet Gynecol 1996;174:1180–1191

95. Rossing K, Jacobsen P, Hommel E, et al. Pregnancy and progression of diabetic nephropathy. Diabetologia 2002;45:36–41

96. Biesenbach G, Stoger H, Zazgornik J. Influence of pregnancy on progression of diabetic nephropathy and subsequent requirement of renal replacement therapy in female type 1 diabetic patients with impaired renal function. Nephrol Dial Transplant 1992;7:105–109

97. Purdy L, Hantsch C, Molitch ME, et al. Effect of pregnancy on renal function in patients with moderate-to-severe diabetic renal insufficiency. Diabetes Care 1996;19:1067–1074

98. Reece EA, Leguizamon G, Homko C. Stringent controls in diabetic nephropathy associated with optimization of pregnancy outcomes. J Matern Fetal Med 1998;7:213–216

99. Leguizamon G, Reece EA. Effect of medical therapy on progressive nephropathy: influence of pregnancy, diabetes and hypertension. J Matern Fetal Med 2000;9:70–80

100. Neilsen LR, Muller C, Damm, P, Mathiesen ER. Reduced prevalence of early preterm delivery in women with type 1 diabetes and microalbuminuria-possible effect of early antihypertensive treatment during pregnancy. Diabet Med 2006;23:426–431

101. McCance DR, Traub AI, Harley JMG, et al. Urinary albumin excretion in diabetic pregnancy. Diabetologia 1989;32:236–239

102. Sibai BM, Chames J. Hypertension in pregnancy: tailoring treatment to risk. OBG Management 2003;15:58–68

103. Cooper WO, Hernandez-Diaz S, Abrogast PG, et al. Major congenital malformations after first-trimester exposure to ACE inhibitors. N Engl J Med 2006;354:2443–2451

104. Quan A. Fetopathy associated with exposure to angiotensin converting enzyme inhibitors and angiotensin receptor antagonists. Early Hum Dev 2006;82:23–28

105. Alwan S, Polifka JE, Friedman JM. Angiotensin II receptor antagonist treatment during pregnancy. Birth Defects Res A Clin Mol Teratol 2005;73:123–130

106. Cockburn J, Moar VA, Ounsted M, Redman CW. Final report of study on hypertension during pregnancy: the effects of specific treatment on the growth and development of the children. Lancet 1982;1(18273):647–649

107. Knopp RH, Bergelin RO, Wahl PW, Walden CD, Chapman M, Irvine S. Population-based lipoprotein lipid reference values for pregnant women compared to nonpregnant women classified by sex hormone usage. Am J Obstet Gynecol 1982;143:626–637

108. American Academy of Pediatrics Committee on Drugs. The transfer of drugs and other chemicals into human milk. Pediatrics 2001;108:776–789

109. Lapolla A, Cardone C, Negrin P, et al. Pregnancy does not induce or worsen retinal and peripheral nerve dysfunction in insulin-dependent diabetic women. J Diabetes Complications 1998;12:74–80

110. Stellato TA, Danziger LH, Burkons D. Fetal salvage with maternal total parenteral nutrition: the pregnant mother as her own control. JPEN J Parenter Enteral Nutr 1988;23:412–413

111. Macleod AF, Smith SA, Sonksen PH, Lowy C. The problem of autonomic neuropathy in diabetic pregnancy. Diabet med 1990;7:80–82

112. Maschi S, Clavenna A, Campi R, et al. Neonatal outcome following pregnancy exposure to antidepressants: a prospective controlled cohort study. BJOG 2008;115:283–289

113. Montouris G. Gabapentin exposure in human pregnancy: results from the gabapentin pregnancy registry. Epilepsy Behav 2003;4:310–317

114. Kjaer D, Horvath-Puho E, Christensen J, et al. Antiepileptic drug use, folic acid supplementation, and congenital abnormalities: a population-based case-control study. BJOG 2008;115:98–103

115. Larsson A, Palm M, Hansson L-O, Axelsson O. Reference values for clinical chemistry tests during normal pregnancy. BJOG 2008;115:874–881

116. Lippi G, Albiero A, Montagnana M, Salvagno GL, Scevarolli S, Franchi M, Guidi GC. Lipid and lipoprotein profile in physiological pregnancy. Clin Lab 2007;53:173–177

117. Nies BM, Dreiss RJ. Hyperlipidemic pancreatitis in pregnancy: a case report and review of the literature. Am J Perinatol 1990;7:166–169

118. Yamauchi H, Sunamura M, Takeda K, Suzuki T, Itoh K, Miyagawa K. Hyperlipidemia and pregnancy associated pancreatitis with reference to plasma exchange as a therapeutic intervention. Tohoku J Exp Med 1986;148:197–205

119. Brunzell JD, Davidson M, Furberg CD, Goldberg RB, Howard BV, Stein JH, Witztum JL. Lipoprotein management in patients with cardiometabolic risk: consensus statement from the American Diabetes Association and the American college of Cardiology Foundation. Diabetes Care 2008;31:811–822

120. National Cholesterol Education Program expert Panel on Detection, Evaluation and Treatment of High Blood Cholesterol in Adults. Executive summary of the Third Report of the National Cholesterol Education Program (NCEP) Expert Panel on detection, evaluation, and treatment of high blood cholesterol in adults (Adult Treatment Panel III). JAMA 2001;285:2486–2497

121. Hollingsworth DR, Moore TR. Postprandial walking exercise in pregnant insulin-dependent (type 1) diabetic women: reduction of plasma lipid levels but absence of a significant effect on glycemic control. Am J Obstet Gynecol 1987;157:1359–1363

122. Goldberg RB, Jacobson TA. Effects of niacin on glucose control in patients with dyslipidemia. Mayo Clin Proc 2008;83:470–478

123. Aoki Y, Belin RM, Clickner R, Jeffries R, Philips L, Mahaffey KR. Serum TSH and total T4 in the United States population and their association with participant characteristics: National health and Nutrition Examination Survey (NHANES 1999–2002). Thyroid 2007;17:1211–1223

124. Abalovich, M, Amino N, Barbour LA et al. Clinical Practice Guideline - Management of thyroid dysfunction during pregnancy and postpartum: an Endocrine Society clinical practice guideline. J Clin Endocrinol Metab 2007;92:S1–S47

125. Chauhan SP, Perry KG Jr, McLaughlin BN, Roberts WE, Sullivan CA, Morrison JC. Diabetic ketoacidosis complicating pregnancy. J Perinatol 1996;16:173–175

126. Schneider MG, Umpierrez GE, Ramsey RD, Mabie WC, Bennett KA. Pregnancy complicated by diabetic ketoacidosis maternal and fetal outcomes. Diabetes Care 2003;26:958–959

127. Bernstein IM, Catalano PM. Ketoacidosis in pregnancy associated with the parenteral administration of terbutaline and betamethasone. A case report. J Reprod Med 1990;35:818–820

128. Cullen MT, Reece EA, Homko CJ, Sivan E. The changing presentations of diabetic ketoacidosis during pregnancy. Am J Perinatol 1996;13:449–451

129. Carroll ML, Yeomans ER. Diabetic ketoacidosis in pregnancy. Crit Care Med 2005;33:S347

130. Montoro MN, Myers VP, Mestman JH, Xu Y, Anderson BG, Golde SH. Outcome of pregnancy in diabetic ketoacidosis. Am J Perinatol 1992;10:17–20

18

Use of Ultrasound in the Metabolic Management of Gestational Diabetes and Preexisting Diabetes Mellitus in Pregnancy

Schaefer-Graf UM

CONTENTS

ABSTRACT

While in former times pregnancies of women with diabetes often ended unhappily with either intrauterine death or severe postnatal problems for the child, current improved methods of glucose control and fetal surveillance provide the chance of a healthy baby for this high risk group of pregnant women. Management of pregnancies with diabetes has been solely focused on the achievement of very tight glucose control to avoid the negative consequences of maternal hyperglycemia for the fetus, as there is evidence that the development of diabetic fetopathy is linked to maternal glucose values. This has been clearly demonstrated in pregnancies of women with preexisting diabetes with severe hyperglycemia. While in women with gestational diabetes (GDM) who develop only moderate hyperglycemia due to the decreased insulin sensitivity in pregnancy, maternal glucose values seem to be of limited use to identify pregnancies with risk for the fetus. Thus, strategies had been evaluated to include further parameters to target pregnancies with need for intensive metabolic intervention. The first approach, measurement of fetal insulin in amniotic fluid, has been limited due to the invasiveness of amniocentesis but measurement of the fetal abdominal circumference (AC) has become a widely accepted additional tool to guide pregnancies with GDM. Fetal hyperinsulinism leads to accelerated growth primarily of the subcutaneous fat layer of abdomen; excessive growth is the major problem in diabetic pregnancies. Level Ia evidence from four randomized intervention trials supports that metabolic management including fetal ultrasound measurements reduces somatic growth disturbances in diabetic pregnancies.

From: *Diabetes in Women: Pathophysiology and Therapy*
Edited by: A. Tsatsoulis et al. (eds.), DOI 10.1007/978-1-60327-250-6_18
© Humana Press, a part of Springer Science+Business Media, LLC 2009

Key words: Gestational diabetes; Preexisting diabetes;, Pregnancy; Glycemic control; Metabolic therapy; Fetal growth; Ultrasound.

INTRODUCTION

Gestational diabetes (GDM) is defined as glucose intolerance that is first diagnosed in pregnancy. This definition covers a wide spectrum in the degree of glucose intolerance including the possibility of undiagnosed preexisting type 2 diabetes (DM2). GDM is one of the most common disorders in pregnancy. The prevalence varies depending on the ethnic background of the population and the diagnostic strategies and criteria applied. In Caucasians the prevalence is 3–7%, while the frequency of GDM may be up to 20% in populations with a high prevalence of insulin resistance and DM2 as found in Pima Indians and Mexican Americans. Preexisting diabetes complicates about 0.7–1.0% of all pregnancies. Diabetes in pregnancy is associated with neonatal problems such as macrosomia, neonatal hypoglycemia, respiratory problems and hyperbilirubinemia as well as a long-term increased risk of diabetes and obesity for the offspring. Increasing evidence suggests that a disturbed intrauterine metabolic environment produces these short- and long-term complications. Hyperplasia of pancreatic β cells followed by apoptosis *(1)* and dysfunction as well as neuroendocrine disturbances seem to be involved in the predisposition for obesity *(2)*. Being born either small-for-gestational age (SGA) *(3)* or large-for-gestational-age (LGA) *(4–6)* further increases the risk of childhood and adult obesity and metabolic diseases. The obesity rate in children with LGA birth weight approached 40%, while only 19% of the children with birth weight <50th percentile were obese at about age 6 in a study in children from GDM mothers *(4)*. Therefore, normalization of fetal growth is a major goal in the treatment of diabetes in pregnancy.

There is evidence that in diabetic pregnancies increasing maternal hyperglycemia is associated with an increased risk of clinically important morbidity in the offspring. This has been demonstrated impressively in studies in women with preexisting diabetes whose infants are at increased risk for congenital malformation, severe perinatal morbidity and intrauterine death in proportion to the extent of maternal hyperglycemia. Therefore, current therapy of diabetes in pregnancy focuses on tightly controlling maternal glucose levels to achieve "normal" glucose values. This traditional treatment strategy having been successfully applied in pregestational diabetes was then transferred to women with GDM resulting in insulin therapy in up to 50% of women with GDM.

Intensive therapy has lowered the perinatal morbidity in women with GDM; however, the rate of macrosomia and C-sections remains increased despite strict glucose control. Some approaches emphasize universally stricter glucose control aiming for a mean glucose level <90 mg/dl to lower the rate of macrosomia and C-sections. The downside is that this strategy requires insulin therapy accompanied with daily glucose profiles in 50–80% of the patients with GDM *(7, 8)*, and overly aggressive treatment may result in an increased rate of growth-restricted newborns.

In contrast to women with pregestational diabetes not all women with GDM appear to be at risk for accelerated fetal growth and neonatal morbidity *(9)* and, therefore, may not benefit from intensive intervention and surveillance. This chapter reviews one aspect of research aimed at improving current metabolic therapy of diabetes in pregnancy by trying to target women with the need for intensive intervention by investigating the predictive markers that can identify diabetic pregnancies that are at risk for accelerated fetal growth. Two predictive markers are amniotic fluid insulin, which requires an invasive amniocentesis procedure, and measurement of fetal abdominal circumference (AC) early in the third trimester, which has been successfully used to reduce rates of growth disorders and neonatal complications. These fetal-based strategies have been best investigated in pregnancies with GDM but may also be useful in the guidance of the metabolic management in pregnancies with preexisting diabetes.

Features of Fetal Growth in Diabetic Pregnancies

Diabetes-associated accelerated growth, starting in early third trimester when fetal adipocyte proliferation and fetal storage occurs, is the most common problem in pregnancies with diabetes. In the second trimester, the growth of noninsulin-sensitive tissues, e.g., bones, accounts for the main difference in the fetal growth pattern. It has been shown that in this period a previous history of delivery of a macrosomic newborn appears to be the major determinant of growth expressing the strong influence of genetic factors *(10)*, while in the third trimester variation of growth is determined to a greater extent by nutritional supply. Maternal hyperglycemia leads via transport by the placenta to fetal hyperglycemia and consequently to hyperinsulinism (Pedersen hypothesis) *(11)*. Insulin is the strongest growth factor for insulin-sensitive tissue. Thus, a fetus with hyperinsulinism is characterized by asymmetric excessive growth mainly of the AC due to increased subcutaneous fat layers (Fig. 1) and liver size. Diabetic macrosomia (Fig. 2) with disproportion of head and trunk explains the high rate of shoulder dystocia and Erb's palsy, which is an unfortunate complication of deliveries of women with diabetes. Hyperinsulinism also explains other frequent neonatal complications associated with diabetic fetopathy like respiratory distress, hyperbilirubinemia and hypocalcemia.

Long-term observations show a relation between the levels of fetal hyperinsulinism and a predisposition for obesity and diabetes in infants of mothers with GDM or preexisting diabetes *(12, 13)*.

MANAGEMENT OF GDM BASED ON MATERNAL GLUCOSE CONTROL COMBINED WITH FETAL GROWTH

In spring 2004, an advocate of strict metabolic control, Lois Jovanovic (see Chap. 17), suggested in an editorial in Diabetes Care ("Never Say Never in Medicine – Confessions of an Old Dog") *(14)* that there is more and more evidence that successful management of GDM might need more than

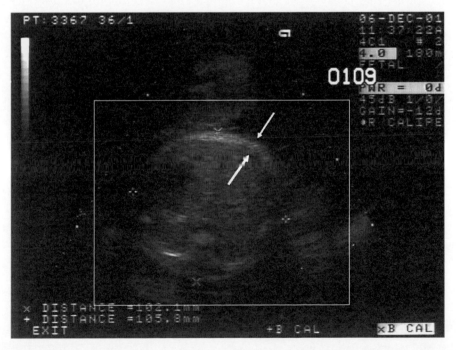

Fig. 1. Fetal abdominal circumference measurement in the third trimester and thickness of subcutaneous fat measured at the ventral abdominal wall.

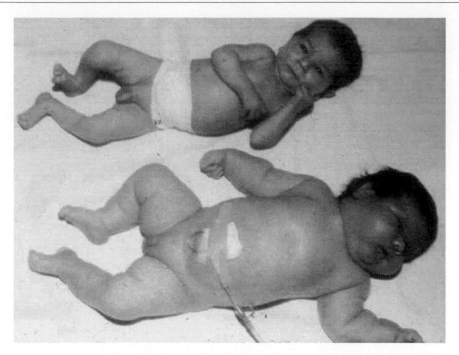

Fig. 2. In front Newborn with diabetes-associated macrosomia.

tight glucose control: "I have religiously clung to the notion that maternal hyperglycemia is the root of all evil in pregnancies complicated by diabetes." What persuaded her to question her opinion and the approach she had practiced for decades?

As mentioned earlier there is evidence that rising maternal glycemia implicates a risk for diabetes-related morbidity for the offspring not only in preexisting diabetes but also in GDM. Blinded evaluation of maternal glucose values has demonstrated a slow and continuous increase in complications, mainly macrosomia and C-section, in the prediabetic glucose range *(15)*. However, while there might be a definable glucose threshold for an increased risk of congenital abnormalities *(16, 17)*, there does not seem to be a clear threshold for macrosomia or other neonatal complications that are the major concerns in GDM. Maternal glucose and excessive growth do not correlate in a linear fashion, and the development of macrosomia seems to be only partly determined by the maternal glucose value *(10, 18)*. Furthermore, because of variations of placental transport and the placenta's own glucose consumption there is a wide range of individual variation to the extent that glucose is transferred from the mother to the fetus. Additionally, Weiss has shown that in pregnancies with fetal hyperinsulinism, glucose transport can be increased, and so maternal hyperglycemia may be masked *(19)*. And last but not least, there is an individual response of each fetus to increased glucose supply shown impressively in twin studies *(20)*. Thus, it is questionable if maternal glycemia by itself can be reliably used for risk assessment in later pregnancy.

The Weiss Concept: Management of Diabetes Based on Maternal Glucose Combined with Amniotic Fluid Insulin

Taking into account all these uncertainties, Weiss had already begun, in the eighties, to implement the first fetal-based strategy of GDM management to target women who would benefit from intensive treatment. Tight glucose control with intensified insulin therapy was limited to pregnancies with fetal hyperinsulinism diagnosed by determination of amniotic fluid insulin *(21)*, which reflects urinary excretion of fetal insulin *(22)*. On the basis of his data it was found that only about 20% of the fetuses have some evidence of fetal hyperinsulinism (insulin levels >90th percentile) *(23)*, and diabetic fetopathy was only seen when third trimester amniotic fluid was above 17 µU/ml. The level of amniotic fluid insulin was also used to adjust the insulin dosage in women with preexisting diabetes resulting in serial amniocentesis in some women. Although the Weiss approach was impressive because of the direct access to the fetus it has not been widely adopted in clinical practice because it requires an invasive and expensive diagnostic strategy.

Management of GDM Based on Maternal Glucose Control Combined with Fetal Growth

The group of Buchanan and Kjos from Los Angeles picked up Weiss' concept of a fetal-based GDM management and investigated if the fetal AC in the third trimester could serve as a noninvasive method to target GDM pregnancies that need intensive treatment. This fetal-growth based strategy uses the diabetes-specific growth pattern of accelerated growth of the abdomen. This is mainly due to increased subcutaneous fat, which determines 63% of the variation of the fetal AC *(24)*. While the measurement of amniotic fluid insulin has a firm pathophysiologic basis, the AC measurement is an indirect approach based on a clinical manifestation of fetal hyperinsulinism. However, studies in type 1 as well as in GDM pregnancies showed a significant association of amniotic fluid insulin and the fetal AC. The AC fails to identify a fetus with moderately elevated amniotic fluid insulin but an AC threshold of the 75th percentile seems to be useful to reliably detect severe hyperinsulinism at a degree that corresponds closely to levels reported by other researchers to be associated with short- and long-term morbidity *(25)* (Fig. 3). The strength of the fetal AC is the exclusion (NPV 100%) or the high sensitivity (100%), respectively, while the low positive predictive value (21.3%) and specificity (66.6%) imply the risk of overtreatment.

The initial study was limited to women with plasma fasting glucose values below 105 mg/dl at diagnosis who would not have qualified for intensive monitoring and insulin therapy if the institutional

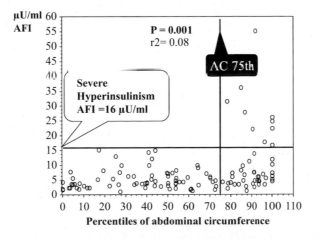

Fig. 3. Correlation of percentiles of the abdominal circumference (AC) according to gestational age and the level of amniotic fluid insulin (AF insulin) in pregnancies with preexisting or gestational diabetes. All cases of severe hyperinsulinism (AF insulin ≥16 µU/ml) were associated with an AC ≥75th percentile (adapted from 25).

criteria had been applied. Ultrasound examination with measurement of the fetal AC was performed between 29 and 33 weeks of gestation for further risk assessment (26). A threshold of the 70th percentile was used to discriminate between low and high risks for neonatal macrosomia. It demonstrated that in women with a fetal AC >70th percentile at entry to diabetes care, who had been randomized to home glucose monitoring and intensive insulin therapy, the macrosomia rate could be almost normalized (13%) in contrast to the diet-only group with a macrosomia rate of 45% (26). Thus, the fetal AC correctly identified the minority of women in this low-risk population based on maternal glycemia who would benefit from intensive treatment to avoid neonatal morbidity.

In contrast to this first report, a later study concentrated on identification of women who are at low risk in a population otherwise considered as at high risk because of fasting glucose values ≥105 mg/dl (27). Women with severe hyperglycemia at entry were excluded (fasting glucose >120 mg/dl, 2-h postprandial >200 mg/dl). In this study measurement of fetal AC was performed at entry and thereafter at 4-week intervals. Insulin was only administered when AC ≥75th percentile or if severe hyperglycemia, defined earlier, occurred in later course of pregnancy. Insulin therapy could be avoided in 33% of the women randomized to the fetal growth-based arm without adverse outcome than in the glycemia-only group with insulin treatment in all women (27). Thus, the fetal AC was an effective parameter for use in identifying pregnancies at low risk in this setting of GDM management, which was based predominately on fetal growth combined with high glycemic goals.

Both of the previous pilot studies had been performed in a population of predominately Mexican-American origin who are characterized by a high rate of insulin resistance and obesity. In a third step, the approach was tested for safety and effectiveness in a population of Caucasians in Northern Europe (28). Additionally the design was modified by avoiding preselection in order to simplify transfer to clinical practice. All women with GDM and fasting glucose values <120 mg/dl and 2-h postprandial values <200 mg/dl in the first profile after 1 week trial of diet were included. According to the prior study in women randomized to the ultrasound group, insulin was only administered when AC >75th percentile at entry or at follow-up, or if the glucose thresholds for severe hyperglycemia were exceeded. In the standard arm, insulin was given based on the recommended glycemia criteria (29). All LGA infants except one were born to mothers on diet only. Similar to the pilot study, the approach was revealed to be safe. There was no adverse outcome in the ultrasound group compared with the standard group in which the glycemia-only strategy had been applied. The fetal growth-based approach resulted in a different treatment assignment for 42% of the women if the maternal glycemia-only strategy had been applied. When subgroups were analyzed, there were three times as many infants with LGA (22%) or delivery by C-section (25%) in the women of the standard group who were not treated with insulin based on maternal glucose values although the fetal AC was >75th percentile. In addition, there were twice as many SGA infants (35.3%) in the standard group when insulin was applied because of maternal hyperglycemia despite normal fetal growth (Table 1). This point might have motivated Lois Jovanovic to reflect upon the strategy of tight glucose control without further risk assessment. Although there had been evidence from prior studies that there is an increased prevalence of SGA infants in programs of tight control – a 20% rate in a study from Langer in the group with mean glucose <86 mg/dl - diabetes care in pregnancy has been so focused on the avoidance of accelerated growth that concern about SGA has been neglected. Similar to excessive growth, growth retardation is known to be associated with a risk of subsequent hypertension and type 2 diabetes (3). Moderate maternal hyperglycemia might be essential in some women to assure the nutritional supply to the fetus, analogous to maternal pregnancy-induced hypertension compensating for disturbed placental vasculature.

Table 1

Outcome of GDM Pregnancies Managed Either Identically or Differentially Based on the Occurrence of Maternal Hyperglycemia and a Fetal Abdominal Circumference >75th Percentile Before 36 Completed Weeks of Gestation

	Maternal hyperglycemia meeting criteria for insulin therapy in ST-group				
	No			Yes	
AC always <75th percentile during study	**A** No insulin in both groups N = 75 (ST = 38, US = 37)			**B** ST-group n = 17 Insulin	US-group n = 18 No insulin
	LGA		2.7%	LGA 5.9%	5.9%
	SGA		20.0%	SGA 35.3%	16.6%
	Hypoglycemia		18.7%	Hypoglycemia 11.8%	11.8%
	NICU		17.3%	NICU 5.9%	5.9%
	Cesarean		14.7%	Cesarean 17.6%	23.5%
AC ever >75th percentile during study	**C**	ST-group n = 32 No insulin	US-group n = 13 Insulin	**D** Insulin in both groups N = 33 (ST = 10, US = 23)	
	LGA	21.9%	8.3%	LGA	26.1%
	SGA	0%	0%	SGA	4.3%
	Hypoglycemia	15.6%	8.3%	Hypo glycemia	18.2%
	NICU	12.5%	8.3%	NICU	24.2%
	Cesarean	25.0%	8.3%	Cesarean	24.2%

In the ST-group hyperglycemia prompted insulin therapy and in the US-Group an AC >75th Percentile. All *p* values for panels B and C >0.05 (adapted from 28)

The maternal glycemic values defined in the studies as severe hyperglycemia prompting insulin therapy independent of fetal growth might be difficult to accept in a clinical setting considering liability and safety aspects. However, a recent study adopting this approach demonstrated that even minor adjustments of glycemic goals dependent on the fetal AC might be useful to concentrate on intensive intervention and to improve the outcome. Glucose targets were fasting values of 80 mg/dl and 1-h postprandial of 120 mg/dl if AC ≥75th percentile or 100/140 mg/dl if AC <75th percentile, respectively *(30)*. Ultrasound was performed every 2 weeks. LGA, macrosomia, and SGA rates were all significantly lower in the group with the adjusted glycemic goals.

The studies evaluating the fetal growth-based approach in GDM generated promising data that more individualized glycemic control is justified when fetal assessment is involved to target pregnancies for intensive intervention. Combining the results from the four existing studies, a total of 484 pregnancies demonstrated that with the modified fetal growth-based approach the LGA rate can be significantly reduced to 8.1% compared with 16.7% (*p* = 0.0017) with the conventional approach solely on maternal glycemia-based strategy (OR 0.44, CI 0.25–0.77) *(31)*. Growth retardation is not as frequent as accelerated growth in GDM pregnancies, thus the number of SGA newborns in the studies were too low to reach a significant difference in the rate of SGA newborns although a reduction of SGA by the modified approach was suggested (11.2 vs. 6.9%, *p* = 0.087; OR 0.59, CI 0.30–1.13).

Figure 4 summarizes the clinical approach of a modified treatment of GDM based on serial ultrasound measurements of the fetal AC.

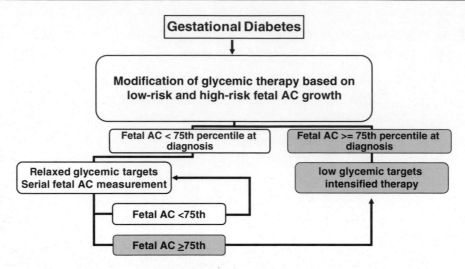

Fig. 4. Flowchart of modified treatment of gestational diabetes (GDM) based on serial ultrasound measurements of the fetal AC [Adapted from *(31)*].

Management of Preexisting Diabetes Based on Maternal Glucose Control Combined with Fetal Growth

In women with preexisting diabetes, ultrasound is considered essential for the detection of congenital malformations. In early pregnancy, maternal hyperglycemia is associated with a high frequency of congenital anomalies. This is a major concern in pregnancies with preexisting diabetes, while in GDM maternal hyperglycemia normally occurs after organogenesis is complete. However, in women with fasting glucose values at diagnosis above 120 mg/dl there is obviously an increased risk of congenital anomalies *(17)*. Maternal obesity in the general population *(32)* as well as in women with GDM per se is known to be associated with an increased risk for multiple anomalies, including neural tube and heart defects. To what extent this high rate of anomalies is caused by undiagnosed type 2 diabetes or at least borderline glucose intolerance before pregnancy can be only speculated, since preconception testing in women with high risk for diabetes is not routinely performed. However, an ultrasound examination at about 20 weeks of gestation performed by highly qualified staff is required in all women with preexisting diabetes and in women with GDM after diagnosis if fasting hyperglycemia is >120 mg/dl.

So far there are no published studies that investigate if protocols incorporating fetal AC or another growth parameter could lower the frequency of growth disturbances in pregnancies with preexisting diabetes. The need for insulin therapy is obvious in women with type 1 or type 2 diabetes but the need to individualize glycemic targets can be debated. Analogous to GDM, in preexisting diabetes, if there are identical glucose targets in every women, then we are faced with the same problem that the same degree of hyperglycemia may have different effects on the fetus. In the absence of vascular diabetes-related complications or pregnancy-induced hypertension that might cause growth retardation by reduced placental flow, a fetal AC <10th percentile could be a sign of undernutrition of the fetus due to strict glucose control. In this case moderate relaxation of glucose control should be considered to prevent further impairment of growth and delivery of a SGA newborn. However, in another woman similar glucose profiles might be associated with a fetal AC in the upper normal or even above the range presumably due to an increased transfer of maternal glucose that caused hyperinsulinism-associated accelerated growth. In contrast to the previous case, in this woman the insulin dosage and diet should be critically reconsidered in search of an approach to lower maternal glucose levels. Testing of the reliability of the glucose meter should not be forgotten.

Level Ia evidence from four randomized intervention trials supports that metabolic management including fetal ultrasound measurements reduces somatic growth disturbances in pregnancies with GDM. This may be valid for pregnancies with preexisting diabetes as well. Further studies need to investigate if the inclusion of additional growth parameters, like the head–abdomen ratio or subcutaneous thickness at the abdominal wall or at the extremities of the fetus, would enhance the specificity of ultrasound parameters to guide therapy and improve discrimination between genetically vs. diabetes-mediated accelerated growth. Percentiles of measured subcutaneous fat at different sites of the body obtained in a population of women with normal glucose tolerance could serve as references (33). On the economic side, further studies should evaluate if the number of ultrasound examinations in GDM could be reduced without missing cases of macrosomia occurring later in pregnancy. The vast majority of fetal macrosomia was diagnosed with the first ultrasound at entry to diabetes care. So far, frequent follow-up examinations have been an essential part of the fetal-growth-based concept; in the study of Bonomo et al. ultrasound had been performed every 2 weeks. It appears that it is not necessarily the frequency but the gestational age of the first ultrasound that determines the success of the intervention. The benefit of early identification and intervention for accelerated growth was demonstrated in a randomized trial with randomization in early (28 plus 32 weeks) vs. late (32 weeks) evaluation of the fetal AC in diet-controlled GDM mothers. The rate of LGA was significantly lower in the group with early evaluation (34). This meets our observations from the last studies (27, 28) that intervention is less successful when macrosomia is already present at the time of diagnosis. This is also an argument for universal screening for GDM at 24 weeks of gestation, which is unfortunately not established in all countries. In Germany, governmental guidelines for prenatal care require an oral glucose tolerance test (OGTT) only in women with risk factors; macrosomia diagnosed with the third (and last) required ultrasound at 30–32 weeks is the most common reason for referral for glucose testing.

Further research on whether home-glucose monitoring could be reduced or even given up in GDM women with normal fetal growth may be warranted. In the existing studies the women in the US arm were asked to perform frequent glucose profiles throughout pregnancy but the values were not used to guide therapy, and none of the women in the latest study had to go on insulin therapy because of the development of severe hyperglycemia.

Research for over a decade showed that use of ultrasound in pregnancies with diabetes can do more than just evaluate for congenital anomalies, fetal growth and estimate fetal weight before delivery. Modified management using high-risk and low-risk AC growth evaluated by ultrasound allows the selection of pregnancies with the need for strict vs. relaxed maternal glucose control.

REFERENCES

1. Holemans K, Aerts L, Van Assche F: Lifetime consequences of abnormal fetal pancreatic development. *J Physiol* 547:11–20, 2003
2. Plagemann A, harder T, Rake A, Janert U, Melchior K, Rohde W, Dörner G: Malformation of hypothalamic nuclei in hyperinsulinaemic offspring of gestational diabetic mother rats. *Int J Dev Neurosci* 17:37–44, 1999
3. Barker D, Hales C, Fall C, Osmond C, Phipps K, Clark P: Type 2 diabetes mellitus, hypertension and hyperlipidaemia (syndrome X): relation to reduced fetal growth. *Diabetologia* 36:62–67, 1993
4. Schaefer-Graf U, Pawliczek J, Passow D, Hartmann R, Rossi R, Bührer C, Harder T, Plagemann A, Vetter K, Kordonouri O: Birth weight and parental BMI predict overweight in children from mothers with gestational diabetes. *Diabetes Care* 28:1745–1750, 2005

5. Vohr B, McGarvey S: Growth patterns of large-for-gestational-age and appropriate-for-gestational-age infants of gestational diabetes mothers and control mothers at 1 year. *Diabetes Care* 20(7):1066–1072, 1997

6. Harder T, Rodekamp E, Schellong K, Dudenhausen J, Plagemann A: Birth weight and subsequent risk of type 2 diabetes: a meta-analysis. *Am J Epidemiol* 165(8):849–857, 2007

7. Jovanovic-Peterson L, Bevier W, Peterson C: The Santa Barbara County Health Services Program: birth weight change concomitant with screening for and treatment of glucose-intolerance of pregnancy: a potential cost-effective intervention? *Am J Perinatol* 14:221–228, 1997

8. Langer O, Levy J, Brustmann L, Anyaegbunam A, Merkatz R, Divon M: Glycemic control in gestational diabetes mellitus – How tight is enough: small for gestational age versus large for gestational age. *Am J Obstet Gynecol* 161:646–653, 1989

9. Crowther C, Hiller J, Moss J, McPhee A, Jeffries W, Robinson J: Effect of treatment of gestational diabetes mellitus on pregnancy outcome. *N Engl J Med* 352:2477–2486, 2005

10. Schaefer-Graf U, Kjos S, Kilavuz Ö, Plagemann A, Brauer M, Dudenhausen J, Vetter K: Determinants of fetal growth at different periods of pregnancies complicated by gestational diabetes or impaired glucose tolerance. *Diabetes Care* 26:193–198, 2003

11. Pedersen J, Osler M: Hyperglycemia as the cause of characteristic features of the foetus and newborn in diabetic mothers. *Dan Med Bull* 8:78, 1961

12. Silverman B, Rizzo T, Cho N, Metzger B: Long-term effects of the intrauterine environment. The Northwestern University Diabetes in Pregnancy Center. *Diabetes Care* 21(Suppl2):142–149, 1998

13. Weiss P, Scholz H, Haas J, Tamussino K, Seissler J, Borkenstein M: Long-term follow-up of infants of mothers with type 1 diabetes: evidence for hereditary and nonhereditary transmission of diabetes and precursors. *Diabetes Care* 23:905–911, 2000

14. Jovanovic L: Never say never in medicine. *Diabetes Care* 27:610–612, 2004

15. Sermer M, Naylor DC, Investigators for the TTHGD: Impact of increasing carbohydrate intolerance on maternal-fetal outcomes in 3637 women without diabetes. *Am J Obstet Gynecol* 173:146–156, 1995

16. Rosenn B, Miodovnik M, Combs C, Khoury J, Siddiqi T: Glycemic thresholds for spontaneous abortion and congenital malformations in insulin-dependent diabetes mellitus. *Obstet Gynecol* 84:515–520, 1994

17. Schaefer UM, Songster G, Xiang A, Berkowitz K, Buchanan TA, Kjos SL: Congenital malformations in offspring of women with hyperglycemia first detected during pregnancy. *Am J Obstet Gynecol* 177:1165–1171, 1997

18. Schaefer-Graf U, Heuer R, Kilavuz Ö, Pandura A, Henrich W, Vetter K: Maternal obesity not maternal glucose values correlates best with high rates of fetal macrosomia in pregnancies complicated by gestational diabetes. *J Perinat Med* 30(4):313–321, 2002

19. Weiss P, Scholz H, Haas J, Tamussino K: Effect of fetal hyperinsulinism on oral glucose tolerance test results in patients with gestational diabetes mellitus. *Am J Obstet Gynecol* 184(3):470–475, 2001

20. Burke B, Sheriff R: Diabetic twins: an unequal result. *Lancet* 1:1372–1373, 1979

21. Weiss P, Hofmann H: Diagnosis and treatment of gestational diabetes according to amniotic fluid insulin levels. *Arch Gynecol* 239:81–91, 1986

22. Weiss P, Hofmann H: Monitoring pregnancy in diabetes: amniotic fluid. *Diabetes Nutr Metab* 3(Suppl. 2):31–35, 1990

23. Hofmann HM: Fructosamine in relation to maternofetal glucose and insulin homeostasis in gestational diabetes. *Arch Gynecol Obstet* 247:173–185, 1990

24. Kehl R, Krew M, Thomas A, Catalano P: Fetal growth and body composition in infants of women with diabetes mellitus during pregnancy. *Matern Fetal Med* 5:273–280, 1996

25. Schaefer-Graf U, Kjos S, Bühling K, Henrich W, Brauer M, Heinze T, Vetter K, Dudenhausen J: Amniotic fluid insulin levels and fetal abdominal circumference at time of amniocentesis in pregnancies with diabetes. *Diabetic Med* 20:349–335, 2003

26. Buchanan TA, Kjos SL, Montoro MN, Wu P, Madrilejo NG, Gonzalez M, Nunez V, Pantoja PM, Xiang A: Use of fetal ultrasound to select metabolic therapy for pregnancies complicated by mild gestational diabetes. *Diabetes Care* 17:275–283, 1994

27. Kjos S, Schaefer-Graf U, Sardesi S, Peters R, Buley A, Xiang A, Byrne J, Sutherland C, Montoro M, Buchanan T: A randomized controlled trial using glycemic plus fetal ultrasound parameters versus glycemic parameters to determine insulin therapy in gestational diabetes with fasting hyperglycemia. *Diabetes Care* 24:1904–1910, 2001

28. Schaefer-Graf U, Kjos S, Fauzan O, Bühling K, Siebert G, Bührer C, Ladendorf B, Dudenhausen J, Vetter K: A randomized trial evaluating a predominately fetal growth-based strategy to guide management of gestational diabetes in Caucasian women. *Diabetes Care* 27:297–302, 2004

29. Metzger BE, Coustan DR: Summary and Recommendations of the 4th International Workshop-Conference on Gestational Diabetes. *Diabetes Care* 21(Suppl.):161–167, 1998

30. Bonomo M, Cetin I, Pisoni M, Faden D, Mion E, Taricco E, Nobile de Santis M, Radaelli T, Motta G, Costa M, Solerte L, Morabito A: Flexible treatment of gestational diabetes modulated on ultrasound evaluation of intrauterine growth: a controlled randomized clinical trial. *Diabetes Metab* 30:237–244, 2004

31. Kjos S, Schaefer-Gra U: Modified therapy for gestational diabetes using high-risk and low-risk fetal abdominal circumference growth to select strict versus relaxed maternal glycemic target. *Diabetes Care* 30:S200–S205, 2007

32. Watkins M, Botto L: Maternal prepregnancy weight and congenital heart defects in offspring. *Epidemiology* 12:439–446, 2001

33. Larciprete G, Valensise H, Vasapollo B, Novelli G, Parretti E, Altomare F, Di Pierro G, Menghini S, Barbati G, Mello G, Arduini D: Fetal subcutaneous tissue thickness in healthy and gestational diabetic pregnancies. *Ultrasound Obstet Gynecol* 22:591–597, 2003

34. Rossi G, Somigliana E, Moschetta M, Bottani M, Vignali M: Adequate timing of fetal ultrasound to guide metabolic therapy in mild gestational diabetes mellitus. Results from a randomized study. *Acta Obstet Gynecol Scand* 79(8):649–654, 2000

19

Preeclampsia

Allison L. Cohen and S. Ananth Karumanchi

ABSTRACT

Preeclampsia is a syndrome of new-onset hypertension and proteinuria after 20-weeks gestation in a previously normotensive woman. Preeclampsia is a leading cause of maternal, fetal, and neonatal morbidity and mortality throughout the world. There are multiple risk factors for preeclampsia, including pregestational diabetes and obesity. Women with preeclampsia have an increased risk of recurrence in subsequent pregnancies and have an increased long-term risk of cardiovascular disease.

Although the etiology of preeclampsia is still unclear, recent studies have elucidated the pathophysiology underlying the disease. All of the clinical features of preeclampsia can be explained as a maternal response to placental-derived toxic factors that lead to generalized endothelial dysfunction. Recent evidence has shown alterations in angiogenic factors, including an increase in soluble fms-like tyrosine kinase 1 (sFlt-1), a naturally occurring circulating vascular endothelial growth factor (VEGF) antagonist, in women with preeclampsia. Soluble endoglin (sEng), a novel placenta-derived soluble anti-angiogenic protein appears to be another mediator of preeclampsia. Abnormalities in these circulating angiogenic proteins are not only present during clinical preeclampsia, but also antedate clinical symptoms by several weeks. There are also immunologic changes and changes in the renin-angiotensin system that may lead to the development of preeclampsia.

Women with pregestational diabetes have an increased risk of preeclampsia, especially those with underlying renal disease. It is especially difficult to diagnose preeclampsia in these women with underlying hypertension and proteinuria. In this chapter, we will discuss the epidemiology and the recent developments in the pathogenesis of preeclampsia. We will also highlight the contribution of pregestational diabetes in preeclampsia and discuss the long term of implications for maternal health in women with a history of preeclampsia.

Key words: Preeclampsia; Vascular endothelial growth factor; Soluble fms-like tyrosine kinase 1 receptor; Placental like growth factor; Endoglin; Diabetes; Proteinuria; Angiogenesis; Gestational hypertension.

From: *Diabetes in Women: Pathophysiology and Therapy*
Edited by: A. Tsatsoulis et al. (eds.), DOI 10.1007/978-1-60327-250-6_19
© Humana Press, a part of Springer Science+Business Media, LLC 2009

EPIDEMIOLOGY OF PREECLAMPSIA

Definition of Preeclampsia (1)

Preeclampsia is a syndrome of new-onset hypertension and proteinuria after 20 weeks of gestation in a previously normotensive female without proteinuria (Table 1). Women with preeclampsia are often asymptomatic, and the onset may be insidious. Early signs and symptoms may include headache, visual changes, epigastric pain, and edema of the hands and face. More severe complications include renal failure, cerebral edema, cerebral hemorrhage, seizures (eclampsia), pulmonary edema, and HELLP - the syndrome of hemolysis, elevated liver enzymes, and low platelets.

Women with severe preeclampsia have at least one of the following findings (Table 2): systolic blood pressure ≥160 (on two occasions at least 6 h apart, while on bedrest), diastolic blood pressure ≥110, proteinuria ≥5 g in 24 h, or 3+ on two random dipsticks >4 h apart, oliguria <500 ml/24 h, cerebral/visual symptoms, pulmonary edema or cyanosis, epigastric or RUQ pain, impaired liver function tests, platelets <100,000 mm^3, or fetal growth restriction.

It is important to distinguish preeclampsia from gestational hypertension. Gestational hypertension is hypertension without proteinuria at >20 weeks, which resolves by 12 weeks postpartum (Table 3).

Table 1
Preeclampsia *(1)*

BP ≥140 mmHg systolic
or ≥90 mmHg diastolic
and proteinuria >300 mg/24 h or ≥1+ on urine dipstick (in woman >20
   weeks gestation with previously normal BP)

Table 2
Severe Preeclampsia *(1)*

SBP ≥160 (on two occasions at least 6 h apart, while on bedrest)
DBP ≥110
Proteinuria ≥5 g in 24 h, or 3+ on two random dipsticks >4 h apart
Oliguria <500 ml/24 h
Cerebral/visual symptoms
Pulmonary edema or cyanosis
Epigastric or RUQ pain
Impaired LFTs
Platelets <100,000 mm^3
Fetal growth restriction

Table 3
Gestational Hypertension *(1)*

SBP ≥140 mmHg
or DBP ≥90 mmHg (in woman >20-weeks gestation with previously normal BP)
and no proteinuria
and BP normal by <12 weeks postpartum

Table 4
Superimposed Preeclampsia *(1)*

New onset proteinuria in a woman with a history of hypertension at <20 weeks
Sudden increase in proteinuria in a woman with baseline proteinuria
Sudden increase in BP
HELLP syndrome
Headache, scotomata, epigastric pain

Women with chronic hypertension have SBP ≥ 140, DBP ≥ 90, or both, that is either present pregestation at <20 weeks or persists greater than 12 weeks postpartum. Women with chronic hypertension can have superimposed preeclampsia when they develop proteinuria >20 weeks. Women with preexisting hypertension and proteinuria are considered to have preeclampsia if there is an increase in blood pressure, increase in proteinuria, severe preeclampsia or HELLP syndrome, or other signs of severe preeclampsia (Table 4).

Prevalence of Preeclampsia

Preeclampsia develops in 3–14% of pregnancies worldwide and in 5–8% in the USA *(1–5)*. Most cases in the US are mild. The incidence in women with pregestational diabetes is threefold to fourfold that of the general population. In a large study of 462 women with pregestational diabetes, 20% developed preeclampsia. The frequency of preeclampsia rose with increasing severity of diabetes, by the White classification (Chap. 16, Table 1) (Class B, 11%; class C, 22%; class D, 21%; Class R and F, 36%) *(6)*.

Preeclampsia Worldwide

Hypertensive disorders of pregnancy are one of the most common direct causes of maternal and neonatal morbidity and mortality. Developing countries have persistently higher rates of maternal and child mortality due to preeclampsia than developed countries. In a study of maternal deaths in South Africa between 2002 and 2004 *(7)*, hypertensive disorders of pregnancy were the most common direct cause of death. Nineteen percent of maternal deaths were due to hypertensive disorders of pregnancy. Cerebral complications, mainly cerebral hemorrhage, were the pathologic cause of death in about 50% of these cases. Eclampsia was the most common clinical condition leading to death from hypertension. Avoidable factors, missed opportunities, and substandard care were found in a majority of these deaths *(7)*. In a retrospective analysis of the World Health Organization's (WHO) Maternal Health and Safe Motherhood Programme *(8)*, morbidity and mortality due to hypertensive disorders of pregnancy were assessed in Africa, Asia, Latin American, and Caribbean countries. Overall estimates of mortality associated with hypertensive disorders of pregnancy were similar in Africa, Latin America, and the Caribbean; however, overall mortality was higher in Africa. In Asia, the estimates of overall maternal mortality and that due to hypertensive disorders varied extensively. These data indicate that overall 10–15% of maternal deaths were associated with hypertensive disorders, and of these deaths, 60–100% were due to eclampsia, thus eclampsia caused 10% of all maternal deaths *(8)*. A WHO systematic review of causes of maternal death from 1997 to 2002 *(9)* noted that hypertensive disorders of pregnancy were responsible for 16.1% of maternal deaths in developing countries, 9.1% in Africa, 9.1% in Asia, and 25.7% in Latin America/

Caribbean. Hemorrhage was the most common etiology of maternal mortality in Africa and Asia. In the USA, racial disparities in pregnancy-related mortality from preeclampsia and eclampsia exist. A study using data from the CDC form 1979 to 1992 found that black women were 3.1 times more likely to die from preeclampsia or eclampsia than white women *(10)*. The UK has developed the preeclampsia community guideline (PRECOG) to help improve screening and detection of preeclampsia in the community setting. They had found that many of the cases of preeclampsia in the UK would have had different outcomes had different management been in place *(11)*. Guidelines such as PRECOG may be useful for other countries in order to improve morbidity and mortality from preeclampsia and eclampsia worldwide.

Risk Factors for Preeclampsia

There are multiple risk factors for preeclampsia (Table 5) *(12)*. First pregnancy is associated with an increase risk in preeclampsia, though it is not clear why this is such an important factor (RR 2.91, 95% CI 1.28–6.61) *(13)*. There are some data suggesting that the risk increases in women who have had limited sperm exposure with the same partner prior to conception *(14–16)*, though this theory has been challenged. A past history of preeclampsia is a very strong risk factor for preeclampsia in a future pregnancy with a relative risk of 7.19 (95% CI 5.85–8.83) *(13)*. A family history of preeclampsia suggests some heritable mechanism, and this includes family history of preeclampsia in the mother, as well as the father. Advanced age in the mother is another independent risk factor (RR 1.96, 95% CI 1.34–2.87 – in multiparous women age >40); however, older women often have other comorbidities that put them at increased risk *(13)*. The risk of preeclampsia also rises with the number of fetuses. Risk of preeclampsia clearly increases with greater body mass index (BMI) *(14, 17)*, and obesity is strongly linked to insulin resistance, which is also a risk factor for preeclampsia *(14, 18)*. There are multiple other risks, as listed in Table 5. The risk in women with diabetes is discussed in the preceding paragraph.

Table 5
Risk Factors for Preeclampsia *(7)*

Nulliparity
Preeclampsia in prior pregnancy
Extremes of maternal age
Family history of preeclampsia
Chronic hypertension
Chronic renal disease
Pregestational diabetes
Antiphospholipid antibody syndrome
Inherited thrombophilia
Vascular/connective tissue disease
Multifetal gestation
Obesity
Maternal low birth weight
Male partner whose prior partner had preeclampsia
Hydrops fetalis
Unexplained fetal growth restriction
Trisomy 13
High-altitude pregnancies

PATHOPHYSIOLOGY OF PREECLAMPSIA

Preeclampsia only occurs in the presence of a placenta, and almost always resolves after delivery of the placenta. Severe preeclampsia is associated with pathologic evidence of placental hypoperfusion and ischemia. Prior to the onset of preeclampsia, abnormal uterine artery Doppler ultrasound results suggest increased uteroplacental resistance to blood flow (19). Thus, placental ischemia may be an early or precipitating event in the development of preeclampsia. Theories of the pathogenesis of preeclampsia are discussed later.

Normal Placental Development (Fig. 1)

Normal placenta development requires cytotrophoblast cells from the placenta to invade the maternal spiral arteries. During cytotrophoblast migration, endothelial cells are destroyed and removed, and cytotrophoblast cells line the lumen (20, 21), which generally occurs around 6–12 weeks of gestation. The trophoblasts then invade the vessel wall, which results in removal of the muscularis layer and disruption of the internal elastic lamina (20, 21), from 14 to 18 weeks of gestation. This remodeling results in maternal spiral arteries that are large-capacitance, low-resistance vessels, allowing increased blood flow to the fetus. Trophoblast invasion involves changes in the expression of certain cytokines, adhesion molecules, extracellular matrix molecules, metalloproteinases, and class Ib major histocompatability complex (MHC), human leukocyte antigen (HLA)-G (22, 23). Trophoblasts alter their adhesion molecule expression from those of epithelial cells (integrin $\alpha6/\beta1$, $\alpha v/\beta5$, and E-cadherin) to those of endothelial cells (integrin $\alpha1/\beta1$, $\alpha5/\beta3$, and VE-cadherin). This process is called "pseudovasculogenesis" (24).

Abnormal Placental Development in Preeclampsia (Fig. 1)

In women who develop preeclampsia, cytotrophoblast endovascular invasion is shallow, infiltrating the decidual portion of the spiral arteries, but not the myometrial portion. This results in narrow vessels, resulting in hypoperfusion, defective uteroplacental circulation, and ischemia (25, 26). Trophoblasts of women with preeclampsia do not undergo adhesion molecule alterations and pseudovasculogenesis (24, 27). The cause of the shallow cytotrophoblast invasion is unclear, though some believe that hypoxia may be the cause, but is still unclear whether hypoxia in preeclamptic placentas is a primary or secondary phenomenon (28).

Maternal Endothelial Dysfunction

All of the clinical features of preeclampsia can be explained as a maternal response to generalized endothelial dysfunction (29, 30), and women with underlying vascular disease may be at higher risk of developing preeclampsia due to preexisting endothelial dysfunction (31). Increased vascular permeability results in proteinuria and edema; disturbed endothelial control of vascular tone leads to hypertension, and abnormal endothelial expression of procoagulants leads to coagulopathy. In the kidney, a characteristic pathologic lesion known as glomerular endotheliosis occurs and is characterized by diffuse, glomerular endothelial cell swelling. This was originally considered pathognomonic for preeclampsia, but a recent study (32) showed that milder glomerular endotheliosis may occur in a significant percentage of normal pregnancies, suggesting that the endothelial dysfunction of pregnancy may be an exaggeration of a process that is present near term in all pregnancies.

Multiple markers of endothelial cell injury have been found to be elevated in the sera of women with preeclampsia, including von Willebrand factor (33), circulating cellular fibronectin (34), soluble

Normal

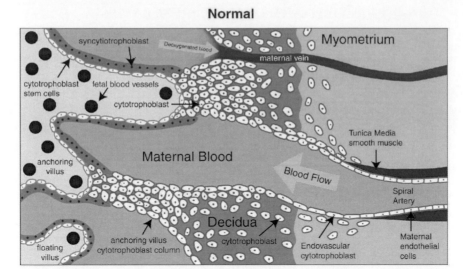

Preeclampsia

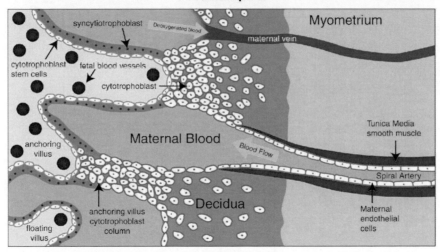

Fig. 1. Placental changes in preeclampsia. Exchange of oxygen, nutrients, and waste products between the fetus and the mother depends on adequate placental perfusion by maternal vessels. In normal placental development, invasive cytotrophoblasts of fetal origin invade the maternal spiral arteries, transforming them from small-caliber resistance vessels to high-caliber capacitance vessels capable of providing placental perfusion adequate to sustain the growing fetus. During the process of vascular invasion, the cytotrophoblasts differentiate from an epithelial phenotype to an endothelial phenotype, a process referred to as "pseudovasculogenesis" (*upper panel*). In preeclampsia, cytotrophoblasts fail to adopt an invasive endothelial phenotype. Instead, invasion of the spiral arteries is shallow and they remain small caliber, resistance vessels (*lower panel*). This may result in the placental ischemia. (Figure reproduced with permission from Lam et al., Hypertension, 2005;46:1077–1085.)

tissue factor, E-selectin, platelet-derived growth factor, endothelin *(35)*, and vascular cell adhesion molecule-1 (VCAM-1) *(36)*. There is evidence of increased oxidative stress *(37)*, increased lipid peroxidation *(38)*, and platelet activation *(39)*, as well as early increases in leptin *(40)*. Studies demonstrate decreased production of endothelial-derived vasodilators, such as nitric oxide (NO) and prostacylin, and increased production of vasoconstrictors, such as endothelins and thromboxanes *(41–43)*. Maternal vascular reactivity to vasopressors including angiotensin II and norepinephrine is increased in preeclampsia (42). In vitro studies of endothelial function of small isolated arteries from subcutaneous fat biopsies from women with and without preeclampsia were performed, and when preconstricted with adrenaline, the dilator response to acetylcholine and bradykinin was blunted in those with preeclampsia than in controls (44, 45). The dilator response to flow, using perfusion myography, in vitro (46), demonstrated a complete absence of flow-mediated dilation (FMD) in the small subcutaneous arteries of affected women.

In vivo assessment of endothelial-dependent vasodilation is performed by using ultrasound monitoring of FMD of the brachial artery after stimulation of intraluminal flow by reactive hyperemia (forearm cuff occlusion). Takase showed that women who are in their second half of pregnancy, but normotensive, have an increase in FMD compared with nonpregnant women (47). He also showed that women who developed preeclampsia had reduced FMD prior to the onset of preeclampsia compared with both the normotensive pregnant controls and nonpregnant women. Similar findings were seen by Garcia (48), with reduced FMD in women who subsequently developed preeclampsia, compared with those who did not, prior to 30 weeks of gestation. Impaired endothelial function 3 years after a preeclamptic pregnancy has also been demonstrated by brachial artery FMD (49).

Circulating Angiogenic Factors

SOLUBLE FMS-LIKE TYROSINE KINASE-1 (sFlt-1) (Fig. 1)

The search for circulating factors that mediate the generalized maternal endothelial function has been the focus of much research, and recent studies have demonstrated an increase in placental expression and secretion of soluble fms-like tyrosine kinase 1 (sFLT-1 or sVEGFR-1), which is a naturally occurring circulating vascular endothelial growth factor (VEGF) antagonist. VEGF has several receptors, including Flt1 (VEGFR1) and Flk1 (VEGFR2), and sFlt1 is a truncated form of Flt1. sFlt1 includes the extracellular binding domain but lacks the transmembrane and intracellular domains, and thus it is secreted. It antagonizes VEGF and placental-like growth factor (PlGF) in the circulation by binding and preventing interactions with their endothelial receptors (50). sFlt1 is made in small amounts by endothelial cells and monocytes; however, the placenta is the main source of sFlt1 during pregnancy, as evidenced by the dramatic fall in circulating levels after removal of the placenta (51). sFlt1 levels are elevated in the serum of women during clinical preeclampsia, and free PlGF and free VEGF are reduced (51–55). Elevated sFlt1 and reduced PlGF and VEGF have been found at least 5 weeks prior to the onset of preeclampsia (56). Another study found that the concentration of sFlt1 correlated with the increasing severity of disease, with higher concentrations in women with early (<34 weeks) preeclampsia than in those with mild or later preeclampsia (54). In vitro studies have shown that the antiangiogenic state in preeclampsia induced by excess production of placenta sFlt1 could be rescued by giving VEGF and PlGF (51). sFlt1 was introduced into pregnant rats by exogenous gene transfer using an adenoviral vector, and this resulted in hypertension, proteinuria, and glomerular endotheliosis. This was also seen in nonpregnant rats, suggesting that the effects of sFlt1 on the maternal vasculature were direct and not dependent on the presence of the placenta (51). When pregnant rats were given soluble VEGFR2 antagonist, which only antagonizes VEGF and not PlGF, the rats did not develop the preeclampsia phenotype. This suggests that preeclampsia requires a reduction in both PlGF and VEGF (51).

SOLUBLE ENDOGLIN (Fig. 2)

Soluble endoglin (sEng) is a novel placental-derived antiangiogenic protein that appears to be another important mediator in preeclampsia (57–60). sEng is a coreceptor for TGF-β and is highly expressed on cell membranes of vascular endothelium and syncytiotrophoblasts and acts by inhibiting

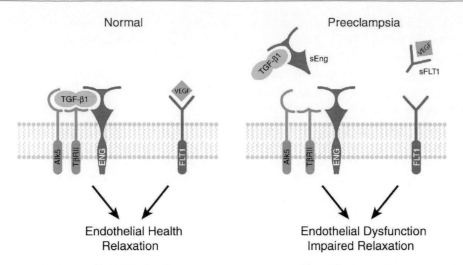

Fig. 2. sFlt1 and sEng causes endothelial dysfunction by antagonizing VEGF and TGF-β1 signaling. There is mounting evidence that VEGF and TGF-β1 are required to maintain endothelial health in several tissues including the kidney and perhaps the placenta. During normal pregnancy, vascular homeostasis is maintained by physiological levels of VEGF and TGF-β1 signaling in the vasculature. In preeclampsia, excess placental secretion of sFlt1 and sEng (two endogenous circulating antiangiogenic proteins) inhibits VEGF and TGF-β1 signaling, respectively, in the vasculature. This results in endothelial cell dysfunction, including decreased prostacyclin, NO production, and release of procoagulant proteins. (Figure reproduced with permission from Karumanchi et al., Kidney International, 2007;71:959–961.)

TGF-β signaling *(58)*. sEng has been found to be elevated in the serum of women with preeclampsia up to 2–3 months prior to the onset of clinical preeclampsia *(57)*. The levels of sEng also seem to correlate with disease severity and fall after delivery *(57)*. In pregnant rats, sEng appears to potentiate the effects of sFlt and induces severe preeclampsia, HELLP syndrome, and restriction of fetal growth *(58)*.

Immunologic Factors

Several epidemiological studies suggest that maternal-fetal (paternal) immune maladaptation is central in the etiology of preeclampsia *(14, 16, 61)*, with prior exposure to paternal/fetal antigens being protective against preeclampsia. The length of sexual cohabitation prior to conception appears inversely related to the risk of preeclampsia, which suggests that prolonged exposure to paternal sperm antigens may be protective *(15, 61–64)*. A review found no clear evidence that one or several specific HLA alleles are involved in the etiology of preeclampsia *(64)*, but rather it might be the interaction of maternal, paternal, and fetal HLA types that may be important in the pathogenesis of preeclampsia.

Renin-Angiotensin System

In normal pregnancy, renin, angiotensinogen, angiotensin II, and aldosterone are increased *(65)*; however, in preeclampsia plasma renin and aldosterone are suppressed, with higher than expected aldosterone levels for the given renin level *(66, 67)*. Normal pregnancy has a decreased vascular responsiveness to angiotensin II, but preeclampsia is associated with an increased sensitivity to angiotensin II *(68)*. This may be due to upregulation of Bradykinin (B2) receptor, which leads to heterodimerization of B2 receptors with angiotensin II type 1 receptors (AT1), and this AT1/B2 increases responsiveness to angiotensin II in vitro *(60)*. Women with preeclampsia have elevated autoantibodies against AT1 receptor *(69)*, and it has been suggested that these autoantibodies may play a role in enhancing vascular responsiveness to angiotensin II in preeclampsia *(69, 70)*.

Genetic Factors

Although preeclampsia is sporadic, genetic factors are thought to play a role in disease susceptibility. Primigravid women with a family history of preeclampsia have a two- to fivefold higher risk of preeclampsia than primigravid women without a family history *(71–74)*. Women who become pregnant by a man whose previous partner had preeclampsia are at higher risk than those who become pregnant by a man whose prior partner was normotensive *(75)*. The spouses of men who were the product of a pregnancy complicated by preeclampsia are also more likely to develop preeclampsia than the spouses of men without a history *(73, 76)*. These data suggest that both maternal and paternal contributions to fetal genes may have a role in subsequent preeclampsia. Though several candidate genes have been linked to preeclampsia (angiotensinogen gene variant T235 and endothelial nitric oxide synthase), larger studies have not found them to be important for disease susceptibility *(77)*. Genome scanning of Icelandic women with preeclampsia revealed a locus at 2p13 *(77)*, and other loci have suggested a gene on chromosome 13 as well. Of note, the gene for sFlt1 is carried on chromosome 13, and fetuses with Trisomy 13 have a much higher rate of preeclampsia in their mothers compared with fetuses with other trisomies and normal pregnancies *(78)*, along with higher ratios of sFlt1 to PlGF *(79)*.

Oxidative Stress and Inflammation

Oxidative stress of the placenta, due to hypoxia, may lead to endothelial dysfunction *(80, 81)*. F2-isoprostanes are considered to be the best in vivo marker of lipid peroxidation, and they are products of free radical attacks on arachidonic acid *(82, 83)*. In a study measuring F2-isoprostanes, they were found to be elevated in women with preeclampsia and remained elevated up to 6 weeks postpartum *(84)*. In preeclampsia, plasma levels of free-8 isoprostanes are elevated compared with those with a normal pregnancy *(85, 86)*. Breath methylated alkanes are measures of oxidative stress and have also been found to be elevated in women with preeclampsia *(87)*. Given the suggestion that oxidative stress may be an underlying etiology of preeclampsia, studies using antioxidants to prevent preeclampsia were performed; however, these found that vitamin C and vitamin E did not reduce the risk of preeclampsia in high- and low-risk women *(88, 89)*.

Normal pregnancy appears to be a mildly inflammatory state, and preeclampsia seems to be an exaggeration of this normal state. Neutrophil counts are elevated in pregnancy and more so in preeclampsia *(90)*. Other markers of inflammation, such as CRP, TNF-α, IL-2, IL-6, IL-12, and IL-18, have been found to be elevated in preeclampsia in some, but not all studies *(91–95)*. Obesity is also associated with elevated inflammatory mediators, and the incidence of preeclampsia is elevated in obese women *(13)*.

Evolution of Preeclampsia

There may also be an evolutionary explanation for the pathogenesis of preeclampsia *(96)*. This hypothesis is based on the evolutionary theory of parent-offspring conflict that what is "best" for a parent is not always "best" for an offspring, and vice versa *(97)*. This conflict is illustrated in the clinical dilemmas of treating preterm preeclampsia: the longer that induction of delivery is delayed, the greater the risk to a mother's health but the greater the benefits to the fetus. On the basis of this theory,

David Haig has hypothesized that the induction of preeclampsia is an adaptation to enhance fetal nutrition when the fetus's uteroplacental blood supply is inadequate by raising the systemic vascular resistance and thus maternal blood pressure to increase maternal blood supply to the fetus. The adaptation need not be simple and could involve the release of multiple placental factors that target different physiological systems of the mother *(98)*. That is, sFlt1 may be just one component, albeit an important component, of a cocktail of substances that are released into maternal blood in nutritionally compromised pregnancies.

PREDICTION AND DIAGNOSIS OF PREECLAMPSIA

Diagnosis of Preeclampsia

Although preeclampsia is usually diagnosed clinically based on clinical criteria as outlined by ACOG, the diagnosis can be a challenge in some patients in differentiating preeclampsia from pregestational diabetes, gestational hypertension, and/or chronic hypertension. In this regard, it has been recently reported in a small pilot study *(99)* that both sFlt1 and sEng may be useful in differentiating preeclampsia from other hypertensive disorders in pregnancy. This study found that the sensitivity and specificity of sFlt1 in differentiating preeclampsia from normal pregnancy were 90% and 90%, respectively, and 90% and 95% for sEng. In differentiating women with preeclampsia from those with gestational hypertension sensitivity and specificity were 79% and 88% for sFlt1 and 84% and 88% for sEng. Finally, in differentiating preeclampsia from chronic hypertension they were 84% and 95% for sFlt1 and 84% and 79% for sEng. Another study *(100)* evaluated the utility of urinary levels of angiogenic proteins to differentiate severe preeclampsia from normal pregnancy, nonpregnant controls, and pregnant women with hypertension and proteinuria who did not meet the diagnosis for severe preeclampsia. They found that severe preeclampsia was associated with an elevated urinary sFlt1 and reduced urinary PlGF, and that the log of urinary (sFlt1/PlGF) had an 88.2% sensitivity and 100% specificity in distinguishing severe preeclampsia from normotensive controls when a cutoff of 2.1 was used. In another small pilot study *(101)*, women with preexisting diabetes were evaluated, comparing a small group of those who did not develop preeclampsia with those who did. Women with preeclampsia had much higher sFlt1 levels at the time of delivery than those who did not [102.99 ± 39.27 vs. 18.13 ± 10.29 ng/ml ($p = 0.01$)]. PlGF was significantly lower in those with diabetes who developed preeclampsia than in those who did not, and the sFlt1/PlGF was significantly higher in those women with diabetes who developed preeclampsia than in those who did not. A case report illustrated that sFlt1 and PlGF may also be helpful to distinguish a flare of lupus in pregnancy from preeclampsia, though baseline values of sFlt1 and PlGF in lupus are not currently known *(102)*. Prospective studies are needed to definitively answer whether angiogenic markers can be used to aid in the diagnosis of preeclampsia.

Predicting Preeclampsia

As the only current treatment for preeclampsia is delivery, a good screening test would be helpful to identify women at risk, diagnose them early, and to provide them with appropriate management that might lead to improved maternal and perinatal outcomes. Women with known risk factors should be assessed early in pregnancy by a physician who is experienced in the management of preeclampsia. Both human and animal data described earlier in "Circulating Angiogenic Factors" suggest that angiogenic factors may be important in the pathogenesis of preeclampsia. Alterations in the levels of VEGF, PlGF, sFlt1, and sEng have been found in the serum of women who develop preeclampsia, and these alterations precede the onset of preeclampsia by weeks to months *(51, 56–60, 103–105)*.

Measurements have also been performed in the urine *(106–108)*, with one of the studies focusing on urinary PlGF. It was found that urinary PlGF increased during the first two trimesters, peaking at 29–32 weeks and then decreasing; however, in the women who went on to develop preeclampsia, they had lower levels of PlGF at each sampling point, beginning at 25 weeks of gestation. At 21–32 weeks, the PlGF of the lowest quartile was predictive of preeclampsia before term (OR 22.5, 95% CI 7.4–67.8), but less predictive of term preeclampsia (OR 2.2, 95% CI 1.2–4.3) *(106)*. Some suggest that using a ratio of sFlt1/VEGF or sFlt1/PlGF is superior than using absolute levels of angiogenic factors to predict preeclampsia *(57, 108)*. A review evaluating sFlt1 and PlGF concluded that after 25 weeks of gestation these factors were predictive of severe preeclampsia, but in the absence of prospective studies there is no evidence to recommend these tests for screening at this time *(109)*.

Diabetic Nephropathy and Superimposed Preeclampsia

Women with diabetes and microalbuminuria or nephropathy are at an increased risk for preeclampsia compared to women with diabetes and no renal disease. In a Danish study *(110)* of 203 women with type 1 diabetes, 85% had normal albumin excretion, 11% had microalbuminuria, and 5% had diabetic nephropathy. Of those with normal albumin excretion 6% developed preeclampsia, and there was preterm delivery in 35%. In those with microalbuminuria, 42% developed preeclampsia and 62% with preterm delivery, and in those with diabetic nephropathy, 64% developed preeclampsia and 91% with preterm delivery. This study illustrated for the first time that urinary albumin excretion rate (AER) was associated with preterm delivery, in addition to preeclampsia, which had been shown in prior studies *(6, 111–113)*. A study comparing women with type 2 (DM2) and type 1 (DM1) diabetes *(114)* found that though the overall rate of hypertension in pregnancy was similar between women with DM2 and women with DM1 (41% vs. 45%); however, women with DM2 had more chronic hypertension but less preeclampsia than women with DM1. Early pregnancy AER were increased more frequently in women with DM2 than in women with DM1, but were less strongly associated with the development of preeclampsia in women with DM2. In women with microalbuminuria or overt albuminuria, 59% of those with DM1 developed preeclampsia, and only 30% of those with DM2 developed preeclampsia ($p = 0.034$). A recent study has also shown that women with a history of preeclampsia and DM1 are at greater risk for future diabetic nephropathy (microalbuminuria, macroalbuminuria, and ESRD) than those with normotensive pregnancies (41.9% vs. 8.9%, $p < 0.001$) *(115)*.

COMPLICATIONS OF PREECLAMPSIA

Preeclampsia may cause both acute complications to the mother and neonate, as well as long term complications for the mother. Usually maternal and perinatal outcomes are more favorable in women with mild preeclampsia that develops after 36 weeks of gestation *(116–118)*. Women who develop preeclampsia prior to 33 weeks who have preexisting medical conditions or who live in developing countries have increased maternal and neonatal morbidity and mortality. Immediate complications for the mother include placental abruption, disseminated intravascular coagulation (DIC)/HELLP syndrome, acute renal failure, eclampsia, liver failure, and extremely rarely stroke and death. Complications for the neonate include preterm delivery, fetal growth restriction, and rarely hypoxia, neurologic injury, and perinatal death (Table 6).

There is accumulating evidence suggesting that preeclampsia confers a risk for long-term maternal cardiovascular disease. A large population-based study of 62,272 births in Norway *(119)* showed that women with preeclampsia had a 1.2-fold higher long-term risk of death than women without preeclampsia. A recent meta-analysis *(120)* found that women with preeclampsia have a relative risk of

Table 6
Complications of Preeclampsia *(7)*

Maternal complications	*Neonatal complications*
Placental abruption	Preterm delivery
DIC/HELLP syndrome	Fetal growth restriction
Pulmonary edema/aspiration	Hypoxia/neurologic injury
Acute renal failure	Perinatal death
Eclampsia	Long-term cardiovascular morbidity associated with low birth weight
Liver failure or hemorrhage	
Stroke	
Death	
Long-term cardiovascular morbidity	

hypertension of 3.70 (95% CI 2.7–5.05) after 14.1 years mean follow-up, a relative risk of ischemic heart disease of 2.16 (95% CI 1.86–2.52) after 11.7 years, a relative risk of stroke of 1.81 (95% CI 1.45–2.27) after 10.4 years, and for venous thromboembolism 1.79 (95% CI 1.05–2.14) after 14.5 years. It is unclear whether the increased risk of cardiovascular disease subsequent to preeclampsia is due to the preeclampsia during pregnancy or due to underlying traits of the mother. In a study of 3,494 women of whom 133 developed preeclampsia, there was a positive association found with prepregnancy levels of triglycerides, total cholesterol, LDL, non-HDL cholesterol, and BP with the risk of preeclampsia, after adjusting for smoking, history of preeclampsia, and socioeconomic status *(121)*. This study suggests that women with cardiovascular risk factors may be predisposed to preeclampsia. Interestingly several studies have suggested that patients with a history of preeclampsia are relatively protected from solid cancers such as breast and ovarian tumors *(122, 123)*. The increased incidence of cardiovascular diseases and a relative protection against cancers may suggest that patients with preeclampsia may have a persistent antiangiogenic state due to increased susceptibility to induce antiangiogenic factors; however, evidence for this hypothesis is lacking.

SUMMARY

Preeclampsia is a leading cause of maternal, fetal, and neonatal morbidity and mortality worldwide. Recent knowledge elucidating the pathogenesis of preeclampsia may be useful in the development of diagnostic tests for preeclampsia as well therapeutics to treat preeclampsia in the future.

Acknowledgments: A.L.C. is funded by the Clinical Investigator Training Program: Beth Israel Deaconess Medical Center - Harvard/MIT Health Sciences and Technology, in collaboration with Pfizer Inc., and Merck & Co. S.A.K. is funded by R01 grants from the National Institute of Diabetes, Digestive and Kidney Diseases (DK 065997) and the National Heart, Lung, and Blood Institute (HL079594).

REFERENCES

1. ACOG practice bulletin. Diagnosis and management of preeclampsia and eclampsia. Int J Gynaecol Obstet 2002;77:67–75
2. Cunningham FG, Lindheimer MD. Hypertension in pregnancy. N Engl J Med 1992;326:927–932
3. Saftlas AF, Olson DR, Franks AL, et al. Epidemiology of preeclampsia and eclampsia in the United States, 1979–1986. Am J Obstet Gynecol 1990;163:460–465
4. Centers for Disease Control and Prevention (CDC). Maternal mortality - United States, 1982–1996. MMWR Morb Mortal Wkly Rep 1998;47:705

5. Sibai BM, Gordon T, Thorn E, et al. Risk factors for preeclampsia in healthy nulliparous women; a prospective multi-center study. The National Institutes of Child Health and Human Development Network of Maternal-Fetal Medicine Units. Am J Obstet Gynecol 1995;172:642–648

6. Sibai BM, Caritis S, Hauth J, et al. Risks of preeclampsia and adverse neonatal outcomes among women with pregestational diabetes mellitus. Am J Obstet Gynecol 2000;182:364–369

7. Moodley J. Maternal deaths due to hypertensive disorders of pregnancy: saving Mothers report 2002–2004. Cardiovasc J Afr 2007;18:358–361

8. Duley L. Maternal mortality associated with hypertensive disorders of pregnancy in Africa, Asia, Latin America, and the Caribbean. Br J Obstet Gynaecol 1992;99:547–553

9. Khan SK, Wojdyla D, Say L, et al. WHO analysis of causes of maternal death: a systematic review. Lancet 2006;367:1066–1074

10. Mackay AP, Berg CJ, Atrash HK. Pregnancy-related mortality from preeclampsia and eclampsia. Obstet Gynecol 2001;97:533–538

11. Milne F, Redman C, Walker J, et al. The pre-eclampsia community guideline (PRECOG): how to screen for and detect onset of pre-eclampsia in the community. BMJ 2005;330:576–580

12. Sibai BM, Dekker G, Kupferminc M. Pre-eclampsia. Lancet 2005;365:785–799

13. Duckitt K, Harrington D. Risk factors for preeclampsia at antenatal booking: systemic review of controlled studies. BMJ 2005;330:565

14. Dekker G, Sibai B. Primary, secondary, and tertiary prevention of preeclampsia. Lancet 2001;357:209–215

15. Einarsson JI, Sangi-Haghpeykar H, Gardner NO. Sperm exposure and the development of preeclampsia. Am J Obstet Gynecol 2003;188:1241–1243

16. Dekker G, Robillary PY. The birth interval hypothesis - does it really indicate the end of the primipaternity hypothesis? J Reprod Immunol 2003;59:245–251

17. O'Brien TE, Ray JG, Chan WS. Maternal body mass index and the risk of preeclampsia: a systematic overview. Epidemiology 2003;14:368–374

18. Wolf M, Sandler L, Munoz K, et al. First trimester insulin resistance and subsequent preeclampsia: a prospective study. J Clin Endocrinol Metab 2002;87:1563–1568

19. Bower S, Schuchter K, Campbell S. Doppler ultrasound screening as part of routine antenatal scanning: prediction of pre-eclampsia and intrauterine growth retardation. Br J Obstet Gynaecol 1993;100:989–994

20. Brosens I, Dixon HG. The anatomy of the maternal side of the placenta. J Obstet Gynaecol Br Commonw 1966;73:357–363

21. Shah DM. Preeclampsia: new insights. Curr Opin Nephrol Hypertens 2007;16:213–220

22. Cross JC, Werb Z, Fisher SJ. Implantation and the placenta: key pieces of the development puzzle. Science 1994;266:1508–1518

23. Lim KH, Zhou Y Janatpour M, et al. Human cytotrophoblast differentiation/invasion is abnormal in preeclampsia. Am J Pathol 1997;151:1809–1818

24. Zhou Y, Damsky CH, Fisher SJ. Preeclampsia is associated with failure of human cytotrophoblasts to mimic a vascular adhesion phenotype. One cause of defective endovascular invasion in this syndrome? J Clin Invest 1997;99:2152–2164

25. Roberts JM, Redman CW. Pre-eclampsia: more than pregnancy-induced hypertension. Lancet 1993;341:1447–1451

26. Meekins JW, Pijnenborg R, Hanssens M, et al. A study of placental bed spiral arteries and trophoblast invasion in normal and severe pre-eclamptic pregnancies. Br J Obstet Gynaecol 1994;101:669–674

27. Zhou Y, Damsky CH, Chiu K, et al. Preeclampsia is associated with abnormal expression of adhesion molecules by invasive cytorophoblasts. J Clin Invest 1993;91:950–960

28. Karumanchi SA, Bdolah Y. Hypoxia and sFlt-1 in preeclampsia: the 'chicken-and-egg' question. Endocrinology 2004;145:4835–4837

29. Redman CW, Sacks GP, Sargent IL. Preeclampsia: an excessive maternal inflammatory response to pregnancy. Am J Obstet Gynecol 1999;180:499–506

30. Roberts JM, Taylor RN, Goldfien A. Clinical and biochemical evidence of endothelial cell dysfunction in the pregnancy syndrome preeclampsia. Am J Hypertens 1991;4:700–708

31. Levine RJ, Qian C, Maynard SE, et al. Serum sFlt1 concentration during preeclampsia and mid trimester blood pressure in healthy nulliparous women. Am J Obstet Gynecol 2006;194:1034–1041

32. Strevens H, Wide-Swensson D, Hansen A et al. Glomerular endotheliosis in normal pregnancy and preeclampsia. BJOG 2003;110:831–836

33. Calvin S, Corrigan J, Weinstein L. Factor VIII: von Willebrand factor patterns in the plasma of patients with pre-eclampsia. Am J Perinatol 1988;5:29–32

34. Lockwood CJ, Peters JH. Increased plasma levels of ED1+ cellular fibronectin precede the clinical signs of preeclampsia. Am J Obstet Gynecol 1990;162:358–362
35. Nova A, Sibai BM, Barton JR, et al. Maternal plasma level of endothelin is increased in preeclampsia. Am J Obstet Gynecol 1991;165:724–727
36. Higgins JR, Papayianni A, Brady HR, et al. Circulating vascular cell adhesion molecule-1 in pre-eclampsia, gestational hypertension, and normal pregnancy: evidence of selective dysregulation of vascular cell adhesion molecule-1 homeostasis in preeclampsia. Am J Obstet Gynecol 1998;179:464–469
37. Davidge ST. Oxidative stress and altered endothelial cell function in preeclampsia. Semin Reprod Endocrinol 1998;16:65–73
38. Hubel CA, McLaughlin MK, Evans RW, et al. Fasting serum triglyerides, free fatty acids, and malondialdehyde are increased in the preeclampsia, are positively correlated, and decrease within 48 hours postpartum. Am J Obstet Gynecol 1996;174:975–982
39. Kolben M, Lopens A, Blaser J, et al. Measuring the concentration of various plasma and placenta extract proteolytic and vascular factors in pregnant patients with HELLP syndrome, pre-eclampsia, and highly pathologic Doppler flow values. Gynakol Geburtshilfliche Rundsch 1995;35(suppl 1):126–131
40. Chappell LC, Seed PT, Briley A, et al. A longitudinal study of biochemical variables in women at risk for preeclampsia. Am J Obstet Gynecol 2002;187:127–136
41. Mills JL, DerSimonian R, Raymond E, et al. Prostacylin and thromboxane changes predating clinical onset of preeclampsia: a multicenter prospective study. JAMA 1999;282:356–362
42. Gant NF, Daley GL, Chand S, et al. A study of angiotensin II pressor response throughout primigravid pregnancy. J Clin Invest 1973;52:2682–2689
43. Clark BA, Halvorson L, Sachs B, et al. Plasma endothelin levels in preeclampsia: elevation and correlation with uric acid levels and renal impairment. Am J Obstet Gynecol 1992;166:962–968
44. Knock GA, Poston L. Bradykinin-mediated relaxation of isolated maternal resistance arteries in normal pregnancy and preeclampsia. Am J Obstet Gynecol 1996,175:1668–1774
45. McCarthy AL, Woolfson RG, Raju SK, et al. Abnormal endothelial cell function of resistance arteries from women with preeclampsia. Am J Obstet Gynecol 1993;168:1323–1330
46. Cockell AP, Posten L. Flow medicated vasodilation is enhanced in normal pregnancy but reduced in preeclampsia. Hypertension 1997;30:247–251
47. Takase B, Hamabe A, Uehata A, et al. Flow-mediated dilation in brachial artery in the second half of pregnancy and prediction of pre-eclampsia. J Hum Hypertens 2003;17:697–704
48. Garcia RG, celadon J, Sierra-Laguado J, et al. Raised C-reactive protein and impaired vasodilation precede the development of preeclampsia. Am J Hypertens 2007;20:98–103
49. Chambers JC, Fusi L, Malik IS, et al. Association of maternal endothelial dysfunction with preeclampsia. JAMA 2001;285:1607–1612
50. Kendall RL, Thomas KA. Inhibition of vascular endothelial cell growth factor activity by an endogenously encoded soluble receptor. Proc Natl Acad Sci U S A 1993;90:10705–10709
51. Maynard SE, Min JY, Merchan J, et al. Excess placental soluble fms-like tyrosine kinase 1 (sFlt1) may contribute to endothelial dysfunction, hypertension, and proteinuria in preeclampsia. J Clin Invest 2003;111:649–658
52. Koga K, Osuga Y, Yoshino O, et al. Elevated serum soluble vascular endothelial growth factor receptor 1 (sVEGFR-1) levels in women with preeclampsia. J Clin Endocrinol Metab 2003;88:2348–2351
53. Tsatsaris V, Goffin F, Munaut C, et al. Overexpression of the soluble vascular endothelial growth factor receptor in preeclamptic patients: pathophysiological consequences. J Clin Endocrinol Metab 2003;88:5555–5563
54. Chaiworapongsa T, Romero R, Espinoza J, et al. Evidence supporting a role for blockade of the vascular endothelial growth factor systerm in the pathophysiology of preeclampsia. Young Investigator Award. Am J Obstet Gynecol 2004;190:1541–1547
55. Taylor RN, Grimwood J, Taylor RS, et al. Longitudinal serum concentrations of placental growth factor: evidence for abnormal placental angiogenesis in pathologic pregnancies. Am J Obstet Gynecol 2003;188:177–182
56. Levine RJ, Maynard SE, Qian C, et al. Circulating angiogenic factors and the risk for preeclampsia. N Engl J Med 2004;350:672–683
57. Levine RJ, Lam C, Qian C, et al. Soluble endoglin and other circulating antiangiogenic factors in preeclampsia. N Engl J Med. 2006;355:992–1005
58. Venkatesha S, Toporsian M, Lam C, et al. Soluble endoglin contributes to the pathogenesis of preeclampsia. Nat Med 2006;12:642–649
59. Luft FC. Soluble endoglin (sEng) joins the soluble fms-like tyrosine kinase (sFlt) receptor as a preeclampsia molecule. Nephrol Dial Transplant 2006;21:3052–3054

60. AbdAlla S, Lother H, el Massiery A, et al. Increased AT(1) receptor heterodimers in preeclampsia mediate enhanced angiotensin II responsiveness. Nat Med 2001;7:1003–1009

61. Wang JX, Knottnerus AM, Schui G, et al. Surgically obtained sperm ad risk of gestational hypertension and pre-eclampsia. Lancet 2002;359:673–674

62. Robillard PY, Hulsey TC, Perianin J, et al. Association of pregnancy-induced hypertension with duration of sexual cohabitation before conception. Lancet 1994;344:973–975

63. Koelman CA, Coumans AB, Nijman HW, et al. Correlation between oral sex and low incidence of preeclampsia: a role for soluble HLA in seminal fluid. J Reprod Immunol 2000;46:155–166

64. Saftlas AF, Beydoun H, Triche E. Immunogenetic determinants of preeclampsia and related pregnancy disorders: a systematic review. Obstet Gynecol 2005;106:162–172

65. Skinner SL, Lumbers Er, Symonds EM. Analysis of changes in the rennin-angiotensin system during pregnancy. Clin Sci 1972;42:479–488

66. Brown MA, Zammit VC, Mitar DA, et al. Renin-aldosterone relationships in pregnancy-induced hypertension. Am J Hypertens 1992;5:366–371

67. Symonds EM, Broughton Pipkin F, Craven DJ. Changes in the renin-angiotensin system in primigravidae with hypertensive disease of pregnancy. Br J Obstet Gynaecol 1975;82:643–650

68. Granger JP, Alexander BT, Bennett WA, et al. Pathophysiology of pregnancy-induced hypertension. Am J Hypertens 2001;14:178S–185S

69. Wallukat G, Homuth V, Fischer T, et al. Patients with preeclampsia develop agonistic autoantibodies against the angiotensin AT1 receptor. J Clin Invest 1999;103:945–952

70. Dechend R, Gratze P, Wallukat G, et al. Agonistic autoantibodies ot the AT1 receptor in a transgenic rat model of preeclmapsia. Hypertension 2005;45:742–746

71. Mogren I, Hogberg U, Winkvist A, et al. Familial occurrence of preeclampsia. Epidemiology 1999;10:518–522

72. Cincotta RB, Brennecke SP. Family history of pre-eclampsia as a predictor for pre-eclampsia in primigravidas. Int J Gynaecol Obstet 1998;60:23–27

73. Skjaerven R, Vatten LJ, Wilcox AJ, et al. Recurrence of pre-eclampsia across generations: exploring fetal and maternal genetic components in a population based cohort. BMJ 2005;331:877

74. Carr DB, Epplein M, Johnson CO, et al. A sister's risk: family history as a predictor of preeclampsia. Am J Obstet Gynecol 2005;193:965–972

75. Lie RT, Rasmussen S, Brunborg H, et al. Fetal and maternal contributions to risk of pre-eclampsia: population based study. BMJ 1998;316:1343–1347

76. Esplin MS, Fausett MB, Fraser A, et al. Paternal and maternal components of the predisposition to preeclampsia. N Engl J Med 2001;344:867–872

77. Arngrimsson R, Sigurard ttir S, Frigge ML, et al. A genome-wide scan reveals a maternal susceptibility locus for pre-eclampsia on chromosome 2p13. Hum Mol Genet 1999;8:1799–1805

78. Tuohy Y, James DK. Pre-eclampsia and trisomy 13. Br J Obstet Gynaecol 1992;99:891–894

79. Bdolah Y, Palomaki GE, Yaron Y, et al. Circulating angiogenic proteins in trisomy 13. Am J Obstet Gynecol 2006;194:239–245

80. Posten L. Endothelial dysfunction in pre-eclampsia. Pharmacol Rep 2006;58:S69–S74

81. Posten L, Raijmakers MT. Trophoblast oxidative stress, antioxidants, and pregnancy outcome - a review. Placenta 2004;25:S72–S78

82. Barden A. Pre-eclampsia: contributions of maternal constitutional factors and the consequences for cardiovascular health. Clin Exp Pharmacol Physiol 2006;33:826–830

83. Cracowksi JL, Durand T, Bessard G. Isoprostanes as a biomarker of lipid peroxidation in humans: physiology, pharmacology, and clinical implications. Trends Pharmacol Sci 2002;23:360–366

84. Barden A, Ritchie J, Walters B, et al. Study of plasma factors associated with neutrophil activation and lipid peroxidation in pre-eclampsia. Hypertension 2001;38:803–808

85. Barden A, Beilin LJ, Ritchie J, et al. Plasma and urinary 8-iso-prostane as an indicator of lipid peroxidation in pre-eclampsia and normal pregnancy. Clin Sci 1996;91:711–718

86. McKinney ET, Shouri R, Hunt Rs, et al. Plasma, urinary, and salivary 8-epi-prostaglandin F2alpha levels in normotensive and preeclamptic pregnancies. Am J Obstet Gynecol 2000;183:874–877

87. Moretti M, Phillips M, Abouzeid A, et al. Increased breath markers of oxidative stress in normal pregnancy and pre-eclampsia. Am J Obstet Gynecol 2004;190:1184–1190

88. Posten L, Briley AL, Seed PT, et al. Vitamin C and vitamin E in pregnant women at risk for pre-eclampsia (VIP trial): randomized placebo controlled trial. Lancet 2006;367:1145–1154

89. Rumbold AR, Crowther CA, Haslam RR, et al. Vitamins C and E and the risk of preeclampsia and perinatal complications. N Engl J Med 2006;354:1796–1806

90. Barden A, Graham D, Beilin LJ, et al. Neutrophil CD11b expression and neutrophil activation in pre-eclampsia. Clin Sci 1997;92:37–44

91. Saito S, Sakai M. Th1/Th2 balance in pre-eclampsia. J Reprod Immunol 2003;59:161–173

92. Conrad KP, Miles TM, Benyo DF. Circulating levels of immunoreactive cytokines in women with preeclampsia. Am J Reprod Immunol 1998;40:102–111

93. Vince GS, Starkey PM, Austgulen R, et al. Interleukin-6, tumour necrosis factor and soluble tumour necrosis factor receptors in women with pre-eclampsia. Br J Obstet Gynaecol 1995;102:20–25

94. Benyo DF, Smarason A, Redman CW, et al. Expression of inflammatory cytokines in the placentas from women with pre-eclampsia. J Clin Endocrinol Metab 2001;86:2505–2512

95. Heyl W, Handt S, Reister F, et al. Elevated soluble adhesion molecules in women with pre-eclampsia. Do Cytokines like tumour necrosis factor-alpha and interleukin-1beta cause endothelial activation. Eur J Obstet Gynecol Reprod Biol 1999;86:35–41

96. Haig D. Genetic conflicts in human pregnancy. Q Rev Biol 1993;68:495–532

97. Trivers RL. Parent-offspring conflict. Am Zool 1974;14:249–264

98. Yuan HT, Haig D, Karumanchi SA. Angiogenic factors in the pathogenesis of preeclampsia. Curr Top Dev Biol 2005;71:297–312

99. Salahuddin S, Lee Y, Vadnais M, et al. Diagnostic utility of soluble fms-like tyrosine kinase 1 and soluble endoglin in hypertensive diseases of pregnancy. Am J Obstet Gynecol 2007;197:28.e1–28.e6

100. Buhimchi CS, Norwitz ER, Funai E, et al. Urinary angiogenic factors cluster hypertensive disorders and identify women with severe preeclampsia. Am J Obstet Gynecol 2005;192:734–741

101. Cohen A, Lim KH, Lee Y, et al. Circulating levels of the antiangiogenic marker soluble FMS-like tyrosine kinase 1 are elevated in women with pregestational diabetes and preeclampsia: angiogenic markers in preeclampsia and preexisting diabetes. Diabetes Care 2007;30:375–377

102. Williams WW, Ecker JL, Thadhani RI, et al. A 29-year-old pregnant woman with nephritic syndrome and hypertension. N Engl J Med 2005;353:2590–2600

103. Lam C, Lim KH, Karumanchi SA. Circulating angiogenic factors in the pathogenesis and prediction of preeclampsia. Hypertension 2005;46:1077–1085

104. Wolf M, Hubel CA, Lam C, et al. Preeclampsia and future cardiovascular disease: potential role of altered angiogenesis and insulin resistance. J Clin Endocrinol Metab 2004;89:6239–6243

105. Chaiworapongsa T, Romero R, Kim YM, et al. Plasma soluble vascular endothelial growth factor receptor-1 concentration is elevated prior to the clinical diagnosis of preeclampsia. J Matern Fetal Neonatal Med 2005;17:3–18

106. Levine RJ, Thadani R, Qian C, et al. Urinary placental growth factor and risk of preeclampsia. JAMA 2005;293:77–85

107. Aggarwal PK, Jain V, Sakhuja V, et al. Low urinary placental growth factor is a marker of preeclampsia. Kidney Int 2006;69:621–624

108. Buhimchi CS, Magloire L, Funai E, et al. Fractional excretion of angiogenic factors in women with severe preeclampsia. Obstet Gynecol 2006;107:1103–1113

109. Widmer M, Villar J, Benigni A, et al. Mapping the theories of preeclampsia and the role of angiogenic factors. A systematic review. Obstet Gynecol 2007;109:168–180

110. Ekbom P, Damm P, Feldt-Rasmussen B, et al. Pregnancy outcome in type 1 diabetic women with microalbuminuria. Diabetes Care 2001;24:1739–1744

111. Reece AE, Leguizaman G, Homko C. Stringent control in diabetic nephropathy associated with optimization of pregnancy outcomes. J Matern Fetal Med 1998;7:213–216

112. Combs CA, Rosenn B, Kitzmiller JL, et al. Early-pregnancy proteinuria in diabetes related to preeclampsia. Obstet Gynecol 1993;82:802–807

113. Ekbom P, and the Copenhagen Preeclampsia in Diabetic Pregnancy Study Group. Pre-pregnancy microalbuminuria predicts preeclampsia in diabetes mellitus (letter). Lancet 1999;353:377

114. Cundy T, Slee F, Gamble G, et al. Hypertensive disorders of pregnancy in women with Type 1 and Type 2 diabetes. Diabet Med 2002;19:482–489

115. Gordin D, Hiilesmaa V, Fagerudd J, et al. Pre-eclampsia but not pregnancy-induced hypertension is a risk factor for diabetic nephropathy in type 1 diabetic women. Diabetologia 2007;50:516–522

116. Report of the National High Blood Pressure Education Program. Working group report on high blood pressure in pregnancy. Am J Obstet Gynecol 2000;183:S1–S22

117. Sibai BM. Diagnosis and management of gestational hypertension and preeclampsia. Obstet Gynecol 2003;102:181–192

118. Hauth JC, Ewell MG, Levine RL, et al. Pregnancy outcomes in healthy nulliparous women who subsequently developed hypertension. Obstet Gynecol 2000;95:24–28

119. Irgens LM. The medical birth registry of Norway. Epidemiological research and surveillance throughout 30 years. Acta Obstet Gynecol Scand 2000;79:435–439

120. Bellamy L, Casas JP, Hingorani AD, et al. Pre-eclampsia and risk of cardiovascular disease and cancer in later life: systemic review and meta-analysis. BMJ 2007;335:974

121. Magnussen EB, Vatten LJ, Ivar T, et al. Prepregnancy cardiovascular risk factors as predictors of preeclampsia: population based cohort study. BMJ 2007;335:978

122. Aagaard-Tillery KM, Stoddard GJ, Holmgren C, et al. Preeclampsia and subsequent risk of cancer in Utah. Am J Obstet Gynecol 2006;195:691–699

123. Xue F, Michels KB. Intrauterine factors and risk of breast cancer: a systematic review and meta-analysis of current evidence. Lancet Oncol 2007;8:1088–1100

20

The Infant of the Diabetic Mother: Metabolic Imprinting

Janet K. Snell-Bergeon and Dana Dabelea

Contents

ABSTRACT

Diabetes during pregnancy is thought to contribute to metabolic changes in the fetus, which predispose the offspring of diabetic mothers to obesity, insulin resistance, diabetes and cardiovascular disease. Altered maternal fuels, including but not limited to glucose, may affect the development of the endocrine pancreas in the fetus, resulting in increased adiposity and decreased beta cell mass and/or function.

Prospective studies in the Pima Indians and at Northwestern University in Chicago have demonstrated increased adiposity among children exposed to diabetes in utero, although not all studies have replicated this relationship. Impaired glucose tolerance (IGT), which can result from either reduced insulin secretion or increased insulin resistance, has also been associated with exposure to diabetes in utero. Type 2 diabetes is more common in offspring of mothers with diabetes than in offspring of nondiabetic and prediabetic women among the Pima Indians. Further, a diabetic intrauterine environment has been shown to induce biochemical alterations in the cardiovascular system, and children born to diabetic mothers have increased cardiovascular risk factors compared with children not exposed to diabetes in utero.

Type 2 diabetes has a known genetic component and tends to cluster in families. As a result, obesity, IGT and type 2 diabetes may be more common in offspring of diabetic mothers due to maternal genes rather than metabolic imprinting during fetal development. In order to disentangle genetic vs. environmental causes of type 2 diabetes, several methods were employed. The offspring of mothers with early onset type 2 diabetes have been compared by exposure to intrauterine diabetes, with a higher prevalence of type 2 diabetes demonstrated in exposed Pima Indian children compared with unexposed children. Adjustment for maternal obesity, which is a marker for genetic predisposition to type 2 diabetes, does not explain the increased risk of obesity in the offspring of diabetic mothers, further supporting an environmental contribution of excess maternal fuel. A comparison of offspring with maternal vs. paternal type 2 diabetes also

From: *Diabetes in Women: Pathophysiology and Therapy*
Edited by: A. Tsatsoulis et al. (eds.), DOI 10.1007/978-1-60327-250-6_20
© Humana Press, a part of Springer Science+Business Media, LLC 2009

allows for the disentangling of genetic and environmental causes, since fathers would transmit the same genetic risk of type 2 diabetes as mothers. However, the strongest evidence for the role of intrauterine diabetes in the development of type 2 diabetes in the offspring of diabetic mothers has come from the comparison of siblings born before and after the development of maternal diabetes.

Animal studies have allowed for the investigation of experimentally manipulated intrauterine environment on metabolism and glucose homeostasis in the offspring. Hyperglycemia can be induced either to a mild degree late in pregnancy to mimic gestational diabetes or to a severe degree early in pregnancy to mimic type 1 diabetes. An additional genetic model of diabetes has been examined using rats selectively bred for IGT. These animal models have allowed for insight into the effects of maternal hyperglycemia on beta cell mass and pancreatic development.

Diabetes prevalence is increasing worldwide, and it is one of the most pressing public health issues due to the increased costs, comorbidity and mortality associated with diabetes. The exposure to diabetes in utero may create a vicious cycle where the offspring of diabetic mothers are more likely to develop obesity and glucose intolerance, leading to an increased risk of developing gestational diabetes or type 2 diabetes during pregnancy themselves, and therefore perpetuate a destructive cycle of metabolic dysfunction. Reducing obesity and type 2 diabetes must be a primary goal of public health organizations and clinicians.

Key words: Diabetes; Pregnancy; Insulin resistance; Obesity; Fetal programming; Gestational diabetes.

DIABETES IN PREGNANCY

Diabetes during pregnancy is a growing problem worldwide. Type 2 diabetes is increasing at an alarming rate *(1)* and is occurring in younger individuals more often than previously *(2)*, and as a result more women are being diagnosed with type 2 diabetes during their reproductive years. In addition, in several recent studies, gestational diabetes has also been shown to be increasing among all ethnic groups in the USA *(3, 4)*. Type 2 diabetes is a disease that clusters in families, and it therefore clearly has a genetic component; however, it is most often a polygenic disease, and the genes that contribute to the development of type 2 diabetes have not been fully identified *(5)*. Chap. 21 presents for further discussion of the genetic aspects. The recent increase in type 2 diabetes and gestational diabetes is greater than the increase that could be attributed to genetic causes, and so it is likely caused by a combination of environmental factors such as obesity, physical inactivity and poor diet. In addition to these postnatal factors, exposure to a diabetic intrauterine environment could be contributing to the increase in both type 2 and gestational diabetes.

In pregnancies complicated by diabetes, it is hypothesized that fetal exposure to excess fuels (glucose) can cause permanent fetal changes, which lead to malformations, macrosomia or increased birth weight, and increased risk of obesity, cardiovascular disease, hypertension and type 2 diabetes in later life. This hypothesis of fuel-mediated teratogenesis *(6, 7)* is now widely accepted, and there are data from both human epidemiologic studies and animal studies to support permanent effects of fetal nutrition on adult health. An excess of maternal transmission of type 2 diabetes *(8, 9)* also supports the hypothesis that the intrauterine environment, independent of genetic transmission, contributes to increased risk of type 2 diabetes in the offspring. Animal studies have demonstrated that the metabolic imprinting caused by the diabetic intrauterine environment can be transmitted across generations *(10–12)*. It has been suggested that a "vicious cycle" results, explaining at least in part the increases in type 2 and gestational diabetes seen over the past several decades.

This chapter reviews the evidence from human epidemiological and animal studies on the effect of maternal diabetes on fetal growth, metabolic imprinting and adult health. Possible mechanisms for these effects are reviewed, and the public health consequences and clinical implications are discussed.

EPIDEMIOLOGICAL STUDIES

Fetal Growth and Metabolic Consequences

Infants of diabetic mothers display excess fetal growth, often resulting in large-for-gestational age (LGA) or macrosomic *(13)* infants, consequently increasing the risk for cesarean delivery and traumatic birth injury *(14)*. Excess fetal growth is caused by increased substrate availability, including but not necessarily limited to glucose. While maternal glucose freely crosses the placenta, maternal insulin does not. As a result, the fetus receives excessive nutrition, and the fetal pancreas responds by producing increased insulin to meet the excessive glucose load. Insulin acts as a fetal growth hormone and promotes growth and adiposity *(7)*.

Alterations in the delivery of amino acids and upregulation of placental transport systems may also contribute to increased fetal growth, even in pregnancies with excellent glycemic control *(14)*. Even short periods of exposure to altered fetal nutrition have been demonstrated to cause persistent changes in placental growth and transport *(15)*.

It is thought that excessive fetal growth and other metabolic changes related to intrauterine exposure to diabetes can lead to increased adiposity in the offspring. There is evidence that increased adiposity is present at birth in infants of mothers with gestational diabetes. Catalano et al. *(16)* studied a group of 195 infants born to mothers with gestational diabetes and 220 infants of mothers with normal glucose tolerance and found that fat mass, but not birth weight or fat-free mass, was 20% higher in the infants exposed to diabetes in utero. Maternal fasting glucose level measured during the oral glucose tolerance test was the strongest correlate of infant adiposity, further supporting the hypothesis that the degree of hyperglycemia determines the metabolic effect on the neonate. The results of this study suggest that, even in the absence of LGA or macrosomia, exposure to the diabetic intrauterine milieu causes alterations in fetal growth patterns, which likely predispose these infants to being overweight and obese later in life.

The long-term effects of exposure to diabetes in utero on childhood growth and obesity have been studied prospectively in two groups: The Pima Indian Study and the Diabetes in Pregnancy Study at Northwestern University in Chicago. The Pima Indian Study *(17–19)* has been prospectively following women with diabetes during pregnancy and their offspring to examine the effects of in utero exposure to diabetes on the development of obesity as well as type 2 diabetes in the offspring. Pettitt et al. reported on relative weight to height in offspring of women with diabetes during pregnancy compared with offspring of nondiabetic and prediabetic women when the offspring were 5–19 years of age. The authors found that the children exposed to diabetes in utero were heavier than the offspring of both diabetic and prediabetic women. However, increased weight relative to height was present in offspring of women with diabetes during pregnancy regardless of birth weight, and the childhood weight was not correlated with birth weight in these children, in contrast to the offspring of nondiabetic and prediabetic women *(20)*.

At the Diabetes in Pregnancy Center at Northwestern University in Chicago, Silverman et al. studied infants born to women with gestational diabetes or preexisting (type 1 and type 2) diabetes during pregnancy from birth to 6 months of age, and then annually through the age of 8 *(21)*. Half of these infants exceeded the 90th percentile for birth weight, although by the age of 1 they were not significantly different from the general population in terms of height and weight. However, by 8 years of age the offspring of pregnancies complicated by diabetes had increased in adiposity again, so that half exceeded the 90th percentile for weight. At least some of this increase in adiposity could be explained by maternal obesity, as the childhood weight was correlated with maternal weight prior to pregnancy. However, obesity among the offspring was also independently correlated with amniotic fluid insulin levels during the third trimester, suggesting that the degree of fetal overnutrition during the prenatal period influenced later development of obesity in childhood.

Not all studies have shown as clear of an association between exposure to gestational diabetes and childhood adiposity (22, 23). Gillman et al. reported on obesity among 9–14-year-old offspring of mothers with gestational diabetes, with all data collected by questionnaire. In the Growing Up Today Study, children and adolescents reported their height and weight by mailed questionnaire, and these data were linked with questionnaire data collected from their mothers as part of the Nurses' Health Study regarding gestational diabetes, maternal weight and child's birth weight. In this study, each 1-kg increase in birth weight was associated with a 40% increased odds of being overweight (>95th percentile) as an adolescent, and even when maternal BMI and other potential mediators were taken into account, there remained a 30% increased odds of being overweight per 1-kg increase in birth weight. Exposure to gestational diabetes while in utero was also associated with a 40% increased odds of being overweight as an adolescent, although these odds were attenuated when further adjustments were made for birth weight (odds ratio 1.3, 95% confidence interval 0.9–1.9) and maternal BMI (odds ratio 1.2, 95% confidence interval 0.8–1.7). While these results suggest that any increase in childhood obesity associated with prenatal exposure to gestational diabetes is not independent of birth weight and maternal obesity, there are important limitations to this study. All data were collected by questionnaire, and so self-reported weight may be inaccurate. In addition, only about half of the mothers with children agreed to have the Study contact their children, and of the eligible children only 68% of the girls and 58% of the boys completed the questionnaires, for an overall response rate of approximately 34%.

In a retrospective chart review study, Whitaker et al. found no difference in the number of overweight (>85th percentile for weight) children ages 5–10 according to maternal gestational diabetes status (23). The inconsistency in these results may be partly explained by differences in exposure prevalence across populations studied, as the Pima Indians are a population with extremely high rates of obesity and diabetes, including during pregnancy. Further studies are needed to evaluate the effect of intrauterine diabetes exposure on fetal and childhood growth among different ethnic groups.

Abnormal Glucose Tolerance, Insulin Sensitivity and Insulin Secretion

Both insulin resistance and impaired insulin secretion can lead to impaired glucose tolerance (IGT), a metabolic abnormality in glucose homeostasis that often presents prior to the onset of type 2 diabetes (24). Several studies have examined whether IGT is more common among children who were exposed to diabetes in utero than in children born to mothers free from diabetes during pregnancy.

Among children aged 1–9 who were born to mothers with pregestational insulin-dependent diabetes or gestational diabetes, IGT was present in a total of 10.8% of children born to insulin-dependent mothers and 13.0% of children born to mothers with gestational diabetes (between groups comparison, NS) (25). The prevalence of IGT increased with age, with IGT found in 17.4% and 20% of children in the older age group (5–9 years of age) for the preexisting and gestational diabetes groups, respectively. Both groups had higher rates of IGT than are present in the general population (usually <5%). Despite similar prevalence of IGT, the authors noted that the offspring of mothers with gestational diabetes displayed reduced insulin secretion, while the offspring of insulin-dependent mothers were more insulin resistant (25).

Similarly, the Diabetes in Pregnancy Study at Northwestern University in Chicago enrolled multiethnic offspring of women with pregestational diabetes (both insulin-dependent and noninsulin-dependent) and gestational diabetes and evaluated them for postload glucose (26). Offspring of diabetic mothers who were 10–16 years old at evaluation (mean age 12.3 years) had a significantly higher prevalence of IGT than the age- and sex-matched control group (19.3% vs. 2.5%) (26). There was no difference in prevalence of IGT by type of diabetes (preexisting or gestational) during the pregnancy. In another study conducted in a lower risk population of primarily Caucasian children (mean age 9.1 years) born to mothers with gestational diabetes, the prevalence of IGT was 6.9% *(27)*, suggesting that IGT is increased by exposure to gestational diabetes in utero even among low-risk ethnic groups.

A smaller study evaluated insulin sensitivity using frequently sampled intravenous glucose tolerance tests among offspring 5–10 years of age born to mothers with type 1 and type 2 diabetes, as well as a group of control children. Reduced insulin sensitivity was seen only in the offspring of mothers with type 2 diabetes *(28)*.

The Pima Indian Study investigated whether insulin secretion and insulin action were associated with maternal diabetes diagnosed before vs. after pregnancy among adult offspring with normal glucose tolerance. While insulin action as measured by hyperinsulinemic euglycemic clamp did not differ, insulin secretion was reduced by 40% as measured by the acute insulin response among adult offspring exposed to diabetes in utero compared with those whose mothers developed diabetes after pregnancy *(29)*.

Type 2 Diabetes

Since 1965, Pima Indian women have had oral glucose tolerance tests during pregnancy, as well as outside pregnancy approximately every 2 years *(18, 30)*. As a result, extensive maternal diabetes information is available for the offspring of women who had diabetes before or during pregnancy (mothers with diabetes during pregnancy), for those mothers who developed diabetes only after pregnancy (prediabetic mothers), as well as for those who remained nondiabetic.

Figure 1 shows the prevalence of type 2 diabetes by age group in offspring of diabetic, prediabetic, and nondiabetic mothers *(31)*. At ages 5–9 and 10–14 years, diabetes was present almost exclusively among the offspring of women with pregnancies complicated by diabetes. In all age groups, there was significantly more diabetes in the offspring who were exposed to diabetes in utero than in the offspring of prediabetic and nondiabetic women. The prevalence of type 2 diabetes did not differ greatly between offspring of prediabetic and nondiabetic women. These small differences may be due to differences in the genes inherited from the mothers, whereas the large difference in prevalence between the offspring of diabetic and prediabetic mothers, who have presumably inherited the same genes from their

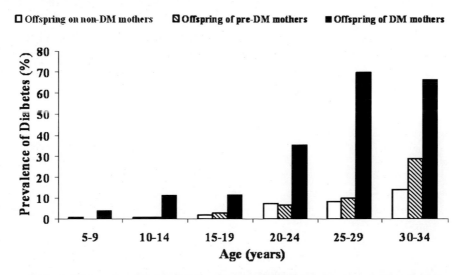

Fig. 1. Prevalence of type 2 diabetes, by mother's diabetes during and following pregnancy in Pima Indians aged 5–34 years. Reprinted from *(31)*. *DM* diabetes, *Open bars* offspring of nondiabetic mothers, *hatched bars* offspring of prediabetic mothers, *solid bars* offspring of diabetic mothers.

mothers, is the consequence of exposure to the diabetic intrauterine environment *(17)*. These differences persisted after adjusting for presence of diabetes in the father, age at onset of diabetes in either parent and obesity in the offspring.

Cardiovascular Abnormalities

There is evidence from animal studies that streptozotocin-induced diabetes during rat pregnancy is associated with cardiovascular dysfunction in adult offspring *(32)*. Diabetes is known to increase the risk of cardiovascular disease *(1)*, and poor intrauterine nutrition or growth appears to result in increased risk of hypertension and cardiovascular disease in adulthood. However, few human studies have examined the effect of a diabetic intrauterine environment on cardiovascular risk factors in the offspring.

Evidence of cardiovascular changes in pregnancies complicated by diabetes is already apparent during the third trimester of pregnancy, with the fetal heart showing reduced left ventricular size, function and contractility in diabetic vs. normal and hypertensive pregnancies *(33)*. These findings suggest that the diabetic intrauterine environment induces biochemical alterations in the cardiovascular system, and these changes are distinct from those caused by other poor uterine environments, such as the hypertensive pregnancy.

Several studies have also reported on the effects of diabetic pregnancy on development of cardiovascular risk factors later in childhood. The Diabetes in Pregnancy follow-up study in Chicago examined cardiovascular risk factors in children 10–14 years of age who were born to mothers with preexisting or gestational diabetes vs. children born to nondiabetic mothers. Children born to mothers with diabetes had significantly higher systolic, diastolic and mean arterial blood pressure than offspring of nondiabetic pregnancies *(21)*. Similarly, the Pima Indian investigators have shown that, independent of adiposity, 7–11-year-old offspring exposed to maternal diabetes during pregnancy have significantly higher systolic blood pressure than offspring of mothers who did not develop type 2 diabetes until after the index pregnancy *(34)*.

Manderson et al. examined cardiovascular risk factors and markers of endothelial dysfunction (ICAM-1, VCAM-1, E-Selectin) among offspring of mothers with type 1 diabetes compared with offspring of nondiabetic pregnancies *(35)*. The children were 5–11 years of age at the time of assessment, and pregnancy records were reviewed retrospectively. The offspring of mothers with type 1 diabetes did not differ significantly from the offspring of nondiabetic mothers on either socioeconomic or anthropometric parameters at the time of their examination. Despite similar levels of adiposity, children exposed to maternal type 1 diabetes in utero had increased insulin-like growth factor-1 (IGF-1), plasminogen activator inhibitor-1 (PAI-1), intercellular adhesion molecule-1 (ICAM-1), vascular cell adhesion molecule-1 (VCAM-1), and E-Selectin, as well as increased total cholesterol, LDL-cholesterol, and cholesterol/HDL-cholesterol ratio. The results of this study suggest that exposure to maternal type 1 diabetes during pregnancy is associated with an increase in dyslipidemia and markers of vascular inflammation in the offspring, both of which are linked with the development of cardiovascular disease in adulthood.

Together, these data suggest that in utero exposure to diabetes confers risks for the development of cardiovascular disease later in life that are independent of adiposity and may be in addition to genetic predisposition to diabetes.

Genetic Factors vs. Environment

Type 2 diabetes is a disease with familial clustering, and clearly there is a genetic component. In particular, early onset (<35 years of age) type 2 diabetes is associated with a more severe insulin secretion defect than older onset diabetes, suggesting that there may be genes associated with both early onset diabetes and more pronounced reduction in glucose-stimulated insulin secretion. As women who develop type 2 diabetes prior to pregnancy often have early onset diabetes, it is possible that these mothers might influence the risk of type 2 diabetes in their offspring through the transmission of this greater genetic susceptibility. Thus, the greater frequency of IGT, diabetes and obesity in the offspring of mothers with preexisting type 2 diabetes might be due to greater genetic susceptibility in such offspring rather than metabolic programing caused by in utero exposure to diabetes.

It is possible to disentangle the effects of genetic susceptibility vs. exposure to diabetes in utero in several ways. First, offspring of mothers who had early onset diabetes either before (diabetic mothers) or after pregnancy (prediabetic mothers) can be compared, as both groups of women will share similar genetic predisposition to type 2 diabetes and so differences in the offspring can be attributed to the diabetic intrauterine environment. Among the Pima Indians, offspring of mothers who were diagnosed with diabetes before the index pregnancy exhibited reduced insulin secretion than offspring born to mothers who developed diabetes at a similar age, but after the index pregnancy (29). In this same high-risk population, children who were exposed to diabetes during pregnancy were more likely to be obese than children born to prediabetic or nondiabetic mothers, and there was no difference in weight relative to height between the offspring of prediabetic vs. nondiabetic mothers (19). Finally, among Pima Indian children born to diabetic mothers, there was a higher prevalence of type 2 diabetes than among children who were not exposed to diabetes in utero, and 40% of the type 2 diabetes in children 5–19 years old could be attributed to the diabetic intrauterine environment (36).

Maternal obesity is a marker for genetic predisposition to type 2 diabetes. A second method to distinguish the effect of intrauterine exposure to diabetes from genetic susceptibility is to examine whether obesity in the offspring exposed to diabetes in utero is independent of maternal obesity. Among the Pima Indians, adjustment for maternal BMI does not explain the excess risk of obesity among children born to mothers with diabetes during pregnancy, supporting the hypothesis that fuel-mediated teratogenesis contributes independently to the development of obesity in offspring of diabetic pregnancy (19, 20).

Third, since fathers with early onset type 2 diabetes should contribute similar genetic susceptibility as mothers with early onset type 2 diabetes, the extent to which maternal transmission exceeds paternal transmission can be attributed to the intrauterine exposure to diabetes. An excess of maternal transmission of type 2 and gestational diabetes has been widely reported, suggesting an epigenetic transmission (8, 37). Further support for excess transmission of diabetes and obesity by mothers beyond what is expected based on genes is found in the results of the Pima Indian Studies, which demonstrate that the offspring of diabetic mothers have excess growth and obesity compared to the offspring of diabetic fathers (38). Additionally, McLean et al. found a twofold excess maternal transmission of gestational diabetes when they compared women with a family history of maternal, paternal, or both maternal and paternal type 2 diabetes and a control group of women with no family history of diabetes (39).

Similarly, the Framingham Offspring Study examined the risk for type 2 diabetes and abnormal glucose tolerance in offspring with maternal, paternal, both maternal and paternal, and no family history of type 2 diabetes. The risks of type 2 diabetes and abnormal glucose tolerance were similarly increased in offspring with maternal [OR 3.4 (2.3–4.9) and OR 2.7 (2.0–3.7), respectively] vs. paternal diabetes history [OR 3.5 (2.3–5.2) and OR 1.7 (1.2–2.4)] and were additive in offspring with both maternal and paternal diabetes [OR 6.1 (2.9–13.0) and OR 5.2 (2.6–10.5)] (5). However, the risk for type 2 diabetes among offspring with maternal early onset type 2 diabetes (<50 years of age) was increased dramatically [OR 9.7 (4.3–22.0)] as was the risk for abnormal glucose tolerance [OR 9.0 (4.2–19.7)] (5). Among offspring with paternal diabetes history, early onset of diabetes did not have the same effect on the odds of abnormal glucose tolerance and type 2 diabetes in the offspring (5).

These results are consistent with the theory that perinatal exposure to diabetes among some of the offspring of mothers with early onset type 2 diabetes is responsible for the dramatically increased odds of developing glucose homeostasis abnormalities in the offspring.

While the methods explored earlier provide strong evidence that genetic confounding does not explain all of the effects of maternal diabetes during pregnancy on the risk of obesity, IGT, and type 2 diabetes in the offspring, there are genetic mutations that have been shown to cause type 2 diabetes and are maternally transmitted *(40)*. Therefore, the ideal way to remove possible confounding by genetic predisposition is to examine sibling pairs in which one sibling is born before and one is born after the onset of their mother's diabetes. The Pima Indian Studies have examined the effect of intrauterine exposure to diabetes on both obesity and type 2 diabetes in discordant siblings *(30)*. Dabelea et al. found that the siblings born after the onset of the mother's diabetes, i.e., exposed to diabetes in utero, had significantly higher BMI (mean BMI difference: 2.6 kg) than their siblings who were not exposed to diabetes in utero. In contrast, there was no significant difference in BMI between siblings born before or after their father was diagnosed with type 2 DM (mean BMI difference: 0.4 kg/m^2) *(30)*. These data further support the hypothesis that the diabetic intrauterine milieu influences growth and body size independently of genetic predisposition.

In a similar study design, the prevalence of type 2 diabetes was compared in Pima Indian siblings born before and after their mother developed diabetes *(30)*. There were 19 nuclear families with sibling pairs (*n* = 28 pairs) discordant for both type 2 diabetes and exposure to a pregnancy complicated by diabetes. In 21 of the 28 sib pairs, the sibling who developed type 2 diabetes was born after the mother's diagnosis of diabetes and in only 7 of the 28 pairs was the sibling with type 2 diabetes born before (OR 3.0, *p* < 0.01). In contrast, among 84 siblings and 39 sib pairs from 24 families of diabetic fathers, the risk for type 2 diabetes was similar in the sib pairs born before and after father's diagnosis of diabetes. Since siblings born before and after a diabetic pregnancy are believed to carry a similar risk of inheriting the same susceptibility genes, the excess risk associated with maternal diabetes likely reflects the effect of intrauterine exposure associated with or directly due to hyperglycemia and/or other fuel alterations of a diabetic pregnancy.

The Growing Up Today Study *(22)*, on the other hand, found that there was a 40% increased odds of being overweight among 9–14-year-old offspring of mothers with gestational diabetes, but this association was no longer significant when adjustment was made for birth weight and reported maternal BMI, which is considered surrogate for genetic susceptibility for obesity. These findings suggest that either shared adverse lifestyle habits among mothers and daughters or maternal transmission of susceptibility genes account for part of the increased risk of obesity among offspring of mothers with gestational diabetes in addition to the intrauterine exposure to diabetes per se.

While most type 2 diabetes is thought to be a polygenic disorder, there are several monogenic types of diabetes such as MODY 3, linked to mutations in the hepatic nuclear factor-1alpha (*HNF-1α*) gene. Stride et al. *(41)* have shown that in persons with MODY 3 associated mutations in the *HNF-1α* gene, offspring of mothers with diabetes before pregnancy developed diabetes at a younger age than offspring of mothers who were diagnosed after the pregnancy (age of onset, 15 vs. 27 years). This suggests that epigenetic effects have an effect on the course of disease development, even in single gene disorders like HNF-1α MODY 3.

Interactions between the prenatal and postnatal environment have been reported to influence the risk of type 2 diabetes in offspring of pregnancies complicated by diabetes as well. An example is the report that among Pima Indians, breastfeeding attenuates the increased risk of developing type 2 diabetes in the offspring of mothers with diabetes (30.1% in children who were breastfed vs. 43.6% in bottle-fed children) *(38)*. These findings suggest that the risk of developing type 2 diabetes is a complex combination of prenatal, postnatal and genetic factors. Targets for prevention, therefore, may include reducing the effects of the diabetic intrauterine environment on fetal programing through stricter glycemic control, as well as encouragement of breastfeeding for infants born to mothers with diabetes during pregnancy.

Thus, there is evidence that exposure to the diabetic intrauterine environment, with alterations of fetal fuels and metabolic imprinting of the fetal beta cells, influences the risk and timing of the development of diabetes later in life. The effect of the intrauterine environment appears to be in addition to that of any inherited susceptibility genes, and the risk can be further modified by infant nutrition and other postnatal environmental factors.

Maternal Diabetes: Does It Matter Which Type?

Several studies have found that the effects of exposure to diabetes in utero on future obesity are similar for pregnancies complicated by preexisting type 1, type 2, or gestational diabetes *(19, 21)*. Weiss et al. *(42)* compared the offspring of women with type 1 diabetes to offspring of women without diabetes, and reported that at age 5–15 years they had significantly higher BMI, greater insulin resistance, and more than a threefold increased odds of type 2 diabetes. Amniotic fluid insulin levels were associated with offspring BMI and insulin resistance, further supporting the influence of the fetal metabolic environment on development of obesity and type 2 diabetes.

In a study of IGT in the offspring of mothers with type 1, type 2 and gestational diabetes, Silverman et al. found that the risk of IGT was not different by type of maternal diabetes *(26)*. Rather, IGT was closely related to the amniotic fluid insulin levels, which are indicative of the degree of fetal hyperinsulinemia. Sobngwi et al. also confirmed that IGT and defective insulin secretory response in adults are associated with exposure to pregestational type 1 diabetes in utero *(43)*. The control population in this study was a group of adult offspring of fathers with type 1 diabetes, in order to control for confounding by genetic susceptibility. These results further support the conclusion that hyperglycemia and other fuel alterations in pregnancies complicated by diabetes, and not the etiology of the mother's diabetes, are the important factors influencing risk of obesity and glucose metabolism abnormalities in the offspring.

In the Pima Indian population, Franks et al. found that maternal glucose levels are associated with excess fetal growth and later risk of diabetes even among women with normal glucose tolerance *(44)*. Birth weight was found to increase significantly with each standard deviation increase in maternal blood glucose level, and the risk of type 2 diabetes in the offspring increased 30% with each standard deviation increase in maternal glucose level. The presence of excess risk of metabolic abnormalities in offspring even in glucose-tolerant mothers suggests that exposure to hyperglycemia is a continuous risk factor, and prevention of long-term consequences in the offspring may require improvement in glycemia even in the absence of frank diabetes during pregnancy.

Animal Data

Animal studies have allowed for the investigation of experimentally manipulated intrauterine environment on metabolism and glucose homeostasis in the offspring, as well as the transmission of epigenetic traits across generations. Hyperglycemia during pregnancy can be easily induced by an injection of streptozotocin early in gestation. Alternatively, late effects of hyperglycemia can be obtained by continuous glucose infusion during the final week of gestation.

The induction of mild hyperglycemia in the rat by glucose infusion late in pregnancy mimics the effect of gestational diabetes in humans, where mild maternal hyperglycemia develops during the third trimester. In studies of the pregnant rat, offspring exposed to mild hyperglycemia while in utero display hyperinsulinism, accompanied by hyperplasia of the fetal pancreatic islet cells *(45, 46)*. Evidence of enhanced glucose-stimulated release of insulin was found *(46)*, suggesting that the fetus exposed to mild hyperglycemia adapted with a more efficient metabolic response, which allows for greater storage of body fat, therefore leading to excess fetal growth. Among adult offspring, pancreatic β-cell mass was not decreased, but an insulin secretion defect was evident *(47, 48)*, resulting in progressive glucose intolerance during adult life.

The induction of severe hyperglycemia by intravenous streptozotocin early in pregnancy has been used in rat models to model the effect of preexisting diabetes on the offspring. In contrast to human studies, animal studies of mothers with severe hyperglycemia during pregnancy generally demonstrate growth-restricted offspring, rather than macrosomic or LGA. Abnormalities in the beta cell development have been reported *(49)*, with increased mass and evidence of beta cell exhaustion likely secondary to overstimulation. In addition, these offspring demonstrate reduced glucose-stimulated insulin secretion, and insulin levels in the pancreas and plasma were reduced. Adult offspring show enhanced beta cell mass *(50)* but increased insulin resistance in response to euglycemic hyperinsulinemic clamp *(51, 52)*.

The development of a model of spontaneous type 2 diabetes in normal weight rats, the Goto–Kakizaki (GK) rat, has allowed for further clarification of genetic and environmental causes of type 2 diabetes. The GK rat was developed by selective breeding of nonobese Wistar rats with glucose tolerance at the upper range of normal. Repeated selective breeding over the course of several generations produced the GK rats, which as adults have lower body weight than Wistar rats and demonstrate mild fasting hyperglycemia *(53)*. Offspring of the GK rat are exposed to mild hyperglycemia during the pregnancy, and a 60% reduction in β-cell mass is found in the adult GK rat. This defect in pancreatic β cells appears to be related to abnormally decreased replication rather than increased apoptosis *(53, 54)*. In the human pancreas, the role of apoptosis vs. decreased replication is not clear, and this may limit the applicability of the GK rat model of type 2 diabetes to the human pancreas *(55)*. Excess maternal transmission of glucose intolerance has been reported in the GK rat *(11)*, confirming the role of intrauterine exposure to diabetes, although hyperglycemia during suckling was shown to have no effect on insulin secretion or β-cell mass in crossed wild-type and GK rats *(56)*.

MECHANISMS

Adipoinsular Axis

The mechanisms behind the metabolic effects of a diabetic intrauterine environment on exposed offspring are not entirely understood. In 1980, Freinkel's Banting Lecture focused on the hypothesis of fuel-mediated teratogenesis *(7)*, which suggests that permanent changes in fetal development occur as a result of exposure to altered maternal fuels in the mother with diabetes. Fetal growth is deranged in pregnancies complicated by diabetes *(57)*, and the excess growth appears to be mainly driven by increased adipose tissue *(16)*. The adipoinsular axis is a proposed endocrine feedback loop that connects the endocrine pancreas with the adipose tissue and the brain to regulate hunger and fat storage through the hormones, insulin and leptin. Insulin promotes fat mass and leptin production, while leptin acts to reduce energy intake and also suppresses insulin secretion via leptin receptors on pancreatic β cells. Abnormal functioning of this feedback loop may, therefore, lead to excess adiposity, hyperphagia, insulin resistance and hyperinsulinism. Hyperinsulinism and elevated leptin levels have been reported in fetuses exposed to diabetes in utero *(58, 59)*, suggesting that changes in the adipoinsular axis may be induced by maternal hyperglycemia.

The fetus exposed to excess maternal glucose produces high levels of insulin from the fetal pancreas, and high amniotic fluid insulin levels are associated with increased obesity and IGT in children exposed to a diabetic intrauterine environment (26, 42). Animal studies have suggested that fetal hyperinsulinism may cause abnormal development of the hypothalamus. In rats born to mothers with gestational diabetes, abnormal growth of the ventromedial hypothalamic nucleus was found, but it was able to be prevented by the restoration of maternal euglycemia by islet cell transplant (60). Dysplasia of the hypothalamus can result in obesity, hyperphagia and reduced insulin secretion, as the hypothalamic centers that control food intake and insulin secretion may be affected.

The degree of fetal hyperinsulinism reflects the maternal fuel excess being provided to the fetus, and so it is difficult to determine whether maternal hyperglycemia or fetal hyperinsulinism is responsible for the observed abnormalities. Studies in rhesus monkeys have been able to examine this question by delivering insulin subcutaneously by use of an implantable minipump in fetal rhesus monkeys born to mothers with normal glucose tolerance (61, 62). Reduced insulin secretion was reported in the offspring during the first several months of life and persisted past the neonatal period (63). This evidence further supports the hypothesis that fetal hyperinsulinism itself is responsible for metabolic changes in the offspring of the diabetic mother.

There is evidence from human studies that the degree of hyperinsulinism during fetal life is related to obesity during childhood. Among the Pima Indians, children who were exposed to abnormal maternal glucose tolerance while in utero had elevated fasting insulin levels at 5–9 years of age compared to children born to mothers with normal glucose tolerance (18). While these differences did not persist into later childhood, fasting insulin levels at 5–9 years of age were positively correlated with later weight gain (64).

The Diabetes in Pregnancy Center at Northwestern University followed women with gestational or preexisting diabetes and their offspring (21). Late in gestation, amniotic fluid was collected and stored for measurement of insulin levels. Amniotic fluid insulin levels reflect fetal insulin production. Offspring were evaluated for symmetry index, which is a measure of weight relative to height with a normal value of 1.0. Childhood obesity at 6–8 years of age as measured by the symmetry index was positively correlated with the amniotic fluid insulin levels in late pregnancy. Measurements of maternal glycemic control during pregnancy, on the other hand, were not related to childhood obesity (21). These results suggest that while fetal insulin secretion is stimulated by maternal glucose levels, it is the degree of fetal hyperinsulinism that is directly correlated with later obesity. There may be additional fuel abnormalities beyond maternal hyperglycemia that contribute to fetal hyperinsulinism in the diabetic intrauterine environment.

In addition to the alterations described in fetal insulin secretion, there is evidence that fetal leptin concentrations are affected by maternal diabetes during pregnancy. Leptin is a hormone that is thought to affect regulation of food intake, body weight and physical activity. Leptin is produced by adipocytes, and blood concentrations correlate with body weight and adiposity (65). Leptin is also produced in the placenta and is thought to play a role in the regulation of fetal growth beyond adiposity. Levels of leptin in cord blood are reported to be higher in neonates born to mothers with type 1 diabetes and gestational diabetes than in neonates born to women without diabetes, although these leptin levels did not correlate with maternal glycemic control or maternal leptin levels (66). In a similar study by Tapanainen et al., infants born to mothers with type 1 diabetes and gestational diabetes had elevated cord leptin levels compared to control infants, and insulin levels were highest in the offspring of mothers with type 1 diabetes and were elevated in the offspring of mothers with gestational diabetes compared to control infants (59). Leptin and insulin levels were correlated among both infants exposed to gestational diabetes and control infants, and birth weight was correlated with cord blood leptin concentrations in all infants studied (59). The results of these studies suggest that the elevated leptin levels found in neonates exposed to diabetes in utero may be related to the excess adipose tissue and hyperinsulinism found in these infants.

Cord blood levels of leptin are also correlated with birth weight in infants who were not exposed to a diabetic intrauterine environment, as demonstrated by Koistinen et al. (65). Leptin levels were compared in a group of infants born LGA, small for gestational age (SGA), and appropriate for gestational age (AGA), and leptin levels were highest in LGA and were reduced in SGA infants compared with AGA infants. Insulin and leptin levels were also correlated in these infants, demonstrating that these hormones are closely tied even among offspring not exposed to diabetes during pregnancy. The mechanism by which leptin is related to fetal growth is unknown, and Christou et al. examined cord leptin and its relationship to both insulin and insulin-like growth factor-I (IGF-I) in a group of AGA and LGA infants *(67)*. Leptin levels were elevated in LGA infants compared to AGA infants and correlated with insulin levels but not IGF-I. As a result, the authors conclude that leptin affects fetal growth independently of the IGF system.

Simmons and Breier examined leptin and insulin levels in infants born to mothers with and without gestational diabetes, among European, South Asian and Polynesian ethnic groups *(68)*. Leptin levels were increased in Polynesian neonates compared to the other ethnic groups studied, and this effect was independent of birth weight. However, among neonates exposed to gestational diabetes in utero, hyperleptinemia was also found, but the higher leptin levels were explained by differences in birth weight between the infants exposed and not exposed to gestational diabetes in utero. As a result, the authors concluded that excess maternal fuels, both glucose and other fuels, may lead to permanent changes to the adipoinsular axis. As a result, the offspring of mothers with diabetes may display leptin resistance, leading to both hyperleptinemia and hyperinsulinism due to the reduced ability of leptin to suppress insulin secretion. This resetting of the adipoinsular axis may then lead to increased fetal adiposity and obesity later in life.

Defective Insulin Secretion

Decreased insulin secretion in offspring of mothers with diabetes has been reported in both animal studies involving the GK rat *(48, 69)*, as well as human studies *(29, 43, 70)*. It is thought that exposure to excess maternal fuels during critical periods in fetal development may lead to permanent changes in physiology, referred to as "programming." In the course of fetal development, the endocrine pancreas begins developing at around 7–8 weeks of gestation, with evidence of insulin, glucagon and somatastatin coproduction *(71)*. Insulin and glucagon are produced by differentiated pancreatic islet cells during the second half of gestation *(72)*. The differentiation, proliferation, innervation and vascularization of the pancreatic islet cells, therefore, could be affected by an altered intrauterine environment during the second half of gestation.

The β-cell mass may be altered in the offspring of mothers with diabetes, dependent on the severity of the hyperglycemia. From animal studies, moderate maternal hyperglycemia has been demonstrated to increase proliferation of β cells, leading to enhanced β-cell mass. Severe hyperglycemia in sheep, on the other hand, is associated with degranulation of the β cell, decreased insulin content and reduced glucose-stimulated insulin secretion *(72)*.

Pancreatic angiogenesis and innervation may also be affected by maternal diabetes in utero. Pancreatic islet development is dependent on a number of growth factors, and vascularization of the islet cells is controlled by vascular endothelial growth factors (VEGFs) expressed by newly differentiated islet cells. Reduced angiogenesis in response to excess maternal fuels is a possible mechanism for reduced β-cell mass, since pancreatic growth is dependent on adequate vascularization. VEGF is regulated by glucose, and there is evidence from animal studies that maternal hyperglycemia can cause defects in angiogenesis in mouse embryos *(73)*. Similarly, the innervation of the pancreas may be altered by the intrauterine fuel availability, leading to changes in the function of the islet cells *(72)* such as glucose-stimulated insulin secretion. A number of other possible mechanisms could be involved in reduced insulin secretion in response to glucose, including altered ion channels, changes in glucokinase and GLUT 2, and reduced prohormone convertase 2 activity.

PUBLIC HEALTH AND CLINICAL IMPLICATIONS

Public Health Consequences

The prevalence of type 2 diabetes has increased dramatically among Pima Indian children, with at least a twofold increase reported over the past three decades *(70)*. During the same period of time, the proportion of offspring exposed to pregnancies complicated by diabetes increased as well, from 18.1% in 1967–1976 to 35.4% in 1987–1996. The proportion of type 2 diabetes among Pima Indian children, attributable to intrauterine exposure to diabetes, also increased approximately twofold between those time periods, accounting now for up to 40% of all type 2 diabetes cases among youth. The epigenetic transmission of diabetes from one generation to the next is evident in this population, where an "epidemic" of type 2 diabetes among children is almost entirely explained, statistically, by greater exposure to diabetic pregnancy in the population.

Increases in gestational diabetes among other ethnic groups have recently been reported as well, suggesting that the epidemic increase in diabetes is not confined to high-risk groups such as Native Americans. From 1991 to 2000, Ferrarra et al. reported a 3.5% per year increase in the incidence of gestational diabetes in Kaiser Permanente of Northern California *(4)*, and similarly a study conducted at Kaiser Permanente in Colorado reported an 11% annual increase in gestational diabetes from 1994 to 2002 *(3)*. Both of these studies found that the increase in gestational diabetes was present among *all* racial/ethnic groups. These findings are important evidences that the "vicious cycle" of diabetes being transmitted from one generation to the next may not be limited to high-risk groups such as the Pima Indians.

Among Pima Indians, the population with the highest prevalence of type 2 diabetes in the world, 70% of adults who were exposed to diabetes in utero developed type 2 diabetes by 25–34 years of age *(36)*. Because of their overall high risk of diabetes, the Pima Indians are perhaps the first group to evidence an increase in type 2 diabetes among children, but this epidemic is becoming apparent worldwide. According to the World Health Organization, it is estimated that diabetes will affect 200–300 million people across the world by 2025 *(1)*. It is widely thought that diabetes is the most pressing public health problem on the horizon, as this disease carries an enormous economic and healthcare burden. Approximately half of type 2 diabetes is thought to be attributable to genetic risk, while the other half is likely due to a combination of lifestyle and environmental factors, including prenatal exposures.

Public health efforts to prevent type 2 diabetes, therefore, should focus not only on adult lifestyle risk factors such as obesity and sedentary lifestyle, but also on prenatal exposure to overnutrition and diabetes in utero. Reduced obesity in women of reproductive age and prevention of excessive weight gain during pregnancy would reduce the risk of developing gestational diabetes in the mother and would likely also reduce the risk of excess fetal growth, high birth weight, and future obesity and diabetes in the offspring. Another potential target for public health policy is the encouragement of breastfeeding and healthy postnatal nutrition for infants, particularly among infants of women whose pregnancy was complicated by diabetes, as better postnatal nutrition can attenuate some of the effects of the diabetic intrauterine environment. More information is needed about the most effective public health measures to combat the worldwide epidemic of type 2 diabetes.

Clinical Health Care Concerns

The hypothesis of fuel-mediated teratogenesis suggests that excess fetal growth caused by maternal fuel abnormalities results in adult disease in the offspring, and so interventions to reduce the transmission of obesity, cardiovascular disease and type 2 diabetes would logically focus on normalizing maternal metabolism and fuel delivery to the infant. There is evidence that hyperglycemia increases fetal growth and also may induce other metabolic changes that are associated with adult chronic disease.

However, there is little information available regarding the optimal level of glycemic control needed to prevent metabolic changes in the offspring. Intensive treatment in women with gestational diabetes reduced birth weight, incidence of LGA, and incidence of macrosomia in infants born to mothers who participated in the intervention compared to in women who received routine care (74). To the extent to which reduced birth weight decreases the risk of long-term metabolic changes in the offspring, stricter glycemic control during pregnancies complicated by both gestational and preexisting diabetes may be an important clinical goal. However, more evidence is needed to determine optimal glucose levels during pregnancy to prevent metabolic disturbances in the offspring.

While excess glucose stimulates fetal insulin production and results in increased fetal growth and adiposity, fetal growth appears to be increased even in well-controlled pregnancies complicated by diabetes. It is, therefore, possible that, in addition to hyperglycemia, alterations in other maternal fuels or derangement in placental transport and metabolism of fuels are involved in fetal overgrowth. There is evidence that increased amino acids and free fatty acids are present in mothers with diabetes. In addition, placental transport and metabolism of amino acids and free fatty acids appear to be altered in diabetic pregnancy, and there may also be upregulation of placental gene expression, resulting in increased leptin and inflammatory markers. In pregnancies complicated by type 1 diabetes, excess fetal growth is associated not only with increased placental transport of glucose and amino acids, but also with increased placental lipoprotein lipase.

The available data suggest that the clinical management of women with diabetes during pregnancy may need to focus not only on achieving tight control of maternal blood glucose levels, but also on additional dietary or other changes, which may be helpful to address given the contribution of other maternal fuel abnormalities such as alterations in amino acids and free fatty acids. In addition, maternal obesity and weight gain during pregnancy contribute to fetal overgrowth, and adjustment for maternal obesity attenuates some of the effects of exposure to intrauterine diabetes on obesity and type 2 diabetes risk in the offspring. In a study of intensive treatment of women with gestational diabetes, women in the intervention group gained significantly less weight during the course of the pregnancy than women who received routine care, and this reduced weight gain probably explains at least part of the lower incidence of LGA and macrosomia in the offspring of intensively treated mothers (74).

Much more information is needed regarding the most effective strategies to address both public health and clinical care concerns regarding exposure to diabetes in utero on the metabolism and risk of chronic diseases in the infant of the diabetic mother. The epidemic of diabetes carries enormous costs, both in terms of economic and health burdens. The development of diabetes and obesity is of great clinical concern, as these disorders not only have a direct impact on an individual's health but are also associated with the development of cardiovascular disease and some cancers. Reducing obesity and type 2 diabetes should therefore be a primary goal of public health organizations and clinicians.

REFERENCES

1. Hussain A, Claussen B, Ramachandran A, Williams R. Prevention of type 2 diabetes: a review. Diabetes Res Clin Pract 2007; 76:317–26
2. Dabelea D, Pettitt DJ, Jones KL, Arslanian SA. Type 2 diabetes mellitus in minority children and adolescents. An emerging problem. Endocrinol Metab Clin North Am 1999; 28:709–29, viii
3. Dabelea D, Snell-Bergeon JK, Hartsfield CL, Bischoff KJ, Hamman RF, McDuffie RS; Kaiser Permanente of Colorado GDM Screening Program. Increasing prevalence of gestational diabetes mellitus (GDM) over time and by birth cohort: Kaiser Permanente of Colorado GDM Screening Program. Diabetes Care 2005; 28:579–84
4. Ferrara A, Kahn HS, Quesenberry CP, Riley C, Hedderson MM. An increase in the incidence of gestational diabetes mellitus: Northern California, 1991–2000. Obstet Gynecol 2004; 103:526–33

5. Meigs JB, Cupples LA, Wilson PW. Parental transmission of type 2 diabetes: the Framingham Offspring Study. Diabetes 2000; 49:2201–7

6. Plagemann A. 'Fetal programming' and 'functional teratogenesis': on epigenetic mechanisms and prevention of perinatally acquired lasting health risks. J Perinat Med 2004; 32:297–305

7. Freinkel N. Banting Lecture 1980. Of pregnancy and progeny. Diabetes 1980; 29:1023–35

8. Dorner G, Mohnike A, Steindel E. On possible genetic and epigenetic modes of diabetes transmission. Endokrinologie 1975; 66:225–7

9. Martin AO, Simpson JL, Ober C, Freinkel N. Frequency of diabetes mellitus in mothers of probands with gestational diabetes: possible maternal influence on the predisposition to gestational diabetes. Am J Obstet Gynecol 1985; 151:471–5

10. Aerts L, Van Assche FA. Animal evidence for the transgenerational development of diabetes mellitus. Int J Biochem Cell Biol 2006; 38:894–903

11. Gauguier D, Nelson I, Bernard C, Parent V, Marsac C, Cohen D, et al. Higher maternal than paternal inheritance of diabetes in GK rats. Diabetes 1994; 43:220–4

12. Gill-Randall RJ, Adams D, Ollerton RL, Alcolado JC. Is human Type 2 diabetes maternally inherited? Insights from an animal model. Diabet Med 2004; 21:759–62

13. Lampl M, Jeanty P. Exposure to maternal diabetes is associated with altered fetal growth patterns: a hypothesis regarding metabolic allocation to growth under hyperglycemic-hypoxemic conditions. Am J Hum Biol 2004; 16:237–63

14. Jansson T, Cetin I, Powell TL, Desoye G, Radaelli T, Ericsson A, et al. Placental transport and metabolism in fetal overgrowth – a workshop report. Placenta 2006; 27(Suppl A):S109–13

15. Ericsson A, Saljo K, Sjostrand E, Jansson N, Prasad PD, Powell TL, et al. Brief hyperglycaemia in the early pregnant rat increases fetal weight at term by stimulating placental growth and affecting placental nutrient transport. J Physiol 2007; 581(3):1323–1332

16. Catalano PM, Thomas A, Huston-Presley L, Amini SB. Increased fetal adiposity: a very sensitive marker of abnormal in utero development. Am J Obstet Gynecol 2003; 189:1698–704

17. Pettitt DJ, Nelson RG, Saad MF, Bennett PH, Knowler WC. Diabetes and obesity in the offspring of Pima Indian women with diabetes during pregnancy. Diabetes Care 1993; 16:310–4

18. Pettitt DJ, Bennett PH, Saad MF, Charles MA, Nelson RG, Knowler WC. Abnormal glucose tolerance during pregnancy in Pima Indian women. Long-term effects on offspring. Diabetes 1991; 40(Suppl 2):126–30

19. Pettitt DJ, Baird HR, Aleck KA, Bennett PH, Knowler WC. Excessive obesity in offspring of Pima Indian women with diabetes during pregnancy. N Engl J Med 1983; 308:242–5

20. Pettitt DJ, Knowler WC, Bennett PH, Aleck KA, Baird HR. Obesity in offspring of diabetic Pima Indian women despite normal birth weight. Diabetes Care 1987; 10:76–80

21. Silverman BL, Rizzo T, Green OC, Cho NH, Winter RJ, Ogata ES, et al. Long-term prospective evaluation of offspring of diabetic mothers. Diabetes 1991; 40(Suppl 2):121–5

22. Gillman MW, Rifas-Shiman S, Berkey CS, Field AE, Colditz GA. Maternal gestational diabetes, birth weight, and adolescent obesity. Pediatrics 2003; 111:e221–6

23. Whitaker RC, Pepe MS, Seidel KD, Wright JA, Knopp RH. Gestational diabetes and the risk of offspring obesity. Pediatrics 1998; 101:E9

24. Petersen JL, McGuire DK. Impaired glucose tolerance and impaired fasting glucose--a review of diagnosis, clinical implications and management. Diab Vasc Dis Res 2005; 2:9–15

25. Plagemann A, Harder T, Kohlhoff R, Rohde W, Dorner G. Glucose tolerance and insulin secretion in children of mothers with pregestational IDDM or gestational diabetes. Diabetologia 1997; 40:1094–100

26. Silverman BL, Metzger BE, Cho NH, Loeb CA. Impaired glucose tolerance in adolescent offspring of diabetic mothers. Relationship to fetal hyperinsulinism. Diabetes Care 1995; 18:611–7

27. Malcolm JC, Lawson ML, Gaboury I, Lough G, Keely E. Glucose tolerance of offspring of mother with gestational diabetes mellitus in a low-risk population. Diabet Med 2006; 23:565–70

28. Hunter WA, Cundy T, Rabone D, Hofman PL, Harris M, Regan F, et al. Insulin sensitivity in the offspring of women with type 1 and type 2 diabetes. Diabetes Care 2004; 27:1148–52

29. Gautier JF, Wilson C, Weyer C, Mott D, Knowler WC, Cavaghan M, et al. Low acute insulin secretory responses in adult offspring of people with early onset type 2 diabetes. Diabetes 2001; 50:1828–33

30. Dabelea D, Hanson RL, Lindsay RS, Pettitt DJ, Imperatore G, Gabir MM, et al. Intrauterine exposure to diabetes conveys risks for type 2 diabetes and obesity: a study of discordant sibships. Diabetes 2000; 49:2208–11

31. Dabelea D, Pettitt DJ. Intrauterine diabetic environment confers risks for type 2 diabetes mellitus and obesity in the offspring, in addition to genetic susceptibility. J Pediatr Endocrinol Metab 2001; 14:1085–91

32. Holemans K, Gerber RT, Meurrens K, De Clerck F, Poston L, Van Assche FA. Streptozotocin diabetes in the pregnant rat induces cardiovascular dysfunction in adult offspring. Diabetologia 1999; 42:81–9

33. Rasanen J, Kirkinen P. Growth and function of human fetal heart in normal, hypertensive and diabetic pregnancy. Acta Obstet Gynecol Scand 1987; 66:349–53

34. Bunt JC, Tataranni PA, Salbe AD. Intrauterine exposure to diabetes is a determinant of hemoglobin A(1)c and systolic blood pressure in pima Indian children. J Clin Endocrinol Metab 2005; 90:3225–9

35. Manderson JG, Mullan B, Patterson CC, Hadden DR, Traub AI, McCance DR. Cardiovascular and metabolic abnormalities in the offspring of diabetic pregnancy. Diabetologia 2002; 45:991–6

36. Dabelea D, Knowler WC, Pettitt DJ. Effect of diabetes in pregnancy on offspring: follow-up research in the Pima Indians. J Matern Fetal Med 2000; 9:83–8

37. Harder T, Franke K, Kohlhoff R, Plagemann A. Maternal and paternal family history of diabetes in women with gestational diabetes or insulin-dependent diabetes mellitus type I. Gynecol Obstet Invest 2001; 51:160–4

38. Pettitt DJ, Knowler WC. Long-term effects of the intrauterine environment, birth weight, and breast-feeding in Pima Indians. Diabetes Care 1998; 21(Suppl 2):B138–41

39. McLean M, Chipps D, Cheung NW. Mother to child transmission of diabetes mellitus: does gestational diabetes program Type 2 diabetes in the next generation? Diabet Med 2006; 23:1213–5

40. Perucca-Lostanlen D, Narbonne H, Hernandez JB, Staccini P, Saunieres A, Paquis-Flucklinger V, et al. Mitochondrial DNA variations in patients with maternally inherited diabetes and deafness syndrome. Biochem Biophys Res Commun 2000; 277:771–5

41. Stride A, Shepherd M, Frayling TM, Bulman MP, Ellard S, Hattersley AT. Intrauterine hyperglycemia is associated with an earlier diagnosis of diabetes in HNF-1alpha gene mutation carriers. Diabetes Care 2002; 25:2287–91

42. Weiss PA, Scholz HS, Haas J, Tamussino KF, Seissler J, Borkenstein MH. Long-term follow-up of infants of mothers with type 1 diabetes: evidence for hereditary and nonhereditary transmission of diabetes and precursors. Diabetes Care 2000; 23:905–11

43. Sobngwi E, Boudou P, Mauvais-Jarvis F, Leblanc H, Velho G, Vexiau P, et al. Effect of a diabetic environment in utero on predisposition to type 2 diabetes. Lancet 2003; 361:1861–5

44. Franks PW, Looker HC, Kobes S, Touger L, Tataranni PA, Hanson RL, et al. Gestational glucose tolerance and risk of type 2 diabetes in young Pima Indian offspring. Diabetes 2006; 55:460–5

45. Bihoreau MT, Ktorza A, Kervran A, Picon L. Effect of gestational hyperglycemia on insulin secretion in vivo and in vitro by fetal rat pancreas. Am J Physiol 1986; 251:E86–91

46. Kervran A, Guillaume M, Jost A. The endocrine pancreas of the fetus from diabetic pregnant rat. Diabetologia 1978; 15:387–93

47. Bihoreau MT, Ktorza A, Kinebanyan MF, Picon L. Impaired glucose homeostasis in adult rats from hyperglycemic mothers. Diabetes 1986; 35:979–84

48. Aerts L, Sodoyez-Goffaux F, Sodoyez JC, Malaisse WJ, Van Assche FA. The diabetic intrauterine milieu has a long-lasting effect on insulin secretion by β cells and on insulin uptake by target tissues. Am J Obstet Gynecol 1988; 159:1287–92

49. Aerts L, Holemans K, Van Assche FA. Maternal diabetes during pregnancy: consequences for the offspring. Diabetes Metab Rev 1990; 6:147–67

50. Aerts L, Vercruysse L, Van Assche FA. The endocrine pancreas in virgin and pregnant offspring of diabetic pregnant rats. Diabetes Res Clin Pract 1997; 38:9–19

51. Holemans K, Aerts L, Van Assche FA. Evidence for an insulin resistance in the adult offspring of pregnant streptozotocin-diabetic rats. Diabetologia 1991; 34:81–5

52. Holemans K, Van Bree R, Verhaeghe J, Aerts L, Van Assche FA. In vivo glucose utilization by individual tissues in virgin and pregnant offspring of severely diabetic rats. Diabetes 1993; 42:530–6

53. Portha B. Programmed disorders of beta-cell development and function as one cause for type 2 diabetes? The GK rat paradigm. Diabetes Metab Res Rev 2005; 21:495–504

54. Serradas P, Gangnerau MN, Giroix MH, Saulnier C, Portha B. Impaired pancreatic beta cell function in the fetal GK rat. Impact of diabetic inheritance. J Clin Invest 1998; 101:899–904

55. Portha B, Lacraz G, Kergoat M, Homo-Delarche F, Giroix MH, Bailbe D, et al. The GK rat beta-cell: a prototype for the diseased human beta-cell in type 2 diabetes? Mol Cell Endocrinol 2009; 297(1–2):73–85

56. Calderari S, Gangnerau MN, Meile MJ, Portha B, Serradas P. Is defective pancreatic beta-cell mass environmentally programmed in Goto-Kakizaki rat model of type 2 diabetes?: insights from crossbreeding studies during suckling period. Pancreas 2006; 33:412–7

57. Pedersen J. Weight and length at birth of infants of diabetic mothers. Acta Endocrinol (Copenh) 1954; 16:330–42

58. Manderson JG, Patterson CC, Hadden DR, Traub AI, Leslie H, McCance DR. Leptin concentrations in maternal serum and cord blood in diabetic and nondiabetic pregnancy. Am J Obstet Gynecol 2003; 188:1326–32

59. Tapanainen P, Leinonen E, Ruokonen A, Knip M. Leptin concentrations are elevated in newborn infants of diabetic mothers. Horm Res 2001; 55:185 90

60. Harder T, Aerts L, Franke K, Van Bree R, Van Assche FA, Plagemann A. Pancreatic islet transplantation in diabetic pregnant rats prevents acquired malformation of the ventromedial hypothalamic nucleus in their offspring. Neurosci Lett 2001; 299:85–8

61. Susa JB, Boylan JM, Sehgal P, Schwartz R. Impaired insulin secretion after intravenous glucose in neonatal rhesus monkeys that had been chronically hyperinsulinemic in utero. Proc Soc Exp Biol Med 1992; 199:327–31

62. Susa JB, Boylan JM, Sehgal P, Schwartz R. Impaired insulin secretion in the neonatal rhesus monkey after chronic hyperinsulinemia in utero. Proc Soc Exp Biol Med 1990; 194:209–15

63. Susa JB, Boylan JM, Sehgal P, Schwartz R. Persistence of impaired insulin secretion in infant rhesus monkeys that had been hyperinsulinemic in utero. J Clin Endocrinol Metab 1992; 75:265–9

64. Odeleye OE, de Courten M, Pettitt DJ, Ravussin E. Fasting hyperinsulinemia is a predictor of increased body weight gain and obesity in Pima Indian children. Diabetes 1997; 46:1341–5

65. Koistinen HA, Koivisto VA, Andersson S, Karonen SL, Kontula K, Oksanen L, et al. Leptin concentration in cord blood correlates with intrauterine growth. J Clin Endocrinol Metab 1997; 82:3328–30

66. Persson B, Westgren M, Celsi G, Nord E, Ortqvist E. Leptin concentrations in cord blood in normal newborn infants and offspring of diabetic mothers. Horm Metab Res 1999; 31:467–71

67. Christou H, Connors JM, Ziotopoulou M, Hatzidakis V, Papathanassoglou E, Ringer SA, et al. Cord blood leptin and insulin-like growth factor levels are independent predictors of fetal growth. J Clin Endocrinol Metab 2001; 86:935–8

68. Simmons D, Breier BH. Fetal overnutrition in Polynesian pregnancies and in gestational diabetes may lead to dysregulation of the adipoinsular axis in offspring. Diabetes Care 2002; 25:1539–44

69. Gauguier D, Bihoreau MT, Picon L, Ktorza A. Insulin secretion in adult rats after intrauterine exposure to mild hyperglycemia during late gestation. Diabetes 1991; 40(Suppl 2):109–14

70. Dabelea D, Hanson RL, Bennett PH, Roumain J, Knowler WC, Pettitt DJ. Increasing prevalence of Type II diabetes in American Indian children. Diabetologia 1998; 41:904–10

71. Polak M, Bouchareb-Banaei L, Scharfmann R, Czernichow P. Early pattern of differentiation in the human pancreas. Diabetes 2000; 49:225–32

72. Fowden AL, Hill DJ. Intra-uterine programming of the endocrine pancreas. Br Med Bull 2001; 60:123–42

73. Pinter E, Haigh J, Nagy A, Madri JA. Hyperglycemia-induced vasculopathy in the murine conceptus is mediated via reductions of VEGF-A expression and VEGF receptor activation. Am J Pathol 2001; 158:1199–206

74. Crowther CA, Hiller JE, Moss JR, McPhee AJ, Jeffries WS, Robinson JS; Australian Carbohydrate Intolerance Study in Pregnant Women (ACHOIS) Trial Group. Effect of treatment of gestational diabetes mellitus on pregnancy outcomes. N Engl J Med 2005; 352:2477–86

21

The Genetic Basis of Diabetes

Hui-Qi Qu and Constantin Polychronakos

CONTENTS

ABSTRACT

Genetic susceptibility to type 1 diabetes (DM1) and type 2 diabetes (DM2) is determined by complex genetic factors. Until recently, only a few loci were known, but this is changing rapidly as a result of the development of high-density genotyping arrays that have permitted genome-wide association studies. Several recent reports of such studies have increased our understanding of the genetics of diabetes by increasing the number of known loci to more than ten for each type of diabetes. The known DM1 genes are mainly involved in central immunotolerance in the thymus and in immune injury in the pancreas. The known DM2 genes are mainly involved in pancreatic β-cell function and peripheral insulin sensitivity. Compared with DM1 and DM2, monogenic diabetes is much rarer, and in most cases these genetics have been elucidated with classical genetic approaches. The novel physiologic insights derived from these new discoveries are discussed.

Key words: Diabetes; Genetics; Metabolism; Hyperglycemia; Pregnancy; Autoimmunity; Insulin.

ABBREVIATIONS

A	adenosine
ABCC8	the gene encoding SUR1, a modulator of K⁺-ATP channels
APC	antigen presenting cell
C	cytosine
c-Cbl	an adaptor protein for receptor protein-tyrosine kinases
CDK2	a gene encoding a member of the Ser/Thr protein kinase family
CDKAL1	the cyclin-dependent kinase 5 regulatory subunit associated protein 1-like 1 gene

From: *Diabetes in Women: Pathophysiology and Therapy*
Edited by: A. Tsatsoulis et al. (eds.), DOI 10.1007/978-1-60327-250-6_21
© Humana Press, a part of Springer Science+Business Media, LLC 2009

CDKN2A	the cyclin-dependent kinase inhibitor 2A gene
CDKN2B	the cyclin-dependent kinase inhibitor 2B gene
CEL	the carboxyl ester lipase gene
GCG	the proglucagon gene
Chr1–22	chromosomes 1–22
CLEC16A	the C-type lectin 16A gene
CTLA4	the cytotoxic T-lymphocyte-associated protein 4 gene
CYP27B1	the cytochrome P450, subfamily XXVIIB, polypeptide 1 gene
Csk	C-terminal Src kinase
DNA	deoxyribonucleic acid
EGFR	epidermal growth factor receptor
ERBB3	a gene encoding a member of the EGFR family of receptor tyrosine kinases
FTO	the fat mass and obesity-associated gene
G	guanine
GCK	the glucokinase gene
GDM	gestational diabetes mellitus
GLP1	glucagon-like peptide 1
GSIS	glucose-stimulated insulin secretion
GvHD	graft versus host disease
GWA	genome-wide association
HHEX	the hematopoietically expressed homeobox gene
HLA	the human leukocyte antigen genes
HNF1A	the hepatocyte nuclear factor-1 (HNF1) homeobox A gene
HNF1B	the hepatocyte nuclear factor-1 (HNF1) homeobox B gene
HNF4A	the hepatocyte nuclear factor 4, alpha gene
IDE	the insulin-degrading enzyme gene
IFIH1	the interferon induced with helicase C domain 1 gene
IGF2BP2	the insulin-like growth factor 2 mRNA binding protein 2 gene
IKZF4	a gene encoding a zinc finger protein specifically expressed in lymphocytes and implicated in the control of lymphoid development
IL2	interleukin-2
IL2RA	the interleukin-2 receptor alpha gene
INS	the insulin gene
INSR	the insulin receptor gene
IPF1	insulin promoter factor 1
ITPR3	the inositol 1,4,5-triphosphate receptor type 3 gene
JIA	juvenile idiopathic arthritis
KCNJ11	the potassium inwardly rectifying channel, subfamily J, member 11 gene
KIAA0350	see *CLEC16A*
KLF11	the Kruppel-like factor 11 gene
LD	linkage disequilibrium
LNK	lymphocyte adaptor protein, also known as SH2B adaptor protein 3
Lyp	lymphoid phosphatase
MODY	maturity-onset diabetes of the young
NEUROD1	the neurogenic differentiation 1 gene
NK	natural killer cell
NOD	nonobese diabetic mouse model

nsSNP	nonsynonymous SNPs
OAS1	the 2′,5′-oligoadenylate synthetase 1 gene
PBMC	peripheral blood mononuclear cell
PCOS	polycystic ovarian syndrome
PDX1	the pancreatic and duodenal homeobox 1 gene
PEP	the mouse ortholog of Lyp
PHTF1	the putative homeodomain transcription factor 1 gene
PNDM	permanent neonatal diabetes mellitus
PPARG	the peroxisome proliferator-activated receptor gamma gene
PRE	peroxisome proliferator response element
PTF1A	the pancreas specific transcription factor 1a gene
PTK	protein tyrosine kinase
PTPN2	the lymphoid protein tyrosine phosphatase, nonreceptor type 2 gene
PTPN22	the lymphoid protein tyrosine phosphatase, nonreceptor type 22 gene
RA	rheumatoid arthritis
RAB5B	a member of the *RAS* oncogene family
RPGRIP1L	the retinitis pigmentosa GTPase regulator interacting protein 1-like gene
RSBN1	round spermatid basic protein 1, also known as *FLJ11220*
RXR	retinoid X receptor
SH2B3	codes for SH2B adaptor protein 3, also known as LNK, lymphocyte adaptor protein
SLC30A8	the solute carrier family 30 (zinc transporter) gene
SLE	systemic lupus erythematosus
SNP	single-nucleotide polymorphism
SUMO4	I kappa B alpha modifier gene
SUOX	a gene encoding a liver-specific sulfite oxidase
SUR1	a modulator of K+-ATP channels
T	thymine
DM1	type 1 diabetes
DM2	type 2 diabetes
TAP2	the transport 2, ATP-binding cassette, subfamily B gene
TCF7L2	the transcription factor 7-like 2 gene
TCR	T cell receptor
TDT	transmission disequilibrium test
TNDM	transient neonatal diabetes mellitus
TZD	thiazolidinediones
VDR	the vitamin D receptor gene
VNTR	variable number tandem repeats

INTRODUCTION

Genetic Variations

Genetic variation in the human population confers varied susceptibilities to genetic diseases on each individual. This is clearly the case for diabetes. For a gene to confer diabetes genetic susceptibility, there are two basic requirements. First, the gene must have a function in the pathogenetic mechanism. Second, there must be deoxyribonucleic acid (DNA) variation(s) changing the gene's function.

DNA is the genetic basis of all living organisms. A DNA molecule comprises a long chain of nucleotides, with each nucleotide containing one of the four bases, that is, adenine (A), cytosine (C), guanine (G), or thymine (T). In human genome, DNA sequences exist in a form of a double-helix structure. All together approximately three billion DNA base pairs *(1)* are distributed in 22 pairs of autosomes and two sex chromosomes (X and Y). Chromosomes are numbered 1 (Chr1) to 22, from longest to shortest. Around 20,000–25,000 protein-coding genes are encoded in human nuclear genome *(2)*. In addition to the nuclear genome, there is the small circular DNA molecule comprising the human mitochondrial genome. The human mitochondrial genome is around 16.6 kilo base pairs (kb) in length, with variable copy numbers in cells of different tissues. Thirty-seven genes encoded by the mitochondrial genome have been described.

The most common form of DNA variation in the human genome is the change of a single base. The frequency of these sequence variants can range from very rare to 50% (in which case the two alleles have equal frequencies). These are called single-nucleotide polymorphisms (SNPs). SNPs with frequencies >1% occur every 100–300 bases along the human genome and are the most studied DNA variations. Most SNPs in the genome have no impact on gene function. SNPs may change the gene's function by causing an amino acid change in a peptide (i.e., a nonsynonymous SNP) or by regulating gene expression and/or alternative splicing. Compared with the original nucleotide, the substituted nucleotide may correspond to either enhanced (gain) or impaired (loss) gene function (Fig. 1).

Besides SNPs, there are other types of common genetic polymorphisms, such as tandem repeat polymorphisms and insertion/deletion polymorphisms. Any type of polymorphism can change the susceptibility to a genetic disease (or a phenotypic trait) through gene function change. In most cases, a polymorphism-associated disease is not inherited in a Mendelian fashion because polymorphisms from many different genes must contribute to the disease (genetically complex disease). Gene function change from a polymorphism can be seen in healthy individuals. On the contrary, a Mendelian inherited (monogenic) disease from a single abnormal gene is usually a rare mutation with dramatic impact on the gene function.

Genetic Variations and Diabetes

There is ample evidence showing that type 1 diabetes (DM1) and type 2 diabetes (DM2) are complex genetic diseases *(3, 4)*. For both DM1 and DM2, the concordance rate of monozygotic twins is much higher than that of dizygotic twins. In DM1, the concordance rate for monozygotic twins is reported to range between 21 and 70% and that for dizygotic twins to range between 0 and 13% *(5)*. In DM2, the concordance rate for monozygotic twins is 63%, and for dizygotic twins it is 43% *(6)*. In addition, for both DM1 and DM2, the sibling of a patient has much higher risk than the general population. The risk to siblings of type 1 diabetic individuals is about 6%, compared to about 0.4% in the general European population *(4)*. Siblings of individuals with DM2 have about fourfold to sixfold higher risk than a random individual *(3)*. However, although the genetic nature of the common types of diabetes is obvious, the pathogenesis is complicated, involving multiple genes, environment

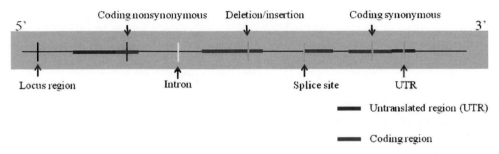

Fig. 1. SNP classification.

factors, and the interaction of genes and environment. At the same time, rare types of diabetes, with Mendelian inheritance from rare mutations, are also known.

There are two general methods used to locate diabetes genes, that is, linkage study and association study. A linkage study examines the genome regions shared by affected relatives, based on the coseg-regation of genes found together in close proximity on a chromosome. An association study examines the coexistence of genetic markers with the disease. There are two types of association study, that is, the population-based study using a case-control format and the family-based study using the transmission disequilibrium test (TDT). Compared with the family-based study, the population-based study has relatively higher statistical power, that is, less demanding on the sample size. However, the population-based study can suffer from bias from population stratification. Population stratification occurs when there are multiple subgroups with different allele frequencies within a population. The different underlying allele frequencies in sampled subgroups might be independent of the disease and can lead to erroneous conclusions of disease relevance *(7)*. The advantage of a family-based study is that it is immune to the bias from population stratification. But in many cases, it is hard to collect complete family samples, especially for, late onset genetic diseases, such as DM2.

Association studies are more powerful, but each marker covers a very small part of the genome and must be well targeted. Marker targeting has been done in three ways: (1) Association studies can follow a linkage study. The genetic regions identified by linkage typically extend over several megabases and include many genes inside the region. Therefore, following the linkage study, an association study is needed to pinpoint the disease causative gene. (2) Association studies can use a candidate gene approach. For a candidate gene implicated in a disease, an association study can address its disease causative effect, no matter whether the gene is located in an interesting region from linkage study. Successful examples of this approach are the DM1 genes *INS(8)*, *PTPN22(9)*, and *IL2RA(10)*. (3) Most recently there are genome-wide association (GWA) studies. Taking advantage of the recent availability of high-throughput genotyping platforms, for example, the *Illumina* Beadarray and the *Affymetrix* GeneChips, researchers are able to screen the whole genome for disease associations with high-density coverage. This has rapidly accelerated diabetes gene discovery in the past year or two. In what follows, we will discuss the genetic basis of different types of diabetes in detail, based largely on recent progress.

TYPE 1 DIABETES

Type 1 diabetes (DM1) is characterized by autoimmune destruction of the pancreatic β cells. The pathogenesis of DM1 involves loss of self-tolerance to pancreatic β-cell autoantigens, either centrally in the thymus or in the periphery, resulting in immune injury in pancreas. Using a national registry in Finland of 5,291 offspring of a parent with DM1, the cumulative incidence of developing DM1 up to the age of 20 was 6.7% *(11)*. The offspring's risk of developing DM1 was higher for offspring of fathers with DM1 (7.8%) than for mothers with DM1 (5.3%). A Colorado study of 1,586 DM1 patients investigated the risks of developing DM1 in siblings and parents of probands with DM1 *(12)*. A sibling had a 4.4% risk of DM1 by age 20; a parent had a 2.6% risk. The risk was higher for fathers than for mothers and was higher if the proband was diagnosed before age 7 *(12)*. The incidence of DM1 world-wide is rising *(13)*. Little is known about what environmental factors may play a role in this development. The genetic mechanisms underlying DM1 are not completely understood either, but much recent progress has been made. We review here the genes that have validated DM1 associations.

The HLA Locus

The major genetic susceptibility of DM1 is from the *HLA* locus. The *HLA* genes locate at Chr6p21.3 (Fig. 2). The *HLA class I* and *class II* genes encode cell-surface antigen-presenting proteins. Antigens

Fig. 2. The *HLA* genes.

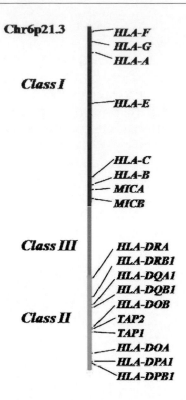

presented by *HLA class I* proteins are from inside the cell, while antigens presented by *HLA class II* proteins are from the cell surroundings. The two classes of *HLA* play essential roles in infectious diseases, autoimmune diseases, graft vs. host disease (GvHD) and cancer, by presenting native or foreign antigens to T lymphocytes. *Class I* proteins play indispensable roles in anti-infection by presenting pathogenic antigens expressed inside the cells, to get the infected cells destroyed; *class II* proteins play key roles in autoimmune diseases by presenting autoantigens to T cells and inducing autoimmune reaction. Among the *HLA* genes, present knowledge suggests that the *HLA class II* genes (*HLA-DR, -DQ* genes) confer the primary effects to DM1 susceptibility *(14–18)*, while *HLA class I* genes (*HLA-A, -B,* and *-C*) may modulate the DM1 susceptibility *(19, 20)*. The genetic susceptibility to DM1 from the *HLA* locus has been found in all the major human populations *(21, 22)*.

The HLA proteins are by far the most polymorphic in the human genome. Multiple amino acid substitutions have been driven by the evolutionary advantage of heterozygosity, permitting the presentation of a wider range of antigens from emerging pathogens. The multiple alleles are classified by a code preceded by an asterisk.

The *HLA class II* genes account for about 50% of the genetic susceptibility to DM1 in the European population *(14)*. For the *HLA-DQ*, the most potent risk is from *DQB1*0302*, and the most protective effect is from *DQB1*0602*. For the *HLA-DR*, the most potent risk is from *DR*0401* (*DR4* in serologic terminology), and the most protective effect is from *DR*15*. Actually, it is difficult to separate the effect of *DQ* from *DR*, as the two are highly correlated, a phenomenon known as linkage disequilibrium (LD). According to the *HLA* genotyping data of 2,298 DM1 nuclear families (11,159 individuals, 5,003 affected) from the Type 1 Diabetes Genetics Consortium (T1DGC, https://www.t1dgc.org), the *DQ*0302-DR*0401* haplotype has the strongest risk effect [OR (95% CI) = 3.877 *(3.480, 4.318)*], and the *DQ*0602-DR*15* haplotype has the most protective effect [OR (95% CI) = 0.037 (0.025, 0.055)]. The frequencies of *DQ, DR* alleles and the *DQ-DR* haplotypes vary dramatically in different populations, reflecting historical exposure to different pathogens. Interested readers may refer to the National Center for Biotechnology Information Major Histocompatibility Complex database (http://www.ncbi.nlm.nih.

gov/mhc) for the frequency of a specific population. Besides DM1, *HLA* variations have also been shown to be associated with other autoimmune diseases, including rheumatoid arthritis (RA) *(23)*, systemic lupus erythematosus (SLE) *(24)*, multiple sclerosis *(25)*, and Graves' disease *(26)*. This suggests that a common mechanism mediated by the *HLA* gene is shared by T-cell mediated autoimmune diseases.

As DM1 is an autoimmune disease, it is not surprising to find that a major genetic risk factor for DM1 is from *HLA class II* genes, as they are responsible for the presentation of autoantigens *(27)*. In the context of a T-cell-mediated autoimmune disease like DM1, CD4+ T-cell recognition of islet autoantigenic epitopes, presented by *HLA class II* proteins, is a key step in the autoimmune cascade *(28)*. However, how the *class II* genes' function influences DM1 risk is not clear. The development of regulatory T cells in the thymus plays a crucial role in immune self-tolerance and autoimmunity *(29)*. Generation of CD4+ CD25+ regulatory thymocytes requires a T-cell receptor (TCR) with high affinity for a self-peptide presented by DQ-β *(30)*. It has been known for a long time that a non-Aspartic acid (asp) at residue 57 of the DQ-β protein confers susceptibility to DM1 *(14)*. By studying the crystal structure of human DQ-β protein and the homologous molecule found in mice, it was discovered that non-Asp57 DQ-β has different crystal structure, which may change the property of autoantigen presentation *(31, 32)*. On the other hand, a study on the crystal structure of the DM1 protective *DQ*0602* disclosed a unique stability of DQ-β and its ability to present expanded peptide repertoire *(33)*. The crystal property of *DQ*0602* may promote thymic selection of regulatory T cells through increased affinity with TCRs. Compared with *DQ*0602*, *DQ*0302* may have poor presentation of ectopic autoantigens in the thymus and thus cause deficient development of regulatory T cells and insufficient immune self-tolerance.

Besides the *HLA class I* and *class II* genes, non-*HLA* genes in the *HLA* locus may participate in the DM1 immunopathogenesis through different mechanisms. Recent studies have shown that the *TAP2* gene (transporter 2, ATP-binding cassette, sub-family B) may contribute to the DM1 susceptibility through genetic control of alternative splicing *(34)*. TAP2 is involved in the transport of antigenic peptides to *HLA* class I molecules. In the human, differential peptide selectivity is conferred by two splicing isoforms with alternative carboxy terminals *(35)*. DM1 association independent of *HLA* was reported from the inositol 1,4,5-trisphosphate receptor type 3 gene (*ITPR3*), which is located at ~500 kb centrometric flanking of the *HLA class II* genes *(36)*. However, this association could not be replicated in later studies with sufficient statistical power *(37, 38)*. It is worth noting that, because of extended LD in the *HLA* locus, any DM1 associations found in the *HLA* locus may be from the LD with the *HLA class II* and *class I* genes, but may not represent independent genetic effect.

The INS Locus

The genetic association between the insulin gene (*INS*) and DM1 has long been recognized and extensively examined using a candidate gene approach *(8)*. The genetic susceptibility for DM1 was mapped to variable number tandem repeats (VNTR) located in the 5′ upstream region of the INS gene *(39–41)*. The *INS*-VNTR has the consensus sequence ACAGGGGTGTGGGG, repeated from 30 to more than 150 times in Caucasian chromosomes *(42)*. About 80% of Caucasian alleles are in the range of 30–44 repeats (class I), and virtually all of the rest are longer than 110 repeats (class III). Intermediate lengths (class II) are rare. The class III alleles are associated with decreased DM1 risk *(8, 39–41, 43)*. Fine mapping of the INS region identified no additional genetic effect besides the VNTR, although two SNPs, -23HphI (rs689) and +1140A/C (rs3842753), in perfect LD with the VNTR, can not be excluded as causative of DM1 susceptibility *(44)*. In different ethnic populations, the *INS*-VNTR has different frequencies, but the DM1 susceptibility is still detectable *(45)*.

Recent studies have provided solid evidence for insulin as the primary autoantigen that initiates the T-cell autoimmune destruction of the pancreatic β cells and results in DM1 in both humans and the nonobese diabetic (NOD) mouse model *(46, 47)*. The mechanism of self-tolerance to insulin and its breakdown in DM1 is incompletely understood, but there is strong evidence in favor of an important role of central tolerance in the thymus. Evidence is mounting that central T-cell tolerance to tissue-specific antigens involves their ectopic expression in the thymus *(48, 49)*. Tolerance to transgenic allo- *(50)* or xeno- *(51)* antigens expressed under the insulin promoter can be transferred by thymus transplant to nontransgenic mice.

Studies of both ours and other groups showed that the *INS*-VNTR genotype has drastic effects on insulin expression levels in thymus, with little or no effect on insulin levels in pancreatic β cells *(52, 53)*. The protective alleles of INS-VNTR have higher ectopic insulin expression in the thymus. The thymus plays a critical role in determining central tolerance by generating regulatory T cells and deleting autoreactive T cells *(54, 55)*. Class I alleles predispose to DM1 through inadequate *INS* expression in the thymus, resulting in less complete deletion of insulin-reactive clones. This hypothesis is supported in a knockout mouse model of thymic insulin deficiency with normal pancreatic expression, in which we found T-cell autoreactivity to insulin, even against a nondiabetes-prone genetic background *(56)*. Against the DM1-prone NOD background, this loss of thymic insulin expression drastically accelerates diabetes *(57)* (Fig. 3).

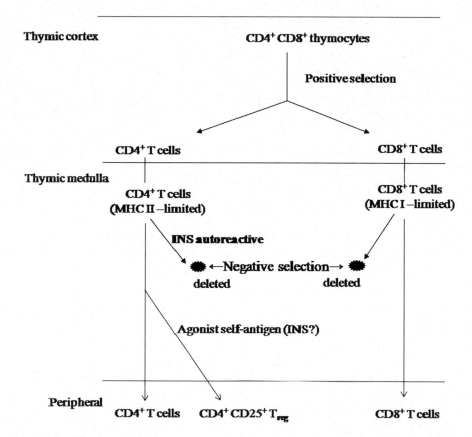

Fig. 3. Ectopic thymic insulin expression and central immune tolerance. Presentation of the insulin autoantigen by MHC II plays an important role in negative selection in thymic medulla. During this process, autoreactive T cells against insulin autoantigen will be deleted. As the deletion of autoreactive CD4+ T cells depends on the presentation of insulin autoantigen, the genetic variation causing higher expression of insulin in thymic medulla will make the negative selection process more efficient, thus being protective against DM1 *(58)*. It is also possible that higher insulin levels in thymus promote the generation of regulatory T cells.

The CTLA4 Locus

The cytotoxic T-lymphocyte-associated protein 4 gene (*CTLA4*) mapping to Chr2q33 was also found to be associated with DM1.

Activation of T lymphocytes by the TCR complex after antigen recognition requires the costimulation by CD28 *(59)*. The protein encoded by *CTLA4* transmits inhibitory signals to attenuate T-cell activation by competing for the B7 ligands with its homologue CD28 *(60, 61)*. In addition, CTLA-4 can inhibit TCR signaling by direct interaction with the TCR complex *(62)*. Blocking CTLA-4 by anti-CTLA-4 mAb can increase IL-2 mRNA expression and IL-2 secretion *(63)* and promote T-cell proliferation *(63, 64)*. Therefore, it is conceivable that genetic variations associated with decreased *CTLA4* expression might increase the risk of autoimmune diseases because of the deficit of inhibiting T-cell activity.

An A–G transition at position 49 (+49G >A, rs231775), which encodes an Ala/Thr substitution in the signal peptide, had been associated with DM1 in a European population *(65)*. Subsequently, this DM1 association was replicated in different populations *(66–70)*. However, controversy remains that some studies did not replicate the DM1 association. The mechanism remains undetermined. Kouti et al. found that the predisposing +49G allele is associated with reduced T-cell proliferation *(64)*, while Maurer et al. found that the predisposing +49G allele is associated with greater proliferative response of T cells *(63)*. Besides DM1, the *CTLA4* gene variation is also associated with RA *(26)*, SLE *(71)*, Graves' disease, and autoimmune hypothyroidism *(72)*. In patients with DM1 and the *CTLA4* gene variation, female gender is a known risk factor for the development of antithyroid antibodies *(73)*. The Ala/Thr substitution from +49G >A maps to the signal peptide and does not exist in the mature protein of CTLA-4. Data from our group showed that the predisposing Ala (+49G) allele can change the efficiency of posttranslational modifications and thus lead to inefficient production of functional CTLA-4 protein *(74)*. However, further fine mapping of the gene region rejected +49G >A as the only causal SNP of DM1 susceptibility, while stronger association was identified from rs3087243, a SNP at the 3′ flanking region of *CTLA4(72)*.

The stronger DM1-associated SNP does not involve an amino acid change, making regulatory effect on gene expression the most likely mechanism. Two CTLA-4 isoforms through alternative splicing are known, that is, the full-length isoform (flCTLA-4) with the transmembrane domain and the soluble isoform (sCTLA-4) lacking the transmembrane domain. The sCTLA-4 is expressed in B cells and nonactivated T cells *(75, 76)*, which may be important to maintain immune homeostasis. In peripheral blood mononuclear cells (PBMCs) of three +49A/G-CT60 A/G heterozygous individuals, the DM1 protective haplotype +49A-CT60A was reported to correspond to higher sCTLA-4 mRNA level than the predisposing haplotype +49G-CT60G *(72)*, although our group could not replicate this finding *(77)*. Therefore, further study is needed to clarify the genetic mechanism of the DM1 association of *CTLA4*. Combined effect of multiple genetic variations from the *CTLA4* locus may explain the DM1 association.

The PTPN22 Locus

The *PTPN22* gene (lymphoid protein tyrosine phosphatase, nonreceptor type 22) was identified to be a DM1 locus by Bottini et al. in 2004 *(9)*. The lymphoid phosphatase (Lyp) encoded by *PTPN22* is a negative regulator of TCR signaling in T cells and a well-established suppressor of T-cell activation, acting alone or interacting with C-terminal Src kinase (Csk) or c-Cbl (an adaptor protein for receptor protein-tyrosine kinases) to inhibit Src family protein tyrosine kinases (PTKs, involved in TCR signal integration) *(78, 79)*. Targeted disruption of PEP, the mouse ortholog of Lyp, results in increased expansion and function of the effector/memory T-cell pool, which was also associated with spontaneous development of germinal centers and elevated serum antibody levels *(80)*.

The DM1 association is with a nsSNP R620W (Arg620Trp, rs2476601) *(9)* and has been confirmed by multiple studies *(9, 81–89)*. The protein encoded by the Trp allele (DM1 predisposing) is unable to bind to its Csk partner *(9)*. The association between Csk and PEP is highly specific. A previous study has shown that disruption of binding to Csk with an induced mutation that mimics the effect of R620W abolishes the inhibitory effect of PEP on TCR signaling *(90)*. As shown by Hasegawa et al., Lyp plays an inhibitory role in positive but not negative selection *(80)*. The predisposing Trp allele of the R620W may cause the loss of inhibition of thymus positive selection and lead to the increase of autoreactive T lymphocytes. Besides DM1, the R620W has also been shown to be associated with other autoimmune disorders, including RA *(91)* and SLE *(92)*, Grave's disease, and juvenile idiopathic arthritis (JIA) *(93)*, which suggests that the Lyp-Csk pathway is involved in a common mechanism of autoimmune diseases.

Although disruption of Lyp-Csk binding suggests that R620W is the causal variation of DM1 susceptibility, another SNP is also interesting. The SNP rs6679677 has the allele frequency identical to that of *PTPN22*-R620W ($r^2 = 1$), which makes it impossible to dissect the effects of these two SNPs on the basis of genetic data alone. This SNP is located in the intergenic region between *RSBN1* (round spermatid basic protein 1, also known as *FLJ11220*) and *PHTF1* (putative homeodomain transcription factor 1). Through bioinformatic models, SNP rs6679677 is predicted to destroy a binding site of promoter CCAAT binding factors, or destroy a site of enhancer CCAAT binding factors, or generate a binding site of the transcription factor, Sox-5 *(86)*. In addition, both R620W and rs6679677 are nonpolymorphic in Asian populations, as shown by both the HapMap data *(94)* and a large-scale study in East Asians *(95)*. The DM1 predisposing Trp allele does not exist in the East Asian population. However, a promoter SNP -1123G-C (rs2488457) was found to be DM1-associated *(95)*. This interesting finding suggests that R620W may not be the sole causative polymorphism.

The IL2RA Locus

Vella et al. identified a novel DM1 locus, interleukin-2 receptor alpha (*IL2RA*), by multilocus association test, based on a candidate gene approach *(10)*. Our study confirmed this DM1 association *(96)*. An association between Graves' disease and *IL2RA* was also found *(97)*. The DM1 association was initially mapped to an LD block encompassing the *IL2RA* gene 5′ side and promoter region *(96)*.

IL2RA encodes the α chain of the IL2 receptor complex (IL2Rα, also known as CD25). Interleukin-2 (IL2) is a powerful growth factor for both T and B lymphocytes *(98)*. It acts through a quaternary receptor signaling complex containing α, β, and common γ ($γ_c$, a common component of many interleukin receptors) chain receptors *(99)*. IL2 receptors can be classified into three types according to the binding ability to IL2 *(100)*. IL2Rα alone is of the low-affinity type; the complex of IL2Rβ and $γ_c$ is of the medium-affinity type, and the high-affinity type is the complex with all three subunits, IL2Rα, IL2Rβ, and $γ_c$ *(101)*. Most biological effects of IL2 were mediated by the high-affinity type *(99)*.

What makes the *IL2RA* association interesting is the increased awareness of the importance of regulatory T cells in recent years. CD4+ CD25+ T cells, naturally occurring in the thymus, are a population of regulatory T cells, which are anergic to TCR signals and potently suppress activated T cells in a contact-dependent and cytokine-independent fashion *(102)*. This active immune suppression mechanism plays an important role in maintaining immune homeostasis and inhibiting autoimmune disease *(103)*. As direct evidence of the protective effect of CD4+ CD25+ T cells in DM1, the transfer of CD4+ CD25+ T cells can prevent diabetes in recipient NOD mice *(104)*. CD4+ CD25+ T cells depend on interleukin-2 (IL-2) for their growth and survival, and the IL-2 signaling effect is mainly mediated by IL2Rα *(105,*

106). Adult IL2Rα-deficient mice develop massive enlargement of peripheral lymphoid organs from impaired T-cell death after activation, and older IL2Rα-deficient mice develop autoimmune disorders, including hemolytic anemia and inflammatory bowel disease *(106).* The association of DM1 with the *IL2RA* gene highlights the role of IL2Rα in the pathogenesis of DM1. There is no common nsSNP in the *IL2RA* region. The regulatory effect of genetic variation on gene expression is suggested. Lower expression of *IL2RA*, which is correlated with the DM1 susceptible allele, may impair the immune inhibition function of IL2Rα, thus contributing to disease development.

The IFIH1 Locus

A large-scale screening of 12,000 nonsynonymous SNPs (nsSNP) across the human genome found association of DM1 with a nsSNP (Ala946Thr, rs1990760) at the "interferon induced with helicase C domain 1" gene *(IFIH1) (107).* The association was replicated in our own dataset *(108).* *IFIH1* is a putative RNA helicase, upregulated by interferons, especially β interferon *(109).* *IFIH1*-deficient mice are highly susceptible to picornavirus infection, which suggests that *IFIH1* is critical for innate antivirus responses *(110).* This is of particular interest given evidence for a role of viral infection in DM1 *(111).* In addition to a proven causal link between DM1 and congenital rubella *(112),* there is evidence suggesting an association with enterovirus and picornavirus infections *(113).* Although the genetic effect was relatively small (OR = 0.85), it suggests a potentially important role of innate immunity and interferon responses in the pathogenesis of DM1 that may reveal therapeutic targets.

The KIAA0350 Locus

DM1 association with *CLEC16A* (C-type lectin 16A, formerly *KIAA0350*) was independently identified by two recent GWA studies *(114–116).* The DM1-associated SNPs map to a large LD block (233 kb); *CLEC16A* is the only identified gene in the region, which makes this gene a prime candidate for harboring the causative variant. The predicted protein product bears similarities to a subset of adhesion and immune function signaling molecules. It contains a calcium-dependent (C-type) lectin-binding domain structure and may be involved with calcium current flux. The C-type lectins are known for their recognition of a diversity of carbohydrates and are critical for a variety of processes ranging from cell adhesion to pathogen recognition *(117).* *CLEC16A* is expressed in B lymphocytes, dendritic antigen-presenting cells, and NK-cells, which is in keeping with a function relevant to an immune-mediated disease such as DM1. The mechanism underlying the genetic effect remains to be elucidated.

The Vitamin D Metabolism Gene CYP27B1

The cytochrome P450, subfamily XXVIIB, polypeptide 1 gene *(CYP27B1)* encodes 25-hydroxy-vitamin D_3-1-α-hydroxylase, which is expressed in the renal proximal tubule and catalyzes metabolic activation of 25-hydroxyvitamin D_3 into 1α, 25-dihydroxyvitamin D_3 [1-α,25-$(OH)_2$ D_3], the active form of vitamin D *(118).* As a key enzyme in vitamin D metabolism, mutations of this gene have been shown to cause type 1 vitamin D-dependent rickets *(119–122).* Two polymorphisms, a promoter region SNP rs10877012 and an intronic SNP rs4646536, were reported to be associated with DM1 by a study of 187 DM1 German families *(123).* Recently, the DM1 association was confirmed by a large-scale study *(124).* Besides DM1, Lopez et al. showed also that the *CYP27B1* promoter SNP is also associated with Addison's disease, Hashimoto's thyroiditis and Graves' disease *(125).* The role of vitamin D goes beyond calcium regulation, and there is increasing evidence that it is also involved in regulation of the immune system *(126)*. There is no evidence for association between the vitamin D receptor gene *(VDR)* polymorphisms and DM1 *(127)*.

DM1 predisposition from vitamin D deficiency and an effect of vitamin D treatment in DM1 prevention have been suggested *(128, 129)*. As a key gene in vitamin D metabolism, the DM1 association of the *CYP27B1* gene variation provides new evidence for the role of vitamin D in DM1. This finding has also potential pharmacogenetic value. As the variants are involved in the production of active form of vitamin D, they could serve as the markers for the clinical administration of vitamin D drugs.

Other Loci

A 250-kb locus at Chr12q13 was also identified by two GWA studies independently *(114, 116, 130)*. Several genes, including five reasonable candidate genes, i.e., *RAB5B*, *SUOX*, *IKZF4*, *ERBB3*, and *CDK2*, are included in this locus, but which gene is causative of DM1 remains unknown. *RAB5B* (MIM:179514) encodes a member of the *RAS* oncogene family, which may be involved in vesicular trafficking at the plasma membrane *(131)*. *SUOX* (MIM:606887) encodes a liver-specific sulfite oxidase involved in the degradation of sulfur-containing amino acids. Neither gene has known function in immunity or pancreatic development. *IKZF4* (MIM:606239) encodes a potential functional candidate, a zinc finger protein specifically expressed in lymphocytes and implicated in the control of lymphoid development. *ERBB3* (MIM:190151) encodes a member of the epidermal growth factor receptor (EGFR) family of receptor tyrosine kinases, which is involved in the regulation of cell proliferation or differentiation *(132)*. *CDK2* (MIM: 116953) encodes a member of the Ser/Thr protein kinase family whose activity is regulated by its protein phosphorylation; members of related gene families have been recently implicated in GWA studies of type 2 diabetes *(133–136)*. Fine mapping and functional studies will be required to identify the causative variant and generate functional insights from this genetic finding.

Three other DM1 loci have also been reported by the Welcome Trust study and Todd et al. *(114, 116)*: (1) One locus at 12q24 contains the *SH2B3* (SH2B adaptor protein 3, also known as LNK, lymphocyte adaptor protein) gene. The protein encoded by *SH2B3* has been known to interact with the protein encoded by *ERBB3* at the DM1 locus 12q13 *(132)*. (2) Another locus at 18p11 contains the lymphoid protein tyrosine phosphatase, nonreceptor type 2 gene *(PTPN2)*. *PTPN2* belongs to the same family as the previously known DM1 gene *PTPN22*, and thus it may contribute to DM1 by a similar mechanism. (3) Another locus at 4q27 contains the interleukin-2 gene *(IL2)*, whose receptor has been associated with DM1. What changes in the function of these genes are determined by these genetic variations is not known yet.

Other DM1 loci, for example, *SUMO4(137)* and *OAS1(138, 139)*, have also been reported but not widely replicated *(137–143)* (Figs. 4–6).

The discovery of these DM1 genes greatly expands the understanding of the etiology of DM1. The genetic susceptibility from the variation of the *INS* gene, which encodes the primary autoantigen that initiates the T-cell autoimmune destruction of the pancreatic β cells, is specific for the development of DM1. Other DM1-associated genes are involved in the activation of autoreactive CD4+ T cell and/or the maintaining of immune homeostasis and may be involved in other autoimmune diseases. These genetic findings will help in disease prediction and identification of potential therapeutic targets for drug development.

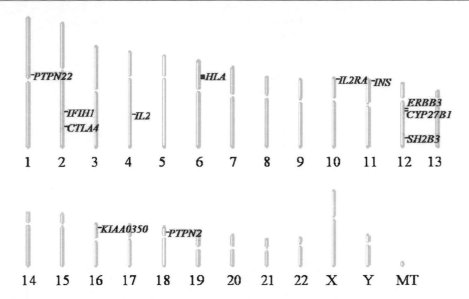

Fig. 4. The known DM1 loci.

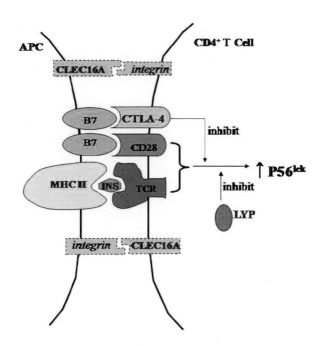

Fig. 5. Roles of DM1 genes in the activation of autoreactive CD4+ T cell. The autoantigen INS is presented by MHC II of antigen presenting cell (APC) to TCR of CD4+ T cell, consequently activating the CD4+ T cell. The activation of CD4+ T cell requires the costimulation by B7-CD28 signaling. CTLA-4 competes with CD28 for the binding of B7, and its cytoplasmic domain has phosphatase-recruiting activity, thus inhibiting the activation of CD4+ T cell in two different ways. LYP encoded by the *PTPN22* gene inhibits Src family protein tyrosine kinases (PTKs), for example, P56lck, thus attenuating TCR signaling for CD4+ T-cell activation. The KIAA0350 protein can promote cell adhesion and enable autoantigen presentation.

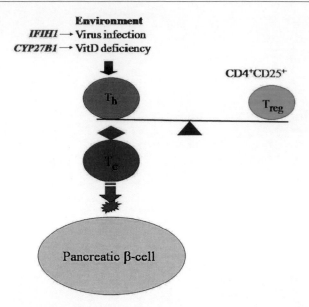

Fig. 6. Roles of DM1 genes in maintaining immune homeostasis. In the process of autoimmune pancreatic β-cell destruction, CD8⁺ cytotoxic T cells (Tc) require the assistance of CD4⁺ helper T cells (T$_h$) to differentiate and activate. CD4⁺ CD25⁺ regulatory T cells antagonize the effect of T$_h$, in order to maintain immune homeostasis. Environmental factors, such as viral infection and vitamin D deficiency, have impact on this balance and may influence the development of cytotoxic β-cell destruction. *IFIH1* variations change the susceptibility to virus infection. *CYP27B1* variations change the efficiency of active vitamin D synthesis, which, in lymphocytes, may be regulated independently of parathyroid hormone *(126)*.

TYPE 2 DIABETES

DM2 results from a progressive insulin secretory defect on the background of insulin resistance *(144)*. Diabetes has a prevalence of 6.8% in the USA *(145)*, and DM2 accounts for 90–95% of those with diabetes *(146)*. Because of the high heritability of DM2, there has been intense research trying to identify DM2 susceptibility loci.

PPARG

The most widely studied DM2 candidate gene is the peroxisome proliferator-activated receptor gamma gene *(PPARG)*. Mutations of *PPARG* can cause lipodystrophy *(147, 148)* and severe insulin resistance *(149)*. DM2 is associated with a nsSNP *PPARG* Pro12Ala (P12A) polymorphism (dbSNP ID rs1801282) *(150, 151)*.

Table 1
The Subtypes of PPARs

Gene	Chr position	Protein
PPARA	22q13	PPAR-α
PPARD	6p21	PPAR-δ
PPARG	3p25	PPAR-γ1
		PPAR-γ2
		PPAR-γ3

The peroxisome proliferator-activated receptors (PPARs) are members of the nuclear hormone receptor subfamily of transcription factors. PPARs form complexes with retinoid X receptors (RXRs), and these PPAR/RXR heterodimers regulate transcription of various genes by binding to peroxisome proliferator response elements (PREs) on target genes *(152)*. PPARs play a central role in mediating the actions of peroxisome proliferators *(153)*. There are three known subtypes, PPAR-α, PPAR-δ (also known as PPAR-β), and PPAR-γ, encoded by different loci (Table 1), with distinct expression patterns, different ligand-binding specificity and metabolic functions *(154)*. They are highly expressed in reproductive tissues and placenta and may play important roles in gestation and fetus development *(155)*.

There are three isoforms of the PPAR-γ protein, that is, PPAR-γ1, PPAR-γ2, and PPAR-γ3 *(152, 156)*. Expression of the three isoforms is regulated by different mechanisms, and each isoform has different tissue distribution. The DM2-associated SNP rs1801282 is located at the first coding exon of PPAR-γ2 but at the intronic region of PPAR-γ1 and PPAR-γ3. Therefore, the amino acid change Pro12Ala caused by rs1801282 is seen only on PPAR-γ2 (Pro12Ala). PPAR-γ2 is highly expressed in adipose tissue and involved in adipocyte differentiation. Activation of PPAR-γ2 improves adipose tissue function and may have a role in preventing progression of insulin resistance *(157)*. Thiazolidinediones (TZD), which are PPAR-γ activating ligands, are used in the treatment of type 2 diabetes mellitus currently because of their insulin-sensitizing effects *(158)*. However, the DM2 protective Ala allele corresponds to reduced transcriptional activity of PPAR-γ2 and has decreased binding to the PPAR-γ-responsive DNA elements on target genes *(159, 160)*. This finding is obviously paradoxical to the beneficial effect of improving insulin resistance by a PPAR-γ agonist TZD. The mechanism of this genetic susceptibility of DM2 still needs much further study.

The *PPARG* Pro12Ala variant may not affect the therapeutic efficacy of TZD *(161, 162)*. But still, some controversy remains *(163)*. Another study showed that Pro12Ala may be related to the side effects of TZD, for example, TZD-induced edema *(164)*. Another controversy related to this variant is whether or not it plays any role in polycystic ovarian syndrome (PCOS) *(165, 166)*. The Ala allele of the *PPARG* Pro12Ala variant has been associated with lower birth weight and a shorter gestation *(167)*; effects on postnatal growth have also been reported *(168, 169)*.

KCNJ11 and ABCC8

DM2 association with the *KCNJ11* (potassium inwardly rectifying channel, subfamily J, member 11) Glu23Lys (E23K) polymorphism (rs5219) has also been widely replicated *(170–174)*. The K allele corresponds to increased DM2 susceptibility.

ATP-sensitive K⁺(K⁺-ATP) channels couple cell metabolism to electrical activity by regulating K⁺ fluxes across the cell membrane. This mechanism plays an important role in regulating insulin secretion from pancreatic β cells *(175)*. The K⁺-ATP channels in the pancreatic β-cell surface are octameric complexes, comprising four inwardly rectifying K⁺ channel subunits (Kir6.2) and four regulatory sulfonylurea receptor subunits (SUR1) *(176)*. KIR6.2 is encoded by *KCNJ11* at Chr11p15, closely linked to *ABCC8*, the gene encoding SUR1, a modulator of K⁺-ATP channels. In the absence of stimulation from high plasma glucose, K⁺-ATP channels are open. K⁺ efflux through K⁺-ATP channels keeps the β-cell membrane hyperpolarized, which prevents opening of voltage-gated Ca²⁺ channels and Ca²⁺ influx. Under the stimulation of elevated plasma glucose, ATP inhibits K⁺-ATP channels and K⁺ efflux and thus produces a membrane depolarization. Consequently, voltage-gated Ca²⁺ channels open, and Ca²⁺ influx triggers insulin secretion through exocytosis of insulin granules. Blockers of Kir6.2/SUR1 K⁺-ATP channels, for example, glibenclamide and repaglinide, stimulate release of insulin and are used for treatment of type 2 diabetes *(177)*.

The DM2 susceptibility conferred by the E23K polymorphism comes from a functional change of Kir6.2 by the amino acid substitution. Empirical evidence shows reduced ATP sensitivity of K⁺-ATP channels in heterozygous (E/K) and homozygous (K/K) state *(178)*. The reduced ATP sensitivity increases the stimulatory threshold of closing K^+-ATP channels and K^+ efflux and inhibits Ca^{2+} influx and insulin secretion.

The E23K variant in KCNJ11 may influence the variability in the response of patients to sulfonylureas, while the DM2 risk K allele may increase the risk of secondary failure to sulfonylurea *(179)*.

TCF7L2

The DM2 association of the transcription factor 7-like 2 (*TCF7L2*) locus was first reported by Grant et al. in 2006 *(180)*. Because of the large effect size (OR ~1.48) of the DM2 susceptibility from this locus, this association is highly replicable in a wide variety of populations *(181–191)* (Fig. 7). This was an important finding that inspired people's enthusiasm for searching more DM2 genetic susceptibility loci. Besides DM2 association, the DM2 susceptibility allele of the *TCF7L2* gene variation was reported to be associated with increased birth weight *(192)*, but some controversy remains *(193)*.

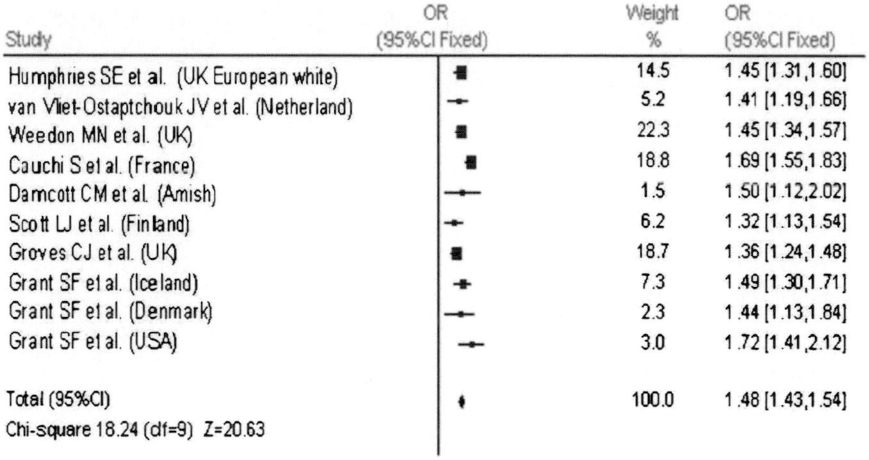

Study	OR (95%CI Fixed)	Weight %	OR (95%CI Fixed)
Humphries SE et al. (UK European white)		14.5	1.45 [1.31,1.60]
van Vliet-Ostaptchouk JV et al. (Netherland)		5.2	1.41 [1.19,1.66]
Weedon MN et al. (UK)		22.3	1.45 [1.34,1.57]
Cauchi S et al. (France)		18.8	1.69 [1.55,1.83]
Damcott CM et al. (Amish)		1.5	1.50 [1.12,2.02]
Scott LJ et al. (Finland)		6.2	1.32 [1.13,1.54]
Groves CJ et al. (UK)		18.7	1.36 [1.24,1.48]
Grant SF et al. (Iceland)		7.3	1.49 [1.30,1.71]
Grant SF et al. (Denmark)		2.3	1.44 [1.13,1.84]
Grant SF et al. (USA)		3.0	1.72 [1.41,2.12]
Total (95%CI)		100.0	1.48 [1.43,1.54]
Chi-square 18.24 (df=9) Z=20.63			

Fig. 7. The highly replicable DM2 association of the *TCF7L2* gene. All ten populations of European descent showed association of DM2 and the *TCF7L2* SNP rs7903146. No publication bias was identified (Egger's regression test $p = 0.441$). The graph was produced using the RevMan4.2 software provided by the Cochrane Collaboration.

The *TCF7L2* gene at Chr10q25.3 encodes a transcription factor, also known as T-cell transcription factor 4 (TCF4), which belongs to a subfamily of TCF7-like HMG box-containing transcription factors *(194)*. TCF4 acts through binding with β-catenin as a complex and consequently activates the expression of TCF4-regulated genes *(195, 196)*. Present studies showed that the DM2 risk allele of the *TCF7L2* gene variation was associated with impaired insulin secretion *(182, 197–199)*. Three mechanisms may be involved in this genetic effect. *(1)* Incretin effects: The *TCF7L2* gene variation is associated with impaired incretin effects and may be involved in the enteroinsular axis *(197)*. Early study showed that *Tcf7l2*-disrupted mice had a phenotype of impaired development of epithelial stem-cell compartments in the small intestine *(200)*. Further study clarified that TCF4 is a component of the Wnt signaling pathway and participates in the tissue-specific regulation of expression of gluca-gon-like peptide 1 (GLP1) *(201)*. GLP1, encoded by the proglucagon gene (*GCG*), is mainly expressed in the intestinal L cells located in the mucosa of distal ileum and colon *(202)*. GLP1 plays a major role in the enteroinsular axis of regulating blood glucose homeostasis, which includes stimulation of insulin secretion and inhibition of glucagon secretion, hepatic glucose production, gastric emptying, and appetite *(203)*. (2) Pancreatic β-cell survival: An in vitro study showed that the *TCF7L2* gene was required for β-cell survival, that is, depleting *TCF7L2* by siRNA resulted in increased β-cell apoptosis, decreased β-cell proliferation, and decreased glucose-stimulated insulin secretion (GSIS), while overexpression of *TCF7L2* protected islets from glucose and cytokine-induced apoptosis and impaired function *(204)*. In vivo, *TCF7L2* may influence the β-cell growth through GLP1. GLP1 has been suggested to promote β-cell growth and differentiation *(205)*. (3) The β-cell proinsulin processing: Prohormone convertases, PC1 and PC2, are the enzymes cleaving the proinsulin peptide to insulin and C-peptide in the β-cell *(206)*. By in silico analysis, both PC1 and PC2 contain TCF-binding sites in their promoters, which raise the possibility that TCF4 may also regulate proinsulin peptide processing through effects on PC1 and PC2 expression *(198)*.

How the *TCF7L2* variation affects the gene function is unclear yet. TCF4 is a 596aa peptide (NP_110383.1), which contains two conserved domains, the CTNNB1_binding domain and the SOX-TCF_HMG-box domain. The CTNNB1_binding domain is located from the 1st to the 236th amino acid, which binds to β-catenin and forms the active complex. The SOX-TCF_HMG-box domain is located from the 330th to the 397th amino acid, which binds to specific DNA motif and regulates gene transcription. Sequencing of all the exons of *TCF7L2* in 184 individuals (93 DM2 cases and 91 controls) has not found a nsSNP *(180)*. The possibility of a protein-sequence polymorphism can be excluded as the basis for the DM2 susceptibility. Therefore, unlike *PPARG* P12A and *KCNJ11* E23K, the DM2 susceptibility could be from the change of gene expression resulting from regulatory gene variations.

Other DM2 Loci

High-density genotyping arrays have recently permitted GWA studies, as a result of which eight novel DM2-associated loci were found since 2007 (Table 2) *(114, 133–135, 207–210)*. These novel loci were well replicated in multiple studies *(114, 133–135, 207, 208, 211–213)*. The discovery of these loci provides a great opportunity to increase the present knowledge of DM2 (Fig. 8). The changes in gene function and the mechanism of DM2 susceptibility of these novel DM2 loci are unclear. Clarification of the molecular mechanism of these new loci in DM2 will promote the development of effective DM2 prevention and therapeutics. (Fig. 9)

To date, no known genetic locus or genetic mechanism is shared by DM1 and DM2, which suggests a genetic distinction of the two diabetes phenotypes. Different from the two main mechanisms of DM1 (central immunotolerance in the thymus and immune injury in the pancreas), the known DM2 genes are mainly involved in two mechanisms, that is, pancreatic β-cell function and peripheral insulin sensitivity. As a special type of DM2, ketosis-prone type 2 diabetes is commonly reported in African descent but also observed in Hispanic and East Asian populations, and it has the clinical characteristics of strong family history and male predominance with a twofold or threefold less prevalence in women *(214)*. The major DM1 susceptibility *HLA* does not play any obvious role in ketosis-prone type 2 diabetes *(214)*, while the role of the DM2 susceptibility loci in ketosis-prone type 2 diabetes is still lacking study.

MONOGENIC DIABETES

A number of monogenic forms of diabetes have been described. Each is relatively rare, and taken together they account for only a small percentage of all cases of diabetes. Recognizing these forms of diabetes is of clinical importance, both for determining the best choices of therapeutic agents and for genetic counseling purposes.

Table 2
Eight Novel DM2 Loci Found in 2007

Locus	Chromosome position	Gene function
IGF2BP2	3q27.2	IGF2BP2 [insulin-like growth factor 2 mRNA binding protein 2] encodes an IGF-II mRNA-binding protein (IMP), which binds to the 5′ UTR of the insulin-like growth factor 2 (IGF2) mRNA and regulates IGF2 translation (215). IGF2 plays important roles in the regulation of metabolism and growth by participating in the insulin/IGF-1 signaling and the insulin action. IGF2BP2 may play important roles in pancreas development (216); DM2-associated variation (134–136)
WFS1	4p16	WFS1 (Wolfram syndrome 1) encodes a transmembrane protein that localizes primarily in the endoplasmic reticulum (ER) (217). Rare mutations of WFS1 cause the autosomal recessive Wolfram syndrome, characterized by insulin-dependent diabetes mellitus and bilateral progressive optic atrophy (218, 219). DM2 risk is associated with a common variant (210, 212, 213)
CDKAL1	6p22.3	CDKAL1 [cyclin-dependent kinase 5 (CDK5) regulatory subunit associated protein 1-like 1] is expressed in human pancreas and skeletal muscle and may be an inhibitor of CDK5 activation (135). The predisposing allele is associated with decreased pancreatic β-cell function (220). CDK5 plays a role in the loss of β-cell function under glucotoxic conditions and CDK5 inhibitors could have therapeutic value for DM2 (221); DM2-associated variation (134–136)
SLC30A8	8q24.11	ZnT-8 encoded by SLC30A8 [solute carrier family 30 (zinc transporter), member 8] may be a major component for providing zinc for insulin maturation and storage processes in insulin-secreting pancreatic β cells (222). The DM2-associated SNP in SLC30A8 is a nonsynonymous SNP (R325W). Zinc is necessary for the formation of insulin peptide hexamers; DM2-associated variation (133–136, 208)
CDKN2A/B	9p21	Two specific inhibitors of cyclin-dependent kinase 4 (CDK4), i.e., p16[INK4a] and p15[INK4b], are encoded by CDKN2A [cyclin-dependent kinase inhibitor 2A (melanoma, p16, inhibits CDK4)] and CDKN2B [cyclin-dependent kinase inhibitor 2B (p15, inhibits CDK4)]. CDK4 is crucial for β-cell proliferation and function. Loss of CDK4 expression causes insulin-deficient diabetes, and CDK4 activation results in β-islet cell hyperplasia (223). Age-induced increase of p16[INK4a] expression limits the regenerative capacity of β cells with ageing (224); DM2-associated variation (134–136)
IDE/HHEX	10q23.33	Two candidate genes, IDE (insulin-degrading enzyme) and HHEX (hematopoietically expressed homeobox), are located in this locus. HHEX encodes a transcription factor involved in pancreatic development. The predisposing allele is associated with decreased pancreatic β-cell function (220); DM2-associated variation (134–136, 208)
FTO/ RPGRIP1L	16q12.2	FTO (fat mass and obesity associated) is associated with obesity (225). The gene function and mechanism are unclear yet. A neighboring gene RPGRIP1L (retinitis pigmentosa GTPase regulator interacting protein 1 like) is highly expressed in pancreatic islet cells and is also a potential DM2 candidate; DM2-associated variation (134, 135)
HNF1B	17cen-q21.3	HNF1B encodes a transcription factor HNF1-β, also known as transcription factor 2 (TCF2). Selective knockout of HNF1-β in pancreatic islets can cause defective insulin release in a mouse model, indicating that HNF1-β is involved in regulating the β-cell transcription factor network and is necessary for glucose sensing or glycolytic signaling (226). Mutations of HNF1B cause MODY5; DM2-associated variation (209, 211)

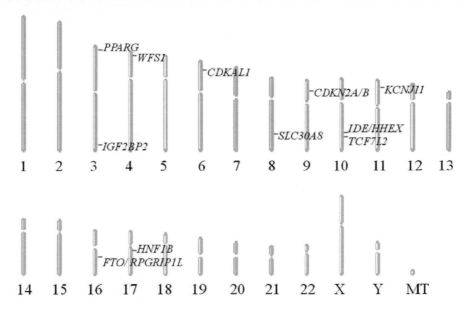

Fig. 8. The known DM2 loci.

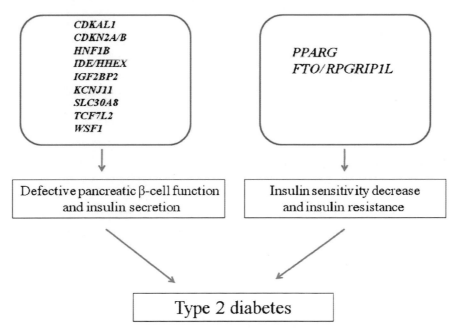

Fig. 9. The known DM2 genes are mainly involved in two mechanisms, that is, pancreatic β-cell function and insulin sensitivity, which are distinct from the genetic mechanisms predisposing to DM1.

Maturity Onset Diabetes of the Young

Maturity-onset diabetes of the young (MODY) is a group of autosomal dominantly inherited diseases, characterized by impaired insulin secretion with minimal or no defects in insulin action. MODY is recognized clinically as type 2 diabetes occurring generally before the age of 25 in individuals with a BMI <25 kg/m²(*144*). MODY accounts for the majority of monogenic diabetes cases and 1–5% of all cases of diabetes (*227*). There are eight syndromes currently described as MODY; however, these eight genes do not appear to account for all cases of clinically diagnosed MODY.

Table 3
MODY Genes

MODY subtype	Gene symbol	Chromosome position	Gene name
MODY1	HNF4A	20q12-q13.1	Hepatocyte nuclear factor 4, alpha
MODY2	GCK	7p15.3-p15.1	Glucokinase (hexokinase 4)
MODY3	HNF1A	12q24.2	Hepatocyte nuclear factor-1 homeobox A
MODY4	PDX1	13q12.1	Pancreatic and duodenal homeobox 1
MODY5	HNF1B	17cen-q21.3	Hepatocyte nuclear factor-1 homeobox B
MODY6	NEUROD1	2q32	Neurogenic differentiation factor 1
MODY7	KLF11	2p25	Kruppel-like factor 11

MODY3 and MODY2 are the two most prevalent forms of MODY. Estimated from a study on 90 MODY families, MODY3 accounts for 63% MODY, and MODY2 accounts for 20% MODY *(228)*. Unlike DM2, patients with MODY are usually nonobese and do not have metabolic syndrome *(227)*. Determining the subtype of MODY is helpful for clinical decision making *(229)*. MODY3 and MODY1 patients are sensitive to sulfonylureas for years before insulin is needed. MODY2 tends to have mild symptoms and often requires only lifestyle interventions. The genetic basis of each subtype of MODY is discussed later (Table 3).

MODY1 is caused by loss-of-function mutations of the *HNF4A* gene. *HNF4A* encodes a nuclear transcription factor HNF4-α and regulates expression of many genes in human liver and pancreatic islets, including *HNF1A* (the MODY3 gene) *(230)*. Acting as a dimer, HNF-4α plays a crucial role in glucose-stimulated insulin secretion, which has been validated in HNF-4α knockout mice, related to the dysfunction of K$^+$-ATP channels *(231)*. Mutated HNF-4α is dominant negative and can not form an active dimer, thus losing its transcriptional activity *(232)*. *HNF4A* mutations are associated with a considerable increase in birthweight and macrosomia, with the natural history of hyperinsulinemia at birth evolving to decreased insulin secretion and diabetes later in life *(233)*.

MODY2 is caused by loss-of-function mutations of the *GCK* gene. *GCK* encodes glucokinase, which catalyzes the phosphorylation of glucose to produce glucose-6-phosphate, and is one of the key enzymes in the regulation of glucolysis and glycogen synthesis. As the rate-limiting enzyme catalyzing the first step and irreversible reaction of glucose metabolism, glucokinase plays a pivotal role as the glucose sensor for β cells *(234)*. Mutations of *GCK* decrease the sensor function and cause a pancreatic β-cell secretory defect, despite normal insulin synthesis *(235)*. MODY2 mutations are correlated with infant birth weight, and special consideration should be taken in the prenatal care and monitoring. MODY2 mutations in infants can decrease the birth weight by ~530 g because of a reduction of fetal insulin secretion, and MODY2 mutations of mothers can increase the infant birth weight by ~600 g because of fetal hyperinsulinemia in response to maternal hyperglycemia *(236)*. These two effects are additive: an affected infant with an unaffected mother has decreased body weight; an affected infant with an affected mother has normal birth weight; an unaffected infant with an affected mother has increased body weight *(236)*. In addition to described MODY2 mutations, some other mutations in GCK have been associated with severe hypoglycemia and abnormalities in fetal growth *(237–240)*.

MODY3 is the most common type of MODY, caused by loss-of-function mutations of the *HNF1A* gene *(228)*. The protein HNF1-α encoded by *HNF1A* is also known as transcription factor 1 (TCF1). HNF1-α regulates expression of many genes in pancreatic islets and liver tissue *(230)*. Although HNF4-α is known to regulate the expression of HNF1-α, HNF1-α plays an essential role in the tissue-specific expression of HNF4-α in pancreatic islets *(241)*. Binding of HNF1-α to a tissue-specific promoter upstream from the *HNF4A* promoter is required to maintain the *HNF4A* expression and pancreatic β-cell function *(242)*. Mutant *HNF1A* causing defective insulin secretion has been validated in a mouse model *(243)*. Like HNF4-α, HNF1-α also acts as a dimer, thus mutated HNF-1α has a dominant-negative effect because of impaired formation of active dimers.

MODY4, caused by a loss-of-function mutation (Glu224Lys) of *PDX1*, has been described in one family. *PDX1* encodes insulin promoter factor 1 (IPF-1), which is needed for islet cell development *(244)*. Homozygosity for the *PDX1* mutation caused pancreatic agenesis *(245)* while the obligatory carrier members of the family had MODY4. In addition, IPF-1 is critical for the maintenance of β-cell function by regulating β-cell-specific gene expression, including insulin *(246)*. The regulation of the tissue-specific expression of *HNF4A* in the pancreatic islets is an important mechanism whereby *PDX1* causes MODY *(241)*.

MODY5 is caused by mutations of *HNF1B*. Different from other MODYs, MODY5 patients have significant cystic renal disease in addition to diabetes *(247, 248)*. Some MODY5 patients have pancreatic atrophy, abnormal liver function tests, and genital tract abnormalities as well *(249)*. *HNF1B* encodes a transcription factor HNF1-β, also known as transcription factor 2 (TCF2). It activates transcription of target genes as a homodimer or as a heterodimer with HNF-1-α *(250)*. Besides, HNF1-β can also regulate the expression of HNF1-α (241). Selective knockout of *HNF1B* in pancreatic islets can cause defective insulin release in a mouse model, indicating that HNF1-β is involved in regulating the β-cell transcription factor network and is necessary for glucose sensing or glycolytic signaling *(226)*. *HNF1B* mutations were also associated with low birth weight *(251, 252)* and renal developmental disorders *(249)*.

MODY6 is caused by mutations of *NEUROD1*. *NEUROD1* encodes neurogenic differentiation 1 (NEUROD1), which belongs to the basic helix-loop-helix (bHLH) family of transcription factors, and is a key regulator of pancreatic islet development and insulin gene transcription. The protein forms heterodimers with other bHLH proteins and regulates insulin gene transcription by binding to the E-box motif on the insulin promoter *(253)*. Mutations of *NEUROD1* disrupt the DNA-binding domain and abolish the E-box binding activity of the NEUROD1 protein, thus causing MODY6, which is characterized by low serum insulin levels *(254)*.

MODY7 is caused by mutations of the Kruppel-like factor 11 gene (*KLF11*), a zinc finger transcription factor. KLF11 plays a role in the regulation of pancreatic β-cell physiology. KLF11 binds to the insulin promoter and regulates glucose-induced expression of the insulin gene. Mutations impairing its transcriptional activity cause MODY7 *(255)*.

In summary, all of the seven known MODY genes are involved in defects in insulin secretion from the pancreatic β cell. Besides the monogenic inheritance, the most striking feature of MODY is normal insulin action, which distinguishes it from DM2. Among the seven MODY genes, six genes (*HNF4A, HNF1A, PDX1, HNF1B, NEUROD1,* and *KLF11*) are members of the transcription factor network that maintains the pancreatic islet β-cell function; the other gene *GCK* is a critical enzyme for glucose metabolism and is necessary for glucose sensing or glycolytic signaling. Besides MODY3 and MODY2 (which accounts for ~83% of MODY), the other types of MODY are rare *(228)*. Some cases with clinical manifestations of MODY have not been linked to the known MODY loci. Novel MODY genes remain to be found. A recent study reported that mutations of the carboxyl ester lipase (bile salt-stimulated lipase) gene (*CEL*) at Chr9q34.3 may be a new type of MODY (MODY8). CEL is excreted by the pancreas and is responsible for the hydrolysis and absorption of cholesterol esters and other dietary esters. Frameshift mutations caused by single-nucleotide deletion can cause defects in the enzyme activity. These patients have both diabetes and exocrine pancreatic dysfunction *(256)*. The pathogenesis of diabetes in MODY8 needs to be clarified by further study. Beside these genes, two missense mutations R46Q and R55C in the *INS* gene were recently reported to cause MODY by impairing the insulin activity or insulin biosynthesis *(257)*.

Other Monogenic Forms of Diabetes

A number of other monogenic forms of early onset diabetes have been reported. These diabetes syndromes can be classified into three main types, that is, congenital pancreatic islet cell dysfunction, congenital insulin resistance, and early autoimmune destruction of pancreatic islet (see Table 4).

Table 4
Monogenic Forms of Congenital Diabetes

Gene	Gene function	Phenotype and mode of inheritance
Pancreatic islet dysfunction		
	1. Transient neonatal diabetes mellitus (TNDM) is a rare type of diabetes (incidence of ~1 in 1 million neonates) that presents soon after birth, resolves by 18 months, and predisposes to type 2 diabetes later in life (262).	
PLAGL1 and *HYMAI*	*PLAGL1* encodes a zinc finger protein Zac1, which regulates apoptosis and cell cycle arrest (263). *HYMAI* generates an untranslated mRNA. Both *PLAGL1* and *HYMAI* are imprinted and expressed only from the paternal chromosome (264). Expression of ZAC or HYMAI inhibits pancreatic development and β-cell function in transgenic mice (265). Overexpression of *PLAGL1* inhibits insulin synthesis and secretion in vitro (unpublished, Qu and Polychronakos)	TNDM1: autosomal dominant with exclusively paternal inheritance when due to paternal duplication or sporadic when due to paternal isodisomy (266). Either condition causes a level of *PLAGL1* expression that is double the physiologic
	2. Permanent neonatal diabetes mellitus (PNDM) is a rare condition (incidence of ~1 in 1 million neonates) characterized by severe hyperglycemia, diagnosed within 3 months from birth and requiring insulin treatment (267)	
GCK	GCK encodes glucokinase, the glucose sensor for β cell (234)	Autosomal recessive inheritance (268)
PTF1A	PTF1A encodes pancreas specific transcription factor 1a and has a role in mammalian pancreatic development (269)	Autosomal recessive inheritance, with cerebellar agenesis (270, 271)
PDX1	PDX1 encodes insulin promoter factor 1 (IPF-1), which is needed for islet cell development (244)	Pancreatic agenesis, autosomal recessive (245) or dominant (272) inheritance
INS	INS encodes preproinsulin	Autosomal dominant inheritance (273, 274)
3. Either TNDM or PNDM		
ABCC8	ABCC8 encodes regulatory sulfonylurea receptors(SUR1) of K+ ATP channels, regulating insulin secretion from pancreatic β cells (175, 176)	TNDM2, autosomal dominant inheritance (275). PNDM: autosomal dominant (275, 276) or recessive (277) inheritance. Responds to high doses of sulfonylureas
KCNJ11	KCNJ11 encodes inwardly rectifying K+ channel subunits, regulating insulin secretion from pancreatic β cells (175, 176)	TNDM3, autosomal dominant inheritance (278). PNDM: autosomal dominant inheritance, with or without neurologic features (267, 279). Often responds to high doses of sulphonylureas, which may improve neurologic function (280)

4. Wolfram syndrome

Gene	Function	Disorder
WFS1	WFS1 encodes a transmembrane protein that localizes primarily in the endoplasmic reticulum (ER) (217)	Wolfram syndrome, an autosomal recessive syndrome characterized by insulin-dependent diabetes mellitus and bilateral progressive optic atrophy (218, 219, 281–284))

5. Mitochondrial diabetes, maternal inheritance (prevalence of 1–3% in diabetic patients (285, 286))

Gene	Function	Disorder
MT-TL1	MT-TL1 encodes the mitochondrial tRNA for leucine	Diabetes-deafness syndrome (287)
MT-TK	MT-TK encodes the mitochondrial tRNA for lysine.	Diabetes-deafness syndrome (288)
MT-TE	MT-TE encodes the mitochondrial tRNA for glutamic acid	Mitochondrial myopathy with diabetes (289)

Insulin resistance syndromes

1. Insulin resistance

Gene	Function	Disorder
INSR	INSR encodes insulin receptor	Type A insulin resistance (290) Donohue syndrome (Leprechaunism) (291, 292) Rabson-Mendenhall syndrome (293)
AKT2	AKT2 encodes a protein kinase that is enriched in insulin-responsive tissues and has been implicated in the metabolic actions of the hormone (294)	Insulin resistance (295)
PPARG and PPP1R3A	PPARG encodes the peroxisome proliferator-activated receptor γ (PPAR-γ). Activation of PPAR-γ improves tissue function and increases insulin sensitivity (157, 158). PPP1R3A encodes protein phosphatase 1, regulatory (inhibitor) subunit 3A (glycogen and sarcoplasmic reticulum binding subunit, skeletal muscle), which promotes glycogen storage and inversely regulates glycogen synthase and glycogen phosphorylase activities (296)	Digenic severe insulin resistance (149)
CD36	CD36 encodes CD36 molecule (thrombospondin receptor). Transgenic expression of CD36 in the spontaneously hypertensive rat (SHR) ameliorates insulin resistance and lowers serum fatty acids (297)	Insulin resistance (298)

2. Inherited lipodystrophic syndromes, characterized by the selective loss of adipose tissue. Affected patients are predisposed to insulin resistance and its attendant complications (299).

(1) Congenital generalized lipodystrophy

Gene	Function	Disorder
AGPAT2	AGPAT2 encodes a 1-acylglycerol-3-phosphate O-acyltransferase, which converts lysophosphatidic acid to phosphatidic acid, the second step in de novo phospholipid biosynthesis	Congenital generalized lipodystrophy type 1 (300)

(continued)

Table 4
(continued)

Gene	Gene function	Phenotype and mode of inheritance
BSCL2	BSCL2 encodes seipin, an integral membrane protein of the endoplasmic reticulum	Congenital generalized lipodystrophy type 2 (301)
(2) Familial partial lipodystrophy		
Unknown		Familial partial lipodystrophy type 1 (302)
LMNA	LMNA encodes lamin A and C. They are structural protein components of the inner nuclear membrane and determine nuclear shape and size	Familial partial lipodystrophy type 2 (303)
PPARG	PPARG encodes the peroxisome proliferator-activated receptor γ (PPAR-γ). Activation of PPAR-γ improves adipose tissue function and increases insulin sensitivity (157, 158)	Familial partial lipodystrophy type 3 (147, 148)
(3) Lipodystrophy associated with mandibuloacral dysplasia		
LMNA	LMNA encodes lamin A and C. They are structural protein components of the inner nuclear membrane and determine nuclear shape and size	Mandibuloacral dysplasia with type A lipodystrophy (304)
ZMPSTE24	ZMPSTE24 encodes a zinc metalloproteinase involved in post-translational proteolytic cleavage of prelamin A to form mature lamin A (305)	Mandibuloacral dysplasia with type B lipodystrophy (305)
Autoimmune destruction of pancreatic islet		
AIRE	AIRE encodes a transcriptional regulator and plays a pivotal role in thymic T-cell tolerance induction by activating ectopic gene expression in the medullary epithelial cells of the thymus (306)	Autoimmune polyendocrinopathy syndrome, type 1 (307, 308)
FOXP3	FOXP3 encodes a member of the forkhead/winged-helix family of transcriptional regulators and controls the development and function of regulatory T cells (309)	Immunodysregulation, polyendocrinopathy, and enteropathy, X-linked syndrome (IPEX) (310, 311)

Except for mitochondrial diabetes, these monogenic forms of diabetes are rarely seen in diabetes cases (<<1%), and the prevalence has not been systematically studied. Most cases of monogenic forms of diabetes are diagnosed in the first few years of life. Wolfram syndrome may present in childhood or early adulthood. In addition, there are a number of recognizable monogenic syndromes in which diabetes is not the primary but rather a secondary manifestation of the disease. These include cystic fibrosis *(258)*, hereditary pancreatitis *(259)*, hemochromatosis *(260)*, and myotonic dystrophy *(261)*. While it is important to recognize these diagnoses as they can have important implications for both genetic counseling and treatment, it is also important to realize that their inherent pathophysiology may also provide important insights into the causes of diabetes.

SPECIAL ISSUES IN WOMEN RELATED TO THE GENETICS OF DIABETES

Gestational Diabetes Mellitus

Gestational diabetes mellitus (GDM) is defined as any degree of glucose intolerance with onset or first recognition during pregnancy *(146)*. GDM complicates 4% of all pregnancies in the USA and represents nearly 90% of all pregnancies complicated by diabetes *(146)*. The heritability of GDM has been demonstrated, suggesting genetic predisposition, although it is unlikely that GDM represents a single disease *(312–315)*. According to the definition of GDM, if a diabetes case is found during pregnancy, regardless of the underlying pathophysiology, the case is diagnosed as GDM. Therefore, it is not surprising to see evidence of DM1 *(312)*, DM2 *(313, 314)*, and MODY *(316)*, all contributing to GDM. Some GDM cases may have genetic predisposition distinct from DM1, DM2 and MODY, but such a hypothesis can be tested only by carefully assuring phenotypic homogeneity or with very large sample sizes.

The Genetics of Polycystic Ovarian Syndrome

PCOS, like diabetes, is a multigenic disorder with clear evidence for familial aggregation *(317)*. There is a 5–10% prevalence of this disorder in women of reproductive age *(318)*. As insulin resistance and hyperinsulinemia are a cause of PCOS, it has been expected that there is some overlap between the genes implicated in PCOS and those for diabetes. However, to date, no DM2-associated genetic variation has been validated for PCOS association. This may not be surprising, as most of the known DM2 loci appear to affect insulin secretion rather than response. A study suggested that the *PPARG* Pro12Ala variant may be a modifier of insulin resistance in Caucasian women with PCOS *(319)*, but controversy remains *(165)*.

CONCLUSION

The ongoing explosion of new knowledge related to the genetics of diabetes and related disorders is staggering. This new knowledge is not merely academic. It lays the ground work for important advances in the prevention and treatment of diabetes in its myriad forms, diabetes complications, autoimmune diseases and metabolic syndrome, not only for the individual patient, but also for the pregnant woman with diabetes and her infant.

REFERENCES

1. Human Genome Sequencing C. Finishing the euchromatic sequence of the human genome. Nature 2004;431(7011):931–45
2. Stein LD. Human genome: end of the beginning. Nature 2004;431(7011):915–6
3. Florez JC, Hirschhorn J, Altshuler D. The inherited basis of diabetes mellitus: implications for the genetic analysis of complex traits. Annu Rev Genomics Hum Genet 2003;4(1):257–91

4. Cordell HJ, Todd JA. Multifactorial inheritance in type 1 diabetes. Trends Genet 1995;11(12):499–504

5. Redondo MJ, Fain PR, Eisenbarth GS. Genetics of type 1A diabetes. Recent Prog Horm Res 2001;56:69–89

6. Poulsen P, Kyvik KO, Vaag A, Beck-Nielsen H. Heritability of Type II (non-insulin-dependent) diabetes mellitus and abnormal glucose tolerance – a population-based twin study. Diabetologia 1999;42(2):139–45

7. Cardon LR, Bell JI. Association study designs for complex diseases. Nat Rev Genet 2001;2(2):91–9

8. Bell GI, Horita S, Karam JH. A polymorphic locus near the human insulin gene is associated with insulin-dependent diabetes mellitus. Diabetes 1984;33(2):176–83

9. Bottini N, Musumeci L, Alonso A, et al. A functional variant of lymphoid tyrosine phosphatase is associated with type I diabetes. Nat Genet 2004;36(4):337–8

10. Vella A, Cooper JD, Lowe CE, et al. Localization of a type 1 diabetes locus in the IL2RA/CD25 region by use of tag single-nucleotide polymorphisms. Am J Hum Genet 2005;76(5):773–9

11. Harjutsalo V, Reunanen A, Tuomilehto J. Differential transmission of type 1 diabetes from diabetic fathers and mothers to their offspring. Diabetes 2006;55(5):1517–24

12. Steck AK, Barriga KJ, Emery LM, Fiallo-Scharer RV, Gottlieb PA, Rewers MJ. Secondary attack rate of type 1 diabetes in Colorado families. Diabetes Care 2005;28(2):296–300

13. Onkamo P, Vaananen S, Karvonen M, Tuomilehto J. Worldwide increase in incidence of Type I diabetes – the analysis of the data on published incidence trends. Diabetologia 1999;42(12):1395–403

14. Todd JA, Bell JI, McDevitt HO. HLA-DQ[beta] gene contributes to susceptibility and resistance to insulin-dependent diabetes mellitus. Nature 1987;329(6140):599–604

15. Baisch JM, Weeks T, Giles R, Hoover M, Stastny P, Capra JD. Analysis of HLA-DQ genotypes and susceptibility in insulin-dependent diabetes mellitus. N Engl J Med 1990;322(26):1836–41

16. Todd JA. Genetic analysis of type 1 diabetes using whole genome approaches. Proc Natl Acad Sci U S A 1995;92(19):8560–5

17. Noble JA, Valdes AM, Cook M, Klitz W, Thomson G, Erlich HA. The role of HLA class II genes in insulin-dependent diabetes mellitus: molecular analysis of 180 Caucasian, multiplex families. Am J Hum Genet 1996;59(5):1134–48

18. she J-X. Susceptibility to type I diabetes: HLA-DQ and DR revisited. Immunol Today 1996;17(7):323

19. Pitkaniemi J, Hakulinen T, Nasanen J, Tuomilehto-Wolf E, Tuomilehto J. Class I and II HLA genes are associated with susceptibility and age at onset in Finnish families with type 1 diabetes. Hum Hered 2004;57(2):69–79

20. Valdes AM, Erlich HA, Noble JA. Human leukocyte antigen class I B and C loci contribute to Type 1 Diabetes (T1D) susceptibility and age at T1D onset. Hum Immunol 2005;66(3):301–13

21. Mbanya JC, Sobngwi E, Mbanya DNS. HLA-DRB1, -DQA1, -DQB1 and DPB1 susceptibility alleles in Cameroonian type 1 diabetes patients and controls. Eur J Immunogenet 2001;28(4):459–62

22. Kawabata Y, Ikegami H, Kawaguchi Y, et al. Asian-specific HLA haplotypes reveal heterogeneity of the contribution of HLA-DR and -DQ haplotypes to susceptibility to type 1 diabetes. Diabetes 2002;51(2):545–51

23. Zanelli E, Breedveld FC, de Vries RRP. HLA class II association with rheumatoid arthritis: facts and interpretations. Hum Immunol 2000;61(12):1254–61

24. Kelly JA, Moser KL, Harley JB. The genetics of systemic lupus erythematosus: putting the pieces together. Genes Immun 2002;3(Suppl 1):S71–85

25. Pender MP, Greer JM. Immunology of multiple sclerosis. Curr Allergy Asthma Rep 2007;7(4):285–92

26. Gough SC. The genetics of Graves' disease. Endocrinol Metab Clin North Am 2000;29(2):255–66

27. Eisenbarth GS. Type I diabetes mellitus. A chronic autoimmune disease. N Engl J Med 1986;314(21):1360–8

28. Di Lorenzo TP, Peakman M, Roep BO. Translational mini-review series on type 1 diabetes: systematic analysis of T cell epitopes in autoimmune diabetes. Clin Exp Immunol 2007;148(1):1–16

29. Lan RY, Ansari AA, Lian ZX, Gershwin ME. Regulatory T cells: development, function and role in autoimmunity. Autoimmun Rev 2005;4(6):351–63

30. Jordan MS, Boesteanu A, Reed AJ, et al. Thymic selection of CD4+ CD25+ regulatory T cells induced by an agonist self-peptide. Nat Immunol 2001;2(4):301–6

31. Corper AL, Stratmann T, Apostolopoulos V, et al. A structural framework for deciphering the link between I-Ag7 and autoimmune diabetes. Science 2000;288(5465):505–11

32. Lee KH, Wucherpfennig KW, Wiley DC. Structure of a human insulin peptide-HLA-DQ8 complex and susceptibility to type 1 diabetes. Nat Immunol 2001;2(6):501–7

33. Siebold C, Hansen BE, Wyer JR, et al. Crystal structure of HLA-DQ0602 that protects against type 1 diabetes and confers strong susceptibility to narcolepsy. Proc Natl Acad Sci U S A 2004;101(7):1999–2004

34. Qu H-Q, Lu Y, Marchand L, et al. Genetic control of alternative splicing in the TAP2 gene: possible implication in the genetics of type 1 diabetes. Diabetes 2007;56(1):270–5

35. Yan G, Shi L, Faustman D. Novel splicing of the human MHC-encoded peptide transporter confers unique properties. J Immunol 1999;162(2):852–9

36. Roach JC, Deutsch K, Li S, et al. Genetic mapping at 3-kilobase resolution reveals inositol 1,4,5-triphosphate receptor 3 as a risk factor for type 1 diabetes in Sweden. Am J Hum Genet 2006;79(4):614–27

37. Nejentsev S, Howson JM, Walker NM, et al. Localization of type 1 diabetes susceptibility to the MHC class I genes HLA-B and HLA-A. Nature 2007;450(7171):887–92

38. Qu HQ, Marchand L, Szymborski A, Grabs R, Polychronakos C. The association between type 1 diabetes and the ITPR3 gene polymorphism due to linkage disequilibrium with HLA class II. Genes Immun 2008;9(3):264–6

39. Owerbach D, Gabbay KH. Localization of a type I diabetes susceptibility locus to the variable tandem repeat region flanking the insulin gene. Diabetes 1993;42(12):1708–14

40. Bennett ST, Lucassen AM, Gough SCL, et al. Susceptibility to human type 1 diabetes at IDDM2 is determined by tandem repeat variation at the insulin gene minisatellite locus. Nat Genet 1995;9(3):284–92

41. Undlien DE, Bennett ST, Todd JA, et al. Insulin gene region-encoded susceptibility to IDDM maps upstream of the insulin gene. Diabetes 1995;44(6):620–5

42. Bell GI, Selby MJ, Rutter WJ. The highly polymorphic region near the human insulin gene is composed of simple tandemly repeating sequences. Nature 1982;295(5844):31–5

43. Vafiadis P, Ounissi-Benkalha H, Palumbo M, et al. Class III alleles of the variable number of tandem repeat insulin polymorphism associated with silencing of thymic insulin predispose to type 1 diabetes. J Clin Endocrinol Metab 2001;86(8):3705–10

44. Barratt BJ, Payne F, Lowe CE, et al. Remapping the insulin gene/IDDM2 locus in type 1 diabetes. Diabetes 2004;53(7):1884–9

45. Kawaguchi Y, Ikegami H, Shen G-Q, et al. Insulin gene region contributes to genetic susceptibility to, but may not to low incidence of, insulin-dependent diabetes mellitus in Japanese. Biochem Biophys Res Commun 1997;233(1):283–7

46. Nakayama M, Abiru N, Moriyama H, et al. Prime role for an insulin epitope in the development of type 1 diabetes in NOD mice. Nature 2005;435(7039):220–3

47. Kent SC, Chen Y, Bregoli L, et al. Expanded T cells from pancreatic lymph nodes of type 1 diabetic subjects recognize an insulin epitope. Nature 2005;435(7039):224

48. Derbinski J, Schulte A, Kyewski B, Klein L. Promiscuous gene expression in medullary thymic epithelial cells mirrors the peripheral self. Nat Immunol 2001;2(11):1032–9

49. Kyewski B, Derbinski J. Self-representation in the thymus: an extended view. Nat Rev Immunol 2004;4(9):688–98

50. Heath WR, Allison J, Hoffmann MW, et al. Autoimmune diabetes as a consequence of locally produced interleukin-2. Nature 1992;359(6395):547–9

51. Smith KM, Olson DC, Hirose R, Hanahan D. Pancreatic gene expression in rare cells of thymic medulla: evidence for functional contribution to T cell tolerance. Int Immunol 1997;9(9):1355–65

52. Pugliese A, Zeller M, Fernandez A, Jr, et al. The insulin gene is transcribed in the human thymus and transcription levels correlated with allelic variation at the INS VNTR-IDDM2 susceptibility locus for type 1 diabetes. Nat Genet 1997;15(3):293–7

53. Vafiadis P, Bennett ST, Todd JA, et al. Insulin expression in human thymus is modulated by INS VNTR alleles at the IDDM2 locus. Nat Genet 1997;15(3):289–92

54. Ashton-Rickardt PG, Bandeira A, Delaney JR, et al. Evidence for a differential avidity model of T cell selection in the thymus. Cell 1994;76(4):651–63

55. Zucchelli S, Holler P, Yamagata T, Roy M, Benoist C, Mathis D. Defective central tolerance induction in NOD mice: genomics and genetics. Immunity 2005;22(3):385–96

56. Chentoufi AA, Polychronakos C. Insulin expression levels in the thymus modulate insulin-specific autoreactive T-cell tolerance: the mechanism by which the IDDM2 locus may predispose to diabetes. Diabetes 2002;51(5):1383–90

57. Thebault-Baumont K, Dubois-Laforgue D, Krief P, et al. Acceleration of type 1 diabetes mellitus in proinsulin 2-deficient NOD mice. J Clin Invest 2003;111(6):851–7

58. Faideau B, Lotton C, Lucas B, et al. Tolerance to proinsulin-2 is due to radioresistant thymic cells. J Immunol 2006;177(1):53–60

59. Alegre M-L, Frauwirth KA, Thompson CB. T-cell regulation by CD28 and CTLA-4. Nat Rev Immunol 2001;1(3):220–8

60. van der Merwe PA, Bodian DL, Daenke S, Linsley P, Davis SJ. CD80 (B7–1) binds both CD28 and CTLA-4 with a low affinity and very fast kinetics. J Exp Med 1997;185(3):393–404

61. Ostrov DA, Shi W, Schwartz J-CD, Almo SC, Nathenson SG. Structure of murine CTLA-4 and its role in modulating T cell responsiveness. Science 2000;290(5492):816–9

62. Lee K-M, Chuang E, Griffin M, et al. Molecular basis of T cell inactivation by CTLA-4. Science 1998;282(5397):2263–6

63. Maurer M, Loserth S, Kolb-Maurer A, et al. A polymorphism in the human cytotoxic T-lymphocyte antigen 4 (CTLA4) gene (exon 1+49) alters T-cell activation. Immunogenetics 2002;54(1):1–8

64. Kouki T, Sawai Y, Gardine CA, Fisfalen ME, Alegre ML, DeGroot LJ. CTLA-4 Gene polymorphism at position 49 in exon 1 reduces the inhibitory function of CTLA-4 and contributes to the pathogenesis of Graves' disease. J Immunol 2000;165(11):6606–11

65. Nistico L, Buzzetti R, Pritchard LE, et al. The CTLA-4 gene region of chromosome 2q33 is linked to, and associated with, type 1 diabetes. Belgian Diabetes Registry. Hum Mol Genet 1996;5(7):1075–80

66. Van Der Auwera BJ, Vandewalle CL, Schuit FC, et al. CTLA-4 gene polymorphism confers susceptibility to insulin-dependent diabetes mellitus (IDDM) independently from age and from other genetic or immune disease markers. Clin Exp Immunol 1997;110(1):98–103

67. Krokowski M, Bodalski J, Bratek A, Machejko P, Caillat-Zucman S. CTLA-4 gene polymorphism is associated with predisposition to IDDM in a population from central Poland. Diabetes Metab 1998;24(3):241–3

68. Takara M, Komiya I, Kinjo Y, et al. Association of CTLA-4 gene A/G polymorphism in Japanese type 1 diabetic patients with younger age of onset and autoimmune thyroid disease. Diabetes Care 2000;23(7):975–8

69. Lee Y-J, Huang F-Y, Lo F-S, et al. Association of CTLA4 gene A-G polymorphism with type 1 diabetes in Chinese children. Clin Endocrinol 2000;52(2):153–7

70. Osei-Hyiaman D, Hou L, Zhiyin R, et al. Association of a novel point mutation (C159G) of the CTLA4 gene with type 1 diabetes in West Africans but not in Chinese. Diabetes 2001;50(9):2169–71

71. Barreto M, Santos E, Ferreira R, et al. Evidence for CTLA4 as a susceptibility gene for systemic lupus erythematosus. Eur J Hum Genet 2004;12(8):620–6

72. Ueda H, Howson JMM, Esposito L, et al. Association of the T-cell regulatory gene CTLA4 with susceptibility to autoimmune disease. Nature 2003;423(6939):506–11

73. Howson JM, Dunger DB, Nutland S, Stevens H, Wicker LS, Todd JA. A type 1 diabetes subgroup with a female bias is characterised by failure in tolerance to thyroid peroxidase at an early age and a strong association with the cytotoxic T-lymphocyte-associated antigen-4 gene. Diabetologia 2007;50(4):741–6

74. Anjos S, Nguyen A, Ounissi-Benkalha H, Tessier M-C, Polychronakos C. A common autoimmunity predisposing signal peptide variant of the cytotoxic T-lymphocyte antigen 4 results in inefficient glycosylation of the susceptibility allele. J Biol Chem 2002;277(48):46478–86

75. Magistrelli G, Jeannin P, Herbault N, et al. A soluble form of CTLA-4 generated by alternative splicing is expressed by nonstimulated human T cells. Eur J Immunol 1999;29(11):3596–602

76. Oaks MK, Hallett KM, Penwell RT, Stauber EC, Warren SJ, Tector AJ. A native soluble form of CTLA-4. Cell Immunol 2000;201(2):144–53

77. Anjos SM, Shao W, Marchand L, Polychronakos C. Allelic effects on gene regulation at the autoimmunity-predisposing CTLA4 locus: a re-evaluation of the 3′ +6230G >A polymorphism. Genes Immun 2005;6(4):305–11

78. Hill RJ, Zozulya S, Lu YL, Ward K, Gishizky M, Jallal B. The lymphoid protein tyrosine phosphatase Lyp interacts with the adaptor molecule Grb2 and functions as a negative regulator of T-cell activation. Exp Hematol 2002;30(3):237–44

79. Siminovitch KA. PTPN22 and autoimmune disease. Nat Genet 2004;36(12):1248–9

80. Hasegawa K, Martin F, Huang G, Tumas D, Diehl L, Chan AC. PEST domain-enriched tyrosine phosphatase (PEP) regulation of effector/memory T cells. Science 2004;303(5658):685–9

81. Gomez LM, Anaya JM, Gonzalez CI, et al. PTPN22 C1858T polymorphism in Colombian patients with autoimmune diseases. Genes Immun 2005;6(7):628–31

82. Kahles H, Ramos-Lopez E, Lange B, Zwermann O, Reincke M, Badenhoop K. Sex-specific association of PTPN22 1858T with type 1 diabetes but not with Hashimoto's thyroiditis or Addison's disease in the German population. Eur J Endocrinol 2005;153(6):895–9

83. Zheng W, She JX. Genetic association between a lymphoid tyrosine phosphatase (PTPN22) and type 1 diabetes. Diabetes 2005;54(3):906–8

84. Zhernakova A, Eerligh P, Wijmenga C, Barrera P, Roep BO, Koeleman BP. Differential association of the PTPN22 coding variant with autoimmune diseases in a Dutch population. Genes Immun 2005;6(6):459–61

85. Ladner MB, Bottini N, Valdes AM, Noble JA. Association of the single nucleotide polymorphism C1858T of the PTPN22 gene with type 1 diabetes. Hum Immunol 2005;66(1):60–4

86. Qu H, Tessier MC, Hudson TJ, Polychronakos C. Confirmation of the association of the R620W polymorphism in the protein tyrosine phosphatase PTPN22 with type 1 diabetes in a family based study. J Med Genet 2005;42(3):266–70

87. Smyth D, Cooper JD, Collins JE, et al. Replication of an association between the lymphoid tyrosine phosphatase locus (LYP/PTPN22) with type 1 diabetes, and evidence for its role as a general autoimmunity locus. Diabetes 2004;53(11):3020–3

88. Viken MK, Amundsen SS, Kvien TK, et al. Association analysis of the 1858C >T polymorphism in the PTPN22 gene in juvenile idiopathic arthritis and other autoimmune diseases. Genes Immun 2005;6(3):271–3

89. Onengut-Gumuscu S, Ewens KG, Spielman RS, Concannon P. A functional polymorphism (1858C/T) in the PTPN22 gene is linked and associated with type I diabetes in multiplex families. Genes Immun 2004;5(8):678–80

90. Cloutier JF, Veillette A. Cooperative inhibition of T-cell antigen receptor signaling by a complex between a kinase and a phosphatase. J Exp Med 1999;189(1):111–21

91. Begovich AB, Carlton VE, Honigberg LA, et al. A missense single-nucleotide polymorphism in a gene encoding a protein tyrosine phosphatase (PTPN22) is associated with rheumatoid arthritis. Am J Hum Genet 2004;75(2):330–7

92. Kyogoku C, Langefeld CD, Ortmann WA, et al. Genetic association of the R620W polymorphism of protein tyrosine phosphatase PTPN22 with human SLE. Am J Hum Genet 2004;75(3):504–7

93. Lee YH, Rho YH, Choi SJ, et al. The PTPN22 C1858T functional polymorphism and autoimmune diseases - a meta-analysis. Rheumatology (Oxford) 2007;46(1):49–56

94. International HapMap Consortium. The International HapMap Project. Nature 2003;426(6968):789–96

95. Kawasaki E, Awata T, Ikegami H, et al. Systematic search for single nucleotide polymorphisms in a lymphoid tyrosine phosphatase gene (PTPN22): association between a promoter polymorphism and type 1 diabetes in Asian populations. Am J Med Genet A 2006;140(6):586–93

96. Qu H-Q, Montpetit A, Ge B, Hudson TJ, Polychronakos C. Toward further mapping of the association between the IL2RA locus and type 1 diabetes. Diabetes 2007;56(4):1174–6

97. Brand OJ, Lowe CE, Heward JM, et al. Association of the interleukin-2 receptor alpha (IL-2Ralpha)/CD25 gene region with Graves' disease using a multilocus test and tag SNPs. Clin Endocrinol (Oxf) 2007;66(4):508–12

98. Lowenthal JW, Zubler RH, Nabholz M, MacDonald HR. Similarities between interleukin-2 receptor number and affinity on activated B and T lymphocytes. Nature 1985;315(6021):669–72

99. Wang X, Rickert M, Garcia KC. Structure of the quaternary complex of interleukin-2 with its alpha, beta, and gamma receptors. Science 2005;310(5751):1159–63

100. Gnarra JR, Otani H, Wang MG, McBride OW, Sharon M, Leonard WJ. Human interleukin 2 receptor beta-chain gene: chromosomal localization and identification of 5′ regulatory sequences. Proc Natl Acad Sci U S A 1990;87(9):3440–4

101. Takeshita T, Asao H, Ohtani K, et al. Cloning of the gamma chain of the human IL-2 receptor. Science 1992; 257(5068):379–82

102. Piccirillo CA, Tritt M, Sgouroudis E, Albanese A, Pyzik M, Hay V. Control of type 1 autoimmune diabetes by naturally occurring CD4+ CD25+ regulatory T lymphocytes in neonatal NOD mice. Ann N Y Acad Sci 2005;1051(1):72–87

103. Shevach EM. Certified professionals: CD4(+)CD25(+) suppressor T cells. J Exp Med 2001;193(11):F41–6

104. Salomon B, Lenschow DJ, Rhee L, et al. B7/CD28 costimulation is essential for the homeostasis of the CD4+ CD25+ immunoregulatory T cells that control autoimmune diabetes. Immunity 2000;12(4):431

105. Randolph DA, Fathman CG. CD4+ CD25+ regulatory T cells and their therapeutic potential. Ann Rev Med 2006; 57(1):381–402

106. Willerford DM, Chen J, Ferry JA, Davidson L, Ma A, Alt FW. Interleukin-2 receptor [alpha] chain regulates the size and content of the peripheral lymphoid compartment. Immunity 1995;3(4):521

107. Smyth DJ, Cooper JD, Bailey R, et al. A genome-wide association study of nonsynonymous SNPs identifies a type 1 diabetes locus in the interferon-induced helicase (IFIH1) region. Nat Genet 2006;38(6):617–9

108. Qu HQ, Marchand L, Grabs R, Polychronakos C. The association between the IFIH1 locus and type 1 diabetes. Diabetologia 2007

109. Kang DC, Gopalkrishnan RV, Wu Q, Jankowsky E, Pyle AM, Fisher PB. MDA-5: an interferon-inducible putative RNA helicase with double-stranded RNA-dependent ATPase activity and melanoma growth-suppressive properties. Proc Natl Acad Sci U S A 2002;99(2):637–42

110. Kato H, Takeuchi O, Sato S, et al. Differential roles of MDA5 and RIG-I helicases in the recognition of RNA viruses. Nature 2006;441(7089):101–5

111. van der Werf N, Kroese FG, Rozing J, Hillebrands J-L. Viral infections as potential triggers of type 1 diabetes. Diabetes Metab Res Rev 2007;23(3):169–83

112. Menser MA, Forrest JM, Bransby RD. Rubella infection and diabetes mellitus. Lancet 1978;1(8055):57–60

113. Haverkos HW, Battula N, Drotman DP, Rennert OM. Enteroviruses and type 1 diabetes mellitus. Biomed Pharmacother 2003;57(9):379–85

114. Wellcome Trust Case Control Consortium. Genome-wide association study of 14,000 cases of seven common diseases and 3,000 shared controls. Nature 2007;447(7145):661–78

115. Hakonarson H, Grant SF, Bradfield JP, et al. A genome-wide association study identifies KIAA0350 as a type 1 diabetes gene. Nature 2007;448(7153):591–4

116. Todd JA, Walker NM, Cooper JD, et al. Robust associations of four new chromosome regions from genome-wide analyses of type 1 diabetes. Nat Genet 2007;39(7):857–64

117. Cambi A, Figdor CG. Levels of complexity in pathogen recognition by C-type lectins. Curr Opin Immunol 2005;17(4):345–51

118. Takeyama K, Kitanaka S, Sato T, Kobori M, Yanagisawa J, Kato S. 25-Hydroxyvitamin D3 1alpha-hydroxylase and vitamin D synthesis. Science 1997;277(5333):1827–30

119. Kitanaka S, Takeyama K, Murayama A, et al. Inactivating mutations in the 25-hydroxyvitamin D3 1alpha-hydroxylase gene in patients with pseudovitamin D-deficiency rickets. N Engl J Med 1998;338(10):653–61

120. Fu GK, Lin D, Zhang MY, et al. Cloning of human 25-hydroxyvitamin D-1 alpha-hydroxylase and mutations causing vitamin D-dependent rickets type 1. Mol Endocrinol 1997;11(13):1961–70

121. Wang JT, Lin CJ, Burridge SM, et al. Genetics of vitamin D 1alpha-hydroxylase deficiency in 17 families. Am J Hum Genet 1998;63(6):1694–702

122. Wang X, Zhang MY, Miller WL, Portale AA. Novel gene mutations in patients with 1alpha-hydroxylase deficiency that confer partial enzyme activity in vitro. J Clin Endocrinol Metab 2002;87(6):2424–30

123. Lopez ER, Regulla K, Pani MA, Krause M, Usadel K-H, Badenhoop K. CYP27B1 polymorphisms variants are associated with type 1 diabetes mellitus in Germans. J Steroid Biochem Mol Biol 2004;89–90:155

124. Bailey R, Cooper JD, Zeitels L, et al. Association of the vitamin D metabolism gene CYP27B1 with type 1 diabetes. Diabetes 2007;56(10):2616–21

125. Lopez ER, Zwermann O, Segni M, et al. A promoter polymorphism of the CYP27B1 gene is associated with Addison's disease, Hashimoto's thyroiditis, Graves' disease and type 1 diabetes mellitus in Germans. Eur J Endocrinol 2004; 151(2):193–7

126. Mathieu C, Jafari M. Immunomodulation by 1,25-dihydroxyvitamin D3: therapeutic implications in hemodialysis and renal transplantation. Clin Nephrol 2006;66(4):275–83

127. Guo SW, Magnuson VL, Schiller JJ, Wang X, Wu Y, Ghosh S. Meta-analysis of vitamin D receptor polymorphisms and type 1 diabetes: a HuGE review of genetic association studies. Am J Epidemiol 2006;164(8):711–24

128. Mathieu C, Gysemans C, Giulietti A, Bouillon R. Vitamin D and diabetes. Diabetologia 2005;48(7):1247–57

129. Luong K, Nguyen LT, Nguyen DN. The role of vitamin D in protecting type 1 diabetes mellitus. Diabetes Metab Res Rev 2005;21(4):338–46

130. Hakonarson H, Qu HQ, Bradfield JP, et al. A novel susceptibility locus for type 1 diabetes, identified by a genome-wide association study. Diabetes 2008;57(4):1143–6

131. Wilson DB, Wilson MP. Identification and subcellular localization of human rab5b, a new member of the ras-related superfamily of GTPases. J Clin Invest 1992;89(3):996–1005

132. Jones RB, Gordus A, Krall JA, MacBeath G. A quantitative protein interaction network for the ErbB receptors using protein microarrays. Nature 2006;439(7073):168–74

133. Steinthorsdottir V, Thorleifsson G, Reynisdottir I, et al. A variant in CDKAL1 influences insulin response and risk of type 2 diabetes. Nat Genet 2007;39(6):770–5

134. Scott LJ, Mohlke KL, Bonnycastle LL, et al. A genome-wide association study of type 2 diabetes in Finns detects multiple susceptibility variants. Science 2007;316(5829):1341–5

135. Zeggini E, Weedon MN, Lindgren CM, et al. Replication of genome-wide association signals in UK samples reveals risk loci for type 2 diabetes. Science 2007;316(5829):1336–41

136. Diabetes Genetics Initiative of Broad Institute of Harvard and MIT, Lund University, and Novartis Institutes of BioMedical Research, Saxena R, Voight BF, et al. Genome-wide association analysis identifies loci for type 2 diabetes and triglyceride levels. Science 2007;316(5829):1331–6

137. Guo D, Li M, Zhang Y, et al. A functional variant of SUMO4, a new I kappa B alpha modifier, is associated with type 1 diabetes. Nat Genet 2004;36(8):837–41

138. Field LL, Bonnevie-Nielsen V, Pociot F, Lu S, Nielsen TB, Beck-Nielsen H. OAS1 splice site polymorphism controlling antiviral enzyme activity influences susceptibility to type 1 diabetes. Diabetes 2005;54(5):1588–91

139. Tessier MC, Qu HQ, Frechette R, et al. Type 1 diabetes and the OAS gene cluster: association with splicing polymorphism or haplotype? J Med Genet 2006;43(2):129–32

140. Smyth DJ, Howson JM, Lowe CE, et al. Assessing the validity of the association between the SUMO4 M55V variant and risk of type 1 diabetes. Nat Genet 2005;37(2):110–1; author reply 2–3

141. Qu H, Bharaj B, Liu XQ, et al. Assessing the validity of the association between the SUMO4 M55V variant and risk of type 1 diabetes. Nat Genet 2005;37(2):111–2; author reply 2–3

142. Park Y, Park S, Kang J, Yang S, Kim D. Assessing the validity of the association between the SUMO4 M55V variant and risk of type 1 diabetes. Nat Genet 2005;37(2):112; author reply 3

143. Smyth DJ, Cooper JD, Lowe CE, et al. No evidence for association of OAS1 with type 1 diabetes in unaffected siblings or type 1 diabetic cases. Diabetes 2006;55(5):1525–8

144. American Diabetes Association. Standards of medical care in diabetes–2007. Diabetes Care 2007;30(Suppl_1):S4–41

145. Valdez R, Yoon PW, Liu T, Khoury MJ. Family history and prevalence of diabetes in the U.S. population: the 6-year results from the National Health and Nutrition Examination Survey (1999 2004). Diabetes Care 2007;30(10): 2517–22

146. American Diabetes A. Diagnosis and classification of diabetes mellitus. Diabetes Care 2007;30(Suppl_1):S42–7

147. Barroso I, Gurnell M, Crowley VE, et al. Dominant negative mutations in human PPARgamma associated with severe insulin resistance, diabetes mellitus and hypertension. Nature 1999;402(6764):880–3

148. Savage DB, Tan GD, Acerini CL, et al. Human metabolic syndrome resulting from dominant-negative mutations in the nuclear receptor peroxisome proliferator-activated receptor-gamma. Diabetes 2003;52(4):910–7

149. Savage DB, Agostini M, Barroso I, et al. Digenic inheritance of severe insulin resistance in a human pedigree. Nat Genet 2002;31(4):379–84

150. Altshuler D, Hirschhorn JN, Klannemark M, et al. The common PPAR[gamma] Pro12Ala polymorphism is associated with decreased risk of type 2 diabetes. Nat Genet 2000;26(1):76–80

151. Ludovico O, Pellegrini F, Di Paola R, et al. Heterogeneous effect of peroxisome proliferator-activated receptor {gamma}2 Ala12 variant on type 2 diabetes risk. Obesity 2007;15(5):1076–81

152. Mukherjee R, Jow L, Croston GE, Paterniti JR, Jr. Identification, characterization, and tissue distribution of human peroxisome proliferator-activated receptor (PPAR) isoforms PPARgamma2 versus PPARgamma1 and activation with retinoid X receptor agonists and antagonists. J Biol Chem 1997;272(12):8071–6

153. Corton JC, Anderson SP, Stauber A. Central role of peroxisome proliferator - activated receptors in the actions of peroxisome proliferators. Annu Rev Pharmacol Toxicol 2000;40(1):491–518

154. Guan Y, Breyer MD. Peroxisome proliferator-activated receptors (PPARs): novel therapeutic targets in renal disease. Kidney Int 2001;60(1):14–30

155. Yang J, Chen L, Zhang X, et al. PPARs and female reproduction: evidence from genetically manipulated mice. PPAR Res 2008;2008:723243

156. Fajas L, Fruchart JC, Auwerx J. PPARgamma3 mRNA: a distinct PPARgamma mRNA subtype transcribed from an independent promoter. FEBS Lett 1998;438(1–2):55–60

157. Sharma AM, Staels B. Peroxisome proliferator-activated receptor {gamma} and adipose tissue - understanding obesity-related changes in regulation of lipid and glucose metabolism. J Clin Endocrinol Metab 2007;92(2):386–95

158. Yki-Jarvinen H. Thiazolidinediones. N Engl J Med 2004;351(11):1106–18

159. Deeb SS, Fajas L, Nemoto M, et al. A Pro12Ala substitution in PPAR[gamma]2 associated with decreased receptor activity, lower body mass index and improved insulin sensitivity. Nat Genet 1998;20(3):284–7

160. Masugi J, Tamori Y, Mori H, Koike T, Kasuga M. Inhibitory effect of a proline-to-alanine substitution at codon 12 of peroxisome proliferator-activated receptor-[gamma] 2 on thiazolidinedione-induced adipogenesis. Biochem Biophys Res Commun 2000;268(1):178–82

161. Snitker S, Watanabe RM, Ani I, et al. Changes in insulin sensitivity in response to troglitazone do not differ between subjects with and without the common, functional Pro12Ala peroxisome proliferator-activated receptor-gamma2 gene variant: results from the Troglitazone in Prevention of Diabetes (TRIPOD) study. Diabetes Care 2004;27(6):1365–8

162. Bluher M, Lubben G, Paschke R. Analysis of the relationship between the Pro12Ala variant in the PPAR-gamma2 gene and the response rate to therapy with pioglitazone in patients with type 2 diabetes. Diabetes Care 2003;26(3):825–31

163. Kang ES, Park SY, Kim HJ, et al. Effects of Pro12Ala polymorphism of peroxisome proliferator-activated receptor gamma2 gene on rosiglitazone response in type 2 diabetes. Clin Pharmacol Ther 2005;78(2):202–8

164. Hansen L, Ekstrom CT, Tabanera YPR, Anant M, Wassermann K, Reinhardt RR. The Pro12Ala variant of the PPARG gene is a risk factor for peroxisome proliferator-activated receptor-gamma/alpha agonist-induced edema in type 2 diabetic patients. J Clin Endocrinol Metab 2006;91(9):3446–50

165. Antoine HJ, Pall M, Trader BC, Chen YD, Azziz R, Goodarzi MO. Genetic variants in peroxisome proliferator-activated receptor gamma influence insulin resistance and testosterone levels in normal women, but not those with polycystic ovary syndrome. Fertil Steril 2007;87(4):862–9

166. Haap M, Machicao F, Stefan N, et al. Genetic determinants of insulin action in polycystic ovary syndrome. Exp Clin Endocrinol Diabetes 2005;113(5):275–81

167. Meirhaeghe A, Boreham CA, Murray LJ, et al. A possible role for the PPARG Pro12Ala polymorphism in preterm birth. Diabetes 2007;56(2):494–8

168. Cecil JE, Fischer B, Doney AS, et al. The Pro12Ala and C-681G variants of the PPARG locus are associated with opposing growth phenotypes in young schoolchildren. Diabetologia 2005;48(8):1496–502

169. Pihlajamaki J, Vanhala M, Vanhala P, Laakso M. The Pro12Ala polymorphism of the PPAR gamma 2 gene regulates weight from birth to adulthood. Obes Res 2004;12(2):187–90

170. Hani EH, Boutin P, Durand E, et al. Missense mutations in the pancreatic islet beta cell inwardly rectifying K+ channel gene (KIR6.2/BIR): a meta-analysis suggests a role in the polygenic basis of Type II diabetes mellitus in Caucasians. Diabetologia 1998;41(12):1511–5

171. Gloyn AL, Weedon MN, Owen KR, et al. Large-scale association studies of variants in genes encoding the pancreatic beta-cell KATP channel subunits Kir6.2 (KCNJ11) and SUR1 (ABCC8) confirm that the KCNJ11 E23K variant is associated with type 2 diabetes. Diabetes 2003;52(2):568–72

172. Nielsen EM, Hansen L, Carstensen B, et al. The E23K variant of Kir6.2 associates with impaired post-OGTT serum insulin response and increased risk of type 2 diabetes. Diabetes 2003;52(2):573–7

173. Florez JC, Sjogren M, Burtt N, et al. Association testing in 9,000 people fails to confirm the association of the insulin receptor substrate-1 G972R polymorphism with type 2 diabetes. Diabetes 2004;53(12):3313–8

174. van Dam RM, Hoebee B, Seidell JC, Schaap MM, de Bruin TW, Feskens EJ. Common variants in the ATP-sensitive K+ channel genes KCNJ11 (Kir6.2) and ABCC8 (SUR1) in relation to glucose intolerance: population-based studies and meta-analyses. Diabet Med 2005;22(5):590–8

175. Ashcroft FM, Rorsman P. Electrophysiology of the pancreatic beta-cell. Prog Biophys Mol Biol 1989;54(2):87–143

176. Ashcroft FM, Gribble FM. Correlating structure and function in ATP-sensitive K+ channels. Trends Neurosci 1998;21(7):288–94

177. Hansen JB. Towards selective Kir6.2/SUR1 potassium channel openers, medicinal chemistry and therapeutic perspectives. Curr Med Chem 2006;13:361–76

178. Schwanstecher C, Meyer U, Schwanstecher M. KIR6.2 polymorphism predisposes to type 2 diabetes by inducing over-activity of pancreatic {beta}-cell ATP-sensitive K+ channels. Diabetes 2002;51(3):875–9

179. Sesti G, Laratta E, Cardellini M, et al. The E23K variant of KCNJ11 encoding the pancreatic beta-cell adenosine 5'-triphosphate-sensitive potassium channel subunit Kir6.2 is associated with an increased risk of secondary failure to sulfonylurea in patients with type 2 diabetes. J Clin Endocrinol Metab 2006;91(6):2334–9

180. Grant SF, Thorleifsson G, Reynisdottir I, et al. Variant of transcription factor 7-like 2 (TCF7L2) gene confers risk of type 2 diabetes. Nat Genet 2006;38(3):320–3

181. Todd JA. Statistical false positive or true disease pathway? Nat Genet 2006;38(7):731–3

182. Florez JC, Jablonski KA, Bayley N, et al. TCF7L2 polymorphisms and progression to diabetes in the Diabetes Prevention Program. N Engl J Med 2006;355(3):241–50

183. Groves CJ, Zeggini E, Minton J, et al. Association analysis of 6,736 U.K. subjects provides replication and confirms TCF7L2 as a type 2 diabetes susceptibility gene with a substantial effect on individual risk. Diabetes 2006;55(9):2640–4

184. Zhang C, Qi L, Hunter DJ, et al. Variant of transcription factor 7-like 2 (TCF7L2) gene and the risk of type 2 diabetes in large cohorts of U.S. women and men. Diabetes 2006;55(9):2645–8

185. Scott LJ, Bonnycastle LL, Willer CJ, et al. Association of transcription factor 7-like 2 (TCF7L2) variants with type 2 diabetes in a Finnish sample. Diabetes 2006;55(9):2649–53

186. Damcott CM, Pollin TI, Reinhart LJ, et al. Polymorphisms in the transcription factor 7-like 2 (TCF7L2) gene are associated with type 2 diabetes in the Amish: replication and evidence for a role in both insulin secretion and insulin resistance. Diabetes 2006;55(9):2654–9

187. Saxena R, Gianniny L, Burtt NP, et al. Common single nucleotide polymorphisms in TCF7L2 are reproducibly associated with type 2 diabetes and reduce the insulin response to glucose in nondiabetic individuals. Diabetes 2006;55(10):2890–5

188. Cauchi S, Meyre D, Dina C, et al. Transcription factor TCF7L2 genetic study in the French population: expression in human beta-cells and adipose tissue and strong association with type 2 diabetes. Diabetes 2006;55(10):2903–8

189. Weedon MN, McCarthy MI, Hitman G, et al. Combining information from common type 2 diabetes risk polymorphisms improves disease prediction. PLoS Med 2006;3(10):e374

190. van Vliet-Ostaptchouk JV, Shiri-Sverdlov R, Zhernakova A, et al. Association of variants of transcription factor 7-like 2 (TCF7L2) with susceptibility to type 2 diabetes in the Dutch Breda cohort. Diabetologia 2006

191. Humphries SE, Gable D, Cooper JA, et al. Common variants in the TCF7L2 gene and predisposition to type 2 diabetes in UK European Whites, Indian Asians and Afro-Caribbean men and women. J Mol Med 2006

192. Freathy RM, Weedon MN, Bennett A, et al. Type 2 diabetes TCF7L2 risk genotypes alter birth weight: a study of 24,053 individuals. Am J Hum Genet 2007;80(6):1150–61

193. Cauchi S, Meyre D, Choquet H, et al. TCF7L2 rs7903146 variant does not associate with smallness for gestational age in the French population. BMC Med Genet 2007;8:37

194. Duval A, Busson-Leconiat M, Berger R, Hamelin R. Assignment of the TCF-4 gene (TCF7L2) to human chromosome band 10q25.3. Cytogenet Cell Genet 2000;88(3–4):264–5

195. Korinek V, Barker N, Morin PJ, et al. Constitutive transcriptional activation by a beta-catenin-Tcf complex in APC−/− colon carcinoma. Science 1997;275(5307):1784–7

196. Morin PJ, Sparks AB, Korinek V, et al. Activation of beta-catenin-Tcf signaling in colon cancer by mutations in beta-catenin or APC. Science 1997;275(5307):1787–90

197. Lyssenko V, Lupi R, Marchetti P, et al. Mechanisms by which common variants in the TCF7L2 gene increase risk of type 2 diabetes. J Clin Invest 2007;117(8):2155–63

198. Loos RJF, Franks PW, Francis RW, et al. TCF7L2 Polymorphisms modulate proinsulin levels and {beta}-cell function in a British Europid population. Diabetes 2007;56(7):1943–7

199. Munoz J, Lok KH, Gower BA, et al. Polymorphism in the transcription factor 7-like 2 (TCF7L2) gene is associated with reduced insulin secretion in nondiabetic women. Diabetes 2006;55(12):3630–4

200. Korinek V, Barker N, Moerer P, et al. Depletion of epithelial stem-cell compartments in the small intestine of mice lacking Tcf-4. Nat Genet 1998;19(4):379–83

201. Yi F, Brubaker PL, Jin T. TCF-4 mediates cell type-specific regulation of proglucagon gene expression by beta-catenin and glycogen synthase kinase-3beta. J Biol Chem 2005;280(2):1457–64

202. Wang Z, Wang RM, Owji AA, Smith DM, Ghatei MA, Bloom SR. Glucagon like peptide-1 is a physiological incretin in rat. J Clin Invest 1995;95(1):417–21

203. Toft-Nielsen M-B, Damholt MB, Madsbad S, et al. Determinants of the impaired secretion of glucagon-like peptide-1 in type 2 diabetic patients. J Clin Endocrinol Metab 2001;86(8):3717–23

204. Shu L, Sauter NS, Schulthess FT, Matveyenko AV, Oberholzer J, Maedler K. Transcription factor 7-like 2 regulates beta-cell survival and function in human pancreatic islets. Diabetes 2008;57(3):645–53

205. Xu G, Stoffers DA, Habener JF, Bonner-Weir S. Exendin-4 stimulates both beta-cell replication and neogenesis, resulting in increased beta-cell mass and improved glucose tolerance in diabetic rats. Diabetes 1999;48(12):2270–6

206. Steiner DF, Rouille Y, Gong Q, Martin S, Carroll R, Chan SJ. The role of prohormone convertases in insulin biosynthesis: evidence for inherited defects in their action in man and experimental animals. Diabetes Metab 1996;22(2):94–104

207. Saxena R, Voight BF, Lyssenko V, et al. Genome-wide association analysis identifies loci for type 2 diabetes and triglyceride levels. Science 2007;316(5829):1331–6

208. Sladek R, Rocheleau G, Rung J, et al. A genome-wide association study identifies novel risk loci for type 2 diabetes. Nature 2007;445(7130):881–5

209. Gudmundsson J, Sulem P, Steinthorsdottir V, et al. Two variants on chromosome 17 confer prostate cancer risk, and the one in TCF2 protects against type 2 diabetes. Nat Genet 2007;39(8):977–83

210. Sandhu MS, Weedon MN, Fawcett KA, et al. Common variants in WFS1 confer risk of type 2 diabetes. Nat Genet 2007;39(8):951–3

211. Winckler W, Weedon MN, Graham RR, et al. Evaluation of common variants in the six known maturity-onset diabetes of the young (MODY) genes for association with type 2 diabetes. Diabetes 2007;56(3):685–93

212. Franks PW, Rolandsson O, Debenham SL, et al. Replication of the association between variants in WFS1 and risk of type 2 diabetes in European populations. Diabetologia 2008;51(3):458–63

213. Florez JC, Jablonski KA, McAteer J, et al. Testing of diabetes-associated WFS1 polymorphisms in the Diabetes Prevention Program. Diabetologia 2008;51(3):451–7

214. Umpierrez GE, Smiley D, Kitabchi AE. Narrative review: ketosis-prone type 2 diabetes mellitus. Ann Intern Med 2006;144(5):350–7

215. Nielsen J, Christiansen J, Lykke-Andersen J, Johnsen AH, Wewer UM, Nielsen FC. A family of insulin-like growth factor II mRNA-binding proteins represses translation in late development. Mol Cell Biol 1999;19(2):1262–70

216. Spagnoli FM, Brivanlou AH. The RNA-binding protein, Vg1RBP, is required for pancreatic fate specification. Dev Biol 2006;292(2):442–56

217. Takeda K, Inoue H, Tanizawa Y, et al. WFS1 (Wolfram syndrome 1) gene product: predominant subcellular localization to endoplasmic reticulum in cultured cells and neuronal expression in rat brain. Hum Mol Genet 2001;10(5):477–84

218. Strom TM, Hortnagel K, Hofmann S, et al. Diabetes insipidus, diabetes mellitus, optic atrophy and deafness (DIDMOAD) caused by mutations in a novel gene (wolframin) coding for a predicted transmembrane protein. Hum Mol Genet 1998;7(13):2021–8

219. Khanim F, Kirk J, Latif F, Barrett TG. WFS1/wolframin mutations, Wolfram syndrome, and associated diseases. Hum Mutat 2001;17(5):357–67

220. Pascoe L, Tura A, Patel SK, et al. Common variants of the novel type 2 diabetes genes, CDKAL1 and HHEX/IDE, are associated with decreased pancreatic {beta}-cell function. Diabetes 2007

221. Ubeda M, Rukstalis JM, Habener JF. Inhibition of cyclin-dependent kinase 5 activity protects pancreatic beta cells from glucotoxicity. J Biol Chem 2006;281(39):28858–64

222. Chimienti F, Devergnas S, Favier A, Seve M. Identification and cloning of a beta-cell-specific zinc transporter, ZnT-8, localized into insulin secretory granules. Diabetes 2004;53(9):2330–7

223. Rane SG, Dubus P, Mettus RV, et al. Loss of Cdk4 expression causes insulin-deficient diabetes and Cdk4 activation results in [beta]-islet cell hyperplasia. Nat Genet 1999;22(1):44–52

224. Krishnamurthy J, Ramsey MR, Ligon KL, et al. p16INK4a induces an age-dependent decline in islet regenerative potential. Nature 2006;443(7110):453–7

225. Frayling TM, Timpson NJ, Weedon MN, et al. A common variant in the FTO gene is associated with body mass index and predisposes to childhood and adult obesity. Science 2007;316(5826):889–94

226. Wang L, Coffinier C, Thomas MK, et al. Selective deletion of the Hnf1{beta} (MODY5) gene in {beta}-cells leads to altered gene expression and defective insulin release. Endocrinology 2004;145(8):3941–9

227. Fajans SS, Bell GI, Polonsky KS. Molecular mechanisms and clinical pathophysiology of maturity-onset diabetes of the young. N Engl J Med 2001;345(13):971–80

228. Frayling TM, Evans JC, Bulman MP, et al. Beta-cell genes and diabetes: molecular and clinical characterization of mutations in transcription factors. Diabetes 2001;50 Suppl 1:S94–100

229. Pearson ER, Liddell WG, Shepherd M, Corrall RJ, Hattersley AT. Sensitivity to sulphonylureas in patients with hepatocyte nuclear factor-1alpha gene mutations: evidence for pharmacogenetics in diabetes. Diabet Med 2000;17(7):543–5

230. Odom DT, Zizlsperger N, Gordon DB, et al. Control of pancreas and liver gene expression by HNF transcription factors. Science 2004;303(5662):1378–81

231. Miura A, Yamagata K, Kakei M, et al. Hepatocyte nuclear factor-4alpha is essential for glucose-stimulated insulin secretion by pancreatic beta-cells. J Biol Chem 2006;281(8):5246–57

232. Stoffel M, Duncan SA. The maturity-onset diabetes of the young (MODY1) transcription factor HNF4alpha regulates expression of genes required for glucose transport and metabolism. Proc Natl Acad Sci U S A 1997;94(24):13209–14

233. Pearson ER, Boj SF, Steele AM, et al. Macrosomia and hyperinsulinaemic hypoglycaemia in patients with heterozygous mutations in the HNF4A gene. PLoS Med 2007;4(4):e118

234. Matschinsky FM. Glucokinase as glucose sensor and metabolic signal generator in pancreatic beta-cells and hepatocytes. Diabetes 1990;39(6):647 52

235. Velho G, Froguel P, Clement K, et al. Primary pancreatic beta-cell secretory defect caused by mutations in glucokinase gene in kindreds of maturity onset diabetes of the young. Lancet 1992;340(8817):444–8

236. Hattersley AT, Beards F, Ballantyne E, Appleton M, Harvey R, Ellard S. Mutations in the glucokinase gene of the fetus result in reduced birth weight. Nat Genet 1998;19(3):268–70

237. Glaser B, Kesavan P, Heyman M, et al. Familial hyperinsulinism caused by an activating glucokinase mutation. N Engl J Med 1998;338(4):226–30

238. Weedon MN, Clark VJ, Qian Y, et al. A common haplotype of the glucokinase gene alters fasting glucose and birth weight: association in six studies and population-genetics analyses. Am J Hum Genet 2006;79(6):991–1001

239. Christesen HB, Jacobsen BB, Odili S, et al. The second activating glucokinase mutation (A456V): implications for glucose homeostasis and diabetes therapy. Diabetes 2002;51(4):1240–6

240. Cuesta-Munoz AL, Huopio H, Otonkoski T, et al. Severe persistent hyperinsulinemic hypoglycemia due to a de novo glucokinase mutation. Diabetes 2004;53(8):2164–8

241. Thomas H, Jaschkowitz K, Bulman M, et al. A distant upstream promoter of the HNF-4alpha gene connects the transcription factors involved in maturity-onset diabetes of the young. Hum Mol Genet 2001;10(19):2089–97

242. Hansen SK, Parrizas M, Jensen ML, et al. Genetic evidence that HNF-1{alpha}-dependent transcriptional control of HNF-4{alpha} is essential for human pancreatic {beta} cell function. J Clin Invest 2002;110(6):827–33

243. Pontoglio M, Sreenan S, Roe M, et al. Defective insulin secretion in hepatocyte nuclear factor 1alpha-deficient Mice. J Clin Invest 1998;101(10):2215–22

244. Jonsson J, Carlsson L, Edlund T, Edlund H. Insulin-promoter-factor 1 is required for pancreas development in mice. Nature 1994;371(6498):606–9

245. Stoffers DA, Zinkin NT, Stanojevic V, Clarke WL, Habener JF. Pancreatic agenesis attributable to a single nucleotide deletion in the human IPF1 gene coding sequence. Nat Genet 1997;15(1):106–10

246. Ahlgren U, Jonsson J, Jonsson L, Simu K, Edlund H. Beta-cell-specific inactivation of the mouse Ipf1/Pdx1 gene results in loss of the beta-cell phenotype and maturity onset diabetes. Genes Dev 1998;12(12):1763–8

247. Horikawa Y, Iwasaki N, Hara M, et al. Mutation in hepatocyte nuclear factor-1 beta gene (TCF2) associated with MODY. Nat Genet 1997;17(4):384–5

248. Bellanne-Chantelot C, Chauveau D, Gautier JF, et al. Clinical spectrum associated with hepatocyte nuclear factor-1beta mutations. Ann Intern Med 2004;140(7):510–7

249. Edghill EL, Bingham C, Ellard S, Hattersley AT. Mutations in hepatocyte nuclear factor-1beta and their related phenotypes. J Med Genet 2006;43(1):84–90

250. Rey-Campos J, Chouard T, Yaniv M, Cereghini S. vHNF1 is a homeoprotein that activates transcription and forms heterodimers with HNF1. EMBO J 1991;10(6):1445–57

251. Mayer C, Bottcher Y, Kovacs P, Halbritter J, Stumvoll M. Phenotype of a patient with a de novo mutation in the hepatocyte nuclear factor 1beta/maturity-onset diabetes of the young type 5 gene. Metabolism 2008;57(3):416–20

252. Edghill EL, Bingham C, Slingerland AS, et al. Hepatocyte nuclear factor-1 beta mutations cause neonatal diabetes and intrauterine growth retardation: support for a critical role of HNF-1beta in human pancreatic development. Diabet Med 2006;23(12):1301–6

253. Naya FJ, Stellrecht CM, Tsai MJ. Tissue-specific regulation of the insulin gene by a novel basic helix-loop-helix transcription factor. Genes Dev 1995;9(8):1009–19

254. Malecki MT, Jhala US, Antonellis A, et al. Mutations in NEUROD1 are associated with the development of type 2 diabetes mellitus. Nat Genet 1999;23(3):323–8

255. Neve B, Fernandez-Zapico ME, Ashkenazi-Katalan V, et al. Role of transcription factor KLF11 and its diabetes-associated gene variants in pancreatic beta cell function. Proc Natl Acad Sci U S A 2005;102(13):4807–12

256. Raeder H, Johansson S, Holm PI, et al. Mutations in the CEL VNTR cause a syndrome of diabetes and pancreatic exocrine dysfunction. Nat Genet 2006;38(1):54–62

257. Molven A, Ringdal M, Nordbo AM, et al. Mutations in the insulin gene can cause MODY and autoantibody-negative type 1 diabetes. Diabetes 2008;57(4):1131–5

258. van den Berg JMW, Morton AM, Kok SW, Pijl H, Conway SP, Heijerman HGM. Microvascular complications in patients with cystic fibrosis - related diabetes (CFRD). J Cyst Fibros 2007;30:1056–1061

259. Rosendahl J, Bodeker H, Mossner J, Teich N. Hereditary chronic pancreatitis. Orphanet J Rare Dis 2007;2:1

260. McDermott JH, Walsh CH. Hypogonadism in hereditary hemochromatosis. J Clin Endocrinol Metab 2005;90(4):2451–5

261. Ristow M. Neurodegenerative disorders associated with diabetes mellitus. J Mol Med 2004;82(8):510–29

262. Temple IK, Gardner RJ, Mackay DJ, Barber JC, Robinson DO, Shield JP. Transient neonatal diabetes: widening the understanding of the etiopathogenesis of diabetes. Diabetes 2000;49(8):1359–66

263. Spengler D, Villalba M, Hoffmann A, et al. Regulation of apoptosis and cell cycle arrest by Zac1, a novel zinc finger protein expressed in the pituitary gland and the brain. EMBO J 1997;16(10):2814–25

264. Arima T, Drewell RA, Oshimura M, Wake N, Surani MA. A novel imprinted gene, HYMAI, is located within an imprinted domain on human chromosome 6 containing ZAC. Genomics 2000;67(3):248–55

265. Ma D, Shield JP, Dean W, et al. Impaired glucose homeostasis in transgenic mice expressing the human transient neonatal diabetes mellitus locus, TNDM. J Clin Invest 2004;114(3):339–48

266. Mackay DJ, Boonen SE, Clayton-Smith J, et al. A maternal hypomethylation syndrome presenting as transient neonatal diabetes mellitus. Hum Genet 2006;120(2):262–9

267. Massa O, Iafusco D, D'Amato E, et al. KCNJ11 activating mutations in Italian patients with permanent neonatal diabetes. Hum Mutat 2005;25(1):22–7

268. Njolstad PR, Sovik O, Cuesta-Munoz A, et al. Neonatal diabetes mellitus due to complete glucokinase deficiency. N Engl J Med 2001;344(21):1588–92

269. Kawaguchi Y, Cooper B, Gannon M, Ray M, MacDonald RJ, Wright CV. The role of the transcriptional regulator Ptf1a in converting intestinal to pancreatic progenitors. Nat Genet 2002;32(1):128–34

270. Hoveyda N, Shield JP, Garrett C, et al. Neonatal diabetes mellitus and cerebellar hypoplasia/agenesis: report of a new recessive syndrome. J Med Genet 1999;36(9):700–4

271. Sellick GS, Barker KT, Stolte-Dijkstra I, et al. Mutations in PTF1A cause pancreatic and cerebellar agenesis. Nat Genet 2004;36(12):1301–5

272. Schwitzgebel VM, Mamin A, Brun T, et al. Agenesis of human pancreas due to decreased half-life of insulin promoter factor 1. J Clin Endocrinol Metab 2003;88(9):4398–406

273. Polak M, Dechaume A, Cave H, et al. Heterozygous missense mutations in the insulin gene are linked to permanent diabetes appearing in the neonatal period or in early infancy: a report from the French ND (Neonatal Diabetes) Study Group. Diabetes 2008;57(4):1115–9

274. Stoy J, Edghill EL, Flanagan SE, et al. Insulin gene mutations as a cause of permanent neonatal diabetes. Proc Natl Acad Sci U S A 2007;104(38):15040–4

275. Babenko AP, Polak M, Cave H, et al. Activating mutations in the ABCC8 gene in neonatal diabetes mellitus. N Engl J Med 2006;355(5):456–66

276. Proks P, Arnold AL, Bruining J, et al. A heterozygous activating mutation in the sulphonylurea receptor SUR1 (ABCC8) causes neonatal diabetes. Hum Mol Genet 2006;15(11):1793–800

277. Ellard S, Flanagan SE, Girard CA, et al. Permanent neonatal diabetes caused by dominant, recessive, or compound heterozygous SUR1 mutations with opposite functional effects. Am J Hum Genet 2007;81(2):375–82

278. Yorifuji T, Nagashima K, Kurokawa K, et al. The C42R mutation in the Kir6.2 (KCNJ11) gene as a cause of transient neonatal diabetes, childhood diabetes, or later-onset, apparently type 2 diabetes mellitus. J Clin Endocrinol Metab 2005;90(6):3174–8

279. Gloyn AL, Pearson ER, Antcliff JF, et al. Activating mutations in the gene encoding the ATP-sensitive potassium-channel subunit Kir6.2 and permanent neonatal diabetes. N Engl J Med 2004;350(18):1838–49

280. Mlynarski W, Tarasov AI, Gach A, et al. Sulfonylurea improves CNS function in a case of intermediate DEND syndrome caused by a mutation in KCNJ11. Nat Clin Pract Neurol 2007;3(11):640–5

281. Hardy C, Khanim F, Torres R, et al. Clinical and molecular genetic analysis of 19 Wolfram syndrome kindreds demonstrating a wide spectrum of mutations in WFS1. Am J Hum Genet 1999;65(5):1279–90

282. Hofmann S, Philbrook C, Gerbitz KD, Bauer MF. Wolfram syndrome: structural and functional analyses of mutant and wild-type wolframin, the WFS1 gene product. Hum Mol Genet 2003;12(16):2003–12

283. Colosimo A, Guida V, Rigoli L, et al. Molecular detection of novel WFS1 mutations in patients with Wolfram syndrome by a DHPLC-based assay. Hum Mutat 2003;21(6):622–9

284. Cryns K, Pfister M, Pennings RJ, et al. Mutations in the WFS1 gene that cause low-frequency sensorineural hearing loss are small non-inactivating mutations. Hum Genet 2002;110(5):389–94

285. Ohkubo K, Yamano A, Nagashima M, et al. Mitochondrial gene mutations in the tRNALeu(UUR) region and diabetes: prevalence and clinical phenotypes in Japan. Clin Chem 2001;47(9):1641–8

286. Maassen JA, t Hart LM, van Essen E, et al. Mitochondrial diabetes: molecular mechanisms and clinical presentation. Diabetes 2004;53(90001):S103–9

287. van den Ouweland JM, Lemkes HH, Ruitenbeek W, et al. Mutation in mitochondrial tRNA(Leu)(UUR) gene in a large pedigree with maternally transmitted type II diabetes mellitus and deafness. Nat Genet 1992;1(5):368–71

288. Kameoka K, Isotani H, Tanaka K, et al. Novel mitochondrial DNA mutation in tRNA(Lys) (8296A→G) associated with diabetes. Biochem Biophys Res Commun 1998;245(2):523–7

289. McFarland R, Schaefer AM, Gardner JL, et al. Familial myopathy: new insights into the T14709C mitochondrial tRNA mutation. Ann Neurol 2004;55(4):478–84

290. Kahn CR, Flier JS, Bar RS, et al. The syndromes of insulin resistance and acanthosis nigricans. Insulin-receptor disorders in man. N Engl J Med 1976;294(14):739–45

291. al-Gazali LI, Khalil M, Devadas K. A syndrome of insulin resistance resembling leprechaunism in five sibs of consanguineous parents. J Med Genet 1993;30(6):470–5

292. Longo N, Wang Y, Smith SA, Langley SD, DiMeglio LA, Giannella-Neto D. Genotype-phenotype correlation in inherited severe insulin resistance. Hum Mol Genet 2002;11(12):1465–75

293. Takahashi Y, Kadowaki H, Ando A, et al. Two aberrant splicings caused by mutations in the insulin receptor gene in cultured lymphocytes from a patient with Rabson-Mendenhall's syndrome. J Clin Invest 1998;101(3):588–94

294. Cho H, Mu J, Kim JK, et al. Insulin resistance and a diabetes mellitus-like syndrome in mice lacking the protein kinase Akt2 (PKBbeta). Science 2001;292(5522):1728–31

295. George S, Rochford JJ, Wolfrum C, et al. A family with severe insulin resistance and diabetes due to a mutation in AKT2. Science 2004;304(5675):1325–8

296. Lerin C, Montell E, Nolasco T, et al. Regulation and function of the muscle glycogen-targeting subunit of protein phosphatase 1 (GM) in human muscle cells depends on the COOH-terminal region and glycogen content. Diabetes 2003;52(9):2221–6

297. Pravenec M, Landa V, Zidek V, et al. Transgenic rescue of defective Cd36 ameliorates insulin resistance in spontaneously hypertensive rats. Nat Genet 2001;27(2):156–8

298. Lepretre F, Vasseur F, Vaxillaire M, et al. A CD36 nonsense mutation associated with insulin resistance and familial type 2 diabetes. Hum Mutat 2004;24(1):104

299. Garg A. Acquired and inherited lipodystrophies. N Engl J Med 2004;350(12):1220–34

300. Agarwal AK, Arioglu E, De Almeida S, et al. AGPAT2 is mutated in congenital generalized lipodystrophy linked to chromosome 9q34. Nat Genet 2002;31(1):21–3

301. Magre J, Delepine M, Khallouf E, et al. Identification of the gene altered in Berardinelli-Seip congenital lipodystrophy on chromosome 11q13. Nat Genet 2001;28(4):365–70

302. Herbst KL, Tannock LR, Deeb SS, Purnell JQ, Brunzell JD, Chait A. Kobberling type of familial partial lipodystrophy: an underrecognized syndrome. Diabetes Care 2003;26(6):1819–24

303. Shackleton S, Lloyd DJ, Jackson SN, et al. LMNA, encoding lamin A/C, is mutated in partial lipodystrophy. Nat Genet 2000;24(2):153–6

304. Novelli G, Muchir A, Sangiuolo F, et al. Mandibuloacral dysplasia is caused by a mutation in LMNA-encoding lamin A/C. Am J Hum Genet 2002;71(2):426–31

305. Agarwal AK, Fryns JP, Auchus RJ, Garg A. Zinc metalloproteinase, ZMPSTE24, is mutated in mandibuloacral dysplasia. Hum Mol Genet 2003;12(16):1995–2001

306. Anderson MS, Venanzi ES, Klein L, et al. Projection of an immunological self shadow within the thymus by the AIRE protein. Science 2002;298(5597):1395–401

307. Nagamine K, Peterson P, Scott HS, et al. Positional cloning of the APECED gene. Nat Genet 1997;17(4):393–8

308. Finnish-German APECED Consortium. An autoimmune disease, APECED, caused by mutations in a novel gene featuring two PHD-type zinc-finger domains. Nat Genet 1997;17(4):399–403

309. Hori S, Nomura T, Sakaguchi S. Control of regulatory T cell development by the transcription factor Foxp3. Science 2003;299(5609):1057–61

310. Wildin RS, Ramsdell F, Peake J, et al. X-linked neonatal diabetes mellitus, enteropathy and endocrinopathy syndrome is the human equivalent of mouse scurfy. Nat Genet 2001;27(1):18–20

311. Bacchetta R, Passerini L, Gambineri E, et al. Defective regulatory and effector T cell functions in patients with FOXP3 mutations. J Clin Invest 2006;116(6):1713–22

312. Dorner G, Plagemann A, Reinagel H. Familial diabetes aggregation in type I diabetics: gestational diabetes an apparent risk factor for increased diabetes susceptibility in the offspring. Exp Clin Endocrinol 1987;89(1):84–90

313. McLellan JA, Barrow BA, Levy JC, et al. Prevalence of diabetes mellitus and impaired glucose tolerance in parents of women with gestational diabetes. Diabetologia 1995;38(6):693–8

314. Martin AO, Simpson JL, Ober C, Freinkel N. Frequency of diabetes mellitus in mothers of probands with gestational diabetes: possible maternal influence on the predisposition to gestational diabetes. Am J Obstet Gynecol 1985;151(4):471–5

315. Freinkel N, Metzger BE, Phelps RL, et al. Gestational diabetes mellitus: a syndrome with phenotypic and genotypic heterogeneity. Horm Metab Res 1986;18(7):427–30

316. Weng J, Ekelund M, Lehto M, et al. Screening for MODY mutations, GAD antibodies, and type 1 diabetes - associated HLA genotypes in women with gestational diabetes mellitus. Diabetes Care 2002;25(1):68–71

317. Unluturk U, Harmanci A, Kocaefe C, Yildiz BO. The genetic basis of the polycystic ovary syndrome: a literature review including discussion of PPAR-gamma. PPAR Res 2007;2007:49109

318. Dunaif A. Insulin resistance and the polycystic ovary syndrome: mechanism and implications for pathogenesis. Endocr Rev 1997;18(6):774–800

319. Hara M, Alcoser SY, Qaadir A, Beiswenger KK, Cox NJ, Ehrmann DA. Insulin resistance is attenuated in women with polycystic ovary syndrome with the Pro(12)Ala polymorphism in the PPARgamma gene. J Clin Endocrinol Metab 2002;87(2):772–5

22

Breastfeeding and Diabetes

Julie Scott Taylor, Melissa Nothnagle, and Susanna R. Magee

CONTENTS

ABSTRACT

As diabetes becomes more prevalent in younger women, diabetes and maternal-child health issues such as breastfeeding coexist with increasing frequency in clinical practice. Women with diabetes of any kind including type 1 diabetes (DM1), type 2 diabetes (DM2) or gestational diabetes (GDM) should be strongly encouraged to breastfeed because of the maternal and pediatric benefits specific to obesity and diabetes that are above and beyond other known benefits of breastfeeding. Many of the benefits of breastfeeding are dose-dependent. Current infant nutrition recommendations for mother-infant dyads include 6 months of exclusive breastfeeding and continued breastfeeding for at least 12 months. In this chapter, we explore in detail the many relationships between breastfeeding and diabetes in a variety of clinical contexts.

Women with diabetes are less likely to breastfeed than women without diabetes, likely due to higher rates of pregnancy-related and neonatal complications among women with diabetes. Medical complications pose significant challenges to breastfeeding, both the inherent clinical issues and the associated hospital protocols. Lactating mothers have increased energy needs that are similar in women with and without diabetes. Breastfeeding may improve postpartum glucose metabolism among women without diabetes and those with GDM but does not appear to reduce the substantial risk of future development of DM2 among women with GDM. Breastfeeding lowers a child's risk of pediatric obesity, DM1 and DM2, regardless of a mother's diabetic status. Some studies have also demonstrated lower rates of obesity and diabetes among the breastfed children of women with diabetes. To date, differences in milk composition of women with diabetes do not preclude them from breastfeeding their infants. Many medications are safe for use among lactating women with diabetes and are not a contraindication to breastfeeding. Contraception for breastfeeding women requires special consideration.

From: *Diabetes in Women: Pathophysiology and Therapy*
Edited by: A. Tsatsoulis et al. (eds.), DOI 10.1007/978-1-60327-250-6_22
© Humana Press, a part of Springer Science+Business Media, LLC 2009

415

Key words: Breast feeding; Lactation; Milk; Human; Obesity; Diabetes; Diabetes mellitus type 1; Diabetes mellitus type 2; Gestational diabetes.

INTRODUCTION

As the prevalence of diabetes increases among younger women *(1, 2)*, diabetes and maternal-child health concerns such as breastfeeding overlap more frequently *(3, 4)*. This chapter explores the many relationships between breastfeeding and diabetes, including type 1 diabetes (DM1), type 2 diabetes (DM2) and gestational diabetes (GDM), from both the maternal and the pediatric perspectives. We begin the chapter with definitions, infant nutrition recommendations and breastfeeding rates. Next, we discuss maternal issues including perinatal complications that may affect breastfeeding, hospital support for breastfeeding mothers, the effect of lactation on maternal energy needs and the impact of breastfeeding on the subsequent glucose tolerance of mothers with diabetes. Our discussion of pediatric issues includes the benefits of breastfeeding for all children in reducing rates of pediatric obesity and diabetes as well as the short- and long-term clinical care, with respect to breastfeeding, of children whose mothers have diabetes. Finally, we include a review of selected medications in the context of breastfeeding and diabetes.

Definitions

Lactation is defined as the process of milk production. Breastfeeding is defined as any breast milk consumption by an infant, either directly from the breast itself or, less commonly, the administration of breast milk that has first been pumped and is then fed to an infant. Exclusive breastfeeding describes an infant who is fed only breast milk and no solids, water or other liquids. Many of the studies discussed in this chapter report only breastfeeding vs. bottle feeding, without more detailed information on exclusivity, frequency or duration. More precise definitions will be extremely important for meaningful interpretation of future breastfeeding research.

Recommendations for Infant Nutrition

Breastfeeding is recommended by numerous health agencies as the preferred method of feeding for infants for at least 1 year because of its multiple immediate- and long-term benefits for both mother and child *(5–8)*. The data supporting the myriad benefits of breastfeeding, increasingly referred to as the "risks of bottle feeding," have recently been rigorously reviewed *(9, 10)*. Maternal benefits of breastfeeding include a lower risk of breast and ovarian cancer and possibly a lower risk of postpartum depression. Pediatric benefits of breastfeeding include significantly lower rates of infections such as otitis media, gastroenteritis and lower respiratory tract diseases as well as lower rates of asthma, leukemia and sudden infant death syndrome. In addition, breastfeeding is associated with improved pediatric cognitive development. Many of these benefits are dose-related. The American Academy of Pediatrics (AAP) and multiple other health organizations recommend that an infant be exclusively breastfed without supplemental foods or liquids for the first 6 months of life, followed by the gradual introduction of complementary foods in conjunction with continued breastfeeding for at least 12 months *(7)*. Cow's milk can be introduced into a child's diet after 1 year.

Healthy People 2010 goals are to have 75% of women breastfeeding at hospital discharge, 50% breastfeeding at 6 months, and 25% still breastfeeding at 12 months *(11)*. In 2007, *Healthy People 2010* expanded its breastfeeding objectives to include targets for breastfeeding exclusivity as well *(12)*. The new objectives are to increase the proportion of mothers who breastfeed exclusively through 3 months to 40% and the proportion of mothers who breastfeed exclusively through 6 months to 17%.

Breastfeeding Rates in the USA

Data from the National Immunization Survey (NIS) show that the percent of children who are breastfed at birth, at 6 months, and at 12 months continues to rise in the USA. In 2004, breastfeeding rates for US mothers were 73.8% and 41.5% at birth and 6 months, respectively *(12)*. Among children born in 2004, 21 states achieved the national *Healthy People 2010* objective of having 75% of mothers initiate breastfeeding, 9 states achieved the objective of having 50% of mothers breastfeeding their infant at 6 months of age; and 12 states achieved the objective of having 25% of mothers breastfeeding their infant at 12 months of age. Six states achieved the objective of having 40% of mothers exclusively breastfeeding their infant through 3 months of age, and five states achieved the objective of having 17% of mothers exclusively breastfeeding their infant through 6 months of age. Consistent with previous national data, the NIS reported lower breastfeeding rates among non Hispanic black women and women from socioeconomically disadvantaged groups.

Breastfeeding Rates Among Women with Diabetes

In the 1980s and 1990s, two small prospective studies of 60 and 37 women, respectively, reported similar rates of breastfeeding initiation and breastfeeding duration among women with diabetes and women without diabetes, in spite of increased medical challenges experienced by mothers with diabetes *(13, 14)*. A more recent German study of 1,560 children born between 1989 and 2004 showed that significantly fewer children of mothers with DM1 were breastfed than children of mothers without diabetes (77% vs. 86%; $p < 0.0001$) *(15)*. That study also demonstrated, among breastfed children, a significantly shorter duration of exclusive breastfeeding (12 weeks vs. 17 weeks; $p < 0.0001$) and nonexclusive breastfeeding (20 weeks vs. 26 weeks, $p < 0.0001$) for children of mothers with DM1 than for children of mothers without diabetes.

Severity of maternal diabetes may also affect breastfeeding practices. In a case series of 530 infants born to 332 women with GDM and 177 women with DM1, higher breastfeeding rates were seen in women with diet-controlled GDM than in women with diabetes complicated by end-organ disease *(16)*.

BREASTFEEDING AND MATERNAL HEALTH

Maternal Obesity, Diabetes and Perinatal Complications

Maternal obesity and diabetes often coexist and are associated with increased perinatal complications, which can interfere with breastfeeding *(17)*. Several studies, including one with more than 120,000 participants, have found an association between maternal obesity and short duration of breastfeeding *(18 20)*. A retrospective analysis of a large British maternity database examining the relationship between maternal obesity and diabetes and adverse pregnancy outcomes in 287,213 pregnancies found that increasing body mass index (BMI) correlated with incidence of GDM *(21)*. This study also found high rates of obstetric and neonatal complications associated with obesity and noted that obese women were significantly less likely to breastfeed their infants at time of hospital discharge [odds ratio (OR) = 0.86 (99% CI 0.84–0.88) for women with BMI 25–30; OR = 0.58 (99% CI 0.56–0.60) for women with BMI ≥ 30].

The most common obstetric complication affecting breastfeeding in women with diabetes is delivery by cesarean section. In one study of 12,303 deliveries from 1997 to 2001, obese and overweight women had a significantly higher risk of cesarean delivery than women with normal BMIs (13.8% and 10.4% vs. 7.7%, respectively, $p < 0.0001$ for each) *(22)*. In addition, women with GDM or DM2 had a twofold to threefold increased risk for cesarean delivery compared with mothers without diabetes, independent of their obesity status. Recovery from cesarean delivery often delays initiation of breastfeeding, in part due to the initial separation of the mother and infant. Furthermore, mothers who undergo a cesarean delivery transfer less milk to their infants in the first 5 days of life despite adequate latch *(23)*. Both of these factors may increase the risk of formula supplementation in the neonatal period.

Independent investigators have consistently found that women with DM1 have a higher risk of delayed lactogenesis *(14, 24–26)*. Delayed onset of milk production could pose an additional challenge for breastfeeding initiation among women with diabetes.

Infants of mothers with DM1, DM2 and GDM have high rates of prematurity, macrosomia, congenital malformations, respiratory distress, hypoglycemia, hypocalcemia, polycythemia and hyperbilirubinemia *(16)*. Many of these conditions also lead to prolonged separation of mother and child immediately following birth, which can adversely affect both the initiation and continuation of breastfeeding.

HOSPITAL SUPPORT FOR BREASTFEEDING AMONG DIABETIC MOTHERS

In light of the medical challenges frequently faced by women with diabetes and their infants, special attention to supporting the initiation of breastfeeding among mothers with diabetes is warranted. The Baby-Friendly Hospital Initiative (BFHI) is a global program sponsored by the World Health Organization (WHO) and the United Nations Children's Fund (UNICEF) to promote breastfeeding at hospitals and birthing centers for all mothers *(27)*. Although each of "The Ten Steps to Successful Breastfeeding" is important for all breastfeeding mothers, the ones most relevant for women with diabetes may be the steps that address the separation of mother and child, specifically steps 4, 5, and 7 (see Table 1 for details). When mothers and infants are separated, breastfeeding "on demand," meaning feeding a baby when it is hungry, becomes very challenging. Missed feeding opportunities can threaten the intrinsic supply and demand mechanism of lactogenesis, resulting in a negative effect on milk production. In light of the complications associated with diabetes that can interfere with lactation, women with diabetes who intend to breastfeed should choose a hospital or birth center that can provide extra support for lactation.

Postpartum Issues for Breastfeeding Women with Diabetes

With respect to the impact of breastfeeding on return to prepregnancy weight for all women, not just those with diabetes, results from seven moderate-quality prospective cohort studies have reported results ranging from none to minimal (less than 1-kg weight change from prepregnancy or first trimester to 1–2 years postpartum). These studies consistently demonstrated that many factors other than breastfeeding, such as diet, had more impact on weight retention or loss than breastfeeding itself *(10)*.

Dietary recommendations for lactating women with diabetes do not differ significantly from recommendations for those without diabetes, aside from the fact that lactating women with diabetes should increase their caloric intake using foods lower in glycemic index *(8)*. During the first 6 months of life, infants receive an average of 500 kcal/day from human milk, which decreases to 400 kcal/day in the second 6 months as other foods are introduced. Women must increase their caloric intake by 330 kcal/day in the first 6 months of breastfeeding (another 170 kcal/day are generated through the metabolism of fat stores) and by 400 kcal/day in the second 6 months of breastfeeding to account for these increased metabolic needs *(28)*.

Effect of Breastfeeding on Maternal Glucose Tolerance and Future Diabetes Risk

Many investigators have attempted to elucidate the metabolic effects of lactation on maternal glucose tolerance. Two small studies suggest that lower levels of estrogen in the postpartum period may be protective with regard to insulin resistance. One cohort study of 23 women without diabetes found that lactating women had significantly lower levels of estradiol, fasting glucose and insulin than

Table 1

The World Health Organization's Ten Steps to Successful Breastfeeding (*(27)*. Adapted from *Protecting, Promoting and Supporting Breastfeeding: The Special Role of Maternity Services,* a Joint WHO/UNICEF Statement Published by the World Health Organization. http://www.unicef. org/programme/breastfeeding/baby.htm#10 (Accessed September 5, 2008))

Every facility providing maternity services and care for newborn infants should

1. Have a written breastfeeding policy that is routinely communicated to all health care staff
2. Train all health care staff in skills necessary to implement this policy
3. Inform all pregnant women about the benefits and management of breastfeeding
4. Help mothers initiate breastfeeding within half an hour of birth
5. Show mothers how to breastfeed and how to maintain lactation even if they should be separated from their infants
6. Give newborn infants no food or drink other than breast milk, unless medically indicated
7. Practice rooming-in - that is, allow mothers and infants to remain together - 24 h a day
8. Encourage breastfeeding on demand
9. Give no artificial teats or pacifiers (also called dummies or soothers) to breastfeeding infants
10. Foster the establishment of breastfeeding support groups and refer mothers to them on discharge rom the hospital or clinic

nonlactating women, suggesting that the low levels of estradiol associated with breastfeeding may confer a protective effect with respect to glucose tolerance *(29)*. Another cohort study of 98 postpartum women without diabetes noted that women treated with estrogens to suppress lactation had higher rates of abnormal glucose tolerance than other postpartum women (both breastfeeding and nonbreastfeeding), again suggesting that estrogen plays an important role in glucose metabolism in the puerperium *(30)*.

Studies of breastfeeding among women with diabetes show inconsistent effects on postpartum glucose tolerance. However, the studies are quite small and the results, therefore, difficult to generalize. For example, one prospective study of 60 women found that postpartum fasting glucose levels were significantly lower at 6 weeks postpartum in breastfeeding women with DM1 than in those who stopped breastfeeding before 6 weeks or who had never breastfed *(13)*. In contrast, another prospective observational study assessing glycemic control in 14 breastfeeding women with DM1 and 25 breastfeeding women without diabetes found that the HgbA1C levels of women with diabetes increased 20% during lactation *(25)*. However, there was no comparison with women with diabetes who were not breastfeeding in this study.

A prospective cohort study of 809 Latina women with GDM found that postpartum glucose values were significantly lower among those who breastfed for 4–12 weeks than among those who did not breastfeed at all ($p = 0.0001$ for mean fasting serum glucose; $p < 0.01$ for mean 2-h glucose level) *(31)*. These differences were significant after adjusting for maternal age, BMI and the use of insulin in pregnancy. Furthermore, nonlactating women in this study were twice as likely to develop postpartum diabetes as lactating women. Another retrospective longitudinal study of 651 women in Nova Scotia, Canada with GDM who then had at least one subsequent pregnancy examined the effect of breastfeeding on the risk of GDM in the subsequent pregnancy. No difference was found in rates of recurrent GDM between women who breastfed or bottle fed after the index pregnancy *(32)*.

A prospective observational cohort study of 83,585 parous women in the Nurses' Health Study (NHS) and a retrospective observational cohort study of 73,418 parous women in the Nurses' Health

Study II (NHS II) examined the relationship between the duration of lactation and the incidence of DM2 *(33)*. Among women without a history of diabetes, after controlling for current BMI and other relevant risk factors for DM2, a longer duration of breastfeeding was associated with a significantly reduced risk of developing DM2 in this study. For each additional year of lactation, NHS participants with a birth in the prior 15 years had a 15% decrease in the risk of diabetes (95% CI 1–27%) and NHS II participants had a 14% decrease in the risk of diabetes (95% CI 7–21%). However, women with a history of GDM had a markedly increased risk of developing DM2 that was not significantly influenced by duration of lactation.

Summary of Maternal Health Issues

The relationship between maternal diabetes and breastfeeding is complex. Among women with diabetes, high rates of cesarean section and neonatal complications often cause separation of mother and infant, which can interfere significantly with breastfeeding. Delayed lactogenesis among women with insulin-dependent diabetes may also contribute to breastfeeding difficulties. Support for early breastfeeding initiation and maintenance of lactation in the context of perinatal complications may improve breastfeeding rates among women with diabetes. Lactating women have increased caloric needs that are similar in women with and without diabetes. Breastfeeding may improve postpartum glucose metabolism among women without diabetes. However, breastfeeding does not appear to reduce the risk of developing DM2 among women with GDM.

BREASTFEEDING AND PEDIATRIC HEALTH

Associations Between Breastfeeding and Pediatric Outcomes

OBESITY

Weight and diabetes are often related conditions. Large, well-designed studies in developed countries suggest that breastfeeding has a protective effect against childhood obesity *(34)*. The many epidemiological studies that have analyzed the impact of breastfeeding on obesity later in life have been summarized in four recent systematic reviews or meta-analyses *(35)*. Breastfeeding has consistently been shown to protect against overweight and obesity in adolescence and adult life. Myriad confounding factors such as maternal obesity may contribute to but do not completely account for these results. An additional 2007 review of 14 studies again confirmed that breastfeeding helps to prevent childhood obesity *(36)*.

TYPE I DIABETES

Both genetic and environmental factors contribute to the development of DM1. The association between breastfeeding and lower rates of DM1 has previously been established *(37)*. The results of two meta-analyses and four case-control studies suggest that breastfeeding for more than 3 months is associated with a reduced risk of DM1 *(10)*. For example, in a multicenter European study of 499 diabetic patients and 1,337 controls, breastfeeding reduced the risk of DM1 by 41% after adjustment for growth pattern *(38)*. Since then, several additional studies in different European nations have reproduced these results *(39–41)*. However, there is still the possibility of both recall bias and suboptimal adjustment for confounders in the primary studies.

The early introduction of formula, cow's milk, and complementary foods seem to increase the risk of DM1 *(42–44)*. Mounting evidence suggests that the biological mechanism for the relationship between infant nutrition and DM1 is immune-mediated, although expert consensus is lacking *(45–50)*.

TYPE 2 DIABETES

Given the well-documented association between breastfeeding and obesity, one would expect that infant nutrition would also affect the incidence of DM2. As discussed in the first systematic review on this topic *(51)*, many but not all individual studies have found a protective association between breast-feeding and DM2 in children *(52, 53)*. The first and only meta-analysis on this subject concluded, based on 23 studies, that having been breastfed as an infant is associated with a 39% reduced risk of DM2 when compared with having been formula fed *(54)*. Breastfeeding was also associated with lower blood glucose and serum insulin concentrations in infancy and marginally lower insulin concentrations in later life. As with DM1, the exact underlying mechanism of this association is still unclear but is hypothesized to be related to the polyunsaturated fatty acids (PUFAs) found in breast milk *(55)*.

GESTATIONAL DIABETES MELLITUS

The only study so far to investigate how women with GDM were themselves fed as infants found no significant differences between women with GDM and women with normal glucose tolerance in pregnancy *(56)*. As part of a larger study on the relationship between GDM and a woman's own birth weight, 138 women with GDM were compared with 100 glucose-tolerant women. Breastfeeding was self-reported in one of five categories (breastfed only, mainly breastfed, equal amounts of breast and bottle, mainly bottle, bottle fed only) for the first 3 months of life. There were no significant differences between women with GDM and glucose-tolerant women with respect to the method by which they were fed as infants ($p = 0.333$). No control for confounding was reported. This result is surprising given that breastfeeding is associated with a reduction in risk of development of DM2. Further study of the relationship between personal infant feeding history and the risk of GDM in adulthood is warranted.

Children of Mothers with Diabetes

BREAST MILK COMPOSITION

A recent review of the biology of human milk provides a summary of our current understanding of the contents of human milk and its benefits for children when compared with infant formula *(57)*. With respect to DM2, one theory is that the long-chain PUFAs (LC-PUFAs) found in breast milk improve the resistance of beta-cells to burning out, thus preventing or postponing the development of diabetes *(58)*. More recently, it has been hypothesized that in children who are breastfed, the insulin-like growth factor axis is programmed to promote higher linear growth velocity later in childhood, resulting in taller children with lower BMIs who are then ostensibly less prone to obesity and diabetes *(35)*.

There has been considerable conflicting research on the similarities and differences in the composition of breast milk of women with and without diabetes. One study comparing the breast milk of six women with tightly controlled insulin-dependent diabetes with that of five women without diabetes found no differences in macronutrient, glucose, cholesterol or fatty acid composition of breast milk, suggesting that glycemic control may modulate differences in breast milk composition between women with and without diabetes *(59)*. Another showed similar levels of vitamin E in the breast milk of mothers with and without diabetes *(60)*. Other studies comparing the biochemical differences between the breast milk of women with and without diabetes have shown higher insulin and glucose content *(61)*, lower prolactin levels *(62)*, and lower LC-PUFA content *(63)* in the breast milk of women with diabetes.

Theoretically, differences in milk composition between mothers with and without diabetes could impact the risk of obesity and diabetes in offspring. A research group in Germany has published several studies comparing the effect of diabetic breast milk (DBM) vs. donor breast milk from mothers without diabetes during the neonatal period on a variety of pediatric outcomes. In this prospective cohort study of 112 mothers with DM1 and GDM, there was a positive correlation between the volume of DBM ingested and risk of overweight at 2 years of age (OR 2.47, 95% CI 1.25–4.87) *(64)*. Therefore, early neonatal ingestion of DBM as compared to donor breast milk from women without diabetes may increase the risk of becoming overweight and, consequently, developing IGT during childhood. Results of another study of a cohort of 242 mothers suggest that infants of mothers with diabetes ingesting DBM in the late neonatal period may have delayed speech development compared with those fed donor breast milk *(65)*.

Breast milk from mothers with and without diabetes is superior to infant formula with respect to pediatric health benefits. Currently, none of the known or potential differences in the breast milk composition of women with diabetes as compared to the breast milk of women without diabetes should preclude them from breastfeeding their own infants *(61, 64)*, although research on this subject is ongoing. Little is known about the effect of glycemic control on breast milk composition among women with diabetes. The International Society for Research in Human Milk and Lactation (ISRHML) regularly posts new developments in research on breast milk composition on the Society's Web site at http://www.isrhml.org *(66)*.

SHORT-TERM ISSUES

A significant concern for infants born to mothers with diabetes is neonatal hypoglycemia. The Academy of Breastfeeding Medicine (ABM), a worldwide organization of physicians dedicated to the promotion, protection, and support of breastfeeding and human lactation, develops clinical protocols for managing common medical problems, such as newborn hypoglycemia, that may impact breastfeeding success. The goals for ABM's 2006 *Guideline for glucose monitoring and treatment of hypoglycemia in breastfed neonates* are "to prevent hypoglycemia in breastfed infants, to monitor blood glucose levels in at risk term and late-preterm breastfed infants, to manage documented hypoglycemia in breastfed infants, and to establish and preserve maternal milk supply during medically necessary supplementation for hypoglycemia." The protocol, available online at http://www.bfmed.org, includes general management recommendations as well as a specific protocol for managing documented hypoglycemia in a breastfeeding infant *(67)*.

In one study of the children of 47 mothers with GDM and 55 matched healthy controls, poorer sucking patterns were found among infants of mothers with GDM who were treated with insulin than among healthy infant controls *(68)*. Newborns of the insulin-treated mothers averaged 5.2 fewer bursts ($p = 0.013$) and 42 fewer sucks ($p = 0.04$) relative to the control group. This preliminary finding, in conjunction with the previously mentioned potential for delayed onset of lactogenesis in diabetic mothers, may be of clinical significance for maternal-infant dyads when establishing lactation.

As of 2003, it is recommended that all exclusively breastfed infants be supplemented with 200 IU of vitamin D per day beginning during the first 2 months of life *(69)*. It is also recommended that an intake of 200 IU of vitamin D per day be continued throughout childhood and adolescence, primarily because adequate sunlight exposure is not easily determined for a given individual. Interestingly, vitamin D deficiency has been associated with an increased risk of both DM1 and DM2 *(70, 71)*.

LONG-TERM ISSUES

Among children of mothers with diabetes, several studies have demonstrated a protective effect of breastfeeding on rates of obesity and diabetes in the next generation. In a study of 324 children of mothers with GDM, breastfeeding for more than 3 months was negatively associated with overweight status in early childhood ($p = 0.008$) *(72)*. In a different large cohort study of the 15,253 offspring in the NHS II, breastfeeding was also inversely associated with childhood obesity regardless of maternal diabetes status or weight status *(73)*. In that study, maternal diabetes and weight status did not diminish the protective effects of breastfeeding on childhood obesity. The BABYDIAB study follows newborn children of parents with DM1. The authors have found that breastfeeding may reduce the risk of development of DM1 autoantibodies in children *(49)*. Finally, in a retrospective cohort study of 572 Pima Indians, among the children of mothers with GDM ($n = 21$), DM2 was less common in the next generation among breastfed children (6.9% vs. 30.1% among offspring of nondiabetic and diabetic women, respectively) than among bottle-fed children (11.9% vs. 43.6%, respectively) *(74)*.

Summary of Pediatric Health Issues

Considerable research has investigated the link between breastfeeding and both obesity and DM1. The protective association between breastfeeding and DM2 has more recently been confirmed. Most studies suggest a dose-response, meaning that longer breastfeeding confers greater benefits. Although the relationship between infant nutrition and glucose control is very complex and easily subject to confounding, the majority of the literature on the pediatric benefits of breastfeeding suggests that breastfeeding lowers rates of obesity, DM1 and DM2 in children, regardless of whether or not the child's mother had diabetes. These effects may not be strong at the individual level but are likely to be of importance at the population level.

In caring for infants of women with diabetes, short-term considerations include establishing an adequate milk supply and the management of hypoglycemia. Milk supply can potentially be threatened by delayed onset of lactation in the mother as well as poor infant suck. Long-term considerations include the future risk of obesity and diabetes, which both appear to be lower among children of women with diabetes who were breastfed for at least 2 months. Despite some biochemical differences between the breast milk of women with and without diabetes, maternal diabetes in and of itself is never a contraindication to breastfeeding.

With the increasing rates of DM2 in both the pediatric and adult populations, any intervention that can potentially decrease risk should be encouraged. Accordingly, the AAP strongly endorses breastfeeding as the primary source of nutrition for infants with a strong family history of diabetes *(7)*. Women should receive information on all the potential benefits of breastfeeding, including the lower risks of obesity and diabetes in children who are breastfed. Although exclusive breastfeeding of a mother's own breast milk is the current clinical recommendation, ongoing research is comparing the effect on children of mothers with diabetes of ingesting their mother's own breast milk vs. donor breast milk from women without diabetes.

PHARMACOLOGIC TREATMENT OPTIONS FOR BREASTFEEDING WOMEN WITH DIABETES

Breastfeeding has significant benefits for all infants, especially infants of women with diabetes, as described earlier. Most maternal medications are transferred to some degree into breast milk. For ethical reasons, we must rely on observational studies and basic knowledge of pharmacology instead of randomized controlled trials to understand the potential risks for breastfed infants of medications taken by their mothers. We do know that most medications are transferred in very small amounts and do not result in a clinically significant dose for the infant. Women are often inappropriately advised to interrupt or discontinue breastfeeding due to misinformation about the safety of medications in lactation. Many medications can be safely taken during breastfeeding without any significant risk to the child.

In this section, we discuss the pharmacokinetics of human milk and provide some general prescribing guidelines. Then, we review individual classes of medicines including drugs used to treat diabetes and its associated diseases. Next, we provide contraceptive recommendations specifically for breastfeeding women with diabetes (please see Chap. 9 for comprehensive coverage of contraceptive options for all women with diabetes). Finally, we provide additional resources for clinicians on medication use for breastfeeding women.

Pharmacokinetics of Human Milk

For the breastfeeding infant to be exposed to a maternal medication, several conditions must be met. First, the medication must reach a sufficiently high concentration in the maternal plasma. Next the medication must be transferred into the milk. Medications enter human milk primarily through diffusion into the alveoli of the breast. Factors that promote transfer into the milk include low molecular weight, low protein binding and high lipid solubility of medications. Finally, the medication must be orally bioavailable in order to be absorbed in the infant gut. Many medications are destroyed or poorly absorbed in the infant gut or metabolized in the liver after absorption.

Relative infant doses of medications can be calculated by dividing the theoretic infant dose received in the milk in mg/kg per day by the maternal dose in mg/kg per day. If the relative infant dose of the medication is less than 10%, most medications are considered safe *(75)*. The vast majority of medications have a relative infant dose of less than 1%. There is a relatively short list of drugs that are absolutely contraindicated in breastfeeding that includes drugs of abuse, excessive alcohol, most antineoplastic drugs and some radioactive isotopes. Please see Table 2 for general guidelines for medication use by breastfeeding women.

Specific Medications Used for Treating Diabetes and Related Conditions

Information on specific medications is derived primarily from the 2006 edition of Thomas Hale's *Medications and Mothers' Milk (75)* unless otherwise specified.

INSULIN

Insulins are among the safest medications for treating maternal diabetes in breastfeeding and therefore the medication of choice for use in women with diabetes who are breastfeeding. Insulin in any form is a very large peptide, which, by virtue of its high molecular weight, will have negligible amounts of transfer into human milk. Because insulin does not cross the placenta like many of the

Table 2
General Guidelines for Medication Use by Breastfeeding Women (Adapted from *(75)*)

1. Avoid unnecessary medications
2. Choose medications with existing data on their effects in breastfeeding over newer medications
3. Use more caution with neonates and preterm infants
4. Remember that the risks of formula feeding instead of breastfeeding are higher than the risks of exposure through breast milk to most medications
5. Choose medications with a shorter half-life, higher protein binding, low oral bioavailability, high molecular weight, and low lipid solubility
6. Avoid medications that may decrease milk production
7. If the medication's half-life is less than 3 h, the medication can be taken at the time of the feeding; by the next feeding the maternal serum level will be declining

oral medications commonly prescribed to women with diabetes, the additional concern that the drug therapy itself is adversely affecting the fetus is completely eliminated. Even if small amounts of insulin were to enter human milk, the molecule would be destroyed in the infant's gastrointestinal tract. Insulin glargine is also considered safe during breastfeeding, although no specifics on its rate of transfer into human milk are available.

METFORMIN

Metformin is considered among the safest oral diabetes medication to prescribe for women who are breastfeeding. Metformin belongs to the biguanide family and works by reducing hepatic glucose production and increasing peripheral insulin sensitivity. It has a low relative infant dose (less than 1%) as well as low oral bioavailability. A recent pharmacology review summarizes the three studies involving a total of 22 women that have measured nonsignificant amounts of metformin in breast milk as well as the one study that has demonstrated no significant long-term differences in height, weight, and motor-social development at 3 and 6 months of age among 111 infants, 61 of whom were breast-fed by mothers taking metformin *(76)*. Metformin is an alternative first-line agent to insulin for treating diabetes among breastfeeding women.

SULFONYLUREAS

Sulfonylureas are oral medications that stimulate insulin secretion from the pancreas. With any sulfonylurea, there would be a theoretical concern for infant hypoglycemia if the medication was transferred into the breast milk in significant levels, but this has not been observed clinically. First-generation sulfonylureas, including chlorpropamide and tolbutamide, are currently rarely used in the USA. Of these two drugs, tolbutamide has a shorter half-life and smaller relative infant dose (less than 1%) and would be preferred. Second-generation sulfonylureas include glyburide, glipizide, and glimepiride. One study of glyburide and glipizide levels in breast milk was unable to detect either of these medications *(77)*. There are no data on the transfer of glimepiride in human milk, but there is significant transfer noted in rodent studies, so this agent is not recommended. The half-lives of glyburide and glipizide depend on their formulation (immediate vs. extended release). Short-acting formulations of glyburide or glipizide are acceptable choices for breastfeeding women with diabetes.

ALPHA-GLUCOSIDASE INHIBITORS

The alpha-glucosidase inhibitors, which include acarbose and miglitol, reduce absorption of carbohydrates in the gut. Although there are no data on acarbose transfer into human milk, it is unlikely that any of this medication reaches the milk due to its very low oral bioavailability. Based on limited data available for miglitol, the estimated relative infant dose is very low - 0.4% of the maternal dose. Both of these agents have half-lives of 2 h or less, making them reasonable choices for treatment of maternal diabetes during lactation.

MEGLITIDINES

Meglitidines are nonsulfonylurea agents that stimulate pancreatic insulin secretion. Available agents in the USA include repaglinide and nateglinide. Rodent studies of repaglinide have suggested that it may cause hypoglycemia in pups via milk. There are no data on the transfer of these medications in human milk, so their safety is unknown. Therefore, it would be prudent to use alternative agents during breastfeeding.

THIAZOLADINEDIONES

The thiazoladinediones, which include pioglitazone and rosiglitazone, act by increasing insulin receptor sensitivity and decreasing hepatic gluconeogenesis. The data on transfer into human milk are not available for either of these agents, so they should be given only if the benefit outweighs the potential risk of infant exposure. Given the history of rare but serous adverse events associated with agents in this class (e.g., hepatotoxicity with troglitazone, cardiovascular events with rosiglitazone), clinicians may be less inclined to prescribe thiazoladinediones to lactating women.

NEW AGENTS FOR DIABETES

Exenatide is an incretin mimetic. Although there are no human studies on transfer to milk, exenatide has a very high molecular weight, making it too large to enter milk in clinically significant quantities. In addition, maternal administration results in low maternal plasma levels, and exenatide has almost no oral bioavailability. In light of these factors, it is unlikely to have any effect on the breastfeeding infant. However, caution is advised given the lack of data.

Pramlintide is an amylin analog. There are no data on its transfer into human milk; however, it has a very high molecular weight and very limited oral bioavailability. Therefore, it is unlikely to be transferred to the infant in any clinically significant quantities. Again, caution is advised given the lack of human data.

ACE INHIBITORS

Many women with diabetes will be prescribed ACE inhibitors for hypertension or microalbuminuria. Because of renal toxicity with fetal exposure to ACE inhibitors, this class of medications should be avoided in pregnant women or in those at risk for pregnancy. Caution should also be used, therefore, in treating women who are breastfeeding premature infants. Enalapril, captopril, quinapril, and benazepril are considered compatible with breastfeeding full-term infants, based on human studies showing nearly undetectable levels in breast milk. Less preferred agents include fosinopril, lisinopril, and ramipril, because they either lack human data or have longer half-lives.

ANGIOTENSIN RECEPTOR BLOCKERS

Like the ACE inhibitor class of medications, angiotensin receptor blockers are associated with renal toxicity in the fetus, so they should not be used in pregnant women or women at risk for conceiving a pregnancy. As with ACE inhibitors, caution is also advised in using angiotensin receptor blockers in mothers who are nursing premature infants. Human studies on transfer of angiotensin receptor blockers into milk are lacking. They should only be used in women who cannot tolerate ACE inhibitors and for whom the benefits outweigh the potential risks.

ASPIRIN

Aspirin prophylaxis is often recommended for cardioprotection in patients with diabetes. Extremely small amounts of aspirin are transferred into breast milk. The major concern with infant exposure to aspirin is the risk of Reye syndrome. Although an 81-mg dose of aspirin in a breastfeeding mother is unlikely to result in significant aspirin exposure to the infant, the dose-response relationship between aspirin and Reye Syndrome is not known. Therefore, aspirin use is not recommended in breastfeeding mothers.

CHOLESTEROL-LOWERING AGENTS

The risks of using lipid-lowering agents while pregnant or breastfeeding may be higher than the short-term risks of hyperlipidemia. Therefore, their use is not usually justified during pregnancy and lactation. Given that atherosclerosis is a chronic process, suspending therapy with lipid-lowering drugs during pregnancy and lactation should not have major impact on long-term management of hypercholesterolemia. In addition, lowering maternal plasma cholesterol may confer a potential risk to infant neurodevelopment by lowering milk cholesterol levels.

The HMG Co-A reductase inhibitor medications (statins) are used frequently for cholesterol lowering in patients with diabetes. Statins are known teratogens and should be avoided in women who are pregnant or may become pregnant. These agents have low oral bioavailability and high protein binding, so they are unlikely to be transferred in clinically relevant amounts into human milk; however, human studies are not available. Use of HMG Co-A reductase inhibitors is not recommended during breastfeeding.

Likewise, there are no data on transfer into human milk of fibric acid derivatives, such as gemfibrozil and fenofibrate, or of ezetimibe, which inhibits intestinal absorption of cholesterol. Therefore, caution is advised with use of these agents in breastfeeding women.

There are little data on levels of nicotinic acid derivatives, such as niacin, in breast milk when used in the high doses (1–2 g per day) needed to achieve cholesterol lowering. Because of the potential risk to the infant of hepatotoxicity with high doses of niacin, breastfeeding women should not exceed the recommended dietary allowance of niacin (17 mg per day for breastfeeding women) *(78)*.

In cases where a woman and her physician determine that treatment of elevated cholesterol during pregnancy and/or lactation is warranted, use of colesevelam, a bile-acid sequestrant, can be considered. This agent is minimally absorbed from the gastrointestinal tract, and therefore it does not enter the maternal bloodstream or the breast milk.

Contraception for Breastfeeding Women with Diabetes

Contraceptive counseling for breastfeeding women with diabetes requires special consideration. Chapter 9 provides comprehensive coverage of contraceptive options for all women with diabetes. Here, we discuss contraceptive methods specifically in the context of establishing or maintaining lactation.

According to the ABM's clinical protocol regarding contraception in the context of breastfeeding *(79)*, first-choice methods for all lactating women include methods that have no effect on lactation. These include the lactational amenorrhea method (LAM), natural family planning and barrier methods. Sterilization for women who have completed childbearing and intrauterine devices (IUDs) are also recommended options, as they have little or no effect on lactation. Because of some reports of possible negative impact on milk production, especially with early postpartum administration, progestin-only hormonal contraceptives are considered second choice by ABM. Progestin-only products currently available in the USA include the progestin-only oral contraceptive pill (containing norethindrone or levonorgestrel), the depo-medroxyprogesterone acetate injection (DMPA) and the progestin implant (containing etonogestrel). Because of concerns about slower hepatic metabolism of progestins by newborns, some authors recommend delaying initiation of progestin-containing contraceptives until 6 weeks postpartum in breastfeeding women *(80)*. Hormonal contraceptives containing both estrogen and progestin such as the combined oral contraceptive pill, the vaginal contraceptive ring and the contraceptive patch are not recommended for breastfeeding women due to significant risks of dose-dependent reduction in milk supply and shorter duration of breastfeeding associated with their use.

Ideal contraceptive choices for mothers with diabetes are methods that are both highly effective in preventing pregnancy and that do not interfere with lactation. Lactational amenorrhea is more than 98% effective in preventing pregnancy when all of the following criteria are met: (1) exclusive frequent breastfeeding (at least every 4 h during the day, every 6 h at night) without supplementation, (2) less than 6 months elapsed since delivery, and (3) no return of menses *(79)*. Higher efficacy can be achieved by combining lactational amenorrhea with a barrier method.

Among the most effective reversible contraceptive methods is the IUD. IUDs currently available in the USA include the Copper T380A IUD and the levonorgestrel-releasing intrauterine system, both of which are more than 99% effective in preventing pregnancy. A randomized controlled trial comparing the effects of the two IUDs in lactating women found no differences in breastfeeding success or infant growth and development *(81)*. The Copper T380A can be inserted immediately postpartum or after 4 weeks postpartum and lasts up to 10 years. The levonorgestrel-releasing IUD can be inserted after 6 weeks postpartum and lasts up to 5 years. Guidelines for patient selection and IUD insertion and monitoring are the same for patients with and without diabetes.

Another highly effective method, the etonogestrel-releasing contraceptive implant, was approved by the US Food and Drug Administration in 2006. A trial comparing its effects on breastfeeding with those of a copper IUD found no differences in volume or content of breast milk or in infant growth *(82)*. The single rod implant can be inserted after the fourth postpartum week and is more than 99% effective in preventing pregnancy for up to 3 years.

Emergency contraception (EC) reduces a woman's risk of pregnancy after unprotected intercourse, sexual assault, or failure or improper use of a birth control method and may be useful to breastfeeding mothers in these circumstances. EC may be used up to 120 h (5 days) after unprotected sex but is more effective if used earlier *(83)*. The best option for EC in breastfeeding women is levonorgestrel administered at a dose of 1.5 mg given either as a single dose or two 0.75 mg doses 12 h apart. This product was approved by the US Food and Drug Administration in 2006 for sale to women of age 18 and over without a prescription.

Current evidence suggests that levonorgestrel EC functions primarily by inhibiting or delaying ovulation. It is not effective after implantation has begun and will not harm an existing pregnancy *(83)*. In light of concerns mentioned earlier regarding immature hepatic metabolism of progestins in the first 6 weeks of life and given the extremely low risk of ovulation in the first 6 weeks postpartum in breastfeeding women, use of levonorgestrel for EC should be delayed until after 6 weeks postpartum.

One study of the pharmacokinetics of levonorgestrel EC recommended that women discard breast milk for the first 8 h after taking levonorgestrel EC in order to avoid exposing their infant to the peak concentrations of the medication *(84)*. However, based on the peak concentrations and estimated total dose received by the infant that were reported in that study, the weight-adjusted relative infant dose in the first 24 h after a maternal dose of 150 mg of levonorgestrel is still much less than 1%. Risks and benefits of interrupting breastfeeding to reduce infant exposure to levonorgestrel from EC should be discussed with patients to help determine the best course of action.

Two studies of breastfeeding Latina women with recent GDM have noted adverse effects of progestin-only contraceptive methods on glucose tolerance. The first study found that, compared with users of nonhormonal contraceptives, Latina women with recent GDM taking progestin-only oral contraceptive pills during breastfeeding had nearly a threefold increased risk of developing diabetes *(85)*. In a second study of the same population, DMPA use was associated with an increased risk of diabetes among women who were breastfeeding *(86)*. The authors recommend avoiding use of progestin-only contraceptive methods in women with prior GDM while they are breastfeeding. Further research is needed to reproduce these findings in other populations. Data are not available regarding the effects of other progestin-only methods, such as the levonorgestrel-releasing IUD or the etonogestrel-releasing implant, on glucose metabolism in women with prior GDM or diabetes. Use of levonorgestrel for EC is unlikely to have long-term effects on glucose metabolism, so EC should not be withheld from breastfeeding women with a history of GDM or diabetes. Since the progestin IUD and implant release lower relative daily doses of progestin than progestin-only pills and DMPA, their effect might be less pronounced. However, in the absence of data, caution is warranted when prescribing these methods for breastfeeding women with prior GDM or diabetes.

Clinical Resources on Medications in Breastfeeding Women

A recent review of resources on drug safety in lactation found five resources that provide citations for their recommendations *(87)*. These include the AAP Committee on Drugs *(88)*, Thomas Hale's *Medications and Mother's Milk (75)*, the online database Lact Med *(80)*, Micro Medex *(89)*, and *Drugs in Pregnancy and Lactation (90)*. Of these resources, the free online database Lact Med contains the most extensive and current citations.

Studies of medication use in lactating women are primarily observational for ethical reasons. As a result, medication package inserts often contain inaccurate or confusing information about medication use during lactation. The *Physicians' Desk Reference* is based on these package inserts, so it is also a poor source of information on medication use during lactation *(91)*. Other drug references such as E-Pocrates *(92)* and Pharmacopoeia *(93)* often include ratings of safety of medication in breastfeeding without citing references. Therefore, these are not preferred sources for clinical information on medication use in lactating women.

Because of conflicting and confusing information from clinicians, pharmacists, and medication package inserts, patients can understandably be unsure about the safety of medications in breastfeeding. Clinicians can help patients by presenting recommendations from the most reliable, evidence-based sources, namely Lact Med and the monographs in Hale's *Medications and Mother's Milk*. When such preferred sources suggest the possibility of harm to the infant from medication exposure through breast milk, clinicians should consider alternative drug choices before recommending that breastfeeding be discontinued or interrupted. If a potentially harmful medication must be used for a short period of time and there is no safe alternative, rather than weaning altogether, a woman can maintain her milk supply by expressing and discarding her breast milk using either a manual or an electric breast pump. In this way, the supply and demand cycle of lactation is not interrupted nor is the child is exposed to the medicine contained in her breast milk. Once the woman finishes taking the medicine and it is has been metabolized, she can return to breastfeeding. The exact timing for resuming breastfeeding safely will depend on the half-life of the medicine that was taken. Finally, the potential risk of medication exposure to the infant must always be weighed against the substantial and well-documented risks to both mother and infant of *not* breastfeeding.

FUTURE RESEARCH

More research is needed on all aspects of breastfeeding in women with diabetes. There are many studies of patients with DM1. As GDM and DM2 reach epidemic proportions, additional studies of women with these conditions are needed. Although some studies of high-risk groups such as Pima Indians and Latinas are fairly large, large studies of more heterogeneous populations are needed. More accurate data collection on breastfeeding frequency and duration as well as exclusivity and formula supplementation is imperative. Because the metabolic environment surrounding glucose tolerance in pregnancy and the postpartum period is extremely complex, studies with more attention to lactation status and with longer follow-up will help clarify the hormonal interactions and subsequent risk. There is also a need to further study the impact of different levels of glycemic control on breast milk composition in women with diabetes. For now, given the well-known significant maternal and pediatric benefits of breastfeeding, it is critical that clinicians universally promote and support breastfeeding for all mothers, especially those with diabetes of any kind.

REFERENCES

1. Kaufman FR. Type 2 diabetes mellitus in children and youth: a new epidemic. J Pediatr Endocrinol Metab 2002;15(Suppl 2):737–744

2. Ludwig DS, Ebbeling CB. Type 2 diabetes mellitus in children: primary care and public health considerations. JAMA 2001;286(12):1427–1430

3. Peterson KA. Diabetes management in the primary care setting: summary. Am J Med 2002;113(Suppl 6A):36S–40S

4. Lunt H. Women and diabetes. Diabet Med 1996;13(12):1009–1016

5. U.S. Department of Health and Human Services. HHS Blueprint for Action on Breastfeeding. Washington, DC: U.S. Department of Health and Human Services, Office on Women's Health, 2000

6. Institute of Medicine. Nutrition During Lactation. Washington, DC: National Academy Press, 1991

7. American Academy of Pediatrics. Work Group on Breastfeeding. Breastfeeding and the use of human milk. Pediatrics 1997;100(6):1035–1039

8. American Academy of Pediatrics. Position of the American Dietetic Association: promotion of breast-feeding. J Am Diet Assoc 1997;97(6):662–666

9. Schack-Nielsen L, Larnkjaer A, Michaelsen KF. Long term effects of breastfeeding on the infant and mother. Adv Exp Med Biol 2005;569:16–23

10. Ip S, Chung M, Raman G, et al. Breastfeeding and Maternal and Infant Health Outcomes in Developed Countries. Rockville, MD: US Department of Health and Human Services, 2007. Available at http://www.ahrq.gov/downloads/pub/evidence/pdf/brfout/brfout.pdf (Accessed December 24, 2007)

11. U.S. Department of Health and Human Services. Healthy People 2010, 2nd edn. With Understanding and Improving Health and Objectives for Improving Health, 2 vols. Washington, DC: U.S. Government Printing Office, 2000

12. Breastfeeding Practices - Results from the 2004 National Immunization Survey. Available at http://www.cdc.gov/breast-feeding/data/NIS_data/data_2004.htm (Accessed December 24, 2007)

13. Ferris AM, Dalidowitz CK, Ingardia CM, Reece EA, Fumia FD, Jensen RG, Allen LH. Lactation outcome in insulin-dependent diabetic women. J Am Diet Assoc 1988;88(3):317–322

14. Webster J, Moore K, McMullan A. Breastfeeding outcomes for women with insulin dependent diabetes. J Hum Lact 1995;11(3):195–200

15. Hummel S, Winkler C, Schoen S, Knopff A, Marienfeld S, Bonifacio E, Ziegler AG. Breastfeeding habits in families with type 1 diabetes. Diabet Med 2007;24(6):671–676

16. Cordero L, Treuer SH, Landon MB, Gabbe SG. Management of infants of diabetic mothers. Arch Pediatr Adolesc Med 1998;152(3):249–254

17. Kjos SL. After pregnancy complicated by diabetes: postpartum care and education. Obstet Gynecol Clin North Am 2007;34(2):335–349

18. Dewey KG, Nommsen-Rivers LA, Heinig MJ, Cohen RJ. Risk factors for suboptimal infant breastfeeding behavior, delayed onset of lactation, and excess neonatal weight loss. Pediatrics 2003;112(3 Pt 1):607–619

19. Li R, Jewell S, Grummer-Strawn L. Maternal obesity and breast-feeding practices. Am J Clin Nutr 2003;77(4):931–936

20. Hilson JA, Rasmussen KM, Kjolhede CL. High prepregnant body mass index is associated with poor lactation outcomes among white, rural women independent of psychosocial and demographic correlates. J Hum Lact 2004;20(1):18–29

21. Sebire NJ, Jolly M, Harris JP, Wadsworth J, Joffe M, Beard RW, Regan L, Robinson S. Maternal obesity and pregnancy outcome: a study of 287,213 pregnancies in London. Int J Obes Relat Metab Disord 2001;25(8):1175–1182

22. Ehrenberg HM, Durnwald CP, Catalano P, Mercer BM. The influence of obesity and diabetes on the risk of cesarean delivery. Am J Obstet Gynecol 2004;191(3):969–974

23. Evans KC, Evans RG, Royal R, Esterman AJ, James SL. Effect of caesarean section on breast milk transfer to the normal term newborn over the first week of life. Arch Dis Child Fetal Neonatal Ed 2003;88(5):F380–F382

24. Neubauer SH, Ferris AM, Chase CG, Fanelli J, Thompson CA, Lammi-Keefe CJ, Clark RM, Jensen RG, Bendel RB, Green KW. Delayed lactogenesis in women with insulin-dependent diabetes mellitus. Am J Clin Nutr 1993;58(1):54–60

25. Murtaugh MA, Ferris AM, Capacchione CM, Reece EA. Energy intake and glycemia in lactating women with type 1 diabetes. J Am Diet Assoc 1998;98(6):642–648

26. Hartmann P, Cregan M. Lactogenesis and the effects of insulin-dependent diabetes mellitus and prematurity. J Nutr 2001;131(11):3016S–3120S

27. The Baby Friendly Hospital Initiative (BFHI). Implementing the UNICEF/WHO Baby Friendly Hospital Initiative in the U.S. Available athttp://www.babyfriendlyusa.org/eng/index.html (Accessed September 5, 2008)

28. Reader D, Franz MJ. Lactation, diabetes, and nutrition recommendations. Curr Diab Rep 2004;4(5):370–376

29. Lenz S, Kuhl C, Hornnes PJ, Hagen C. Influence of lactation on oral glucose tolerance in the puerperium. Acta Endocrinol (Copenh) 1981;98(3):428–431

30. Job D, Eschwege E. Estrogens, lactation and oral glucose tolerance test in the early puerperium. J Perinat Med 1976;4(2):95–99

31. Kjos SL, Henry O, Lee RM, Buchanan TA, Mishell DR Jr. The effect of lactation on glucose and lipid metabolism in women with recent gestational diabetes. Obstet Gynecol 1993;82(3):451–455

32. MacNeill S, Dodds L, Hamilton DC, Armson BA, VandenHof M. Rates and risk factors for recurrence of gestational diabetes. Diabetes Care 2001;24(4):659–662

33. Stuebe AM, Rich-Edwards JW, Willett WC, et al. Duration of lactation and incidence of type 2 diabetes. JAMA 2005;294(20):2601–2610

34. Martorell R, Stein AD, Schroeder DG. Early nutrition and later adiposity. J Nutr 2001;131(3):874S–880S

35. Schack-Nielsen L, Michaelsen KF. Breast feeding and future health. Curr Opin Clin Nutr Metab Care 2006;9(3):289–296

36. Ryan AS. Breastfeeding and the risk of childhood obesity. Coll Antropol 2007;31(1):19–28

37. Dosch HM, Becker DJ. Infant feeding and autoimmune diabetes. Adv Exp Med Biol 2002;503:133–140

38. EURODIAB Substudy 2 Study Group. Rapid early growth is associated with increased risk of childhood type 1 diabetes in various European populations. Diabetes Care 2002;25(10):1755–1760

39. Sadauskaite-Kuehne V, Ludvigsson J, Padaiga Z, Jasinskiene E, Samuelsson U. Longer breastfeeding is an independent protective factor against development of type 1 diabetes mellitus in childhood. Diabetes Metab Res Rev 2004;20(2):150–157

40. Malcova H, Sumnik Z, Drevinek P, Venhacova J, Lebl J, Cinek O. Absence of breast-feeding is associated with the risk of type 1 diabetes: a case-control study in a population with rapidly increasing incidence. Eur J Pediatr 2006;165(2):114–119

41. Rosenbauer J, Herzig P, Kaiser P, Giani G. Early nutrition and risk of type 1 diabetes mellitus - a nationwide case-control study in preschool children. Exp Clin Endocrinol Diabetes 2007;115(8):502–508

42. Davis MK. Breastfeeding and chronic disease in childhood and adolescence. Pediatr Clin North Am 2001;48(1):125–141, ix

43. Knip M, Akerblom HK. Early nutrition and later diabetes risk. Adv Exp Med Biol 2005;569:142–150

44. Gerstein HC. Cow's milk exposure and type I diabetes mellitus. Diabetes Care 1994;17:13–19

45. Schrezenmeir J, Jagla A. Milk and diabetes. J Am Coll Nutr 2000;19(2 Suppl):176S–190S

46. Cavallo MG, Fava D, Monetini L, Barone F, Pozzilli P. Cell-mediated immune response to beta casein in recent-onset insulin-dependent diabetes: implications for disease pathogenesis. Lancet 1996;348(9032):926–928

47. Gerstein HC, VanderMeulen J. The relationship between cow's milk exposure and type 1 diabetes. Diabet Med 1996;13(1):23–29

48. Borch-Johnsen K, Joner G, Mandrup-Poulsen T, Christy M, Zachau-Christiansen B. Relation between breast-feeding and incidence rates of insulin-dependent diabetes mellitus. A hypothesis. Lancet 1984;2(8411):1083–1086

49. Ziegler AG, Schmid S, Huber D, Hummel M, Bonifacio E. Early infant feeding and risk of developing type 1 diabetes-associated autoantibodies. JAMA 2003;290(13):1721–1728

50. Holmberg H, Wahlberg J, Vaarala O, Ludvigsson J; ABIS Study Group. Short duration of breast-feeding as a risk-factor for beta-cell autoantibodies in 5-year-old children from the general population. Br J Nutr 2007;97(1):111–116

51. Taylor JS, Kacmar JE, Nothnagle M, Lawrence RA. A systematic review of the literature associating breastfeeding with type 2 diabetes and gestational diabetes. J Am Coll Nutr 2005;24(5):320–326

52. Pettitt DJ, Forman MR, Hanson RL, Knowler WC, Bennett PH. Breastfeeding and incidence of non-insulin-dependent diabetes mellitus in Pima Indians. Lancet 1997;350(9072):166–168

53. Young TK, Martens PJ, Taback SP, Sellers EAC, Dean HJ, Cheang M, Flett B. Type 2 diabetes mellitus in children: prenatal and early infancy risk factors among native Canadians. Arch Pediatr Adolesc Med 2002;156(7):651–655

54. Owen CG, Martin RM, Whincup PH, Smith GD, Cook DG. Does breastfeeding influence risk of type 2 diabetes in later life? A quantitative analysis of published evidence. Am J Clin Nutr 2006;84(5):1043–1054

55. Das UN. Breastfeeding prevents type 2 diabetes mellitus: but, how and why? Am J Clin Nutr 2007;85(5):1436–1437

56. Knights S, Davis WS, Coleman KJ, Moses RG. Are women with gestational diabetes more likely to have been bottle-fed? Diabetes Care 1999;22(10):1747

57. Schack-Nielsen L, Michaelsen KF. Advances in our understanding of the biology of human milk and its effects on the offspring. J Nutr 2007;137(2):503S–510S

58. Das UN. Can perinatal supplementation of long-chain polyunsaturated fatty acids prevent diabetes mellitus? Eur J Clin Nutr 2003;57(2):218–226

59. van Beusekom CM, Zeegers TA, Martini IA, Velvis HJ, Visser GH, van Doormaal JJ, Muskiet FA. Milk of patients with tightly controlled insulin-dependent diabetes mellitus has normal macronutrient and fatty acid composition. Am J Clin Nutr 1993;57(6):938–943

60. Lammi-Keefe CJ, Jonas CR, Ferris AM, Capacchione CM. Vitamin E in plasma and milk of lactating women with insulin-dependent diabetes mellitus. J Pediatr Gastroenterol Nutr 1995;20(3):305–309

61. Neubauer SH. Lactation in insulin-dependent diabetes. Prog Food Nutr Sci 1990;14(4):333–370

62. Ostrom KM, Ferris AM. Prolactin concentrations in serum and milk of mothers with and without insulin-dependent diabetes mellitus. Am J Clin Nutr 1993;58(1):49–53

63. Jackson MB, Lammi-Keefe CJ, Jensen RG, Couch SC, Ferris AM. Total lipid and fatty acid composition of milk from women with and without insulin-dependent diabetes mellitus. Am J Clin Nutr 1994;60(3):353–361

64. Plagemann A, Harder T, Franke K, Kohlhoff R. Long-term impact of neonatal breast-feeding on body weight and glucose tolerance in children of diabetic mothers. Diabetes Care 2002;25(1):16–22

65. Rodekamp E, Harder T, Kohlhoff R, Dudenhausen JW, Plagemann A. Impact of breast-feeding on psychomotor and neuropsychological development in children of diabetic mothers: role of the late neonatal period. J Perinat Med 2006;34(6):490–496

66. International Society for Research in Human Milk and Lactation. Available at http://www.isrhml.org (Accessed December 30, 2007)

67. Wight N, Marinelli KA, and the Academy of Breastfeeding Medicine Protocol Committee. ABM Clinical Protocol #1: guidelines for glucose monitoring and treatment of hypoglycemia in breastfed neonates. Breastfeed Med 2006;1(3):178–184. Available at:http://www.bfmed.org/ace-files/protocol/hypoglycemia.pdf (Accessed December 30, 2007)

68. Bromiker R, Rachamim A, Hammerman C, Schimmel M, Kaplan M, Medoff-Cooper B. Immature sucking patterns in infants of mothers with diabetes. J Pediatr 2006;149(5):640–643

69. Gartner LM, Greer FR; Section on Breastfeeding and Committee on Nutrition. American Academy of Pediatrics. Prevention of rickets and vitamin D deficiency: new guidelines for vitamin D intake. Pediatrics 2003;111(4 Pt 1):908–910

70. Mathieu C, Badenhoop K. Vitamin D and type 1 diabetes mellitus: state of the art. Trends Endocrinol Metab 2005;16(6):261–266

71. Pittas AG, Lau J, Hu FB, Dawson-Hughes B. The role of vitamin D and calcium in type 2 diabetes. A systematic review and meta-analysis. J Clin Endocrinol Metab 2007;92(6):2017–2029

72. Schaefer-Graf UM, Hartmann R, Pawliczak J, Passow D, Abou-Dakn M, Vetter K, Kordonouri O. Association of breast-feeding and early childhood overweight in children from mothers with gestational diabetes mellitus. Diabetes Care 2006;29(5):1105–1107

73. Mayer-Davis EJ, Rifas-Shiman SL, Zhou L, Hu FB, Colditz GA, Gillman MW. Breast-feeding and risk for childhood obesity: does maternal diabetes or obesity status matter? Diabetes Care 2006;29(10):2231–2237

74. Pettitt DJ, Knowler WC. Long-term effects of the intrauterine environment, birth weight, and breast-feeding in Pima Indians. Diabetes Care 1998;21(Suppl 2):B138–B141

75. Hale TW. Medications and Mothers' Milk, 12th edn. Amarillo, TX: Hale Publishing, 2006

76. Feig DS, Briggs GG, Koren G. Oral antidiabetic agents in pregnancy and lactation: a paradigm shift? Ann Pharmacother 2007;41(7):1174–80. Epub 2007 May 29

77. Feig DS, Briggs GG, Kraemer JM, Ambrose PJ, Moskovitz DN, Nageotte M, Donat DJ, Padilla G, Wan S, Klein J, Koren G. Transfer of glyburide and glipizide into breast milk. Diabetes Care 2005;28(8):1851–1855

78. Food and Nutrition Board, Institute of Medicine. Niacin. Dietary Reference Intakes: Thiamin, Riboflavin, Niacin, Vitamin B_6, Vitamin B_{12}, Pantothenic Acid, Biotin, and Choline. Washington, DC: National Academy Press, 1998, pp. 123–149

79. The Academy of Breastfeeding Medicine Protocol Committee. ABM Clinical Protocol #13: Contraception During Breastfeeding, 2005. Available at http://www.bfmed.org/ace-files/protocol/finalcontraceptionprotocolsent2.pdf (Accessed December 24, 2007)

80. LactMed: Drugs and Lactation Database. Available at http://toxnet.nlm.nih.gov/cgi-bin/sis/htmlgen?LACT (Accessed November 11, 2007)

81. Shaamash AH, Sayed GH, Hussien MM, Shaaban MM. A comparative study of the levonorgestrel-releasing intrauterine system Mirena versus the Copper T380A intrauterine device during lactation: breast-feeding performance, infant growth and infant development. Contraception 2005;72(5):346–351

82. Reinprayoon D, Taneepanichskul S, Bunyavejchevin S, Thaithumyanon P, Punnahitananda S, Tosukhowong P, Machielsen C, van Beek A. Effects of the etonogestrel-releasing contraceptive implant (Implanon) on parameters of breastfeeding compared to those of an intrauterine device. Contraception 2000;62(5):239–346

83. Stewart F, Trussell J, Van Look P. Emergency contraception. In: Hatcher R, Trussell J, Stewart F, Nelson A, Cates W, Guest F, Kowal D (eds.) Contraceptive Technology. New York: Ardent Media, 2004, pp. 279–298

84. Gainer E, Massai R, Lillo S, Reyes V, Forcelledo ML, Caviedes R, Villarroel C, Bouyer J. Levonorgestrel pharmacokinetics in plasma and milk of lactating women who take 1.5 mg for emergency contraception. Hum Reprod 2007;22(6):1578–1584

85. Kjos SL, Peters RK, Xiang A, Thomas D, Schaefer U, Buchanan TA. Contraception and the risk of type 2 diabetes mellitus in Latina women with prior gestational diabetes mellitus. JAMA 1998;280(6):533–538

86. Xiang AH, Kawakubo M, Kjos SL, Buchanan TA. Long-acting injectable progestin contraception and risk of type 2 diabetes in Latino women with prior gestational diabetes mellitus. Diabetes Care 2006;29(3):613–617

87. Akus M, Bartick M. Lactation safety recommendations and reliability compared in 10 medication resources. Ann Pharmacother 2007;41(9):1352–1360

88. American Academy of Pediatrics Committee on Drugs. The transfer of drugs and other chemicals into human milk. Pediatrics 2001;108:776–789

89. Thompson Micromedex. Available at http://www.micromedex.com (Accessed November 11, 2007)

90. Briggs G, Freeman R, Yaffe S. Drugs in Pregnancy and Lactation, 7th edn. Philadelphia, PA: Lippincott, Williams, and Wilkins, 2005

91. 2006 Physicians' Desk Reference, 60th edn. Montvale, NJ: Thomson PDR, 2005

92. Epocrates Rx drug reference. Available at http://www.epocrates.com (Accessed November 11, 2007)

93. Green SM. Tarascon Pocket Pharmacopoeia 2008 Classic Shirt-Pocket Edition. Lompoc, CA: Tarascon, 2007

23 Management of Disease in Women with Diabetes

Catherine Kim

CONTENTS

ABSTRACT

Diabetes management in women consists of controlling cardiovascular risk factors such as smoking, hypertension, hypercholesterolemia and for selected women, aspirin use. Better glycemic control reduces microvascular disease incidence. Screening for comorbidities such as nephropathy, retinopathy, and neuropathy followed by appropriate treatment can lead to effective disease-specific therapies, including angiotensin-converting enzyme inhibitors, photocoagulation and prophylactic footcare.

Key words: Macrovascular; Microvascular; Risk; Interventions; Screening; Diabetes.

INTRODUCTION

The management of women with diabetes is aimed at reducing the incidence and progression of macrovascular and microvascular disease associated with diabetes. Therefore, optimal management involves addressing cardiovascular (CVD) risk factors and screening and treatment for end-organ damage, as well as management of blood glucose. This chapter will review recommended management strategies and evidence for these strategies, with attention to specific differences between women and men as they exist.

From: *Diabetes in Women: Pathophysiology and Therapy*
Edited by: A. Tsatsoulis et al. (eds.), DOI 10.1007/978-1-60327-250-6_23
© Humana Press, a part of Springer Science+Business Media, LLC 2009

MACROVASCULAR OR CARDIOVASCULAR DISEASE

As discussed in Chap. 3, CVD is the primary cause of mortality for both women and men with diabetes *(1)*. Diabetes is a stronger risk factor for fatal ischemic heart disease in women than in men *(2)*. While CVD mortality has declined over time, comparisons of CVD mortality rates between 1971 and 2000 demonstrate reductions for men with diabetes but not for women with diabetes *(1)*. The United Kingdom Prospective Diabetes Study (UKPDS), a cohort of over 3,000 people with type 2 diabetes, identified several modifiable risk factors for CVD disease, including cigarette smoking, hypertension and dyslipidemia *(3)*.

Cigarette and Tobacco Abuse

PREVALENCE

In 2001–2002, 17–19% of individuals with diabetes reported smoking *(4)*. The prevalence of cigarette smoking is higher among persons with diabetes than among persons without diabetes, even after adjustments for age, sex, race and educational level *(5)*. Despite their higher risk of CVD, women with diabetes have similar rates of smoking compared with women without diabetes *(5)*. These rates have remained fairly constant over the past decade, although the percentage of persons with diabetes who attempted to quit increased by approximately 19% from the 1990s to later in the decade *(6)*. Population-based surveys from a decade ago indicated that as many as 41% of diabetic patients did not recall physician advice to quit smoking, although comparisons between 1974, 1985, and 1990 showed positive trends in the recall of such advice *(7)*.

ASSOCIATION WITH DISEASE

Prospective cohort analyses of women in the Nurses Health Study have suggested that smoking is associated with the development of diabetes *(8)*. After controlling for multiple risk factors, the relative risk of type 2 diabetes among women who smoked more than 25 cigarettes a day was approximately 1.5 times that of women who did not smoke *(8)*. For women with known diabetes, smoking and mortality have a dose-response relationship, with smoking cessation of 10 years or more associated with elimination in risk due to smoking *(9)*. Smokers with diabetes have excess macrovascular complications as well; among women with type 2 diabetes, former smokers were more likely to be diagnosed with coronary disease *(10)* or stroke *(11)*. Smokers with diabetes also have excess microvascular complications, particularly nephropathy as measured by microalbuminuria *(12)* and neuropathy *(13)*, although the association with retinopathy is more equivocal *(14)*.

IMPACT OF SMOKING CESSATION AND EFFECTIVENESS OF SMOKING CESSATION INTERVENTIONS

Meta-analyses of CVD risk reduction trials suggest that smoking cessation had a greater effect on survival and CVD events than most other interventions *(15)*. The magnitude of reduction was greater among persons with diabetes than among persons without diabetes *(15)*. Not surprisingly, an extensive review and meta-analysis of randomized smoking cessation interventions documented reductions in macrovascular disease, as well as malignancy *(16)*. The majority of these interventions have been conducted for the population at large, rather than specifically for women or men with diabetes. Published interventions typically consist of single-session counseling, although repetition of cessation messages in multiple sessions is probably more effective *(16)*. The type of healthcare professional does not seem to influence effectiveness; in fact, delivery by multiple providers may increase effectiveness *(16)*. Individual or group counseling may be more effective than self-help interventions, and supplementation with pharmacotherapy, using combination or single-agent approaches such as nicotine replacement, bupropion or varenicline also increase quit rates *(16, 17)*.

Among persons with diabetes, there is minimal literature regarding interventions for smoking cessation *(18)*. One randomized controlled trial compared 15 min of unstructured physician advice vs. intensive behavioral therapy over 10 weeks; quit rates were similar in these two groups, although the mean number of cigarettes decreased in the behavioral therapy group *(18)*. To our knowledge, no studies have examined the impact of pharmacotherapy upon quit rates or other diabetes endpoints among diabetic smokers, and none among women specifically. It is possible that smoking cessation may be harder to achieve among women due to issues of weight gain with smoking cessation. Using the 1982–1984 National Health and Nutrition Examination Survey (NHANES), Williamson et al. found that weight gain attributable to smoking cessation averaged 6–10 pounds, with women gaining more weight than men and women more often having greater than 25 pounds of weight gain *(19)*. Results suggesting concerns about weight gain with smoking cessation were common in women with type 1 diabetes, and almost half of smokers were reluctant to quit because of fear of weight gain with cessation *(20)*. Women are also more vulnerable to depression, thus making them more vulnerable to smoking relapse *(21)*.

RECOMMENDATIONS

Assessment of tobacco use and periodic smoking cessation counseling and pharmacotherapy are recommended for diabetes management *(22)*, but further studies are needed to optimize effectiveness of these strategies, specifically for women concerned about weight gain or those affected by depression.

Hypertension

PREVALENCE

Hypertension, defined as blood pressures $\geq 140/90$ mmHg, affected over 60% of persons with diabetes in 2001, a 1.5- to 3-fold difference compared with adults without diabetes *(23)*. Between 1998 and 2002, approximately 28% of individuals with diabetes under the age of 65 years achieved lower blood pressures through lifestyle and/or medication *(6)*. Rates of control were much worse in the elderly, who are predominantly women *(6)*.

ASSOCIATION WITH DISEASE

Hypertension acts as a comorbid risk factor for diabetes and, increases the risk for both microvascular and macrovascular complications. To some extent, it can also be a product of the nephropathy that is a complication of diabetes, particularly in individuals with type 1 diabetes *(24)*. In some populations, hypertension may precede the eventual onset of glucose intolerance *(25)*. While typically defined as a dichotomous risk factor, increases in diastolic or systolic blood pressure by 5 mmHg are associated with concomitant increases in CVD and retinopathy, even when blood pressures are below 140/90 mmHg *(26)*. Several large prospective studies have demonstrated the benefits of lowering blood pressure well below 140/90, with benefits seen at pressure as low as 115/75 mmHg *(27)*.

EFFECTIVENESS OF INTERVENTIONS

Multiple randomized trials have demonstrated the benefit of blood pressure reduction on coronary disease events, stroke and nephropathy among individuals with diabetes *(28)*. For CVD risk reduction, reduction in blood pressure levels to targets is more beneficial than reductions in hemoglobin A1c (HbA1c) to targets *(29)*. Behavioral treatments, particularly sodium restriction, along with weight reduction and physical activity, are generally recommended initially for a trial of 3 months, although the success of these strategies alone in persons with diabetes is not well studied. These strategies can lead to reductions in blood pressure, in the order of 1–3 mmHg in diastolic blood pressure and 5 mmHg in systolic blood pressure *(30)*.

The effectiveness of these interventions among persons with diabetes has not been reported in either subgroup or primary analyses. Rather, for persons with diabetes, the primary comparisons have examined pharmacologic therapy vs. placebo. A recent review of hypertensive treatments in individuals with diabetes found absolute risk reductions in the order of 0.02–0.08% for total CVD events over 10 years, meaning that 12.5–50 persons with diabetes and hypertension would need to be treated with an agent over a 10-year period to avert one CVD event *(28)*. Risk reductions in mortality were suggested but were only significant in one trial *(28)*.

Regarding blood pressure targets, participants in the Hypertension Optimal Treatment (HOT) study assigned to a group with a target for diastolic blood pressures of 80 mmHg had fewer events and CVD death than those assigned to a target of 90 mmHg *(31)*. In the UKPDS, lower targets were similarly associated with lower event rates, although the lower targets were as high as 150/85 mmHg *(32)*. Of note, intensive hypertension control (mean diastolic blood pressure, 87 mmHg vs. 82 mmHg) had greater benefits than intensive glucose control (mean HbA1c 7.9% vs. 7.0%) for all diabetes outcomes, including microvascular endpoints such as nephropathy. Achieved blood pressures were generally at least five points higher than target blood pressures, demonstrating the difficulty of attaining lower blood pressure even in randomized populations under close surveillance and even with the use of multiple agents.

Regarding the choice of agents, multiple trials have compared angiotensin-converting enzyme (ACE) inhibitors to other agents. Several randomized studies suggested that diabetic participants assigned to ACE inhibitors may have a slightly lower risk for myocardial infarction than diabetic participants assigned to calcium channel blockers, although differences in total mortality were not seen *(33–35)*. The effects of ACE inhibitors may extend beyond that of blood pressure control *(36)*. In contrast, the Antihypertensive and Lipid-lowering Treatment to Prevent Heart Attack Trial (ALLHAT) found that thiazide diuretics were associated with the lowest risk for heart failure compared with ACE inhibitors or calcium channel blockers *(37)*. Beta-blocker therapy and ACE inhibitor comparisons have been less consistent, although event rates may be similar *(32)*. Of note, greater hypoglycemia unawareness in the beta-blocker group was not observed, although weight gain and addition of hypoglycemic agents was observed. Angiotensin II receptor blockers (ARB) and calcium channel blocker comparisons demonstrated that diabetic participants assigned to ARB progressed to renal disease more slowly, with lower rates of microalbuminuria and end-stage renal disease, and perhaps to CVD mortality *(38, 39)*.

These studies did not support the use of different targets or agents for women outside of pregnancy. During pregnancy in women with chronic hypertension, aggressive lowering of blood pressures may impair fetal growth, so recommended targets are generally higher during pregnancy. In addition, the use of specific blood pressure agents such as ACE inhibitors and ARBs is contraindicated due to fetal damage, and diuretic use is not recommended due to restricted maternal plasma volume, which theoretically can affect placental perfusion. Agents considered safe for blood pressure management during pregnancy include methyldopa, labetalol and diltiazem. However, these agents are not considered first-line management for hypertension outside of pregnancy, so women with diabetes may require changes in their hypertension regimen during preconception and after delivery. There is little information on the effectiveness of these drugs on outcomes, but another alpha antagonist, doxazosin, may yield worse outcomes than diuretics in nonpregnant women *(40)*.

RECOMMENDATIONS

Regular assessment of blood pressure is needed, with the primary emphasis on adequate blood pressure control *(22)*. Recommended targets are ≤130/80 mm Hg, with pharmacologic therapy in addition to lifestyle and behavioral therapy as necessary. The choice of the initial agent is usually an ACE inhibitor or an ARB, due to the fact that persons with diabetes may have concomitant conditions such as nephropathy that benefit from these agents. This choice is not as clear-cut for persons who may not achieve targets with these agents. As persons with diabetes will generally require more than one agent, thiazide agents are usually recommended next, followed by other agents.

Dyslipidemia

PREVALENCE

In 2001, 53% of adults with diabetes reported physician-diagnosed lipid abnormalities *(23)*. In population-based cohorts such as the NHANES, approximately 43% of adults with diabetes achieved low-density lipoprotein (LDL) levels <130 mg/dl in 1999–2002, an increase from approximately 20% from the previous decade *(6)*. Only 40% of women with diabetes attained these lower LDL levels, a slightly lower but not significant difference from the 46% of men with diabetes who attained lower levels *(6)*. Only 75–80% reported having their lipids measured in the past year, although this figure is higher in other reports from earlier this decade *(23)*.

ASSOCIATION WITH DISEASE

The lipid abnormalities that may accompany diabetes increase the risk of macrovascular disease *(41)*. As with hypertension, the lipid abnormalities may present before the onset of overt hyperglycemia *(42)*. Levels of high-density lipoprotein cholesterol (HDL) are decreased and triglycerides are increased, and levels of LDL and other atherogenic particles [lipoprotein (a), intermediate-density lipoprotein, and very-low-density lipoprotein] are increased *(43)*. The quality of those components is also affected, resulting in smaller and denser LDL particles *(43)*. The link between elevated lipids and coronary disease is well established, through randomized trials as well as prospective studies, and reduction in lipid levels to targets may reduce CVD events to a greater extent than reduction in HbA1c to targets *(29)*. However, no studies of lipid-lowering therapy that reported CVD outcomes were conducted solely in patients with diabetes, although subgroup analyses were performed for these participants. These studies are reported in greater detail later.

EFFECTIVENESS OF INTERVENTIONS

A recent meta-analysis examined the results of studies of lipid lowering in participants with diabetes *(41)*. Four trials focused on primary prevention or on patients who had not yet developed CVD; six trials focused on secondary prevention or on patients who had developed CVD at the time of entry, and two presented data on both. In four of the primary prevention trials, persons placed on statins or gemfibrozil had a reduced risk of coronary events, although in diabetes subgroup analysis, this finding was not statistically significant, possibly because the studies were not powered to examine persons with diabetes separately. In one of the primary prevention trials, both persons with and without diabetes placed on statins had a reduced risk of coronary events. In the final primary prevention study, Prospective Study of Pravastatin in the Elderly at Risk (PROSPER) *(44)*, patients with diabetes who were placed on a statin actually did worse than those on the placebo arm.

In secondary prevention trials for persons with diabetes who had already experienced a CVD event, treatment with a statin led to reduced CVD events in several randomized controlled trials *(45–48)*. In the Post-Coronary Artery Bypass Graft (POST-CABG) trial *(49)* and the Long-Term Intervention with Pravastatin in Ischemic Disease (LIPID) trial *(50)*, risk reduction of similar magnitude was seen, but was not statistically significant. Again, in the PROSPER study, patients with diabetes randomized to pravastatin did worse than those in the placebo group, despite their previous history of CVD *(44)*. A meta-analysis of these studies found a pooled relative risk for CVD events of 0.78 (95% CI 0.67–0.89), among diabetic patients without CVD, with a number needed to treat of 34.5 diabetic persons to avert one event over approximately 4 years *(41)*. Among diabetic patients with a history of CVD, the relative risk was similar, but the number needed to treat was only 13.8 over 5 years.

Extrapolating these trials to the formation of a single guideline for lipid lowering was not straightforward. Either the studies did not set specific LDL targets, set differing targets, or found that coronary events did not differ by target. The current National Cholesterol Education Panel guidelines state that diabetes should be treated as a CVD equivalent, that is, targets should be a LDL cholesterol level of 100 mg/dl with initiation of drug therapy at levels >130 mg/dl *(51)*. Lower levels of LDL, such as those of 70–75 mg/dl, may be of benefit in the acute setting, such as in patients with acute coronary syndromes *(52)*. However, these low levels may not be achievable in clinical practice as levels this low were not commonly achieved in the trial setting, and the magnitude of benefit was relatively small compared to (1) placement on a statin or (2) lowering to <130 mg/dl. The role of additional agents such as gemfibrozil is less clear, though theoretically they may provide added benefit for some persons already on a statin.

Recommendations for lipid lowering are slightly different among women. First, statin therapy is contraindicated in pregnancy due to lack of proof of benefit. Outside of pregnancy, HDL targets of >50 mg/dl were recommended due to prospective cohort studies such as the Women's Health Study, which found that HDL was more highly predictive of CVD events than LDL, along with elevated (>400 mg/dl) levels of triglycerides *(53)*. The value of these different targets has not been evaluated in primary prevention randomized studies in women, particularly among women with diabetes. However, women's lipid profiles respond to statins as well as men's profiles, and statin use is associated with reduction in CVD events *(54)*.

RECOMMENDATIONS

Testing for lipid disorders is recommended annually and more often as needed to achieve goals, although the degree of benefit for repeat testing may be smaller if patients are already on statin therapy. Measurement of lipid fractions aside from HDL, LDL, and triglycerides is not currently recommended in routine clinical care *(55)*.Goals for women are an LDL <100 mg/dl, with perhaps a target of <70 in the acute coronary setting, HDL >50 mg/dl, and triglycerides <150 mg/dl *(51)*. Lifestyle modification focusing on reduction of saturated fat, trans fat, cholesterol intake, increased physical activity, and weight loss can lead to an improved lipid profile and can be attempted first. Combination therapy beyond statins may assist in reaching these goals, although such combinations have not been evaluated.

Physical Activity or Exercise

PREVALENCE

In 2003, only 39% of adults with diabetes in the USA reported significant physical activity, defined as moderate or vigorous activity for at least 30 min, three times per week, compared with 58% of adults without diabetes *(56)*. Another study from 2005 examined the proportion of persons with diabetes who reported certain types of activities typically associated with increases in heart rate and found that only 44% of women with diabetes met physical activity recommendations *(57)*. Moreover, among adults with diabetes, 31% of NHANES III participants affected by diabetes reported no activity while 38% responded to suboptimal activity *(58)*.

ASSOCIATION WITH DISEASE

Lack of physical activity is associated with onset of diabetes *(59)*, incident macrovascular disease among women with diabetes *(60)*, and mortality among women with diabetes *(61)*. Regarding diabetes prevention, several prospective cohort studies, including cohorts of women, have shown a decreased risk of approximately 30% associated with regular walking or participation in moderate-intensity activities *(59)*. Among women who had already developed diabetes in the Nurses Health Study, women who walked or performed moderate activity at least 4 h per week had a lower risk of developing any CVD, even after adjustment for BMI *(60)*. In another study, adults with diabetes who reported regular activity (defined as walking for at least 2 h per week) had decreased incidence of fatal CVD

(HR 0.66, 95% CI 0.45–0.96), and persons who walked more frequently had an even greater reduction in mortality *(61)*.

EFFECTIVENESS OF INTERVENTIONS

One possible mechanism of the association between exercise and macrovascular disease is improved glycemic control. A meta-analysis of interventions for exercise found that exercise reduced HbA1c levels from 8.31 to 7.65%, even without changes in BMI *(62)*. These benefits of exercise may depend less on the type of exercise rather than the duration of exercise *(63)*. Activity improves peripheral insulin sensitivity in women with diabetes, even without significant weight loss *(64)*.

While exercise has beneficial effects on lipid metabolism *(65)* and blood pressure *(66)* in adults without diabetes, beneficial effects of exercise, independent of medication and diet, have been more difficult to demonstrate among adults with diabetes. The benefits of medical nutritional therapy are covered in Chaps. 14 and 17. The lifestyle interventions successfully resulting in weight loss have usually incorporated both an exercise and dietary component. In the Diabetes Prevention Program, adults with impaired glucose tolerance who were randomized to intensive lifestyle intervention, consisting of individual and group counseling on activity and diet, increased activity and decreased weight *(67)*. While diabetes risk was not associated with activity independent of weight loss, activity was an integral component of weight loss *(68)*. In the Look AHEAD (Action for Health in Diabetes) trial, overweight adults with type 2 diabetes were randomized to intensive lifestyle intervention, aimed at decreasing caloric intake and increasing physical activity vs. diabetes support and education *(69)*. Participants randomized to intensive lifestyle intervention lost more weight, gained in fitness, and had greater reductions in diabetes, hypertension, and lipid-lowering medication *(69)*.

Unfortunately, exercise regimens are difficult for persons with diabetes to maintain; follow-up after one randomized trial showed that at year 1, only 20% of participants reported exercising regularly *(70)*.

RECOMMENDATIONS

On the basis of benefits for both glycemic control and associations with macrovascular disease, ADA guidelines recommend at least 30 min of moderate or more intense activity, several days a week. This may consist of 90 min per week of intense activity or 150 min of moderate activity *(71)*. Women with type 1 diabetes should coordinate their activity carefully with meals and insulin injections, as exercise of longer duration can decrease insulin requirements, and insulin uptake may be affected by the site of injection *(72)*. While the benefits of stress testing before initiation of an exercise regimen have not been established in adults with diabetes, women aged greater than 35 years might consider such testing *(73)*. On the basis of preliminary results from the Look AHEAD trial, it is concluded that successful lifestyle interventions should involve both a physical activity component and a medical nutritional component for successful weight loss and reduction in medication use *(69)*.

Aspirin

PREVALENCE

Because of the coagulation abnormalities and endothelial dysfunction covered in Chap. 3, anticoagulants such as aspirin are generally recommended for patients with known CVD disease and for those at highest risk for coronary disease. However, analysis of Behavioral Risk Factor Surveillance System (BRFSS) data from 2001 has demonstrated that aspirin use in women with diabetes is relatively lower than in men, even among women older than 50 years. In 2001, 74.2% of diabetic adults with CVD, but only 37.9% of those without CVD, used aspirin regularly, including less than 40% with diagnosed hypertension, hypercholesterolemia, or cigarette use *(74)*. Among women at high risk for CVD events, aspirin was relatively underused *(74)*.

ASSOCIATION WITH DISEASE AND EFFECTIVENESS OF INTERVENTIONS

Reasons for aspirin underuse may include perceptions of lower effectiveness in reducing CVD events in persons with diabetes or perception of greater side effects than in the general population. As with other interventions, studies of primary prevention of CVD show less benefit than studies enrolling persons with known CVD. For men, the Physicians' Health Study found that aspirin led to significant reduction in primary CVD event rates, although not mortality (75). Randomized primary prevention trials in women have been more equivocal. In the Women's Health Study, aspirin did not effect CVD death or MI (76). Among women with diabetes, there was no significant reduction in CVD events. However, aspirin was associated with a decreased risk of first stroke in the overall study, and aspirin was effective in reducing MI among women at highest risk for events, that is, women over 65 years of age. The Primary Prevention Project, a randomized study involving over 1,000 diabetic participants, showed that low-dose aspirin only marginally reduced the risk of major CVD events [RR 0.90 (95% CI 0.50–1.62)]; in contrast, significant reductions were seen among participants without diabetes (77). Meta-analyses of primary prevention studies have also not reported significant reductions in risk among patients with diabetes (78). In the Early Treatment of Diabetic Retinopathy Study, consisting of persons both with and without a history of coronary disease, the risk reduction for CVD events and death was not significant for patients with diabetes (79). However, the common concerns of increased risk of retinal bleeding, hemorrhagic stroke and gastrointestinal bleeding were not seen. Also of note, primary prevention studies may enroll participants at a wide range of CVD risk, and it is possible that participants at high risk but with no history of CVD events may benefit compared with participants at lower risk and with no history of CVD events. Therefore, aspirin may have benefited higher risk groups.

Among secondary prevention studies, reductions in CVD are statistically significant, including the subgroup of people with diabetes (78). The dosage of aspirin has not been established, as the dosages in these studies varied widely. The Antiplatelet Trialists' collaboration, a meta-analysis of 145 secondary prevention trials, did not find evidence that higher dosages were more effective than lower dosages.

RECOMMENDATIONS FOR ASPIRIN

Aspirin is recommended at dosages ranging from 75 to 162 mg/day as a secondary prevention strategy and for primary prevention for individuals with elevated CVD risk (22). Use for primary prevention, particularly for women aged greater than 30 but who are at lower CVD risk, is somewhat controversial but can be considered. The exception is among young persons who are under the age of 21 years due to the risk of Reye's syndrome.

Glycemic Control

PREVALENCE

Although optimal glucose targets are still a matter of debate, HbA1c levels greater than 9.0% are considered above target. In the early 1990s, approximately 27% of adults with diabetes under the age of 65 years reported above-target HbA1c levels and approximately 19% of adults greater than 65 reported above-target HbA1c levels; these figures had not significantly improved a decade later (6).

RANDOMIZED STUDIES OF GLYCEMIC C

The benefits of glucose control are determined by diabetes type as well as degree of initial glucose dysregulation. The Diabetes Control and Complications Trial (DCCT), a randomized trial of persons with type 1 diabetes, found lower rates of microvascular complications (retinopathy, nephropathy, and neuropathy) with each 1% drop in HbA1c (80). The goal of tighter control was an HbA1c of 6.0, although the actual HbA1c achieved was approximately 7%, as opposed to 9% with conventional therapy. Follow-up of the cohort found that tighter control was associated with a reduction in CVD events as well (81). Intensive therapy was more effective for prevention of disease rather than prevention of progression, and therefore this highlights the importance of intensive therapy as early as possible after diagnosis. However, intensive therapy was associated with a greater rate of hypoglycemic events, in the order of 105 compared with 25 episodes per 100 patient-years for mean HbA1c values of 5.5 and 10.5%.

The UKPDS, a randomized trial of persons with type 2 diabetes (82), and the Kumamoto study, another randomized trial in persons with type 2 diabetes (83), found improvements in microvascular complication rates but not macrovascular complication rates with HbA1c lowering. In the UKPDS, those assigned to the intensive therapy arm achieved HbA1c levels of 7.0, compared with 7.9 in the conventional therapy group (82), a smaller difference than seen in the DCCT. Moreover, the rates of retinopathy were not as strongly associated with HbA1c lowering as in the DCCT study. As in the DCCT, more intensive therapy was associated with more hypoglycemia and more weight gain due to the use of insulin. Weight gain was approximately 4 kg in those receiving insulin vs. oral agents. In the UKPDS, metformin as opposed to other hypoglycemic agents was associated with a reduction in CVD events, although this finding was of only borderline significance (82). At this point, these agents are not recommended for CVD risk reduction alone, although they may be beneficial as first-line agents for glycemic control per se.

Prospective cohort studies, including follow-up studies in the UKPDS, consistently support associations between HbA1c levels and CVD disease, but the effectiveness of an intervention to lower CVD events by lowering glucose alone among participants with type 2 diabetes has not been shown (84). Therefore, it is difficult to identify optimal levels of control and the point at which these are balanced by the risks of hypoglycemia and other adverse effects.

RECOMMENDATIONS

Current recommendations for glucose control targets vary. The American Diabetes Association recommends a target HbA1c of 7.0%, while other subspecialty organizations recommend lower thresholds (22). Accordingly, HbA1c is to be measured twice yearly among patients who are meeting treatment goals and more frequently as needed for patients who require adjustments to therapy. To achieve these goals, patients are encouraged to engage in self-monitoring of blood glucose and lifestyle modification as well as pharmacologic therapy as needed (22).

MICROVASCULAR COMPLICATIONS

Nephropathy Screening and Treatment

PREVALENCE

Diabetic nephropathy occurs in 20–40% of persons with diabetes (85). Nephropathy ranges from the early stages of persistent microalbuminuria (30–299 mg/24 h) to end-stage renal disease. Once persons with diabetes develop macroalbuminuria (300 mg/24 h), they are likely to progress to end-stage renal disease (86). While approximately one-third of persons with type 1 diabetes will have microalbuminuria after 15 years, only half progress to overt nephropathy (87). Rates among persons with type 2 diabetes are significantly lower, with 0.5% progressing to end-stage renal disease over a 10-year period (88).

EFFECTIVENESS OF INTERVENTIONS

The rationale for nephropathy screening is that effective therapies exist. ACE inhibitors and ARB agents lower urinary protein excretion and slow the rate of nephropathy progression, beyond their antihypertensive effects *(38, 89)*. While the relationship between microalbuminuria and progression is stronger in type 1 diabetes than in type 2 diabetes, these agents are recommended even in patients with microalbuminuria in the absence of other macro- or microvascular risk factors. As mentioned in previous discussions of randomized studies, reduction in blood pressure, independent of the agent used, and intensive glycemic control may also delay nephropathy progression. While difficult to achieve, dietary protein restriction may help slow the decline in the glomerular filtration rate *(90)*.

Once a person with diabetes is already on therapy, particularly an ACE inhibitor or an ARB, the role of repeated microalbumin measurement is less clear, particularly if patients are on maximum dose and other risk factors such as blood pressure are controlled. Strategies comparing period reassessment and adjustment of therapy have not been examined.

RECOMMENDATIONS

Measurement of the albumin–creatinine ratio in a random spot collection is sensitive but repetition is recommended to due to the high number of false positives *(22)*. Early referral to a nephrologist may increase options for management, such as opportunities for peritoneal dialysis. In persons with type 1 diabetes, screening may be deferred several years after diagnosis since microalbuminuria is relatively uncommon at diagnosis, although in type 2 diabetes, screening is often initiated earlier due to a longer average length of time between onset of hyperglycemia and recognition of diabetes *(22)*.

Retinopathy Screening and Treatment

PREVALENCE

Persons with diabetes are at increased risk for premature visual loss due to diabetic retinopathy, a highly specific vascular complication, and also earlier onset of glaucoma, cataracts, macular edema, and other eye disorders *(91)*. The incidence of blindness is 25 times higher in persons with diabetes than in the general population *(91)*. As with nephropathy, the severity of disease varies over a wide range. While over half of the DCCT participants (who had an average diabetes duration of less than 5 years) had retinopathy at baseline, only 0.4% had preproliferative retinopathy and none required laser photocoagulation *(92)*. However, significant racial/ethnic variation may exist, particularly for type 2 diabetes. Among a cohort of veterans, moderate and worse retinopathy was more common among Hispanics (36%) and African-Americans (29%) than for non-Hispanic whites (22%); similar prevalence data for women were not available *(93)*.

EFFECTIVENESS OF INTERVENTIONS

Simulated models for retinopathy screening in type 1 diabetes *(94)* as well as type 2 diabetes *(95)* have suggested that significant cost savings would occur with regular screening. Annual screening was assumed, although it is possible that among persons with excellent HbA1c control, less frequent screening could occur with minimal increases in morbidity *(96)*.

The rationale for screening includes the availability of effective therapies for progression as well as treatment. For persons with type 1 diabetes, the DCCT demonstrated that better glycemic control and hypertension can delay progression of retinopathy *(80)*. The DCCT also noted that retinopathy may temporarily worsen with pregnancy, but that the risk of severe disease can be reduced in women with appropriate screening and photocoagulation as necessary *(97)*. For persons with type 2 diabetes, the UKPDS demonstrates that better control of hypertension decreased retinopathy progression, although the association with glycemic control was less pronounced *(32)*.

Once identified, retinopathy can be treated with laser photocoagulation surgery. The Diabetic Retinopathy Study *(98)* and the Early Treatment Diabetic Retinopathy Study *(99)* demonstrated that photocoagulation for proliferative diabetic retinopathy and macular edema significantly reduced the incidence of severe visual loss. Treatment was not successful in restoring visual acuity.

RECOMMENDATIONS

Screening, consisting of a dilated and comprehensive eye exam, is indicated for persons with diabetes. Screening frequency may be based on risk, that is, may occur less frequently for people with optimal blood pressure and glucose control and more frequently among persons whose retinopathy is progressing. Because of the transient worsening of retinopathy with pregnancy, women with type 1 diabetes and type 2 diabetes who are planning pregnancy should undergo a comprehensive eye exam *(22)*.

Neuropathy

PREVALENCE

Diabetic neuropathy presents in a wide range of forms, but most common are chronic sensorimotor distal peripheral neuropathy and autonomic neuropathy *(100)*. In the Rochester Diabetic Retinopathy Study, approximately 54% of adults using insulin had a polyneuropathy and 7% had an autonomic neuropathy; among participants with type 2 diabetes, approximately 45% had a polyneuropathy and about 5% had an autonomic neuropathy *(100)*. However, only 13–15% of the polyneuropathies were symptomatic. While foot inspection and monofilament testing are recommended, performance varies widely *(101)*. The pain that may result can interfere with diabetes self-management activities *(102)*.

EFFECTIVENESS OF INTERVENTIONS AND TREATMENT

Duration of diabetes and degree of glycemic control are the major risk factors for progression *(103)*. In the DCCT, the incidence of diabetic neuropathy was reduced by 60% over 10 years among participants randomized to the tight control arm *(104)*. Reduced neuropathy was seen in the UKPDS as well when neuropathy was examined as a component of a composite microvascular endpoint *(82)*. In the Steno type 2 trial, intensive multifactorial intervention reduced progression of autonomic neuropathy (30% in the intervention arm vs. 54% in the control arm), but did not slow peripheral neuropathy *(105)*.

Once neuropathy is present, pain may spontaneously remit, but a broad range of agents may assist with painful symptoms *(22)*. None of these are approved in the USA for the treatment of painful diabetic neuropathy but are used on an off-label basis based on efficacy studies. Agents include antidepressants and seizure medications, such as tricyclic antidepressants, duloxetine, pregabalin, venlexafine, carbamazepine and lamotrogine. Topical therapies may also be tried, such as capsaicin and lidocaine.

Neuropathy with loss of protective sensation, combined with other conditions common in diabetes such as peripheral vascular disease, increases the risk of ulceration and amputations *(106)*. Therefore, careful assessment of skin integrity, footwear and patient education on foot self-care may delay amputation *(107)*.

RECOMMENDATIONS

Persons with diabetes are to be screened for distal symmetric polyneuropathy using simple clinical tests such as foot inspection combined with monofilament testing *(22)*. Simple preventive measures such as counseling about self-care and referral for assessment and tailored footwear may reduce progression to ulceration. Inquiring about pain and treatment of pain may have a beneficial effect on macrovascular risk factors as well as quality of life.

OTHER DISEASE MANAGEMENT RECOMMENDATIONS

Vaccinations

Since persons with diabetes are relatively immunocompromised, annual influenza vaccination and an initial pneumococcal vaccination are recommended, with a pneumococcal booster if the initial vaccination is prior to the age of 65. Because of the increased risk of skin breakdown, tetanus boosters are also recommended *(22)*.

Preconception Care

Preconception care and family planning are covered in greater detail in Chaps. 9 and 15. To briefly summarize, glycemic control prior to conception, discontinuation of teratogenic agents such as statins and ACE inhibitors, and use of effective family planning until these goals are achieved are necessary *(22)*.

Depression and Anxiety

Affective disorders are more common in adults with diabetes, as depression is a risk factor for incident diabetes and because diabetes is also associated with incident depression *(108)*. Affective disorders are covered in greater detail in Chap. 7. Because of the high prevalence of depression among patients with diabetes, reportedly three times more common in people with diabetes than in healthy controls for a prevalence of about 15% *(109)*, screening for these conditions are recommended.

Eating Disorders

The association between the eating disorders and diabetes, particularly type 1 diabetes, has been discussed in Chap. 7. To briefly summarize, mortality is high in the type 1 diabetic population with anorexia; in a Danish series, the mortality rate was 2.2 per 1,000 person-years for type 1 diabetes, 7.3 for women with anorexia nervosa only, and 34.6 for women with both disorders *(110)*. Less is known about eating disorders in women of reproductive age with type 2 diabetes. Crow et al. noted that 26% of patients with type 2 diabetes engaged in binge eating *(111)*. As the average age at diagnosis for type 2 diabetes continues to drop, eating disorders may become more common and may have more severe metabolic repercussions. Further study is needed of the prevalence of eating disorders and tertiary complications, particularly for women with type 2 diabetes of reproductive age, and screening for these disorders is recommended.

HEALTHCARE DELIVERY FOR DIABETES

Multifactorial Interventions

The high risk of macrovascular and microvascular disease, along with other complications, among persons with diabetes along with the complexity of the management of risk factors supports a long-term, individualized, multifactorial approach. In the Steno-2 study, participants with type 2 diabetes and microalbuminuria were randomized to an intensive intervention vs. conventional management *(105)*. Goals in the intensive therapy arm were lower than in the conventional therapy arm and targeted systolic and diastolic blood pressure, HbA1c, total cholesterol, triglycerides, treatment with ACE inhibitors irrespective of blood pressure, and treatment with aspirin. Participants in the intensive therapy arm were offered consultations every 3 months during the 8-year follow-up, overseen by a project team consisting of a physician, nurse and dietician. After approximately 8 years, those in the intervention arm had a significant lower risk of CVD events, as well as individual microvascular events. Steno-2 suggests that particular attention to the multifactorial nature of CVD risk factor management, as well as long-term continuous care, may assist in reducing CVD events. Unfortunately, as noted in studies examining risk factor control, the majority of participants with diabetes do not achieve these goals.

Health System Characteristics

Steno-2 highlights the importance of diabetes education and the potential impact of a team approach to diabetes management. In a 2006 meta-analysis by Shojania et al. *(112)*, interventions involving team changes and case management reduced HbA1c values by 0.22–0.33% more than interventions without such changes. Specifically, case management interventions that empowered the nurse or pharmacist case manager to make medication changes were significantly more effective than those that did not (0.96%, 95% CI: 0.52%, 1.41% vs. 0.41%, 5% CI: 0.20%, 0.62%). Similarly, interventions involving multidisciplinary teams were more effective than team interventions without this feature.

Other health system delivery elements can also contribute to improved diabetes care. Mangione et al. found that disease management programs that included a greater number of quality improvement elements (such as physician reminders, performance feedback, and care management) were associated with better processes of care than programs that contained fewer elements *(101)*. In addition to measurement of HbA1c, these process measures included measurement of lipid and proteinuria. Fleming et al. noted that greater infrastructure (registries, automated reminders, academic detailing, quality improvement work groups) was associated with better performance of diabetes-related Health Plan Employer Data Information Set (HEDIS) measures *(113)*.

Individual Interventions

Interventions aimed at improving diabetes self-care skills, or diabetes self-management, may also improve diabetes care. In a 2002 meta-analysis by Norris et al. *(114)*, self-management interventions improved HbA1c levels by 0.76% (95% CI 0.34%, 1.18%) more than the control group, although effects tended to wane slightly over time. Other meta-analyses by Warsi et al. *(115)* and Ellis et al. *(116)* also found that diabetes education led to significant reductions in HbA1c. Of note, improvement in other risk factors, particularly hypertension, was not as marked. Chodosh et al. *(117)* found that diabetes self-management interventions had no significant effect on weight reduction or hypertension, even as the interventions were associated with reductions in fasting glucose and HbA1c.

Common features of these interventions include the greatest improvement in those with the worst risk factor control at baseline and the minimal improvement in risk factors other than glycemic control. Thus, greater focus on risk factors aside from glycemic measures is needed in persons with diabetes. Effective interventions for those with intermediate, but not ideal, control are needed. Comprehensive programs that cover aspects of care unique to women, such as preconception care, and morbidities more common in women, such as eating disorders, are also needed. Ideally, such programs would involve changes in healthcare delivery at the health system, provider and individual levels.

REFERENCES

1. Gregg E, Gu Q, Cheng Y, Narayan K, Cowie C. Mortality trends in men and women with diabetes, 1971 to 2000. Ann Intern Med 2007;147:149–55
2. Barrett-Connor E, Wingard D. Sex differential in ischemic heart disease mortality in diabetics: a prospective population-based study. Am J Epidemiol 1983;118:489

3. Turner R, Millns H, Neil H, et al. Risk factors for coronary artery disease in non-insulin dependent diabetes mellitus: United Kingdom Prospective Diabetes Study (UKPDS: 23). BMJ 1998;316(7134):823–8

4. Saaddine J, Engelgau M, Beckles G, Gregg E, Thompson T, Narayan K. A diabetes report card for the United States: quality of care in the 1990s. Ann Intern Med 2002;136(8):565–74

5. Ford E, Mokdad A, Gregg E. Trends in cigarette smoking among U.S. adults with diabetes: findings from the Behavioral Risk Factor Surveillance System. Prev Med 2004;39(6):1238–42

6. Saaddine J, Cadwell B, Gregg E, et al. Improvements in diabetes processes of care and intermediate outcomes: United States, 1988–2002. Ann Intern Med 2006;144(7):465–74

7. Malarcher A, Ford E, Nelson D, et al. Trends in cigarette smoking and physicians' advice to quit smoking among people with diabetes in the U.S. Diabetes Care 1995;18(5):694–7

8. Rimm E, Manson J, Stampfer M, et al. Cigarette smoking and the risk of diabetes in women. Am J Public Health 1993;83(2):211–4

9. Al-Delaimy W, Willett W, Manson J, Speizer F, Hu F. Smoking and mortality among women with type 2 diabetes: The Nurses' Health Study cohort. Diabetes Care 2001;24(12):2043–8

10. Meigs J, Singer D, Sullivan L, et al. Metabolic control and prevalent cardiovascular disease in non-insulin dependent diabetes mellitus (NIDDM): The NIDDM Patient Outcome Research Team. Am J Med 1997;102(1):38–47

11. Tuomilehto J, Rastenyte D, Jousilahti P, Sarti C, Vartiainen E. Diabetes mellitus as a risk factor for death from stroke. Prospective study of the middle-aged Finnish population. Stroke 1996;27(2):210–5

12. Chase H, Garg S, Marshall G, et al. Cigarette smoking increases the risk of albuminuria among subjects with type 1 diabetes. JAMA 1991;265(5):614–7

13. Sawicki P, Didjurgeit U, Muhlhauser I, Bender R, Heinemann L, Berger M. Smoking is associated with progression of diabetic nephropathy. Diabetes Care 1994;17(2):126–31

14. Klein R, Klein B, Moss S. Epidemiology of proliferative diabetic retinopathy. Diabetes Care 1992;15(12):1875–91

15. Yudkin J. How can we best prolong life? Benefits of coronary risk factor reduction in non-diabetic and diabetic subjects. BMJ 1993;306(6888):1313–8

16. Clinical Practice Guideline Treating Tobacco Use and Dependence 2008 Update Panel. A clinical practice guideline for treating tobacco use and dependence: 2008 update. Am J Prev Med 2008;35(2):158–76

17. Gonzales D, Rennard S, Nides M, et al. Varenicline, an alpha4beta2 nicotinic acetylcholine receptor partial agonist, vs. sustained-release bupropion and placebo for smoking cessation: a randomized controlled trial. JAMA 2006;296(1):47–55

18. Sawicki P, Didjurgeit U, Muhlhauser I, Berger M. Behaviour therapy versus doctor's anti-smoking advice in diabetic patients. J Intern Med 1993;234:407–9

19. Williamson D, Madans J, Anda R, Kleinman J, Giovino G, Byers T. Smoking cessation and severity of weight gain in a national cohort. N Engl J Med 1991;324(11):739–45

20. Haire-Joshu D, Heady S, Thomas L, Schechtman K, Fisher E, Jr. Beliefs about smoking and diabetes care. Diabetes Educ 1994;20(5):410–5

21. Fant R, Everson D, Dayton G, Pickworth W, Henningfield J. Nicotine dependence in women. J Am Med Womens Assoc 1996;51(102):19–24

22. American Diabetes Association. Standards of medical care in diabetes (Position Statement). Diabetes Care 2007;30(Suppl):S4–41

23. Okoro C, Mokdad A, Ford E, Bowman B, Vinicor F, Giles W. Are persons with diabetes practicing healthier behaviors in the year 2001? Results from the Behavioral Risk Factor Surveillance System. Prev Med 2004;38(2):203–8

24. Mathiesen E, Ronn B, Jensen T, Storm B, Deckert T. Relationship between blood pressure and urinary albumin excretion in development of microalbuminuria. Diabetes 1990;39(2):245–9

25. Hypertension in Diabetes Study (HDS). Prevalence of hypertension in newly presenting type 2 diabetic patients and the association with risk factors for cardiovascular and diabetic complications. J Hypertens 1993;11:309–17

26. Adler A, Stratton I, Neil H, et al. Association of systolic blood pressure with macrovascular and microvascular complications of type 2 diabetes (UKPDS 36): prospective observational study. BMJ 2000;321(7258):412–9

27. Chobanian A, Bakrisk G, Black H, et al. The Seventh Report of the Joint National Committee on Prevention, Detection, Evaluation, and Treatment of High Blood Pressure: the JNC 7 report. JAMA 2003;289(19):2560–72

28. Vijan S, Hayward R. Treatment of hypertension in type 2 diabetes mellitus: blood pressure goals, choice of agents, and setting priorities in diabetes care. Ann Intern Med 2003;138(7):593–602

29. Huang E, Meigs J, Singer D. The effect of interventions to prevent cardiovascular disease in patients with type 2 diabetes mellitus. Am J Med 2001;111(633–42)

30. Sacks F, Svetkey L, Vollmer W, et al. Effects on blood pressure of reduced dietary sodium and the Dietary Approaches to Stop Hypertension (DASH) diet. DASH-Sodium Collaborative Research Group. N Engl J Med 2001;344(1):3–10

31. Hansson L, Zanchetti A, Carruthers S, et al. Effects of intensive blood-pressure lowering and low-dose aspirin in patients with hypertension: principal results of the Hypertension Optimal Treatment (HOT) randomised trial. HOT Study Group. Lancet 1998;351(9118):1755–62

32. Tight blood pressure control and risk of macrovascular and microvascular complications in type 2 diabetes: UKPDS 38. UK Prospective Diabetes Study Group. BMJ 1998;317(7160):703–13

33. Estacio R, Jeffers B, Gifford N, Schrier R. Effect of blood pressure control on diabetic microvascular complications in patients with hypertension and type 2 diabetes. Diabetes Care 2000;23(Suppl 2):B54–64

34. Tatti P, Pahor M, Byington R, et al. Outcome results of the Fosinopril vs. Amlodipine Cardiovascular Events Randomized Trial (FACET) in patients with hypertension and NIDDM. Diabetes Care 1998;21(4):597–603

35. Lindholm L, Hansson L, Ekbom T, et al. Comparison of antihypertensive treatments in preventing cardiovascular events in elderly diabetic patients: results from the Swedish Trial in Old Patients with Hypertension-s. Stop Hypertension-2 Study Group. J Hypertens 2000;18(11):1671–5

36. Effects of ramipril on cardiovascular and microvascular outcomes in people with diabetes mellitus: results of the HOPE study and MICRO-HOPE substudy. Lancet 2000;355:253–9

37. The ALLHAT Officers and Coordinators for the ALLHAT Collaborative Research Group. Major outcomes in high-risk hypertensive patients randomized to angiotensin-converting enzyme inhibitor or calcium channel blocker vs. diuretic: the Anti-hypertensive and Lipid-Lowering Treatment to Prevent Heart Attack Trial (ALLHAT). JAMA 2002;288:2981–97

38. Lewis E, Hunsicker L, Clarke W, et al. Renoprotective effect of the angiotensin-receptor antagonist irbesartan in patients with nephropathy due to type 2 diabetes. N Engl J Med 2001;345(12):851–60

39. Lindholm L, Ibsen H, Dahlof B, et al. Cardiovascular morbidity and mortality in patients with diabetes in the Losartan Intervention for Endpoint reduction in hypertension study (LIFE): a randomised trial against atenolol. Lancet 2002;359(9311):1004–10

40. Staessen J, Wang J, Thijs L. Cardiovascular protection and blood pressure reduction: a meta-analysis. Lancet 2001;358(9290):1305–15

41. Vijan S, Hayward R. Pharmacologic lipid-lowering therapy in type 2 diabetes mellitus: background paper for the American College of Physicians. Ann Intern Med 2004;140(8):650–8

42. Hu F, Stampfer M, Haffner S, CG S, Willett W, Manson J. Elevated risk of cardiovascular disease prior to clinical diagnosis of type 2 diabetes. Diabetes Care 2002;25:1129–34

43. Beckman J, Creager M, Libby P. Diabetes and atherosclerosis: epidemiology, pathophysiology, and management. JAMA 2002;287(19):2570–81

44. Shepherd J, Blauw G, Murphy M, et al. Pravastatin in elderly individuals at risk of vascular disease (PROSPER): a randomised controlled trial. Lancet 2002;360(9346):1623–30

45. Pyorala K, Pederson T, Kjekshus J, Faergemann O, Olsson A, Thorgeirsson G. Cholesterol lowering with simvastatin improves prognosis of diabetic patients with coronary heart disease. A subgroup analysis of the Scandinavian Simvastatin Survival Study (4S). Diabetes Care 1997;20(4):6174–20

46. Sacks F, Pfeffer M, Moye L, et al. The effect of pravastatin on coronary events after myocardial infarction in patients with average cholesterol levels. Cholesterol and Recurrent Events Trial Investigators. N Engl J Med 1996;335(14):1001–9

47. Serruys P, de Feyter P, Macaya C, et al. Fluvastatin for prevention of cardiac events following successful first percutaneous coronary intervention: a randomized controlled trial. JAMA 2002;287(24):3215–22

48. Rubins H, Robins S, Collins D, et al. Diabetes, plasma insulin, and cardiovascular disease: subgroup analysis from the Department of Veterans Affairs high-density lipoprotein intervention trial (VA-HIT). Arch Intern Med 2002;162(22):2597–604

49. Hoogwerf B, Waness A, Cressman M, et al. Effects of aggressive cholesterol lowering and low-dose anticoagulation on clinical and angiographic outcomes in patients with diabetes: the Post Coronary Artery Bypass Graft Trial. Diabetes 1999;48(6):1289–94

50. LIPID Study Group. Prevention of cardiovascular events and death with pravastatin in patients with coronary heart disease and a broad range of initial cholesterol levels. N Engl J Med 1998;339:1349–57

51. Expert Panel on Detection, Evaluation, and Treatment of High Blood Cholesterol in Adults. Executive summary of the third report of the National Cholesterol Education Program (NCEP) Expert Panel on Detection, Evaluation, and Treatment of High Blood Cholesterol in Adults (Adult Treatment Panel III). JAMA 2001;285(19):2486–97

52. Cannon C, Braunwald E, McCabe C, et al. Intensive vs. moderate lipid-lowering with statins after acute coronary syndromes. N Engl J Med 2004;350(15):1495–504

53. Everett B, Kurth T, Buring J, Ridker P. The relative strength of C-reactive protein and lipid levels as determinants of ischemic stroke compared with coronary heart disease in women. J Am Coll Cardiol 2006;48(11):2235–42

54. Herrington D, Fong J, Sempos C, et al. Comparison of the Heart and Estrogen/Progestin Replacement Study (HERS) cohort with women with coronary disease from the National Health and Nutrition Examination Survey III (NHANES III). Am Heart J 1998;136(1):115–24

55. Ingelsson E, Schaefer E, Contois J, et al. Clinical utility of different lipid measures for prediction of coronary heart disease in men and women. JAMA 2007;298(7):776–85

56. Morrato E, Hill J, Wyatt H, Ghushchyan V, Sullivan P. Physical activity in U.S. adults with diabetes and at risk for developing diabetes, 2003. Diabetes Care 2007;30(2):203–9

57. Zhao G, Ford E, Li C, Mokdad A. Compliance with physical activity recommendations in U.S. adults with diabetes. Diabet Med 2008;25(2):221–7

58. Nelson K, Reiber G, Boyko E. Diet and exercise among adults with type 2 diabetes: findings from the Third National Health and Nutrition Examination Survey (NHANES III). Diabetes Care 2002;25(10):1722–8

59. Jeon C, Lokken R, Hu F, van Dam R. Physical activity of moderate intensity and risk of type 2 diabetes: a systematic review. Diabetes Care 2007;30(3):744–52

60. Hu F, Stampfer M, Solomon C, et al. Physical activity and risk for cardiovascular events in diabetic women. Ann Intern med 2001;134(2):96–105

61. Gregg E, Gerzoff R, Caspersen C, Williamson D, Narayan K. Relationship of walking to mortality among U.S. adults with diabetes. Arch Intern Med 2003;163(12):1440–7

62. Boule N, Hadded E, Kenny G, Wells G, Sigal R. Effects of exercise on glycemic control and body mass in type 2 diabetes mellitus: a meta-analysis of controlled clinical trials. JAMA 2001;286(10):1218–27

63. Snowling N, Hopkins W. Effects of different modes of exercise training on glucose control and risk factors for complications in type 2 diabetic patients: a meta-analysis. Diabetes Care 2006;29(11):2518–27

64. Duncan G, Perri M, Theriaque D, Hutson A, Eckel R, Stacpoole P. Exercise training, without weight loss, increases insulin sensitivity and postheparin plasma lipase activity in previously sedentary adults. Diabetes Care 2003;26(3):557–62

65. Kraus W, Houmard J, Duscha B, et al. Effects on the amount and intensity of exercise on plasma lipoproteins. N Engl J Med 2002;347(19):1483–92

66. Whelton S, Chin A, Xin X, He J. Effect of aerobic exercise on blood pressure: a meta-analysis of randomized, controlled trials. Ann Intern Med 2002;136(7):493–503

67. Knowler W, Barrett-Connor E, Fowler S, et al. Reduction in the incidence of type 2 diabetes with lifestyle intervention or metformin. N Engl J Med 2002;346:393–403

68. Kriska A, Edelstein S, Hamman R, et al. Physical activity in individuals at risk for diabetes: the Diabetes Prevention Program. Med Sci Sports Exerc 2006;38(5):826–32

69. Look AHEAD Research Group. Reduction in weight and cardiovascular disease risk factors in individuals with type 2 diabetes: one-year results of the Look AHEAD trial. Diabetes Care 2007;30(6):1374–83

70. Schneider S, Khachadurian A, Amorosa L, Clemow L, Ruderman N. Ten-year experience with an exercise-based outpatient life-style modification program in the treatment of diabetes mellitus. Diabetes Care 1992;15(11):1800–10

71. Buse J, Ginsberg H, Bakris G, et al. Primary prevention of cardiovascular diseases in people with diabetes mellitus: a scientific statement from the American Heart Association and the American Diabetes Association. Circulation 2007;115(1):114–26

72. Koivisto V, Felig P. Alterations in insulin absorption and in blood glucose control associated with varying insulin injection sites in diabetic patients. Ann Intern Med 1980;92:59–61

73. Mittleman M, Maclure M, Tofler G, Sherwood J, Goldberg R, Muller J. Triggering of acute myocardial infarction by heavy physical exertion. Protection against triggering by regular exertion. Determinants of Myocardial Infarction Onset Study Investigators. N Engl J Med 1993;329(23):1677–83

74. Kim C, Beckles G. Cardiovascular risk reduction practices in men and women in the Behavioral Risk Factor Surveillance System. Am J Prev Med 2003;27(1):1–7

75. Final report on the aspirin component of the ongoing Physicians' Health Study. Steering Committee of the Physicians' Health Study Research Group. N Engl J Med 1989;321(3):129–35

76. Ridker P, Cook N, Lee I, et al. A randomized trial of low-dose aspirin in the primary prevention of cardiovascular disease in women. N Engl J Med 2005;352(13):1293–304

77. Sacco M, Pellegrini F, Roncaglioni M, et al. Primary prevention of cardiovascular events with low-dose aspirin and vitamin E in type 2 diabetic patients: results of the Primary Prevention Project (PPP) trial. Diabetes Care 2003;26(12):3264–72

78. Collaborative meta-analysis of randomized trials of antiplatelet therapy for prevention of death, myocardial infarction, and stroke in high-risk patients. BMJ 2002;324:71–86

79. Aspirin effects on mortality and morbidity in patients with diabetes mellitus. Early Treatment Diabetic Retinopathy Study report 14. ETDRS Investigators. JAMA 1992;268(10):1292–300

80. Retinopathy and nephropathy in patients with type 1 diabetes four years after a trial of intensive therapy. The Diabetes Control and Complications Trial/Epidemiology of Diabetes Interventions and Complications Research Group. N Engl J Med 2000;342(6):381–9

81. Nathan D, Cleary P, Backlund J, et al. Intensive diabetes treatment and cardiovascular disease in patients with type 1 diabetes. N Engl J Med 2005;353(25):2643–53

82. Intensive blood-glucose control with sulphonylureas or insulin compared with conventional treatment and risk of complications in patients with type 2 diabetes (UKPDS 33). UK Prospective Diabetes Study (UKPDS) Group. Lancet 1998;352(9131):837–53

83. Ohkubo Y, Kishikawa H, Araki E, et al. Intensive insulin therapy prevents the progression of diabetic microvascular complications in Japanese patients with non-insulin-dependent diabetes mellitus: a randomized prospective 6-year study. Diabetes Res Clin Pract 1995;28(2):103–17

84. Selvin E, Marinopoulos S, Berkenblit G, et al. Meta-analysis: glycosylated hemoglobin and cardiovascular disease in diabetes mellitus. Ann Intern Med 2004;141(6):421–31

85. Nelson R, Knowler W, Pettit D, Bennett P. Kidney disease in diabetes. In: Diabetes in America. Bethesda, MD: National Institutes of Health; 1995:349–400

86. Eknoyan G, Hostetter T, Bakris G, et al. Proteinuria and other markers of chronic kidney disease: a position statement of the National Kidney Foundation (NKF) and the National Institute of Diabetes and Digestive and Kidney Diseases (NIDDK). Am J Kidney Dis 2003;42(4):617–22

87. Orchard T, Dorman J, Maser R, et al. Prevalence of complications in IDDM by sex and duration. Pittsburgh Epidemiology of Diabetes Complications Study II. Diabetes 1990;39(9):1116–24

88. Cowie C, Port F, Wolfe R, Savage P, Moll P, Hawthorne V. Disparities in incidence of diabetic end-stage renal disease according to race and type of diabetes. N Engl J Med 1989;321(16):1074–9

89. Lewis E, Hunsicker L, Bain R, Rohde R. The effect of angiotensin-converting enzyme inhibition on diabetic nephropathy. The Collaborative Study Group. N Engl J Med 1993;329(20):1456–62

90. Kasiske B, Lakatua J, Ma J, Lois T. A meta-analysis of the effects of dietary protein restriction on the rate of decline in renal function. Am J Kidney Dis 1998;31(6):954–61

91. Klein R, Klein B. Vision disorders in diabetics. In: Diabetes in America. Bethesda, MD; 1985

92. Malone J, Morrison A, Pavan P, Cuthbertson D, Diabetic Control and Complications Trial. Prevalence and significance of retinopathy in subjects with type 1 diabetes of less than 5 years; duration screened for the Diabetes Control and Complications Trial. Diabetes Care 2001;24(3):522–6

93. Emanuele N, Sacks J, Klein R, et al. Ethnicity, race, and baseline retinopathy correlates in the Veterans Affairs Diabetes Trial. Diabetes Care 2005;28(8):1954–8

94. Javitt J, Aiello L, Bassi L, Chiang Y, Canner J. Detecting and treating retinopathy in patients with type 1 diabetes mellitus. Savings associated with improved implementation of current guidelines. American Academy of Opthalmology. Opthalmology 1991;98(10):1565–73

95. Javitt J, Aiello L, Chiang Y, Ferris F, III, Canner J, Greenfield S. Preventive eye care in people with diabetes is cost-saving to the federal government. Implications for health-care reform. Diabetes Care 1994;17(8):909–17

96. Vijan S, Hofer T, Hayward R. Cost-utility analysis of screening intervals for diabetic retinopathy in patients with type 2 diabetes mellitus. JAMA 2000;283(7):889–96

97. Pregnancy outcomes in the Diabetes Control and Complications Trial. Am J Obstet Gynecol 1996;174(4):1343–53

98. Photocoagulation treatment of proliferative diabetic retinopathy. Clinical application of Diabetic Retinopathy Study (DRS) findings, DRS Report Number 8. The Diabetic Retinopathy Study Research Group. Opthalmology 1981;88(7):583–600

99. Early photocoagulation for diabetic retinopathy. ETDRS report number 9. Early Treatment Diabetic Retinopathy Study Research Group. Opthalmology 1991;98(5 Suppl):766–85

100. Dyck P, Kratz K, Karnes J, et al. The prevalence by staged severity of various types of diabetic neuropathy, retinopathy, and nephropathy in a population-based cohort: the Rochester Diabetic Neuropathy Study. Neurology 1993;43(4):817–24

101. Mangione C, Gerzoff R, Williamson D, et al. The association between quality of care and the intensity of diabetes disease management programs. Ann Intern Med 2006;145:107–16

102. Krein S, Heisler M, Piette J, Makki F, Kerr E. The effect of chronic pain on diabetes patients' self-management. Diabetes Care 2005;28(1):65–70

103. Dyck P, Davies J, Wilson D, Service F, Melton L, III, O'Brien P. Risk factors for severity of diabetic polyneuropathy: intensive longitudinal assessment of the Rochester Diabetic Neuropathy Study cohort. Diabetes Care 1999;22(9):1479–86

104. The effect of intensive diabetes therapy on the development and progression of neuropathy. The Diabetes Control and Complications Trial Research Group. Ann Intern Med 1995;122(8):561–8

105. Gaede P, Vedel P, Larsen N, Jensen G, Parving H, Pedersen O. Multifactorial intervention and cardiovascular disease in patients with type 2 diabetes. N Engl J Med 2003;348(5):383–93

106. Pecoraro R, Reiber G, Burgess E. Pathways to diabetic limb amputation. Basis for prevention. Diabetes Care 1990;13(5):513–21

107. Mayfield J, Reiber G, Sanders L, Janisse D, Pogach L, American Diabetes Association. Preventive foot care in diabetes. Diabetes Care 2004;27(Suppl 1):S63–4

108. Golden S, Lazo M, Carnethon M, et al. Examining a bidirectional association between depressive symptoms and diabetes. JAMA 2008;299(23):2751–9

109. Gavard J, Lustman P, Clouse R. Prevalence of depression in adults with diabetes. An epidemiological evaluation. Diabetes Care 1993;16(8):1167–78

110. Nielsen S, Emborg C, Molbak A. Mortality in concurrent type 1 diabetes and anorexia nervosa. Diabetes Care 2002;25:309–12

111. Crow S, Kendall D, Praus B, Thuras P. Binge eating and other psychopathology in patients with type 2 diabetes mellitus. Int J Eat Disord 2001;30:222–6

112. Shojania K, Ranji S, McDonald K, et al. Effects of quality improvement strategies for type 2 diabetes on glycemic control. JAMA 2006;296:427–40

113. Fleming B, Silver A, Ocepek-Welikson K, Keller D. The relationship between organizational systems and clinical quality in diabetes care. Am J Manag Care 2004;10:934–44

114. Norris S, Lau J, Smith S, Schmid C, Engelgau M. Self-management education for adults with type 2 diabetes. Diabetes Care 2002;25:1159–71

115. Warsi A, Wang P, LaValley M, Avorn J, Solomon D. Self-management education programs in chronic disease. A systematic review and methodological critique of the literature. Arch Intern Med 2004;164:1641–9

116. Ellis S, Speroff T, Dittus R, Brown A, Pichert J, Elasy T. Diabetes patient education: a meta-analysis and meta-regression. Patient Educ Couns 2004;52(1):97–105

117. Chodosh J, Morton S, Mojica W, et al. Meta-analysis: chronic disease self-management programs for older adults. Ann Intern Med 2005;143:427–38

Index